LONG-TERM INTERVENTION IN CHRONIC OBSTRUCTIVE PULMONARY DISEASE

LUNG BIOLOGY IN HEALTH AND DISEASE

Executive Editor

Claude Lenfant

Former Director, National Heart, Lung, and Blood Institute
National Institutes of Health
Bethesda, Maryland

ADDITIONAL VOLUMES IN PREPARATION

The opinions expressed in these volumes do not necessarily represent the views of the National Institutes of Health.

LONG-TERM INTERVENTION IN CHRONIC OBSTRUCTIVE PULMONARY DISEASE

Edited by

Romain A. Pauwels
University Hospital
Ghent, Belgium

Dirkje S. Postma
University Hospital Groningen
Groningen, The Netherlands

Scott T. Weiss
Channing Laboratory
Brigham and Women's Hospital
Boston, Massachusetts

MARCEL DEKKER

NEW YORK

Library of Congress Cataloging-in-Publication Data
A catalog record for this book is available from the Library of Congress.

ISBN: 0-8247-5438-7

This book is printed on acid-free paper.

Headquarters
Marcel Dekker, Inc., 270 Madison Avenue, New York, NY 10016, U.S.A.
tel: 212-696-9000; fax: 212-685-4540

Distribution and Customer Service
Marcel Dekker, Inc., Cimarron Road, Monticello, New York 12701, U.S.A.
tel: 800-228-1160; fax: 845-796-1772

World Wide Web
http://www.dekker.com

The publisher offers discounts on this book when ordered in bulk quantities. For more information, write to Special Sales/Professional Marketing at the headquarters address above.

Current printing (last digit):

10 9 8 7 6 5 4 3 2 1

PRINTED IN THE UNITED STATES OF AMERICA

INTRODUCTION

The year 2004 celebrates the fortieth anniversary of the publication of the first Surgeons General's Report on Smoking. "Smoking and Health," was presented to the public on January 11, 1964. It documented that "cigarette smoking is the most important of the causes of chronic bronchitis in the United States and increases the risk of dying from chronic bronchitis and emphysema. . . ."

Ever since then, a new Surgeon General's report has appeared almost annually. The most recent report—still titled "Smoking and Health"—was presented on May 27, 2004, by Surgeon General Richard H. Carmona. It revealed for the first time that smoking causes diseases in nearly every organ of the body, not just the lungs and heart.

The 1964 report initiated an extraordinary movement about, and against, smoking that even today remains in newspaper headlines in the United States and in many other countries as well. Where did all this take us? On the positive side, in the United States cigarette smoking rates have decreased from 46% of the 1964 population to about 23% today. Not bad—though the preponderance of smokers has shifted, ominously, from adult males to women and young girls and boys.

On the negative side, we are seeing an astonishing increase in the number of deaths from chronic obstructive pulmonary disease (COPD). In 1964, about 32,000 people died of COPD; in 2002, the number of deaths exceeded 120,000. This increase is not explained entirely by the increase of the U.S. population, or by its aging, as the COPD age-adjusted rate rose from about 20.0/100,000 in 1964 to 42.2/100,000 in 2002.

What happened? we are all asking. Many explanations have been advanced, but the reality is that today's situation is the result of many unmet expectations. Since 1964, the message has been, "quit smoking and COPD will disappear." In response, as the editors of the volume note in their Preface, COPD has been viewed as an "orphan disease." True enough, but there are orphans . . . and orphans! Some become full members of the environment in which they exist, while others are just simply ignored and neglected. The latter has been the fate of COPD as a disease.

Today, however, the winds have shifted and we are witnessing an increased attention to COPD that is apparent nearly worldwide. The research community is becoming more active, the pharmaceutical industry is participating and joining the effort as a full partner, the public is concerned, and the patients are coalescing to claim respect and attention. Wonderful examples of such societal interest are the U.S. COPD Coalition and the Global Initiative for Chronic Obstructive Lung Disease (GOLD), which has had an impact throughout the world. Indeed, in many countries, programs have been developed to raise awareness of COPD, implement programs of early diagnosis, provide better care and management, and encourage prevention.

Since its first publication in 1976, this series of monographs has presented COPD many times. Ten volumes have been published, devoted exclusively to COPD, and 14 more have included significant chapters about COPD. This volume—conceived, edited, and written by a cast of international scientific leaders—is a strong expression of the scientific interest in COPD and a wake-up call for many more researchers to recognize that COPD is a fertile area for investigation.

Dr. Romain Pauwels has been the force behind the creation of the international scientific movement against COPD: it was he who launched the GOLD in 1998. Dr. Pauwels and editorial colleagues, Dr. Dirkjie S. Postma and Dr. Scott T. Weiss, conceived this volume—ultimately made possible by the contributions of a group of brilliant and forward-thinking investigators.

As the Executive Editor of the series of monographs, *Lung Biology in Health and Disease*, I cannot say enough to express my enthusiasm for *Long-Term Intervention in Chronic Obstructive Pulmonary Disease* and my gratitude to its editors and contributors. I believe that this monograph provides exciting new dimensions that will bring hope to patients with COPD.

Claude Lenfant, M.D.
Gaithersburg, Maryland

PREFACE

Chronic Obstructive Pulmonary Disease (COPD) has been an "orphan disease" for most of the twentieth century. In the last decade of that century and now into the twenty first, it became clear that COPD had to be recognized world-wide as a chronic disease that has a large impact on the lives of many patients, their families and care takers as well as on health care expenditure and world economics at large. COPD is the fourth leading cause of death and the most rapidly rising cause of death in those over age 65. This has led to the greater interest in the disease and its underlying pathophysiology as well as its management. This book aims to contribute to a better understanding of the epidemiology, pathology and pathophysiology, diagnosis, management and outcome of COPD.

COPD comprises a heterogeneous group of conditions, characterized by chronic airflow limitation and destruction of lung parenchyma with clinical manifestations of dyspnea, cough, sputum production and impaired exercise tolerance. In the US, COPD encompasses chronic bronchitis, chronic obstructive bronchitis, emphysema, or combinations of these conditions. The epidemiology of COPD shows that smoking is the main risk factor for its development. Breathing in other kinds of lung irritants, like pollution, dust, or chemicals over a long period of time may also cause or contribute to COPD. With increasing cumulative pack years of smoking, the risk of COPD increases. However, the risk is never 100% and only 10–20% of smokers develops COPD, providing evidence that a genetic component is present as well. Furthermore, cigarette smoking can only explain about 5% of the variation in level of FEV1. Finally, recent studies suggest that COPD development likely begins in early childhood perhaps even in utero. In such a scenario growth, maximally attained level of lung function and rate of decline all may be pertinent to disease risk.

Since COPD develops slowly, and it may be many years before an individual notices symptoms like feeling short of breath, most of the time COPD is diagnosed in middle-aged or older people. A medical history, physical examination and breathing tests are the most important tests to determine if one has COPD. Spirometry is the most sensitive and commonly used test of lung function. It can detect COPD long before significant symptoms exist. This book shows which physiologic alterations occur in COPD and how they relate to its pathology.

The clinical course of COPD is one of gradual progressive impairment, which may eventually lead to respiratory failure. With continued exposure to cigarette smoke, the disease progresses that can only be changed to some extent by smoking cessation, although even then the inflammatory process that underlies the disease seems to perpetuate. So far, no treatment can prevent the accelerated lung function loss in COPD. Therefore it is of great importance to better understand the pathology and pathophysiology of COPD, with the hope that this leads to new avenues for future treatments. Much attention is therefore paid in the current book towards the underlying mechanisms of COPD, i.e., inflammation, mechanisms of tissue degeneration like the imbalance in proteases and anti-proteases, oxidative stress and anti-oxidants, as well as defective tissue repair.

What can we do about COPD? International guidelines have put forward that the goals of treatment are to:

- Relieve symptoms with no or minimal side effects of treatment
- Slow the progress of the disease
- Improve exercise tolerance
- Prevent and treat complications and sudden onset of problems
- Improve overall health.

Current national and international guidelines advocate the use of bronchodilators for the treatment of all degrees of severity of chronic obstructive pulmonary disease. While anticholinergics are preferred as initial therapy in some countries, the combination of beta-adrenoceptor agonists and anticholinergic drugs with a short or long duration of action are preferred and also more effective (GOLD update 2003) for moderate disease, sometimes supplemented with the use of theophylline. Bronchodilators are the mainstay of current therapy in COPD and while providing relatively little improvement in spirometric lung function compared to asthma, they may significantly reduce symptoms of dyspnea by reducing the increased lung volumes, and may also improve exercise tolerance. Bronchodilators are generally prescribed to symptomatic patients with COPD either for relief of their persistent or worsening symptoms on a p.r.n. basis, or regularly to prevent or to reduce the development of symptoms, especially dyspnea during exercise. In the past years, it has become apparent that further improvements by long-acting bronchodilators may include the reduction of mild exacerbations and the possible need for hospitalization and improvement of health status. This book addresses therefore the effects, benefits and side effects of all types of bronchodilators in COPD.

Given the inflammatory background of COPD, many studies have set out to assess the role of the anti-inflammatory inhaled steroids in COPD. Therefore this book devotes a chapter to the outcomes of the studies so far. Overall, it is clear that inhaled steroids do not reduce the accelerated lung function loss in COPD. However, there are benefits in more advanced disease with respect to quality of life, some symptoms and the frequency of exacerbations.

Pulmonary rehabilitation is a co-ordinated program of exercise, disease management training, and counselling that can help stay more active and carry out day-to-day activities. It may include exercise training, nutrition advice, education about your disease and how to manage it, and counseling. The different parts of the rehabilitation program are managed by different types of health care professionals (doctors, nurses, physical therapists, respiratory therapists, exercise specialists, and dieticians) who work together to develop an individually tailored program.

In summary, this book presents updated, and significant information concerning different aspects of COPD, pathology, pathophysiology, diagnosis, heterogeneity of the disease, management and future perspectives on new therapies. This book offers an overview for pulmonologists, medical students and provides non-specialist researchers in the pulmonary field up-to date information on virtually all aspects of COPD.

The meeting on which this book is based took place in Amsterdam, The Netherlands, and we are grateful to Astra Zeneca Pharmaceuticals, which graciously hosted the event. Finally, we would like to thank the editor of this series, Dr Claude Lenfant, the former director of the National Heart Lung and Blood Institute who has unfailingly supported our efforts.

Romain Pauwels
Dirkje S. Postma
Scott T. Weiss

CONTRIBUTORS

William C. Bailey, M.D. Director, UAB Lung Health Center, and Professor, Department of Medicine, University of Alabama at Birmingham, Birmingham, Alabama, U.S.A.

Peter J. Barnes, D.M., D.Sc., F.R.C.P. Professor and Head of Thoracic Medicine, National Heart and Lung Institute, Imperial College, London, England.

Michael Brunson, M.D. Department of Medicine, University of Alabama at Birmingham, Birmingham, Alabama, U.S.A.

A. Sonia Buist, M.D. Professor, Division of Pulmonary and Critical Care Medicine, Department of Medicine, Oregon Health & Science University, Portland, Oregon, U.S.A.

Antoine Cuvelier, M.D., Ph.D. Division of Pulmonology and Respiratory Intensive Care, Rouen University Hospital, Rouen, France.

Jacob Dankert, M.D., Ph.D.[†] Professor, Department of Medical Microbiology, Academic Medical Center, Amsterdam, The Netherlands.

Nicholas J. Gross, M.D., Ph.D. Professor, Department of Medicine, Stritch-Loyola School of Medicine, Chicago, Illinois, U.S.A.

James C. Hogg, M.D., Ph.D., F.R.S.C. Emeritus Professor, Department of Pathology and Laboratory Medicine, University of British Columbia, Vancouver, British Columbia, Canada.

Huib A. M. Kerstjens, M.D., Ph.D. Professor, Department of Respiratory Medicine, University of Groningen, and University Hospital Groningen, Groningen, The Netherlands.

Todd A. Lee, Pharm.D., Ph.D. Pharmaceutical Outcomes Research and Policy Program, University of Washington, Seattle, Washington, U.S.A.

[†]Deceased.

William W. MacNee, M.B.Ch.B., M.D., F.R.C.P.(G), F.R.C.P.(E) Professor of Respiratory and Environmental Medicine and Honorary Consultant Physician, ELEGI Colt Laboratory, Medical Research Council Centre for Inflammation Research, University of Edinburgh, Edinburgh, Scotland.

Jean-François Muir, M.D., F.C.C.P. Professor and Head of Division of Pulmonology and Respiratory Intensive Care, Rouen University Hospital, Rouen, France.

Sarika Ogale, M.S. Pharmaceutical Outcomes Research and Policy Program, University of Washington, Seattle, Washington, U.S.A.

Romain Pauwels, M.D., Ph.D. Professor, Department of Respiratory Diseases, Ghent University Hospital, Ghent, Belgium.

John R. Pepper, M.D., M.Chir., F.R.C.S. Professor, Department of Surgery, National Heart and Lung Institute, Imperial College, and Royal Brompton Hospital, London, England.

Dirkje S. Postma, M.D., Ph.D. Professor, Department of Pulmonary Diseases, University Hospital Groningen, Groningen, The Netherlands.

N. B. Pride, M.D. Emeritus Professor of Respiratory Medicine, Department of Thoracic Medicine, National Heart and Lung Institute, Imperial College, London, England.

Klaus F. Rabe, M.D., Ph.D. Professor, Department of Pulmonology, Leiden University Medical Center, Leiden, The Netherlands.

Irfan Rahman, Ph.D. Lecturer, ELEGI Laboratory, Medical Research Council Centre for Inflammation Research, University of Edinburgh, Edinburgh, Scotland.

Stephen Rennard, M.D. Larson Professor of Medicine, Division of Pulmonary and Critical Care Medicine, Department of Medicine, University of Nebraska Medical Center, Omaha, Nebraska, U.S.A.

Steven D. Shapiro, M.D. Parker B. Francis Professor of Medicine, Division of Pulmonary and Critical Care Medicine, Department of Medicine, Harvard Medical School and Brigham and Women's Hospital, Boston, Massachusetts, U.S.A.

Nikolaos Siafakas, M.D., Ph.D., F.R.C.P. Professor, Department of Thoracic Medicine, University of Crete Medical School, and University Hospital, Heraklion, Crete, Greece.

Edwin K. Silverman, M.D., Ph.D. Assistant Professor, Division of Pulmonary and Critical Care Medicine, Department of Medicine, Harvard Medical School, and Channing Laboratory, Brigham and Women's Hospital, Boston, Massachusetts, U.S.A.

Robert A. Stockley, M.D., D.Sc., F.R.C.P. Professor, Department of Medicine, University of Birmingham NHS Trust, and Queen Elizabeth Hospital, Edgbaston, Birmingham, England.

Sean D. Sullivan, R.Ph., M.S., Ph.D. Professor, Department of Pharmaceutical Outcomes Research and Policy Program, University of Washington, Seattle, Washington, U.S.A.

Philip Tønnesen, M.D., Dr.Med.Sci. Chair, Department of Pulmonary Medicine, Gentofte University Hospital, Hellerup, Copenhagen, Denmark.

M. Tsoumakidou, M.D., Department of Thoracic Medicine, University Hospital of Heraklion Crete, Heraklion, Crete, Greece.

Eleni Tzortzaki, M.D., Ph.D., F.C.C.P. Lecturer, Department of Thoracic Medicine, University of Crete Medical School, and University Hospital, Heraklion, Crete, Greece.

Loek van Alphen, Ph.D. Product Manager, Meningococcal and Pneumococal Vaccines, Netherlands Vaccine Institute, The Netherlands.

Muriel van Schilfgaarde, Ph.D. Department of Vaccine Research, Netherlands Vaccine Institute, Bilthoven, The Netherlands.

Peter van Ulsen, Ph.D. Department of Molecular Microbiology, Utrecht University, Utrecht, The Netherlands.

Scott T. Weiss, M.D., M.S. Professor of Medicine, Harvard Medical School, and Director, Respiratory, Environmental and Genetic Epidemiology, Channing Laboratory, Brigham and Women's Hospital, Boston, Massachusetts, U.S.A.

Contents

1

Definitions of Chronic Obstructive Pulmonary Disease

N. B. PRIDE

National Heart and Lung Institute, Imperial College
London, England

I. Present Definitions

Until the 1940s ventilatory capacity was assessed by using a spirometer to measure maximum voluntary ventilation. This test reflected both inspiratory and expiratory flows and was reduced by obstructive and restrictive lung disorders, respiratory muscle disorders, and poor motivation. When this test was displaced by the single breath forced expiratory spirogram, expiratory airflow obstruction was swiftly adopted as the dominant functional abnormality in breathless patients with chronic bronchitis and emphysema—and indeed with asthma. The recognition of airflow obstruction led to attempts, staring productively at the Ciba symposium in 1958 (1), to incorporate this concept with the older terminology of chronic bronchitis and emphysema. There was a brief flurry of largely synonymous terms being proposed, but insidiously chronic obstructive pulmonary disease (COPD) became the preferred English-language term and has been used in guidelines worldwide with definitions that differ slightly in detail (as will be discussed through this chapter), but not in concept (Table 1) (2–6). So far the term has not been widely adopted by affected patients or the lay public (7).

1

Table 1 Current Definitions

A. European Respiratory Society (ERS) consensus statement 1995.[a]

Chronic obstructive pulmonary disease (COPD) is a disorder characterized by reduced maximum expiratory flow and slow forced emptying of the lungs; features which do not change markedly over several months. Most of the airflow limitation is slowly progressive and irreversible. The airflow limitation is due to varying combinations of airway disease and emphysema; the relative contribution of the two processes is difficult to define in vivo.

Emphysema is defined anatomically by permanent, destructive enlargement of airspaces distal to the terminal bronchioles without obvious fibrosis.

Chronic bronchitis is defined by the presence of chronic or recurrent increases in bronchial secretions sufficient to cause expectoration. The secretions are present on most days for a minimum of 3 months a year, for at least 2 successive years, and cannot be attributed to other pulmonary or cardiac causes. Hypersecretion can occur in the absence of airflow limitation.

B. Global Initiative for Chronic Obstructive Lung Disease (GOLD) workshop report.[b]

Chronic obstructive pulmonary disease is a disease state characterized by airflow limitation that is not fully reversible. The airflow limitation is usually both progressive and *associated with an abnormal inflammatory response of the lungs to noxious particles or gases.*[c]

[a]*Source*: Ref. 2.
[b]*Source*: Ref. 6.
[c]The new features in the GOLD guidelines are italicized; despite the abbreviation chosen to provide a suitable acronym, the report refers throughout to chronic obstructive pulmonary disease.

Currently, the only positive requirement for diagnosis of COPD is based on the forced expiratory spirogram—a persistent reduction in postbronchodilator forced expiratory volume in one second (FEV_1) and a low FEV_1: forced vital capacity (FVC) ratio (2–6). The staging based on the degree of abnormality of the forced expiratory spirogram proposed by the Global Initiative for Chronic Obstructive Lung Disease (GOLD) (6), and recently revised, has been widely adopted (Table 2). All guidelines remark that the airflow obstruction should be mainly irreversible and slowly progressive over time, but no precise criteria have been developed to ensure this. At one level relying simply on spirometry is strikingly simple and practical, analogous to hypertension or diabetes, and highly suitable for epidemiological use. But there are many other causes of expiratory airflow obstruction, which have to be excluded. The term is only applied to widespread obstruction of the intrathoracic airways,

Table 2 Global Initiative for Obstructive Lung Disease (GOLD)[a]

Stage	Symptoms	FEV$_1$ (% pred)	FEV$_1$/FVC (%)
0, at risk	Present	Normal	Normal
I, mild	—	≥ 80	< 70[b]
II, moderate	—	50–80	< 70
III, severe	—	30–50	< 70
IV, very severe	—	< 30 or < 50 plus chronic respiratory failure [PaO$_2$ < 60 mmHg]	< 70

[a]Revised staging 2003 using postbronchodilator FEV$_1$, www.goldcopd.com.
[b]Using age-independent FEV$_1$/FVC % exaggerates prevalence of abnormality in older subjects.

excluding obstruction of the extrathoracic airway and more localized causes of intrathoracic airway obstruction such as scarring and distortion following sarcoidosis, tuberculosis, or tumors. An early definition of COPD in 1964 described it as "of obscure aetiology" (8) and that is confirmed by the convention of excluding most of the known specific causes of widespread obstruction of the intrathoracic airways such as cystic fibrosis, the grosser forms of bronchiectasis, byssinosis, and uncommon causes of obliterative bronchiolitis (such as those associated with irritant gas inhalation, severe viral infections, lung or bone marrow transplantation, and other causes). The main exception is α_1-antitrypsin deficiency, which is usually regarded as a subcategory of COPD, perhaps because the pulmonary effects are clearly accelerated by smoking and emphysema is a predominant feature, which is not the case for the other disorders above. No doubt other unrecognized diseases are included under the present umbrella of COPD.

Although all these exclusions might surprise a newcomer to the field, in practice they are accepted without difficulty by workers within respiratory medicine, for whom COPD carries a mental image of a more specific form of airflow obstruction, based on the historical association with chronic bronchitis and emphysema. Most of the conditions excluded from COPD are relatively uncommon in adults, except in countries where bronchiectasis remains prevalent. Asthma of course is another matter and a major source of controversy. Surprisingly, the early descriptions of COPD did not specify whether asthma was included or not, but in 1987 the American Thoracic Society (ATS) statement on definitions of COPD and asthma (3) explicitly excluded asthma in principle, whatever the difficulties in practice, particularly in older subjects. Subsequently the ERS (2) and

GOLD (6) guidelines continued to regard asthma and COPD as separate diseases, which may co-exist. The 1995 ATS guidelines were more ambiguous (4); while stating it was "prudent and practical" to separate asthma and COPD, in an accompanying Venn diagram, patient with "unremitting asthma" are classified as having COPD. The British Thoracic Society (BTS) guidelines (5) also include "some patients with asthma" within COPD. The increasing recognition of overlap features, particularly enhanced airway constrictor responses to challenge, mucosal inflammation, and airway remodeling, could be used to support the correctness of the Dutch—or more precisely the Groningen—hypothesis (9), but nevertheless, worldwide, COPD and asthma are still more commonly regarded as separate conditions which *should* be separated. Proponents of separation suspect that the pathogenesis and prognosis of COPD and asthma are radically different and that different types of treatment might be required in the future for COPD.

The definition of chronic bronchitis is unchanged and that of emphysema has been only slightly modified since the Ciba Symposium (Table 1).

All the statements indicate that two processes, primary airway disease and alveolar disease, contribute to the development of chronic expiratory airflow limitation. For practicing doctors over the last few decades this distinction has been of limited importance because the drug management has been similar (the same of course applies for the distinction from asthma); however, with the advent of lung volume reduction surgery for emphysema and continuing evidences that the pathogenesis and tissue response (destruction or proliferation) differ in the two sites, there are increasing arguments for continuing to try to separate out these two processes leading to COPD.

II. How Might the Definitions Be Improved?

Although there is remarkable agreement among the definitions of COPD, emphysema, and chronic bronchitis used in the statements of national societies throughout the world, that probably reflects a lack of interest and expertise in nosology—the science of the classification of disease (10)—rather than satisfaction with the current nonspecific functional definition. The two major problems are our poor knowledge of pathogenesis and our continuing inability to define reliably the respective roles of primary disease of the airways and of emphysema in causing disability. If, following Scadding (11), there is a hierarchy of specifying characteristics of a disease that reflect increasing knowledge—clinical features being displaced by altered structure or function and ultimately by etiology—then the established terms used in airflow obstruction are a mixture of clinical features (chronic bronchitis), altered structure (emphysema), and altered function (COPD), with only the small subset of patients with α_1-antitrypsin deficiency specified by etiology. Modifications have been suggested predominantly in the description of structural (microscopic or gross pathology) and functional features.

A. Pathological (Structural) Features

Obviously most information would come from biopsy of the periphery of the lung, which would allow assessment of structural and inflammatory changes in both major sites of disease, the peripheral airways and alveoli. Such an invasive procedure can only be done as part of another procedure, e.g., lobectomy for bronchial carcinoma or lung volume reduction surgery. A more easily applied procedure, already included in present definitions of asthma, is biopsy of central airways (12) to define a type of inflammation specific to COPD. Originally this specificity was proposed in terms of *lack* of basement membrane thickening, mast cells, and eosinophils characteristic of asthma; more recently, positive characteristics related to proportions of subsets of lymphocytes have been proposed. The obvious drawback to this approach is that the major sites of the *obstructive* changes in COPD are in the lung periphery (13,14). While there is accumulating evidence that the specific cellular characteristics of the inflammation are similar in central airways (15), peripheral airways (16), and alveoli (17), there is no guarantee that these cellular changes are accompanied by significant structural changes. Mucosal inflammation might occur in smokers whether or not they have—or are destined to develop—airflow obstruction. We have known for a long time that chronic bronchitis and even emphysema can be present in the absence of the airflow obstruction necessary for the diagnosis of COPD. It seems more likely that the intensity of the inflammatory response will be related to progressive airflow obstruction (15,17) than that the inflammation will prove to have specific feature(s) predicting such progression. Inflammation may also be inferred less directly from analysis of bronchoalveolar lavage, induced sputum, expired air or condensates, or even by clinical symptoms, because chronic bronchitis—as used in all current definitions (2,4–6) to describe chronic airway hypersecretion—is now believed to be associated with active mucosal inflammation. But inflammatory changes in the small bronchi and bronchioles might well not be associated with chronic sputum production.

Apart from biopsy, emphysema can be detected by imaging and inferred from tests of lung function. Computed tomography (CT) was originally used to detect gross destructive changes (using a densitometry "mask" to highlight all areas with lower density than an arbitrary threshold) in a manner analogous to scoring of whole-lung pathological sections, but a complete analysis of density distribution can be made, potentially allowing progression to be monitored in large regions of the lungs (18–20). Recent pathological interest has focused on microscopic emphysema, which presumably predates the development of destruction visible to the naked eye in whole lung sections. One approach defines microscopic emphysema by increases in established morphometric indices such as mean linear intercept (Lm) (or related measurements such as alveolar wall area), which reflect average alveolar dimensions, rather than destruction of alveolar walls per se (21). The original definition of emphysema proposed by the Ciba symposium allowed the increased size of distal airspaces to arise "either from dilatation or from destruction of their walls" (1), but all subsequent definitions removed dilatation. This was done to ensure that emphysema truly represented an irreversible change (at least before the days of retinoid treatment), to facilitate recognition by pathologists, and because changes in Lm with normal aging (or in fatal exacerbation of asthma) were uncertain (22). In the 1985 NHLBI workshop on the definition of emphysema (23), the phrase "without obvious fibrosis" was added (Table 1). However, it is now recognized that collagen is increased within alveolar walls, and Snider (10) has suggested this phrase should be deleted; emphysema that occurs in COPD could be distinguished from the airspace enlargement associated with obvious fibrosis that is found in many granulomatous and fibrotic diseases by describing such changes as "scar emphysema." In the NHLBI workshop, simple airspace enlargement was also classified separately from emphysema; examples were given of congenital (Down syndrome, congenital lobar overinflation) and acquired causes (aging and compensatory overinflation, secondary to lung resection or persistent lobar collapse) of uniform airspace enlargement, but these could be excluded relatively easily. In humans, destruction is defined as "non-uniformity in the pattern of respiratory airspace enlargement," whereas an animal model of emphysema is defined simply in terms of "enlargement of airspaces" without reference to nonuniformity of such changes or other indicators of destruction (23). The second recent approach to detecting milder degrees of emphysema has been to quantify abnormal breaks in the alveolar wall on histological sections and to describe these by a destructive index (24). Comparing such measurements with Lm, it has been suggested that destructive changes occur before the development of airspace enlargement (24). The pathological definition of microscopic emphysema and the use of precise morphometric criteria to distinguish it from normal aging changes may need to be reviewed if imaging and pulmonary function surrogates come into wider use.

B. Pulmonary Function

An abnormal forced expiratory spirogram forms the current basis for diagnosis and definition of COPD. If the specific features of a maximum expiratory flow-volume (MEFV) curve were included, it would be possible to exclude most patients with obstruction of the extrathoracic airway, but not other specific causes of intrapulmonary airflow obstruction, so the gain would be small. Simple pulmonary function tests (Table 3) have proved disappointing in defining differences in the site of airflow obstruction or in distinguishing the airway from the alveolar component. While a combination of tests may be used to infer the early stages of obstruction of the peripheral airways, distinctive features are lost as obstruction progresses. Measuring total airways resistance has no particular advantage compared to spirometry, and measuring resistance of the peripheral airways requires bronchial intubation (25,26), although potentially this *could* be combined with bronchoscopy and biopsy of the central airways. Even when airflow obstruction is thought to be caused entirely by alveolar disease (loss of lung recoil and loss of alveolar wall attachment to the airway perimeter), this cannot be demonstrated easily. However, loss of lung recoil and carbon monoxide transfer (particularly when expressed per liter of ventilated lung volume) do relate to the presence of emphysema, although the strength of the association varies; lung function tests differ from pathological and imaging methods in reflecting the surviving ventilated lung tissue and not the gross

Table 3 Pulmonary Function—Possibilities for Further Characterizing COPD

Site of airflow obstruction
    Use MEFV curve to exclude obstruction of extrathoracic airway
    Intrabronchial catheter to measure peripheral/central resistance
Nature of airflow obstruction
    Relate lung recoil pressure to resistance or maximum expiratory flow
Airway responsiveness
    Constrictor
    Dilator
    Spontaneous variability
Alveolar disease
    Increased total lung capacity
    Reduced lung recoil pressure
    Reduced carbon monoxide transfer

areas of destruction. This may explain why carbon monoxide transfer is more closely correlated with the extent of microscopic emphysema than with macroscopic emphysema (21). An increased total lung capacity also suggests emphysema. An additional functional characterization is to measure airway responses to constrictor and dilator stimuli. These responses are defining features of asthma, but enhanced responsiveness to inhaled histamine (27) and to methacholine (28) is also found in COPD, albeit at a lesser intensity than in asthma. The intensity of this hyperresponsiveness predicts subsequent accelerated decline in airway function (29), and the possible presence of airway hyperreactivity is included in the ATS definition of COPD (3,4). A more useful distinction would be made if there were specific differences between the hyperreactivity of asthma and COPD, as has been claimed for the response to adenosine inhalation (30). A priori, there is no reason to anticipate a particular degree of bronchodilator response in COPD even if much of the airflow obstruction has a structural basis; in practice, the airflow obstruction commonly is found to be "poorly reversible," and large clinical studies such as the Lung Health Study in North America (31) and Euroscop (32) have used a maximum increase after bronchodilators of 10% of predicted FEV_1 to exclude patients at the more reversible "asthmatic" end of the spectrum. But the distribution of bronchodilator responsiveness is unimodal, so any chosen boundary is arbitrary; furthermore, although measuring the response to a combination of a β_2-adrenergic agonist and muscarinic antagonist would be widely accepted, at the practical level responsiveness shows considerable day-to-day variability.

C. Etiology

Exogenous insults clearly have a major role in COPD, and a frequent proposal is that a history of smoking should be added to the definition (as is sometimes done in clinical trials); but while smoking is involved currently in the pathogenesis of COPD in a very high proportion of sufferers in developed countries (33,34), this may not be the case in all parts of the world (35) and probably was not the case in Britain before the second world war (36,37). The GOLD report has recently met this objection by describing COPD as being "due to an abnormal inflammatory response of the lungs to noxious particles or gases" (6).

III. Practical Possibilities

Presuming definitions have to remain at the intermediate level of describing pathological, structural, and functional changes, there are 3 accepted features to describe: inflammation (of airways and alveoli), airflow obstruction, and structural changes (narrowing of airways, destruction/dilatation of airspaces). By analogy with the amplification of the definition of asthma in recent years, the addition of typical biopsy features from the central airways seems most practical, but of course we are only beginning to explore which inflammatory changes are found in all smokers and which only in smokers destined to develop progressive obstruction [as indicated by the use of "abnormal inflammatory response" in the GOLD report (6)], nor do we know the changes in patients with features intermediate between the polar groups of asthma and COPD so far studied.

Instead of relying on pathological examination for diagnosing emphysema (which in life can only be biopsy of part of one lung), CT and lung function criteria for diagnosing emphysema in vivo could be developed which would reflect better the total amount of disease in the lungs. In practice the gross changes on CT are already used for this purpose, but the subtler changes in lung density on CT and changes in pulmonary function (loss of elastic recoil and reduced CO transfer) occur also with over-distension, which might not be accompanied by destruction. As discussed above, any use of surrogates for emphysema implies that quantitative assessment of milder degrees of distension and destruction might need to be extended.

Problems in describing the airway component of COPD (Table 4) relate to the need to distinguish inflammatory from obstructive components. The idea that chronic mucus hypersecretion was usually an irritative response without overt inflammation, popular from Laennec's day, has been discarded in the last 20 years, so that the presence of chronic cough and sputum can now be regarded as evidence of airway inflammation. But of course many smokers who have chronic hypersecretion never develop troublesome airflow obstruction [reducing the predictive value (38) of stage 0 ("at risk") in the GOLD staging], which is unfortunate because worldwide there is much more information

Table 4 Airway Disease—Possible Refinements in Terminology

Need to distinguish inflammatory from obstructive components
Promote "chronic bronchitis" to a pathological diagnosis?
define as airway inflammation with characteristics that distinguish it from asthma: new adjective required
Invent a term for obstruction and luminal narrowing due to primary ("intrinsic") disease of airways?

on prevalence in the community of chronic cough and secretions than of airflow obstruction. Perhaps chronic bronchitis should be defined pathologically rather than clinically, although this would require a precise description to distinguish it from the airway inflammation of asthma. Surprisingly, for a topic normally associated with redundancy, there is no widely accepted term for primary or intrinsic *obstructive* disease of the intrapulmonary (and especially peripheral) airways. Since the dropping of "chronic obstructive bronchitis" and "small airway disease," chronic bronchitis is again the only term widely used to describe the airway component. In Britain before the Ciba symposium, (chronic) bronchitis was the most common label used in morbidity and mortality studies (37); subsequently this was discarded because of the observed dissociations between chronic mucous hypersecretion and the presence of airflow obstruction in smokers (39). This earlier usage of chronic bronchitis was revived in the 1995 ATS guidelines (4), where COPD was defined as "due to chronic bronchitis or emphysema." Presumably, in this case chronic bronchitis embraced all manifestations of airway disease in COPD. Some years ago "chronic obstructive bronchiolitis" was suggested (40), but this term has since been appropriated by pathologists to describe several other diseases of the peripheral airways which are not included in COPD (41).

The question arises as to how important definitions and diagnostic criteria are for clinical practice. An accepted definition provides a shorthand label which is useful for communication for health professionals and their patients but plays only a small part in decisions about treatment. Agreed-upon definitions and diagnostic criteria are much more important for investigators—in particular, for epidemiologists who have to interpret the various diagnoses recorded in the morbidity and mortality statistics provided by doctors and who may rely on patient-recorded diagnoses in community surveys (7,42).

Some encouragement for future improvements comes from history. Individual disorders have been discovered that would formerly have been included with COPD—the most striking examples being α_1-antitrypsin deficiency and cystic fibrosis—and these discoveries of etiology have made all the conventional approaches to definition of COPD and dependence on spirometry redundant in these subgroups. Other major causes of intrapulmonary airflow obstruction in the presence of smoking or other environmental insults probably remain to be discovered. If COPD today is a miscellaneous collection of disorders held together only by their similar effect on FEV_1, our present difficulties with definition might not be due to incompetence, but rather an accurate reflection of the contemporary lack of knowledge.

References

1. Ciba Guest Symposium. Terminology, definitions and classification of chronic pulmonary emphysema and related conditions. Thorax 1959; 14:286–299.
2. European Respiratory Society. Consensus Statement. Optimal assessment and management of chronic obstructive pulmonary disease (COPD). Eur Respir J 1995; 8:1398–1420.
3. American Thoracic Society. Standards for the diagnosis and care of patients with chronic obstructive pulmonary disease (COPD) and asthma. Am Rev Respir Dis 1987; 139:225–244.
4. American Thoracic Society. Standards for the diagnosis and care of patients with chronic obstructive pulmonary disease. Am J Respir Crit Care Med 1995; 152:S77–S120.
5. British Thoracic Society. Guidelines for the management of chronic obstructive pulmonary disease. Thorax 1997; 52(suppl 5):S1–28.
6. Pauwels RA, Buist AS, Calverley PM, Jenkins CR, Hurd SS. Global strategy for the diagnosis, management, and prevention of chronic obstructive pulmonary disease. NHLBI/WHO Global Initiative for Chronic Obstructive Lung Disease (GOLD) Workshop summary. Am J Respir Crit Care Med 2001; 163:1256–1276. An updated version issued in 2003 with revised staging of severity is available at www.goldcopd.com
7. Rennard S, Decramer M, Calverley PM, Pride NB, Soriano JB, Vermeire PA, Vestbo J. Impact of COPD in North America and Europe in 2000: subjects' perspective of Confronting COPD International Survey. Eur Respir J 2002; 20:799–805.
8. Mitchell RS, Filley GF. Chronic obstructive bronchopulmonary disease. 1. Clinical features. Am Rev Respir Dis 1964; 89:360–371.
9. Sluiter HJ, Köeter GH, de Monchy JGR, Postma DS, de Vries K, Orie NGM. The Dutch hypothesis (chronic non-specific lung disease) revisited. Eur Respir J 1991; 4:479–489.
10. Snider GL. Nosology for our day: its application to chronic obstructive pulmonary disease. Am J Respir Crit Care Med 2003; 167:678–683.
11. Scadding JG. Meaning of diagnostic terms in bronchopulmonary disease. Br Med J 1963; 2:1425–1430.
12. Jeffery PK. Bronchial biopsies and airway inflammation. Eur Respir J 1996; 9:1583–1587.
13. Hogg JC, Macklem PT, Thurlbeck WM. Site and nature of airway obstruction in chronic obstructive lung disease. N Engl J Med 1968; 278:1355–1360.
14. Verbeken EK, Cauberghs M, Mertens I, Lauweryns JM, Van de Woestijne KP. Tissue and airway impedance of excised normal, senile and emphysematous lungs. J Appl Physiol 1992; 72:2343–2353.
15. Di Stefano A, Capelli A, Lusuardi M. Balbo P, Vecchio C, Maestrelli P, Mapp CE, Fabbri LM, Donner CF, Saetta M. Severity of airflow limitation is associated with severity of airway inflammation in smokers. Am J Respir Crit Care Med 1998; 158:1277–1285.

16. Saetta M, Di Stefano A, Turato G, Facchini FM, Corbino CE, Mapp P, Maestrelli P, Ciaccia A, Fabbri LM. CD8+ T-lymphocytes in peripheral airways of smokers with chronic obstructive pulmonary disease. Am J Respir Crit Care Med 1998; 157:822–826.

17. Saetta M, Baraldo S, Corbino L, Turato G, Braccioni F, Rea F, Cavallesco G, Tropeano G, Mapp CE, Maestrelli P, Ciaccia A, Fabbri LM. CD8+ve cells in the lungs of smokers with chronic obstructive pulmonary disease. Am J Respir Crit Care Med 1999; 160:711–717.

18. Gould GA, Macnee W, Mclean A, Warren PM, Redpath A, Best JJK, Lamb D, Flenley DC. CT measurements of lung density in life can quantitate distal airspace enlargement—an essential defining feature of human emphysema. Am Rev Respir Dis 1988; 137:380–392.

19. Dirksen A, Friis M, Olesen KP, Skovgaard LT, Sorensen K. Progress of emphysema in severe α_1-antitrypsin deficiency as assessed by annual CT. Acta Radiologica 1997; 38:826–832.

20. Coxson HO, Rogers RM, Whittal KP, D'Yachkova Y, Paré PD, Sciurba FC, Hogg JC. A quantification of the lung surface area in emphysema using computed tomgraphy. Am J Respir Crit Care Med 1999; 159:851–856.

21. McLean A, Warren PM, Gillooly M, MacNee W, Lamb D. Microscopic and macroscopic measurements of emphysema: relation to carbon monoxide gas transfer. Thorax 1992; 47:144–149.

22. Thurlbeck WM, Wright JL. Emphysema: Classification, morphology, and associations. In: Thurlbeck's Chronic Airflow Obstruction. 2nd ed. Hamilton, Ontario: B C Decker Inc, 1999:85–144.

23. National Heart, Lung and Blood Institute. The definition of emphysema. Am Rev Respir Dis 1985; 321:182–185.

24. Saetta M, Ghezzo H, Kim WD, King M, Angus GE, Wang N-S, Cosio MG. Loss of alveolar attachments in smokers. Am Rev Respir Dis 1985; 132:894–900.

25. Wagner EM, Bleecker ER, Permutt S. Liu MC. Peripheral airways resistance in smokers. Am Rev Respir Dis 1992; 146:92–95.

26. Yanai M, Sekizawa K, Ohrui T, Sasaki H, Takishima T. Site of airway obstruction in pulmonary disease: direct measurement of intrabronchial pressure. J Appl Physiol 1992; 72:1016–1023.

27. Taylor RG, Joyce H, Gross E, Holland F, Pride NB. Bronchial reactivity to inhaled histamine and annual rate of decline in FEV_1 in male smokers and ex-smokers. Thorax 1985; 40:9–16.

28. Tashkin, DP, Altose MD, Bleecker ER, Connett JE, Kanner RE, Lee WW, Wise R for the Lung Health Study Research Group. Airway responsiveness to inhaled methacholine in smokers with mild to moderate airflow limitation. Am Rev Respir Dis 1992; 145:301–310.

29. Tashkin DP, Altose MD, Connett JE, Kanner RE, Lee WW, Wise RA for the Lung Health Study Research Group. Methacholine reactivity predicts changes in lung function over time in smokers with early chronic obstructive pulmonary disease. Am J Respir Crit Care Med 1996; 153:1802–1811.

30. Polosa R, Rorke S, Holgate ST. Evolving concepts on the value of adenosine hyperresponsiveness in asthma and chronic obstructive pulmonary disease. Thorax 2002; 57:649–654.

31. Anthonisen NR, Connett JR, Kiley JP, Altose MD, Bailey WC, Buist AS, Conway WA, Enright PL, Kanner RE, O'Hara P, Owens G, Scanlon PD, Tashkin Wise RA for the Lung Health Study Research Group. Effects of smoking intervention, and the use of an inhaled anticholinergic bronchodilator on the rate of decline in FEV1. The lung Health Study. J Am Med Assoc 1994; 272:1497–1505.

32. Pauwels RA, Lofdahl C-G, Laitinen L, Schouten JP, Postma DS, Pride NB, Ohlsson, SV. Long-term treatment with inhaled budesonide in persons with mild chronic obstructive pulmonary disease who continue smoking. N Engl J Med 1999; 340:1948–1953.

33. Doll R, Peto R, Wheatley K, Gray R, Sutherland I. Mortality in relation to smoking: 40 years' observation on male British doctors. Br Med J 1994; 309:901–911.

34. Peto R, Lopez AD, Boreham J, Thun M, Heath C. Mortality from smoking in developed countries, 1950–2000. Oxford: Oxford University Press, 1994.

35. Lui B-Q, Peto R, Chen Z-M, Boreham J, Wu Y-P, Li J-Y, Campbell TC, Chen J-S. Emerging tobacco hazards in China: 1. Retrospective proportional mortality study of one million deaths. Br Med J 1998; 317:1411–1422.

36. Marks GB, Burney PGJ. Diseases of the respiratory system. In: Charlton J, Murphy M, eds. Health of Adult Britain: 1841 to 1994 Part II. London: HMSO, 1997: 93–113.

37. Pride NB, Soriano JB. Chronic obstructive pulmonary disease in the United Kingdom: trends in mortality, morbidity, and smoking. Curr Opin Pulm Med 2002; 8:95–101.

38. Vestbo J, Lange P. Can GOLD Stage 0 provide information of prognostic value in chronic obstructive pulmonary disease? Am J Respir Crit Care Med 2002; 166:329–332.

39. Fletcher C, Peto R, Tinker CM, Speizer FE. The Natural History of Chronic Bronchitis and Emphysema. Oxford: Oxford University Press, 1976, p. 272.

40. Fletcher CM, Pride NB. Definitions of emphysema, chronic bronchitis, asthma, and airflow obstruction: 25 years on from the CIBA symposium (editorial). Thorax 1984; 39:81–85.

41. Myers JL, Colby TV. Pathological manifestations of bronchiolitis, constrictive bronchiolitis, cryptogenic organizing pneumonia and diffuse panbronchiolitis. Clin Chest Med 1993; 14:611–622.

42. Mannino DM, Gagnon RC, Petty TL, Lydick E. Obstructive lung disease and low lung function in adults in the United States: data from the National Health and Nutrition Examination Survey, 1988–1994. Arch Intern Med 2000; 160:1683–1689.

2

COPD: Worldwide Prevalence

A. SONIA BUIST

Oregon Health & Science University
Portland, U.S.A.

Imprecise and variable definitions have made it hard to quantify the prevalence and burden of chronic obstructive pulmonary disease (COPD) in both developed and developing countries (1). A number of different approaches have been used to estimate the prevalence of COPD. Historically, most of these have been surveys based on symptoms and/or diagnosed conditions. Few have included lung function. A different approach has been used by the Global Burden of Disease (GBD) Study, sponsored by the World Health Organization (WHO) and the World Bank (2,3). This study is described below and essentially involves finding all published and unpublished data and filling in the gaps with best estimates. These different approaches will inevitably provide widely varying estimates of COPD prevalence. All estimates, however, provide useful information that helps to complete the picture of the burden of COPD, so the three approaches will be discussed briefly.

Prevalence estimates depend on the definition of COPD used, and many definitions have been used over the years. Most of the definitions include the terms "chronic bronchitis" and "emphysema," the two major components of the spectrum of diseases that make up COPD. Only one of these (chronic bronchitis) has a definition that can be operationalized since it only requires a history of chronic cough and sputum. Emphysema is an anatomical definition and cannot be diagnosed clinically without sophisticated tests such as high-resolution computed tomography (CT) scans. Given the difficulty of performing spirometry in large surveys, most studies done over the past 30 years have not included lung function tests, so have not reported on the prevalence of airflow limitation, now considered essential for the diagnosis of COPD (4,5). The most recent definition of COPD from the Global Initiative on Chronic Obstructive Lung Disease (GOLD) (6) does not mention chronic bronchitis and emphysema but does emphasize the importance of measuring lung function in diagnosing COPD. In GOLD, COPD is defined as: "A disease state characterized by airflow limitation that is not fully reversible. The airflow limitation is usually progressive and associated with an abnormal response of the lungs to noxious particles or gases."

GOLD also provides a new (and probably better) staging of COPD that includes a new stage (Stage 0) when symptoms are present but lung

Table 1 Classification of Severity of COPD

Stage	Characteristics
0: At Risk	• normal spirometry • chronic symptoms (cough, sputum production)
I: Mild COPD	• $FEV_1/FVC < 70\%$ • $FEV_1 \geq 80\%$ predicted • with or without chronic symptoms (cough, sputum production)
II: Moderate COPD	• $FEV_1/FVC < 70\%$ • $50\% \leq FEV_1 < 80\%$ predicted • with or without chronic symptoms (cough, sputum production)
III: Severe COPD	• $FEV_1/FVC < 70\%$ • $30\% \leq FEV_1 < 50\%$ predicted • with or without chronic symptoms (cough, sputum production)
IV: Very Severe COPD	• $FEV_1/FVC < 70\%$ • $FEV_1 \leq 30\%$ predicted or $FEV_1 < 50\%$ predicted plus chronic respiratory failure

FEV_1: forced expiratory volume in one second; FVC: forced vital capacity.
Arterial partial pressure of oxygen (PaO_2) less than 8.0 kPa (60 mm Hg) with or without.
Arterial partial pressure of CO_2 ($PaCO_2$) greater than 6.7 kPa (50 mm Hg) while breathing air at sea level.
Source: Ref. 6.

function is still normal (Table 1). The importance of this is that it emphasizes that symptoms of chronic cough and sputum are not normal but, in some, indicate the early stage of a disease that may progress to clinically significant COPD. This validates the use of symptoms as a way to estimate the potential pool of COPD in a population. Symptoms will overestimate the burden of COPD but provide an outer bound to the COPD prevalence. Using lung function, the earliest stage of airflow limitation (Stage I) is defined as $FEV_1/FVC\% < 70\%$ and $FEV_1 > 80\%$ predicted. Stage II (moderate COPD) is defined as $FEV_1/FVC < 70\%$ together with an $FEV_1 \geq 50\%$ and $<80\%$ predicted. Stage III (severe COPD) is defined as $FEV_1/FVC < 70\%$ together with an $FEV_1 \geq 30\%$ predicted and $<50\%$ predicted. Stage IV (very severe COPD) is defined as an $FEV_1/FVC < 70\%$ together with an $FEV_1 < 30\%$ predicted or $FEV_1 < 50\%$ predicted plus chronic respiratory failure.

On the principle that each of the approaches to estimating prevalence provides useful information, the different approaches will be described briefly.

I. Prevalence Based on Symptoms

The history of the evolution of the methodology of estimating COPD prevalence is interesting and worth relating. Most of the early surveys for COPD used standardized respiratory symptom questionnaires to estimate the prevalence of the classic symptoms of COPD: chronic cough and phlegm production. These surveys used the definition of chronic bronchitis developed in the United Kingdom in the 1950s (7). Chronic bronchitis was defined as a disease characterized by the presence of cough and sputum production for at least 3 months a year for at least 2 or 3 years (the definitions vary). Chronic bronchitis was often further defined as being with airflow obstruction or without airflow obstruction (defined by an abnormal FEV_1).

The simple definition of chronic bronchitis as a disease characterized by the presence of chronic cough and chronic sputum production has proved both useful and controversial. It has proved useful because it has been possible to develop standardized questionnaires that ask about the presence of these symptoms in language that is usually understandable in most countries and most cultures. It has been controversial because some have argued (7) that individuals who have persistent cough and sputum should not be regarded as having a disease since they are not disabled. Fletcher, in the late 1950s (6) argued persuasively that "persistent expectoration is an abnormality of function and merits description as a disease just as much as any other abnormality or function which may not at first cause disability." An additional argument might be that putting emphasis on the symptoms of chronic cough and chronic phlegm production before lung function becomes abnormal, and dyspnea becomes apparent, focuses attention on the early stages of disease when many of the changes may be reversible. This is essentially the argument used by GOLD when Stage 0 COPD was included.

The development of standardized questionnaires was an important step in developing accurate prevalence data. The earliest standardized questionnaire was the British Medical Research Council (MRC) Questionnaire developed in the 1950s (8). Later, the American Thoracic Society/ Division of Lung Disease Respiratory Symptom Questionnaire was developed (4), based largely on experience with the MRC Questionnaire, and this is probably now the most widely used of the respiratory symptoms questionnaires. The usefulness of these standardized questionnaires has been primarily to estimate the prevalence of a number of well-recognized symptoms, such as cough, sputum, and shortness of breath, and the duration of symptoms. Also, since chronic bronchitis is defined as chronic cough and sputum of at least 3 months per year for at least 2 years, the questionnaires have been able to provide estimates of the prevalence of chronic bronchitis. They also provide a standardized approach to obtaining information about smoking and occupation. Their value in separating chronic bronchitis, emphysema, and asthma is limited, however.

In the 1950s and 1960s COPD prevalence surveys using respiratory symptom questionnaires were carried out and reported from the United States. (9), the United Kingdom (10), Denmark (11), and Papua New Guinea (12). In the 1970s additional studies were reported from the same countries (13–15), and prevalence data were reported from Africa (16), Micronesia (17), India (18), the Caribbean (19), and Canada (20). In the 1980s data from France were added (21), and in the 1990s data from Italy (22,23) and Sweden (24) were reported and surveys that specifically focused on the elderly in the United States (25) and the United Kingdom were reported (26).

The studies of COPD prevalence based on respiratory symptoms, taken in aggregate, clearly showed that chronic bronchitis varies by age, gender, smoking, occupational and environmental exposures, and country/ region. This will be discussed in the following sections.

A.   Gradient in Respiratory Symptoms by Age

There is no clear consensus among the many prevalence surveys as to whether there is an age-related gradient for chronic cough and sputum.

The reason for this lack of consensus seems to lie primarily in whether the data were reported as crude data, or whether they were adjusted for age and smoking. Differences are also related to where the surveys were carried out. For example, a comparison of two early major U.S. and U.K. surveys, reported by Reid and coworkers in 1964 (27), did not find a clear-cut age gradient in either men or women in the restricted age group of 45–64 years. This study reported the prevalence of chronic cough and phlegm for 2 years or more in a random sample of men and women in the United Kingdom drawn from practice lists of 92 doctors working in urban and country areas of Britain, and a probability sample of residents in Berlin, New Hampshire. Prevalences of chronic cough and phlegm were remarkably high: 45% in the United States and 43% in the United Kingdom for men; 22% and 18% for women. For the age group 55–64 years, the prevalence of chronic cough and phlegm was 47% for the United States and 52% for the United Kingdom in men; 17% and 27%, respectively, for the women. A more recent, population-based survey (13), carried out in Glenwood Springs, Colorado, also showed no age-related gradient until age 60 years in men and no gradient in women (Table 2).

In marked contrast, studies from developing countries tell a different story. Pandey (28) reported on the prevalence of chronic bronchitis in a rural community in the hill region of Nepal in 1984 (Table 2). In that survey, the prevalence of chronic bronchitis increased appreciably with age in both men and women, reaching very high prevalences (41% in both men and women) over age 60 years.

As the statistical approach to data analysis has become more sophisticated, care has been taken to adjust for potentially confounding factors.

Table 2 Prevalence of Chronic Bronchitis by Age and Gender, United States and Nepal

Age (yr)	United States[a]	Nepal[b]	United States	Nepal
20–29	24	2.2	28	4.8
30–39	25	14.2	22	14.2
40–49	22	19.1	20	21.1
50–59	25	29.0	17	34.4
60–69	33	41.0	27	41.2
>70	39.1		33.9	
Overall	25	17.6	22	18.9

[a]Glenwood Springs, Colorado; 53% of men, 41% of women were current smokers.
[b]Hill region of Nepal; 68% overall were current smokers, not further separated by gender. Women were reported to be very light smokers.
Source: Ref. 32.

Table 3 Odds Ratios (95% CI) from Logistic Regression for Risk Factors for Chronic Cough and Chronic Bronchitis by Gender—French Cooperative Study (PAARC)

	Chronic cough		Chronic bronchitis	
	Men	Women	Men	Women
Occupational exposure	1.36[a]	1.37	1.53	2.09
	(1.18–1.57)	(1.09–1.73)	(1.27–1.8)	(1.41–3.12)
Age (× 10 years)	1.40	1.39	1.30	1.32
	(1.30–1.52)	(1.24–1.55)	(1.17–1.43)	(1.11–1.57)
Current tobacco use				
1–9 g/day[a]	1.51	1.74	1.30	0.76
	(1.09–2.09)	(1.23–2.47)	(0.88–1.92)	(0.39–1.52)
10–19 g/day[a]	2.93	3.14	2.47	2.21
	(2.26–3.80)	(2.26–3.80)	(1.86–3.29)	(1.86–3.29)
>20 g/day[a]	7.46	9.95	4.56	5.58
	(5.96–9.34)	(7.55–13.12)	(3.61–5.77)	(3.67–8.49)

[a]Versus 0 g/day.
Source: Adapted from Ref. 29.

When this has been done, for example, in the large French Cooperative (PAARC) Study that involved 23,715 residents aged 25–59 years from 24 areas and seven cities throughout France (29), age was found to be a significant factor both for chronic cough and chronic bronchitis [odds ratios from logistic regression for men for chronic cough was 1.40 (95% CI 1.30–1.52) and for chronic bronchitis 1.30 (95% CI 1.17–1.43)]. The equivalent odds ratios and 95% CI for women for chronic cough and chronic bronchitis were chronic cough 1.39 (95% CI 1.24–1.55) and for chronic bronchitis 1.32 (95% CI 1.11–1.57) (Table 3).

One way of interpreting the age-related gradient in chronic cough and chronic phlegm is to consider it as a response to the cumulative burden of respiratory insults from inspired particulates and gases over a lifetime.

B. Gradient in Respiratory Symptoms by Gender

Most surveys show a clear gender-related difference in the prevalence of symptoms of chronic cough and chronic phlegm, with men having appreciably higher prevalence than women in developed countries and equal or lower prevalence in some areas of developing countries. The gender gradient in developed countries can be attributed to the gender-related differences in smoking habits and occupational exposures to particulates and gases. In developing countries, such as Nepal and the northern regions of India, the high prevalences of chronic cough and sputum in women have been attributed to heavy indoor air pollution from cooking and heating in dwellings with unvented cooking and heating stoves (30). This results in huge exposures to particulates and gases described in greater detail below.

C. Gradient in Respiratory Symptoms by Smoking

There is complete consensus among the many prevalence surveys that there is a strong gradient in the prevalence of respiratory symptoms and conditions both by smoking habits and amounts smoked. The prevalence of chronic cough and sputum in nonsmokers is generally very low, next lowest in ex-smokers, and next highest in smokers. Table 4 shows the prevalence of chronic cough and sputum in three cities in North America (31) by smoking habits. For both men and women, the prevalence of both chronic cough and chronic sputum was severalfold higher in smokers than nonsmokers or ex-smokers.

The French PAARC Study (29) looked at the dose-response relationship for chronic cough and chronic bronchitis with amount smoked, adjusting for age, occupational exposures, education, and socio-occupational class (Table 3). The odds ratios for chronic cough increased from 1.51 for 1–9 g/day of tobacco to 2.93 for 10–19 g/day and 7.46 for >20 g/day. All of the 95% confidence intervals were highly significant.

Table 4 Prevalence of Chronic Cough and Sputum by Smoking and Gender for Three North American Cities

	Men			Women		
	Non-smoker	Ex-smoker	Current smoker	Non-smoker	Ex-smoker	Current smoker
Chronic cough						
Portland	4	7	28	6	9	27
Montreal	0	5	24	7	7	26
Winnepeg	3	2	30	6	5	14
Chronic sputum						
Portland	5	10	30	2	6	19
Montreal	14	9	22	2	4	24
Winnepeg	3	4	34	4	0	2

Source: Ref. 31.

D. Gradient in Prevalence of Respiratory Symptoms by Occupation

A number of studies have focused   cifically on the role of occupational exposures to particulates and gases   . increasing the prevalence of chronic cough and sputum. These studies have been able to demonstrate the additional contribution of occupational exposures over and above personal or environmental exposures. Two examples of such studies are the French PAARC Study (29) and a study carried out in the Po River Delta area in northern Italy (22,23). Both found a significant contribution of occupational exposure to current respiratory symptoms or chronic bronchitis after adjusting for confounding factors (Table 3).

E. Gradient in Prevalence of Respiratory Symptoms by Indoor Environment

The major studies that have demonstrated the important contribution of indoor air pollution to the burden of respiratory symptoms and conditions have been carried out in developing countries, such as India, Nepal, and Papua New Guinea. The evidence is compelling that in regions such as the northern areas of India and Nepal where women have heavy exposure to particulates as a result of cooking and heating in poorly vented dwellings, the prevalence of chronic cough and sputum and chronic bronchitis may be very high. An example of such a study was reported by Pandey from the hill region of Nepal (28,32). In that area, domestic smoke is produced by burning biomass fuel for cooking and heating, such as firewood and straw. Cooking is done by the women on traditional stoves in the corner of one of the rooms in the morning and evenings. The dwellings have no chimneys and are very poorly ventilated. Pandey assessed the prevalence of chronic bronchitis in men and women according to the hours per day spent near the fireplace. He reported a marked gradient in the age-adjusted prevalence in chronic bronchitis in both men and women with increasing time spent near the fireplace (32) (Table 5). Pandey did not provide data on smoking by gender in his study population, but did note that the women who smoked were very light smokers.

II. Comparison of Prevalence of Chronic Bronchitis Across Countries

Table 6 shows a comparison of the prevalence of chronic bronchitis across several countries from population-based surveys that used standardized questionnaires (4,6,33–38). There is a striking range of prevalences, with

Table 5 Age-Adjusted Prevalence of Chronic Bronchitis in Nepal by Smoking, Gender, and Hours per Day Spent Near Fireplace

Average hr/day near fireplace	Men	Women
Nonsmokers		
0.09	8.4	7.8
1–1.9	28.9	13.4
2–3.9	31.1	24.3
≥ 4	34.5	28.6
Ex-smokers		
0–0.9	1.9	
1–1.9	40.2	13.9
2–3.9	45.4	34.0
≥ 4	58.8	62.9
Smokers		
0–0.9	8.4	7.8
1–1.9	28.9	13.4
2–3.9	31.0	24.3
≥ 4	34.5	28.6

Source: Ref. 32.

Table 6 Prevalence of Chronic Bronchitis in Several Countries Based on Standardized Questionnaires

Country (Ref.)	Year reported	Place	Age (yr)	n	Prevalence/100 Men	Women
United Kingdom (33)	1961	National Survey	40–64	1569	17	8
United States (9)	1962	Berlin, NH	25–74	1139	21.6	9.4
Sweden (34)	1968	Uppsala	30–64	41679	2.2	1.5
Japan (35)	1977	Summary of Several Surveys	50–59	22590	5.8	3.1
India (36)	1977	Delhi	35–74	300	12	5
(37)	1977	Madras	50–60+	523	2.4	1.5
Africa (38)	1977	Nigeria	31–70+	1544	0.27	0.24
(16)	1978	Zimbabwe	> 20	4994	1.2	2.8
Nepal (28)	1984	Hill Region	≥ 20	2826	17.6	18.9

Chronic bronchitis defined as phlegm for days/week, 3 months/yr for 3 years or more.
Source: Adapted from Ref. 28.

very low prevalences in two African countries (Nigeria and Zimbabwe), Sweden, and South India. The highest prevalences among these surveys were in the United States and Nepal.

III. Studies Based on a Physician Diagnosis

Studies based on diagnoses rely on the individual's self-report of a doctor diagnosis of the condition in question. This clearly presents a problem for conditions, such as COPD, which are poorly understood by patients and often by physicians (6). For example, physicians are often unclear on whether the term COPD does or does not include asthma. The lay public is unfamiliar with the term chronic obstructive pulmonary disease or COPD and is generally more familiar with the term emphysema. Physicians often, therefore, use terms that they think their patients will understand, such as emphysema rather than COPD. Consequently, misclassification with respect to COPD is inevitable and is much more of a problem for COPD than for many other conditions that are better understood. Also, as noted above, since COPD is not recognized and diagnosed until the disease is clinically apparent and moderately advanced—often not until lung function is appreciably reduced—the prevalence is appreciably underestimated. Nevertheless, surveys based on awareness of diagnoses are helpful because they can identify the burden of diagnosed and clinically significant diseases.

The United States has the most extensive database of population-based surveys of doctor-diagnosed chronic condition, and these are useful for illustration (39,40). However, these cannot be extrapolated globally since risk factors operating in different countries, in particular smoking and indoor and outdoor air pollution, have different temporal patterns.

The most comprehensive database in the United States derives from large representative samples of the civilian noninstitutionalized population of the United States who have participated in the National Health Interview Surveys (NHIS) (39,40). These surveys, carried out every few years, use standardized questions about the prevalence of chronic conditions. To assess the prevalence of chronic respiratory disease, for example, the question used is: During the past 12 months, did anyone in the family have: bronchitis? asthma? or emphysema? In this question, bronchitis refers to chronic bronchitis, and the interviewer is specifically instructed to obtain information about a *chronic* condition. It should be emphasized, therefore, that the large U.S. population-based surveys on which estimates of the prevalence of COPD are based use the term "bronchitis" for *chronic* bronchitis; there is no mention of COPD. These surveys, therefore, rely on

Table 7 Estimated Annual Prevalence* of Self-Reported, or Self-Reported, Physician-Diagnosed Lifetime Emphysema or Chronic Bronchitis During the Preceding 12 Months by Race, Sex, and Age Group—United States, National Health Interview Survey, 1997–2000

Variable	1997	1998	1999	2000
Race[a]				
White	65.7	62.4	59.4	63.6
Black	63.2	47.4	40.8	50.4
Other	40.0	31.0	33.0	31.4
Sex[a]				
Male	50.3[b]	45.4[b]	43.3[b]	45.5[b]
Female	76.7[b]	71.5[b]	67.3[b]	73.2[b]
Age (yr)				
25–44	44.0	38.2	37.4	38.5
45–54	61.1	59.8	50.9	59.2
55–64	85.9	78.4	74.9	79.5
65–74	111.2	103.8	92.0	96.4
≥ 75	97.4	92.0	98.1	106.0
Total	64.2	59.1	55.9	60.0

[a]Age-adjusted to 2000 U.S. population.
[b]Represents a statistically significant difference between blacks and whites or males and females for that year.
*Per 1000 population.
Source: Ref. 41.

recognition of the terms "bronchitis" or "emphysema," and no attempt is made to check the accuracy of the diagnoses or whether there is under- or overreporting. Although these data are useful in estimating the burden of clinically diagnosed and clinically significantly COPD, they seriously underestimate the total burden of COPD.

These surveys show that the prevalence of COPD (defined as positive responses to the questions on bronchitis and emphysema) increases with age, is higher in men than women, and is higher in whites than blacks or other races (Table 7).

IV. Worldwide Prevalence Estimates from the Global Burden of Disease Study

The Global Burden of Disease (GBD) Study (2,3) was initiated in 1992 by the World Bank in an effort to foster an independent evidenced-based approach to public health. The study was designed to develop internally consistent estimates of mortality from 107 major causes of death, disaggregated by age and sex, from eight major geographic areas of the world. One of the major objectives of the GBD was to focus attention on nonfatal outcomes and on disability. Quantifying disability for the world posed a huge challenge since the data on the epidemiology of important nonfatal health conditions are extremely limited for some regions of the world. The main metric used to quantify the burden of nonfatal health outcomes in the GBD study was years lived with a disability (YLD). To derive this, methodology was developed to fill in the gaps where no data existed. In order to calculate YLD, the incidence, average age of onset, duration, and disability severity weight need to be known. This requires, therefore, that incidence and prevalence data be identified or estimated. Since valid population-based epidemiological studies do not exist for many nonfatal health outcomes in many regions, a methodology based on an iterative process was developed.

The first step was to identify and convene disease experts from a number of international agencies and many countries. Next, first-round estimates of the prevalence, incidence, duration, case-fatality and death rates were made on the basis of published and unpublished studies. Where few data for a region were available, experts made informed estimates. Where no information was available, preliminary estimates were based on data or information from other regions that purport to have similar epidemiological patterns. The first-round estimates were then critically reviewed for internal consistency and revised as necessary. These revised estimated were extensively reviewed by international health experts and further revised to insure internal consistency.

Using this process, incidence and prevalence data for eight regions/ countries around the world were published (Table 8). The worldwide prevalence of COPD was estimated to be 9.34/1000 in men and 7.33/1000 in women. The lowest prevalences were for the Middle Eastern Crescent for men (2.69/1000) and other Asia and Islands for women (1.79/1000). The male-female gradient in all of the regions/countries, except for the Middle Eastern Crescent, is very notable. Also very striking are the extraordinarily high prevalences for China (26.2/1000 for men, 23.7/1000 for women). The incidence data for women for China are also very striking, with a severalfold difference in incidence between China and most of the other regions.

Given the striking dearth of population-based data for COPD for many regions/countries of the world, the prevalences in Table 8 should not be viewed as very firm. Nevertheless, the pattern of COPD prevalence with (apart from China) highest prevalences in countries where cigarette smoking has been, or still is, very common and the lowest prevalences in countries where smoking is less common or total tobacco

Table 8 COPD Around the World

Region or country	1990 Prevalence per 1000 males/females
Established market economies	6.98/3.79
Former socialist economies of Europe	7.35/3.45
India	4.38/3.44
China[a]	26.20/23.70
Other Asia and Islands	2.89/1.79
Sub-Saharan Africa	4.41/2.49
Latin America and Caribbean	3.36/2.72
Middle Eastern Crescent	2.69/2.83
World	9.34/7.33

[a]The prevalence of COPD in China reported in this study has been questioned based on recent publications from China.
Source: Ref. 6.

consumption per capita per individuals is still low, is likely to change as smoking becomes more prevalent and heavier in developing countries. The outliers in these data are clearly the prevalence and incidence data for men and women in China.

V. Estimates Based on Lung Function

Surveys based on questionnaires or a doctor diagnosis are much easier to do but provide very crude estimates of COPD prevalence. As pointed out above, these may err seriously on the side of underestimating if based on a doctor diagnosis and on the side of overestimating if based on respiratory symptoms. Clearly, estimates based on lung function are likely to be more accurate since COPD is now defined as characterized by airflow limitation, assuming that the lung function testing is performed with appropriate attention to quality control. Population-based surveys that have used spirometry have been done in very few countries, largely because of the expense and difficulty of doing high-quality spirometry in field studies. Some data are available, however, and provide estimates of COPD prevalence that are enormously useful in estimating the burden of this common and costly disease.

VI. U.S. Data

Probably the best prevalence data (most extensive and population-based for a whole country) are those from the U.S. National Health and Nutrition

Table 9 Estimated Prevalence (%) Mild and Moderate Airflow Limitation by Race, Sex, and Age—U.S. National Health and Nutrition Examination Survey 3, 1988–1994

Mild airflow limitation, FEV$_1$/FVC < 70% and FEV$_1$/FVC ≥ 80% pred.		Moderate airflow limitation, FEV$_1$ < 70% pred. and FEV$_1$ < 80% pred.
Sex[a]		
Male	9.1	7.4
Female	4.9	5.8
Race[a]		
White	7.1	6.7
Black	5.0	5.6
Age (yr)		
25–44	3.7	2.3
45–54	8.7	7.2
55–64	12.6	14.1
65–74	17.8	22.9
Total	6.9	6.6

[a]Age-adjusted to 2000 U.S. population.
Source: Adapted from Ref. 41.

Surveys (NHANES) (41,42). These surveys were probability samples of the civilian, noninstitutionalized population of the United States. Spirometry was done on 13,869 adults in the NHANES 3 survey (1988–1994). Quality control was strictly maintained. Reference values for nonsmokers were derived from the asymptomatic nonsmokers. A modification of the GOLD criteria was used in the analysis. Mild COPD (Stage I) was defined as FEV$_1$/FVC < 70% together with FEV$_1$ >80% predicted. Moderate COPD (Stage II) was defined as FEV$_1$/FVC < 70% together with FEV$_1$ > 30% and < 80% predicted. Severe COPD (Stage III) was defined as FEV$_1$/FVC < 70% together with FEV$_1$ < 30% predicted. The prevalence of mild and moderate airflow limitation in NHANES 3 is shown in Table 9 by sex, age, and race.

VII. Data from Spain

Data are available from a population-based survey carried out in seven different geographic areas in Spain between 1996 and 1997, the IBERPOC Study (43). A total of 4035 men and women aged 40–69 years (3978 for spirometry) were studied out of a target population of 236,412 noninstitutionalized inhabitants. Every attempt was made to use standardized methods and identical equipment. The criteria used to define COPD included no prior diagnosis of asthma, together with airflow limitation defined as $FEV_1/FVC < 88\%$ predicted in men and $< 89\%$ predicted in women, using the predicted values of Roca et al. (44).

Significant differences were found in COPD prevalence across the seven geographic areas (Table 10) and between men and women (presumably reflecting the difference in smoking between men and women in Spain). The expected gradient by smoking (active smokers > ex-smokers > nonsmokers) was reported as well, together with a strong dose-response relationship with cumulative consumption of cigarettes. The overall prevalence of COPD was 9.1%, with a range of 6.1–18%—an enormous range. No obvious reasons for this wide range of prevalences have emerged, although differences in response rate across the areas may account for some of the differences.

VIII. How Different Criteria for COPD Affect Prevalence Estimates

As noted above, prevalence estimates depend inevitably on the criteria used to define COPD. As illustrated above, estimates based on respiratory symptoms will *overestimate* COPD prevalence, whereas estimates based on a physician diagnosis will *underestimate* prevalence. Similarly, different criteria for airflow limitation will provide widely different estimates of COPD prevalence.

This is beautifully illustrated by Viegi and coworkers, who used data from a survey of a general population sample living in the Po Delta area of northern Italy (22) carried out between 1988 and 1991. This survey used standardized interviewer-administered respiratory symptom questionnaires and lung function tests. The authors compared three criteria for COPD: the ERS lung function criterion (FEV_1/slow VC $< 88\%$ predicted in men and $< 89\%$ predicted in women); the ERS "clinical" criterion ($FEV_1/FVC < 70\%$); and the ATS criterion from 1986 ($FEV_1/FVC < 75\%$).

The differences in the estimates of COPD prevalence using these three criteria are astonishing (Table 11). The highest prevalence of airflow limitation (by far) was seen using the ATS criterion, and the lowest with the ERS lung function criterion. There was a small difference between the ERS lung function and "clinical" criteria. The main reason for the surprisingly high prevalence using the ATS criteria was the large prevalence of mild

Table 10 Prevalence of COPD Stratified by Sex, Tobacco Consumption, and Age Group

Prevalence	Oviedo	Burgos	Caceres	Madrid	Manlleu	Seville	Biscay	Total
COPD prevalence,	6.1[a]	10.3	4.9	9.8	18[b]	6.3[c]	8.2	9.1
95% CI OR (95% CI)	4.4–8.3	7.6–12.7	3.2–7.0	7.4–12.7	14.8–21.2	4.5–8.6	6.1–10.7	8.1–9.9
	1.2	2.2	1	2.1	4.7	1.3	1.7	
	(0.7–2.1)	(1.4–3.5)		(1.3–3.4)	(2.7–6.6)	(0.8–2.2)	(1.1–2.8)	
Prevalence in smokers	10.2[a]	16.2	12.5	20.8[a]	25.3[b]	9.0[a]	18.5	15.0
								(12.8–17.1)
Prevalence in ex-smokers	9.7	11.8	4.7[b]	15.9	28.0[b]	8.5[c]	11.9	12.8
								(10.7–14.8)
Prevalence in nonsmokers	2.3	7.1[a]	0.4[b]	1.6[a]	11.9[b]	2.8	1.0[a]	4.1
								(3.3–5.1)
Percentage of nonsmokers among COPD cases	18.4	36.9[a]	3.7[a]	8[a]	39.1[b]	18.4	6.25[a]	23.4
Percentage of women among COPD cases	23.7	29	3.7[c]	14	28.9	21.1	16.7	22

Data are presented as % or % (95% CI) unless otherwise indicated.

[a] < 0.01 with respect to total numbers.

[b] < 0.001 with respect to total numbers.

[c] < 0.05 with respect to total numbers.

Source: Ref. 44.

Table 11 Prevalence of Obstructed Subjects by Age Group with Abnormal Levels of FEV$_1$ % by ERS, Clinical, and ATS Criteria

Variables	ERS (%)	Clinical (%)	ATS (%)
Subjects ≥ 46 yr (*n* = 772)			
Possible physiological variant	0.5	5.3	16.7
Mild	8.1	19.0	35.1
Moderate	2.6	—	2.3
Moderately severe	—	4.4	1.7
Severe	1.0	—	1.2
Very severe	—	—	—
Any abnormal level	12.2	28.7	57.0
All subjects (*n* = 1727)			
Possible physiological variant	1.0	3.1	12.0
Mild	8.1	13.0	25.8
Moderate	1.4	—	1.3
Moderately severe	—	2.1	0.8
Severe	0.5	—	0.5
Very severe	—	—	—
Any abnormal level	11.0	18.3	40.4

ERS criteria = FEV$_1$/slow VC < 88% pred. men, < 8% pred. women; clinical criteria = FEV$_1$/FVC% < 70%; ATS criteria = FEV$_1$/FVC% < 75%.
Source: Ref. 22.

abnormalities. This suggests that the ATS 1986 criterion (still commonly used) is too stringent.

Viegi et al. also analyzed the sensitivity, specificity, predictive power, and overall accuracy of the three criteria with respect to the presence or absence of respiratory symptoms. The ERS criteria had the highest specificity and positive predictive value; the ATS criteria had the lowest. Conversely, the ATS criteria had the highest sensitivity, and the ERS the lowest. This analysis is helpful since it again emphasizes that criteria must be used carefully and comparisons of prevalence across countries or regions must take into account the use of different criteria, as well as more obvious differences, such as methodological differences in equipment, procedures, and questionnaires.

IX. Summary

Several different approaches have been used to estimate prevalence of COPD. Not surprisingly, these give very different answers. Estimates based on respiratory symptoms overestimate the prevalence of COPD. Estimates based on doctor diagnoses appreciably underestimate the total burden of disease since COPD is not diagnosed until moderately advanced. The most accurate estimates are based on measurements of lung function and the presence of airflow limitation.

COPD prevalence varies by age, gender, smoking, environmental exposures, and region/country. COPD prevalences are likely to increase markedly in developing countries as smoking and life expectancy increases. The key to decreasing the burden of COPD lies in reducing exposure to inhaled particulates and gases, the most important of which worldwide is clearly tobacco smoke. In those parts of the world where indoor pollution is a particular problem, attention needs to be paid to the design of dwellings and cleaner cooking methods.

References

1. Higgins MW, Thom T. Incidence, prevalence, and mortality: intra-and inter-country differences. In: Clinical Epidemiology of Chronic Obstructive Pulmonary Disease. New York: Marcel Dekker, 1989:23–43.
2. Murray CJL, Lopez AD. The Global Burden of Disease. Published by the Harvard School of Public Health on Behalf of the World Health Organization and the World Bank. Distributed by Harvard University Press.
3. Murray JF, Nadel JA. Textbook of Respiratory Medicine. Philadelphia: WB Saunders, 1994: 1259–1287.
4. American Thoracic Society. Standards for the diagnosis and care of patients with chronic obstructive pulmonary disease. Am J Respir Crit Care Med 1995; 152:S77–S120.
5. Siafakas NM, Vermeire P, Pride NB, Paoletti P, Gibson J, Howard P, Yernault JC, Decramer M, Higenbottam T, Postma DS, Rees. Optimal assessment and management of chronic obstructive pulmonary disease (COPD). European Respiratory Society Consensus Statement. Eur Respir J 1995; 8:1398–1420.
6. Global Strategy for the Diagnosis, Management, and Prevention of Chronic Obstructive Pulmonary Disease. Executive Summary. NIH Publication No. 2701A. March 2001 (updated 2003).
7. Fletcher CM. Chronic bronchitis: Its prevalence, nature and pathogenesis. Am Rev Respir Dis 1959; 80:483–494.
8. Medical Research Council. Standardized questionnaires on respiratory symptoms. Br Med J 1960; 2:1665.
9. Ferris BG, Anderson DO. The prevalence of chronic respiratory disease in a New Hampshire town. AARD 1962; 165–177.
10. Higgins ITT. Respiratory symptoms, bronchitis, and ventilatory capacity in random sample of an agriculture population. Br Med J 1957; 1198–1203.

11. Olsen HC, Gilson JC. Respiratory symptoms, bronchitis, and ventilatory capacity in men. An Anglo-Danish comparison, with special reference to differences in smoking habits. Br Med J 1960; 450–456.

12. Anderson HR. Respiratory abnormalities, smoking habits and ventilatory capacity in a highland community in Papua New Guinea: prevalence and effect on mortality. IJE 1979; 8:127–135.

13. Mueller RE, Keble DL, Plummer J, Walker SH. The prevalence of chronic bronchitis, chronic airway obstruction, and respiratory symptoms in a Colorado city. ARRD 1971; 103:209–228.

14. Mitchell CA, Schilling RSF, Bouhuys A. Community studies of lung disease in Connecticut: organization and methods. AJE 1976; 103:212–225.

15. Lebowitz MD, Knudson RJ, Burrows B. Tucson epidemiologic study of obstructive lung disease. AJE 1975; 102:137–152.

16. Cookson JB, Mataka G. Prevalence of chronic bronchitis in Rhodesian Africans. Thorax 1978; 33:328–334.

17. Brown P, Gajduser DC. Acute and chronic pulmonary airway disease in Pacific Island Micronesians. AJE 1978; 108:266–273.

18. Joshi RC, Madan RN, Brash AA. Prevalence of chronic bronchitis in an industrial population in North India. Thorax 1975; 30:61–67.

19. Miller GJ, Ashcroft MT. A community survey of respiratory disease among East Indian and African adults in Guyana. Thorax 1971; 26:331–338.

20. Manfreda J, Nelson N, Cherniack RM. Prevalence of respiratory abnormalities in a rural and an urban community. ARRD 1978; 117:215–224.

21. Krzyzanowski M, Kauffmann F. The relation of respiratory symptoms and ventilatory function to moderate occupational exposure in a general population. Results from the French PAARC study of 16,000 adults. Int J Epidemiol 1988; 17:397–406.

22. Viegi G, Paoletti P, Prediletto R, Carrozzi L, Fazzi P, Di Pede F, Pistelli G, Giuntini C, Lebowitz MD. Prevalence of respiratory symptoms in an unpolluted area of northern Italy. Eur Respir J 1988; 1:311–318.

23. Viegi G, Paoletti P, Carrozzi L, Vellutini M, Ballerin L, Biavati P, Nardini G, Di Pede F, Sapigni T, Lebowitz MD, Giuntini C. Effects of home environment on respiratory symptoms and lung function in a general population sample in north Italy. Eur Respir J 1991; 4:580–586.

24. Lundbäck B, Stjernberg N, Nyström, Lundbäck K, Jönsson E, Rosenhall L. Epidemiology of respiratory symptoms, lung function and important determinants. Tubercle Lung Dis 1994; 75:116–126.

25. Enright PL, Kronmal RA, Higgins MW, Schenker MB, Haponik EF. Prevalence and correlates of respiratory symptoms and disease in the elderly. Chest 1994; 106:827–834.

26. Dow L, Coggon D, Osmond C, Holgate ST. A population survey of respiratory symptoms in the elderly. Eur Respir J 1991; 4:267–272.

27. Reid D, Anderson DO, Ferris BG, Fletcher CM. An Anglo-American comparison of the prevalence of bronchitis. BMJ 1964; 1487–1491.

28. Gendra MR, Pandey RAJ. Prevalence of chronic bronchitis in a rural community of the hill region of Nepal. Thorax 1984; 39:331–336.
29. Krzyzanowski M, Kauffmann F. The relation of respiratory symptoms and ventilatory function to moderate occupational exposure in a general population. Results from the French PAARC study of 16,000 adults. Intl J Epidemiol 1988; 17:397–406.
30. Malik SK. Profile of chronic bronchitis in north India — the PGI experience (1972–1985). Lung India 1986; 89–100.
31. Buist AS, Ghezzo H, Anthonisen NR, Cherniack RM, Ducic S, Macklem PT, Manfreda J, Martin RR, McCarthy D, Ross BB. Relationship between the single-breath N_2 test and age, sex, and smoking habit in three North American cities. ARRD 1979; 120:305–318.
32. Pandey, MR. Domestic smoke pollution and chronic bronchitis in a rural community of the hill region of Nepal. Thorax 1984; 39:337–339.
33. College of General Practitioners. Chronic bronchitis in Great Britain: a national survey carried out by the respiratory disease study group of the college of general practitioners. Br Med J 1961; ii:973–9.
34. Irnell L, Kiviloog J. Bronchial asthma and bronchitis in Swedish urban and rural population. Scand J Respir Dis 1968; (suppl 66):1–86.
35. Toyama T, Kagawa J. Prevalence of chronic bronchitis in Japan. In: Viswanathan R, Jaggi OP, eds. Advances in Chronic Obstructive Lung Disease: Proceedings of the World Congress on Asthma, Bronchitis and Allied Conditions (1974). Delhi: Asthma and Bronchitis Foundation of India, 1977:5–19.
36. Viswanathan R, Singh K. Chronic bronchitis and asthma in urban and rural Delhi. In: Viswaranthan R, Jaggi OP, eds. Advances in Chronic Obstructive Lung Disease: Proceedings of the World Congress on Asthma, Bronchitis and Allied Conditions (1974). Delhi: Asthma and Bronchitis Foundation of India, 1977:44–48.
37. Thiruvenagadam KV, Raghava TP, Krisnaswamy KV. Survey of the prevalence of chronic bronchitis in Madras city. In: Viswanathan R, Jaggi OP, eds. Advances in Chronic Obstructive Lung Disease: Proceedings of the World Congress on Asthma, Bronchitis and Allied Conditions (1974). Delhi: Asthma and Bronchitis Foundation of India, 1977:59–69.
38. Sofowora EO. Chronic bronchitis and asthma in a Nigerian community. In: Viswanathan R, Jaggi OP, eds. Advances in Chronic Obstructive Lung Disease: Proceedings of the World Congress on Asthma, Bronchitis and Allied Conditions (1974). Delhi: Asthma and Bronchitis Foundation of India, 1977: 36–43.
39. Centers for Disease Control and Prevention, 1998. Vital and Health Statistics: Current Estimates from the National Health Interview Survey, 1995. DHHS Publication No. (PHS) 96–1527.
40. National Center for Health Statistics. National Hospital Interview Survey. Vital and Health Statistics: series 13:(1970–1998).

41. Centers for Disease Control and Prevention. Chronic Obstructive Pulmonary Disease Surveillance—United States, 1971–2000. MMWR 2002; 51 (No. SS06).

42. Mannino DM, Gagnan RC, Petty TL, Lydrick E. Obstructive lung disease and low lung function in adults in the United States: data from the National Health and Nutrition Examination Survey, 1988–1994. Arch Intern Med 2000; 160:1683–1689.

43. Sobradillo Peña V, Miravitlles M, Gabriel R, Jiménez-Ruiz CA, Villasante C, Masa JF, Viego JL, Fernández-Fau L. Geographic variations in prevalence and underdiagnosis of COPD. Chest 2000; 118:981–989.

44. Roca J, Sanchis J, Agusti-Vidal A, et al. Spirometric reference values from a Mediterranean population. Bull Eur Physiopathol Respir 1986; 22:217–224.

3

Worldwide Mortality from COPD

JEAN-FRANÇOIS MUIR and ANTOINE CUVELIER

CHU de Rouen
Rouen, France

Chronic obstructive pulmonary disease (COPD) is a very common disease around the world, especially in the aged and in the industrialized countries (1), afflicting as many as 600 million people (2). In 1996 COPD was the fifth leading cause of death, and current trends suggest that it will become the third leading cause of death (3) by the year 2020 (4). The primary trigger for COPD is cigarette smoking (5); other potential risk factors for developing COPD including childhood asthma, occupational exposure, and air pollution. The vast majority of patients with COPD are current or former smokers, and it is estimated that 80–90% of all COPD cases are caused by smoking. The likelihood of dying as a result of COPD is 10 times higher for a smoker than for a nonsmoker (6).

The task of comparing mortality rates from COPD and allied conditions is complicated by the fact that they vary widely among countries and also within countries. Rates are also likely to be underestimated because of frequent co-morbidity resulting in failure to code for COPD and availability of heterogeneous data among the different countries (7). In comparison, during this century both COPD and lung cancer have constantly increased as causes of death in industrialized countries, while deaths from tuberculosis and infectious diseases have shown a decreasing trend (8,9).

I. Mortality Evaluation: Difficulties and Limits

The lack of reliability of death certificates, which indicate that an important proportion of patients die with chronic respiratory disease, has consequences on determining the real role of COPD in the general death rate of the population (10). Using death certificate data for epidemiological studies has certain limitations, as they are not validated and some degree of misclassification inevitably occurs (11). They also do not contain data on the severity of chronic diseases or risk factors for COPD, which are an important cause of mortality around the world, leading to their underestimation. The use of mortality statistics to explore the epidemiology of COPD is impaired by the fact that COPD is not a clearly standardized diagnosis. The subsequent changes of the rules for coding the underlying cause of death using successive International Classification of Diseases (ICD) releases also introduces limits to appreciate the real evolution of deaths related to COPD and the international comparisons, since different countries do not use the same versions (9,12,13). This problem does not exist for lung cancer, being clearly identified by code 162 in the ICD 9th revision (ICD-9). COPD does not, in fact appear as a specific single category in any revision of the ICD used to classify mortality data, but is derived from subgroups comprising primarily chronic bronchitis and emphysema. However, a category of "chronic airway obstruction not elsewhere classified" was introduced into the ninth revision of the ICD in 1979 (14) (Table 1). If the successive ICD releases have been responsible for a diagnostic transfer from the chronic

Table 1 Classification of Chronic Obstructive Pulmonary Disease and Allied Conditions in the Ninth Revision of the International Classification of Diseases

Code	Description
490	Bronchitis, not specified as acute or chronic
491	Chronic bronchitis
492	Emphysema
493	Asthma
494	Bronchiectasis
495	Extrinsic allergic alveolitis
496	Chronic airways obstruction, not elsewhere classified

Source: Ref. (14).

Table 2 Classification of Chronic Obstructive Pulmonary Disease and Allied Conditions in the Tenth Revision of the International Classification of Diseases

Code	Description
J40	Bronchitis (not specified acute or chronic)
J41	Simple chronic bronchitis
J42	Chronic bronchitis
J43	Emphysema
J44	Other obstructive disease
J45	Asthma
J46	Acute asthma
J47	Bronchiectasis

Source: Tenth Revision of the International Classification of Diseases.

bronchitis to the chronic airway obstruction categories (the latter having been introduced in 1979), the extent of variation from year to year in the total number of deaths attributed to COPD appears to be in fact relatively small. Unfortunately, the tenth classification (Table 2) does not help in the ascertainment of the disease, as it separates bronchitis (unspecified), simple chronic bronchitis, chronic bronchitis, emphysema, and other obstructive diseases. Several recent studies have demonstrated that reduced levels of FEV_1 (i.e., COPD-related) predict subsequent mortality from a range of nonrespiratory diseases, particularly coronary heart disease (15,16) and stroke (17). Indeed, it is arguable that the greater part of the burden of mortality attributable to these conditions is concealed among deaths attributed to other causes, notably coronary artery disease.

II. COPD Mortality Around the World

A. Introduction

The total number of deaths involved confirms that in most developed countries, COPD is a major cause of death in adult populations (8). France, the United States, Japan, and the United Kingdom have similar age-adjusted COPD mortality rates (9.5 for France, 8.9 for the United Kingdom, 8.8 for the United States, and 10/100,000 for Japan). In these four countries the mortality rate is more elevated in men than in women. In Europe, France has the lowest rate, 9.8, versus 16 for Germany, 21 for Italy, 18 for Poland, 39.6 for Hungary, and 40 for Russia (Fig. 1) (8,18,19). While differences between countries in level and trend of mortality are apparent (20), the highest mortality for COPD, as for lung cancer, during

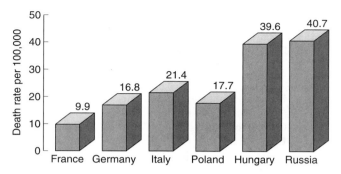

Figure 1 Annual mortality related to COPD per 100,000 inhabitants in Europe and Russia, 1995. (From Ref 7.)

the 1980s occurred in eastern European countries, Ireland, and the United Kingdom, and the lowest in southern Europe, Japan, and Israel (12). At the same time, mortality had a diminishing trend only for subjects aged 45–64 years, while it has been stable in those aged 65–74 years and has increased in those aged >75 years in the United States, the United Kingdom, France, West Germany, Israel, Canada, Belgium, and Australia (Fig. 2). Mortality from COPD is consistently seen to be greater in older age groups and in males than in females, with age-adjusted mortality being clearly more elevated in men (14). Countries with relatively high mortality rates in males also tend to have relatively high mortality rates in females, though not exclusively so. In females there is a dramatic 125% increase linked to the increasing tobacco usage in women. Ethnic differences are also present, with a mortality rate in white patients 1.5 times higher than in nonwhite ethnies. Between 1979 and 1993, age-adjusted mortality increased 10% for white men and 35% in black men (21). The main cause is tobacco; smokers die more often from COPD than nonsmokers, with a higher proportion of documented emphysema on necropsy, the corresponding lesions being proportional to the duration of the exposure to tobacco smoke (14).

B. United States and Canada

In 1993, the overall U.S. death rate adjusted for age was 20/100,000, COPD being the fourth leading cause of mortality, with nearly 96,000 deaths (8). Of 31 million deaths in 1979–1993, approximately 1% of all deaths below the age of 44 years were caused by obstructive lung disease (22). In the age

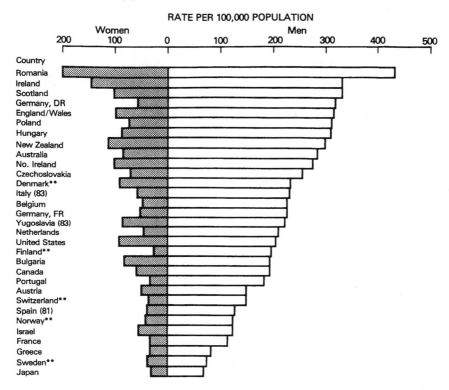

Figure 2 Death rates for COPD and allied conditions by sex, age 65–74, and by country in 1984. **ICD-8 Codes 490–493. (From Ref. 12.)

group 55–84 years, approximately 8% of all death certificates contained a diagnosis of obstructive lung disease (22). However, only 43% of the death certificates with obstructive lung disease (22) listed had obstructive lung disease as the primary underlying cause of death (11). The mortality rate due to COPD is two to three times lower in females than in males. It was reported in 1994 that 16 million Americans were suffering from COPD, an increase of 60% from 1982 (8). In 1985, COPD was estimated as the underlying cause for 3.6% of all U.S. deaths, and a contributory cause in an additional 4.3%. Obstructive lung diseases (OLD), including COPD and asthma, are leading causes of mortality among both men and women in the United States (23), and OLD-related mortality rates have been increasing in the United States, as in other countries (9,12). A relatively persistent overall trend in mortality was observed over a 35-year period

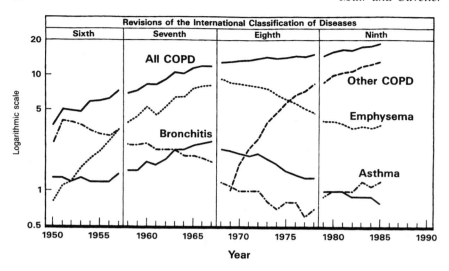

Figure 3 Mortality from COPD and its subcategories standardized to the total U.S. population in 1940. (From Ref. 9.)

from 1950 to 1985 (14), during which time the overall mortality from all COPD increased approximately fourfold (Fig. 3). Absolute mortality rates in males and females aged 55–84 years in 1985 were approximately 200/100,000 males and 80/100,000 females. The effect of specific ICD revisions on the overall trend in mortality during this period appears to have been small during that period (9). In another study of mortality trends among people who died with a diagnosis of obstructive lung disease from 1979 through 1993, using death certificate reports of 31,314,160 decedents in the Multiple-Cause Mortality Files compiled by the U.S. National Center for Health Statistics, 8.2% had a diagnosis of obstructive lung disease (ICD-9 490 to 493.9, 496) listed on their death certificates (11). Only 43.3% had obstructive lung disease listed as the underlying cause of death. The global age-adjusted mortality rate increased 47.3%, from 52.6/100,000 in 1979 to 77.5/100,000 in 1993. The age-adjusted mortality rate increased 17.1% among men, from 96.3%/100,000 in 1979 to 112.8/100,000 in 1993, whereas this rate increased 126.1% among women, from 24.5/100,000 in 1979 to 55.4/100,000 in 1993. Over the study period, white males had the highest mortality rates (98.8–115.5/100,000), followed by black males (77.5–100.2/100,000), males of other races (38.1–58.6/100,000), white females (25.5–57.7/100,000), black females (14.9–38.5/100,000), and females of other races (10.9–20.9/100,000). It was concluded that mortality related to obstructive lung disease is underestimated in studies that look at only the underlying cause of death. Mortality rates of obstructive lung disease have started to stabilize among men since the mid-1980s, although they are still increasing among men older than 85 years, but they continue to increase among women, reflecting smoking trends in these populations. These different patterns are probably related both to trends of current and former smoking rates and to patterns of occupational exposures among men and women (24,25). Women may also have a different susceptibility to the effects of continued cigarette smoking or smoking cessation than men (26,27). In studies of lung cancer mortality rates, it was found that black males had the highest rates, mirroring their higher rates of current smoking (28). In spite of the fact that tobacco use is the most important risk factor for the development of COPD, it was listed on only 2.8% of the death records that listed COPD (29). Although this proportion increased from 0.5% in 1979 to 5.1% in 1993, tobacco-use disorder remains underreported. These findings support the observation that OLD are diseases of aging and increase as the population ages.

Information drawn from the Canadian National Mortality Database regarding the mortality and morbidity of COPD (including asthma) in Canada (30) previously established between 1950 and 1984 suggested that the increase in mortality from COPD had leveled off among men but was still increasing among women. For the 750,000 Canadians having chronic bronchitis or emphysema diagnosed by a health professional, prevalence rates were for (a) age 55–64 years, 4.6%, (b) age 65–74 years, 5.0%, (c) age ≥75 years, 6.8%. From 1980 to 1995, the total number of deaths from COPD increased from 4438 to 8583. Although the age-standardized mortality rate remained stable throughout this period in men (around 45/100,000 population), it doubled in women (8.3/100,000 in 1980 to 17.3/100,000 in 1995). There were 55,782 hospital separations in 1993–1994 with COPD as the primary discharge diagnosis (compared to 42,102 in 1981–1982). In people ≥ 65 years, the age-specific hospital separation rate increased over this period, especially in women ≥ 75 years (from 504/100,000 to 1033/100,000). The average in-hospital length of stay was 9.6 days in 1981–1982 and 8.3 days in 1993–1994. Age-adjusted obstructive lung disease–related mortality rates of 77.5/100,000 were reported in 1993 in the United States (11) versus 20.4/100,000 in Canada when obstructive lung disease was cited as the primary cause of death; however, using death records that specified obstructive lung disease as the underlying cause of death, mortality rates in the United States and Canada were quite similar (U.S. 1995 mortality 3.6%; Canada 1995 mortality 4.1%). Thus, COPD is a major health issue in Canada and will remain so for decades (Fig. 4).

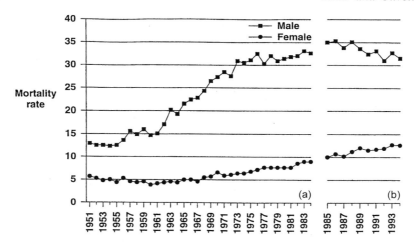

Figure 4 Age-standardized mortality rates per 10,000 population for COPD (including asthma) in Canada, 1951–1994. All mortality rates were adjusted for the 1971 Canadian population. (Left) Mortality rate, 1951–1983. (Right) Mortality rate, 1984–1994. (From Ref. 30.)

C. Asia

In Asia, China is now the largest tobacco-producing country in the world, and it has the most smokers—over 300 million (31). Smoking prevalence in China has increased rapidly in recent decades, but, compared with the West, China is only at the early stage of the epidemic. Data from a large case-control study in China estimated deaths from smoking at about 500,000 per year (32).

Few prospective studies of smoking and mortality in China have been published (33,34). All had a short duration of follow-up (4–13 years), and some were limited to men only (34). One study compared tobacco-related mortality in Shanghai and the United States and concluded the risk of mortality in the Chinese was lower (33). The study from Shanghai described only the early stage of the Chinese epidemic, and the risk estimates might have been underestimated (33).

A cohort study was conducted in Xi'an (31) to examine the relationship between smoking and mortality in men and women after 20 years of follow-up involving 1696 people aged 35 years or older (1124 men, 572 women) examined in May 1976. A total of 56% of the men and 12% of the women were never-smokers at baseline. Through August 31, 1996, 218 persons (173 men, 45 women) had died. The relative risks (95% confidence intervals for ever-smoking after adjusting for age, marital status, occupation, education, diastolic blood pressure, and triglyceride and cholesterol levels) for deaths resulting from all causes, all cancer, and coronary heart disease were, respectively, 2.42 (95% CI 1.72–3.42), 2.50 (95% CI 1.41–4.43), and 3.61 (95% CI 1.35–9.67) in men and 2.32 (95% CI 1.18–4.56), 1.98 (95% CI 0.50–7.92), and 4.67 (95% CI 0.78–27.8) in women.

D. Europe

The total population of 54 European countries is approximately 750 million according to the World Health Organization (WHO). The countries with the highest COPD rates include those in eastern Europe, the United Kingdom, and Ireland (22). Lower rates are observed in the countries of southern and northern Europe. When codes other than ICD 490–496 are used for COPD, the distribution of mortality rates caused by COPD changes considerably among European countries (12). There are also considerable differences in mortality rate trends among the European countries, increasing among females in northern European countries such as Denmark and the United Kingdom and decreasing in the countries of central and eastern Europe such as Czechoslovakia and Bulgaria. Overall mortality due to chronic pulmonary disease will most probably increase in Europe owing to an increasing proportion of smoking females as well as increased aging of the population. Data from other countries collected by WHO confirm marked variation in overall rates of mortality from COPD between countries (12,21) (Fig. 2) within a range of more than fourfold between the extremes of > 400 deaths/100,000 males aged 65–74 years in Romania and <100/100,000 in Japan. Projections suggest a further worldwide increase in the COPD death rate in future years (35).

In the Flemish region of Belgium (36), age-standardized mortality by COPD in men was 87/100,000 in 1997, causing in the age group 1–74 years a loss of 2.0 potential years of life per 1000 person-years. Only four other diseases caused a larger overall loss of years of life: lung cancer (8.5), ischemic heart disease (7.6), cerebro-vascular disease (2.7), and colorectal cancer (2.2). In females COPD caused a loss of 0.7 potential years of life per 1000 person-years, and it was the eighth cause of such loss by disease.

In Italy from 1979 to 1990, using data from the Italian Central Statistical Institute (ISTAT), mortality from lung cancer appeared to increase in all age groups except for those aged 45–64 years after 1985 (8). Respiratory diseases showed a consistent reduction; in particular, mortality from emphysema decreased slowly, and mortality from chronic bronchitis showed a significant reduction in all age groups. In 1990, data stratified for age group and gender indicated a higher mortality rate in males that tended to be age-dependent, with the highest rate ratio male/female in those aged 65–74 years.

Chronic bronchitis, together with bronchitis not specified as either acute or chronic (ICD-9 490–491), represented a large part of the whole mortality from respiratory diseases. These analyses have confirmed data collected in the 1970s (37), and respiratory diseases continued to rank third among the most frequent causes of death in Italy in the period 1979–1990, after circulatory disorders and tumors. The same gender difference was found by other authors in 1980–1985 (12) and 1988–1991 (38). The fact that the highest ratios male/female were found in 65- to 74-year-olds might be due to the longer lifetime of females.

Mortality figures for England and Wales during the period 1971–1990 reveal relatively static overall COPD mortality during this period at 250–300 deaths/100,000 persons aged 65–84 years per annum (Fig. 5), though sex-specific mortality in those aged > 65 years in England and Wales in 1990–1992 was 482 and 225/100,000 males and females, respectively, approximately twice that reported for comparable age groups in the United States during the 1980s (9,39).

The evolution of these trends may reflect diagnostic transfer, changes in use of hospital services (particularly for asthma), or improvements in domiciliary care of COPD (10). The analyses differ in the effect shown for period of death on chronic respiratory disease mortality. This is because there has been a very substantial downward trend in age-specific mortality

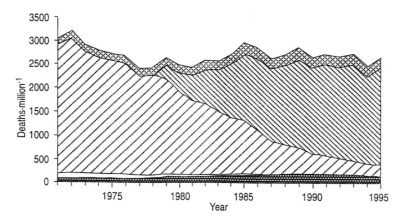

Figure 5 Mortality of COPD in England and Wales, 1975–1995, in males and females, combined ages 65–84 years. □: bronchitis not specified as acute or chronic; ▓: asthma; ▨: chronic bronchitis; ▧: chronic airways obstruction; ▨: emphysema. *Source*: Ref. 39.

rates since the second world war and it is statistically impossible to assign this with confidence to a generation or to a period of death effect or to some combination of the two. However, the downward drift started in the late nineteenth century in all age groups simultaneously and therefore is perhaps more likely to be a period-of-death effect. It continued throughout the 1970s, a period during which there were substantial reductions in urban smoke and sulfur dioxide air pollution in Britain. COPD represents a major burden on healthcare services in these countries.

It is estimated in France that 2–3 million people suffer from chronic bronchitis corresponding to a prevalence of 5–10%. In 1991 (40,41) 7792 deaths in men were attributed to COPD, and 4763 in women in 1998, corresponding to an overall mortality of 28/100,000 in men and 16.3/100,000 in women (42). The number of patients corresponding to the ERS definition (14) has been estimated at between 700,000 and 1 million; men are predominantly represented (70–75%). Hypoxemic bronchitis patients in France are estimated at 60,000–100,000, in the United Kingdom at 60,000. In France, overall mortality was estimated in 1985 as 2.3% of the total mortality (11,000–12,000), the fifth leading cause of mortality. As this diagnosis is underevaluated in France 15,000–20,000 deaths per year seems an acceptable estimate (43).

III. Future Trends

Other factors with prognostic value include nutritional depletion, which is an independent risk factor for mortality and hospitalization in patients with COPD receiving long-term oxygen therapy (LTOT) (44). Similar results were observed in other studies, such as the National Mortality Survey where low weight was associated with COPD mortality (45) and the Copenhagen City Heart Study (46) concerning malnutrition. It seems that midthigh muscle cross-sectional area is a better predictor of mortality than body mass index in patients with COPD (47).

Health studies using questionnaires such as the St. Georges's Respiratory Questionnaire have shown quality of life (QOL) to be significantly correlated with mortality (48,49). Just as lower QOL is a powerful predictor of hospitalization and all-cause mortality, brief, self-administered COPD–specific QOL measures such, as the Seattle Obstruction Lung Disease Questionnaire, provide an opportunity to identify patients who could benefit from preventive interventions facing hospitalization and mortality risks due to COPD (50).

Worldwide mortality secondary to COPD varies greatly from one country to another, being linked to the poor reliability of death certificate information and successive ICD revisions. Although mortality trends are decreasing in the United States, this is not the case in other countries because of the continued importance of tobacco-related diseases. COPD morbidity and mortality could be more efficiently prevented on a worldwide level if screening were improved, and it remains an underdiagnosed disease (51).

References

1. Bourier MH, Guideraux M. Mortality from disorders of the respiratory system throughout the world between 1950 and 1972. World Health Stat Q 1979; 32(3):174–197.
2. World Health Statistics Annual 1998, WHO, Geneva.
3. World Health Statistics Annual 1999, WHO, Geneva.
4. Murray CJL, Lopez AD. The Global Burden of Disease and Injury.1. Cambridge, MA: Harvard University Press, 1996.
5. American Thoracic Society. Standards for the diagnosis and care of patients with COPD. Am J Respir Crit Care Med 1995; 152:S77–S120.
6. American Lung Association. COPD. American Lung Association fact sheet, Sept. 1988.
7. Snider GL. Facteurs de risque et populations à risque. Rev Mal Respir 1998; 15:2S5–2S9.
8. Desideri M, Viegi G, Carrozzi L, Pedreschi M, Pistelli F, Magiorelli F, Fornai E, Paoletti P, Giuntini C. Mortality rates for respiratory disorders in Italy. Monaldi Arch Chest Dis 1997; 52:212–216.
9. Feinleib M, Rosemberg HM, Collins JG, Delozier JE, Pokras R, Chevariey FM. Trends in COPD morbidity and mortality in the United States. Am Rev Respir Dis 1989; 140:S9—S18.
10. Strachan DP. Epidemiology: a British perspective. In: Calverley PM, Pride NB, eds. Chronic Obstructive Pulmonary Disease. London: Chapman & Hall, 1995: 47–68.
11. Mannino DM, Brown C, Giovino GA. Obstructive lung disease in the United States from 1979 through 1993. An analysis using multicause mortality data. Am J Respir Crit Care Med 1997; 156:814–818.
12. Thom TJ. International comparisons in COPD mortality. Am Rev Respir Dis 1989; 140:S27—S34.
13. Manfreda J, Mao Y, Litven W. Morbidity and mortality from chronic obstructive pulmonary disease. Am Rev Respir Dis 1989; 140:S19—S26.
14. Rijcken B, Britton J. Epidemiology of COPD. Eur Respir Monogr 1998; 7:41–73.
15. Cook DG, Shaper AG. Breathlessness, lung function, and risks of a heart attack. Eur Heart J 1988; 9:1215–1222.
16. Ebi-Kryston AL. Respiratory symptoms and pulmonary function as predictors of 10-years mortality from respiratory disease, cardiovascular disease, and all causes in the Whitehall study. J Epidemiol Community Health 1986; 41: 251–260.

17. Strachan DP. Ventilatory function as a predictor of fatal stroke. Br Med J 1991; 302:84–87.
18. Annuaire De Statistiques Sanitaires Mondiales, 1995. Organisation Mondiale De Santé, Genève, 1996.
19. Trends in chronic bronchitis and emphysema: Morbidity and Mortality. Epidemiology and Statistics Unit, American Lung Association, New York, September 1996.
20. Cooreman J, Thom TJ, Higgins MW. Mortality from chronic obstructive pulmonary disease and asthma in France, 1969—1983. Comparisons with the US and Canada. Chest 1990; 97:2 13—219.
21. Higgins MW, Thom T. Incidence, prevalence and mortality: infra- and inter-country differences. In: Hensley MJ, Saunders NA, eds. Clinical Epidemiology of Chronic Obstructive Pulmonary Disease. New York: Marcel Dekker, 1989; 23–43.
22. Gulsvik A. Mortality in and prevalence of COPD in different parts of Europe. Monaldi Arch. Chest Dis 1999; 54:160–162.
23. Mortality patterns—United States, 1993. 1996. MMWR 45:161–164.
24. Giovino GA, Schooley MW, Zhu BP, Chrismon JH, Tomar SL, Peddicord JP, Merritt RK, Husten CG, and Eriksen MP. Centers for Disease Control and Prevention—surveillance for selected tobacco-use behaviors—United States, 1900—1994. MMWR C.D.C. Surveill Summ 1994; 43(No. SS-3):1–43.
25. Becklake MR. Occupational exposures: evidence for a causal association with chronic obstructive pulmonary disease. Am Rev Respir Dis 1989; 140:S85–S91.
26. Paoletti P, Carrozzi L, Viegi G, Modena P, Ballerin L, DiPede F, Grado L, Baldacci S, Pedreschi M, Vellutini M. Distribution of bronchial responsiveness in a general population: effect of sex, age, smoking and level of pulmonary function. Am J Respir Crit Care Med 1995; 151:1770–1777.
27. Sherrill DL, Holberg CJ, Enright PL, Lebowitz MD, Burrows B. Longitudinal analysis of the effects of smoking onset and cessation on pulmonary function. Am J Respir Crit Care Med 1994; 149:591–597.
28. Mannino DM, Ford E, Giovino GA, Thun M. Lung cancer deaths in the United States from 1979 through 1992: an analysis using multiple-cause mortality data (abst). Am Rev Respir Dis 1996; 153: A658.
29. Bartecchi CE, MacKenzie TD, Schrier RW. The human costs of tobacco use. N Engl J Med 1994; 330:907–912.
30. Lacasse Y, Brooks D, Goldstein RS, and Rehabilitation Committee of the Canadian Thoracic Society. Trends in epidemiology of COPD in Canada, 1980 to 1995. Chest 1999; 116:306–313.
31. Tai Hing Lam, Yao He, Lan Sun Li, Liang Shou Li, Shu Fang He, Bao Qing Liang. Mortality attributable to cigarette smoking in China. JAMA 1997; 278:1505–1508.
32. Peto R, Lopezs DA, Boreham J, Thun M, Heath C Jr. Mortality from Smoking in Developed Countries 1950–2000 Oxford, England: Oxford University Press, 1994, pp. 35–55.

33. Yuan JM, Ross RK, Wang XL, Gao YT, Henderson BE, Yu MC. Morbidity and mortality in relation to cigarette smoking in Shanghai, China: a prospective male cohort study. JAMA 1996; 275:1646–1650.

34. Wu XG, Wan SY, He JS. A prospective study on risk factors of coronary heart disease in male workers in Beijing Capital Steel Company: relationship between blood pressure, serum cholesterol, smoking, and coronary heart disease. Chin Circ J 1991; 6:127–130.

35. Murray C, Lopez A. Alternative projections of mortality and disability by cause 1990–2020: global burden of disease study. Lancet 1997; 349: 1498–1504.

36. Aelvoet W, Komitzer M, DeBacker G. Gezondheidsindicatoren 1997. Flemish Ministry of Public Health 1999.

37. Giuntini C, Paoletti P. Epidemiologia delle malattie polmonari in Italia. Aggiorn Med 1983; 3:333–339.

38. Siafakas NM, Vermeire P, Pride NB, Parletti P, Gibson J, Howard P, Yernault JC, Decramen M, Higenbottam T, Postman DL on behalf of the ERS Task Force. Optimal assessment and management of COPD. Eur Respir J 1995; 8: 1398–1420.

39. Lung and Asthma Information Agency. Trends in asthma mortality in the elderly. New York, 1992; 92/1.

40. Pharmametrics. DIP-Base Disease segment: subcategories of chronic bronchitis 1994; (suppl):1–18. www.pharmiq.com.

41. Pharmametrics DIP-Base. Disease segment: COPD. 1994; 1:44–70. www.pharmiq.com

42. INSERM: Causes mèdicales de dècès. Annèe 1991. Rèsultats dèfinitifs.France.

43. Weitzenblum E, Chaouat A, Faller M, Kessler R. L'insuffisance respiratoire chronique: evaluation, èvolution, pronostic. Bull Acad Natle Mèd., 1998; 182: 1123–1137.

44. Chailleux E, Laaban JP, Veale D. Prognostic value of nutritional depletion in patients with COPD treated by long-term oxygen therapy: data from the ANTADIR observatory. Chest 2003; 123(5): 1460–1466.

45. Meyer PA, Manino DM, Redd SC, Olson DR. Characteristics of adults dying with COPD. Chest 2002; 122(6): 2003–2008.

46. Prescott E, Almdal T, Mikkelsen KL, Tofteng CL, Vqestbo J, Lange P. Pronostic value of weight change in chronic obstructive pulmonary disease: results from the Copenhagen City Heart Study. Eur Respir J 2002; 20(3): 539–544.

47. Marquis K, Debigare R, Lacasse Y, Leblanc P, Jobin J, Carrier G, Maltais F. Midthigh muscle cross-sectional area is a better predictor of mortality than body mass index in patients with chronic obstructive pulmonary disease. Am J Respir Crit Care Med 2002; 166(6): 809–813.

48. Oga T, Nishimura K, Tsukino M, Sato S, Hajiro T. Analysis of the factors related to mortality in chronic obstructive pulmonary disease: role of exercise capacity and health status. Am J Respir Crit Care Med 167(4): 544–549.

49. Domingo-Salvany A, Lamarca R, Ferrer M, Garcia-Aymerich J, Alonso J, Felez M, Khalaf A, Marrades RM, Monso E, Serra-Batlles J, Anto JM.

Health-related quality of life and mortality in male patients with chronic obstructive pulmonary disease. Am J Respir Crit Care Med 2002; 166(5): 680–685.

50. Fan VS, Curtis JR, Tu SP, McDonell MB, Fihn SD, Ambulatory Care Quality Improvement Project Investigators. Using quality of life to predict hospitalisation and mortality in patients with obstructive lung diseases. Chest 2002; 122(2): 429–436.

51. Mannino DM, Homa DM, Akinbami LJ, Ford ES, Redd SC. Chronic obstructive pulmonary disease surveillance—United States, 1971–2000. Respir Care 2002; 47(10): 1148–1149.

4

Risk Factors for the Development of COPD

SCOTT T. WEISS and EDWIN K. SILVERMAN

Harvard Medical School
and Brigham and Women's Hospital
Boston, Massachusetts, U.S.A.

I. Introduction and Definitions

Chronic obstructive pulmonary disease (COPD) is a syndrome characterized by abnormal tests of expiratory airflow (FEV_1 and FEV_1/FVC) that do not change markedly over several months of observations (1). Different levels of fixed airflow obstruction have been utilized to define COPD. No universally accepted thresholds for these continuous pulmonary function variables exist in the clinical literature. Some studies incorporate a decrease in the FEV_1/FVC ratio into the definition, while other studies rely only on reduction in FEV_1. It is important to recognize that the physiological definition of disease occurrence can be contrasted with the clinical criteria for the definition of chronic bronchitis, which traditionally utilizes cough and phlegm production for 3 months per year for 2 consecutive years (2). Pathological correlates of these physiological and epidemiological definitions are the presence of emphysema (defined as abnormal enlargement and destruction of airspaces beyond the terminal bronchiole) and inflammation at the level of the respiratory bronchiole (1). These disease-defining characteristics are not perfectly correlated. Airflow obstruction is more likely with greater severity of anatomical emphysema, but a substantial fraction of subjects with airflow obstruction do not have significant emphysema, and some subjects with significant emphysema do not have airflow obstruction (3,4). To date, it remains unclear what genetic, environmental, and pathobiological factors contribute to this less than perfect correlation.

This chapter will focus on environmental and genetic risk factors for the development of COPD. The intent is to take a life cycle approach to this disorder and to emphasize the importance of early life events, genetics, and intermediate phenotypes to disease occurrence. Attention will be paid to the fetal origins of disease hypothesis and the potential for gene-by-environment interaction early in life. Finally, the concept that the dose and timing of environmental exposures (particularly cigarette smoke) is essential will be introduced, with consideration of the potential influences of dose and timing on disease progression and occurrence.

The importance of COPD as a public health problem is obvious. Entering the year 2000, 13% of the U.S. population (35 million people) were over the age of 65 years. This is the most rapidly growing segment of the population, and COPD is the most rapidly rising cause of death in this age group. There are estimated to be 14 million individuals in the United States with chronic bronchitis, and more than 100,000 people die each year from COPD (5,6).

II. Cigarette Smoking

It is well known that only 10–15% of cigarette smokers will ever develop COPD (2). Several factors likely contribute to the variable influence of cigarette smoking on the development of COPD. The first factor is competing risks. Cigarette smokers may die from early myocardial infarction, stroke, or cancer prior to the development of COPD. However, a second and more intriguing reason is genetic susceptibility. It is well known, from the data of Burrows, that within a given level of smoking exposure, the level of FEV_1 varies substantially (7) (Fig. 1). Part of this variation is likely due to differential genetic susceptibility to cigarette smoke. At the present time, the gene or genes responsible for this postulated gene-by-environment interaction are unknown.

Genetic susceptibility is, however, not the whole story. Cunningham et al. (8) estimated that maternal smoking during pregnancy resulted in a 1.3% reduction in FEV_1 when those children reach the ages of 8–12 years. Tager and coworkers examined the effect of actively smoking cigarettes during adolescence; individuals who smoke cigarettes from age 15–20 years

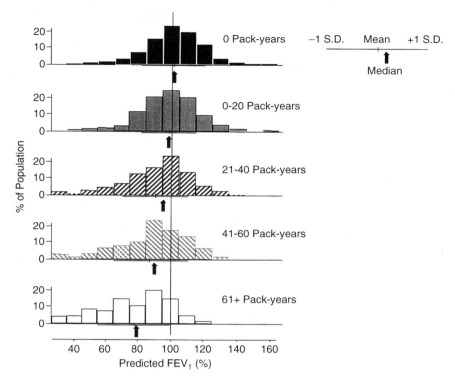

Figure 1 Distributions of FEV_1 (percent predicted) values with varying pack-years of smoking among adult subjects. Mean, median, and ± 1 standard deviation are shown for each group. Many heavy cigarette smokers have FEV_1 values within the normal range. (From Ref. 7.)

were estimated to have an 8% reduction in FEV_1 (9). Xu and colleagues, with data from the Vlagtwedde/Vlaardingen Study, demonstrated that there is a large effect of cigarette smoking to decrease maximal level of lung function in individuals less than 20 years that far exceeded the effect of cigarette smoking on decline in lung function in older age groups (10) (Fig. 2). Table 1 details the dose-effect relationship between in utero, adolescent, and adult cigarette smoke exposure and its relationship to FEV_1. This table clearly demonstrates that dose and timing of exposure can have a profound impact on disease expression at different stages of the life cycle. Indeed, small amounts of cigarette smoking in utero or in adolescence have far greater effect on reduction in pulmonary function many years later than active smoking after the age of 35.

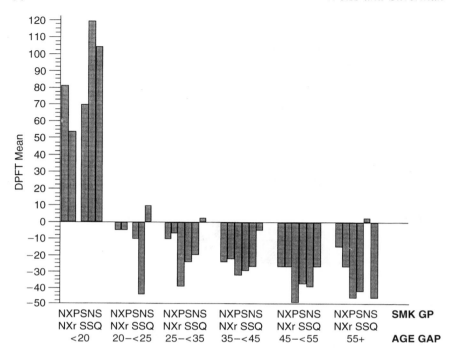

Figure 2 Mean change in FEV_1 (mL/yr) stratified by age and smoking status. Growth in FEV_1 is demonstrated in subjects below age 20 years; decline is demonstrated for subjects aged 25–35, 35–45, 45–55, and > 55 years. Smoking code is S = smoker, P = pipe and cigar, I = intermittent, Q = quit smoking, X = ex-smoker, N = nonsmoker. First initial refers to status at the beginning of the interval. Second refers to status at the end of the interval. (From Ref. 10.)

III. Early Life Events and the Impact on COPD Development

In western industrialized countries the most common chronic lung disease in children is asthma. Epidemiolgical estimates of wheeze prevalence in early childhood reveal that 40% of children wheeze in the first year of life, and this percentage rapidly drops to 20% by age 6 (11). Of those 20% of children wheezing at age 6, only one half were also wheezing in the first year of life. Martinez described four groups of children: never wheezers, transient early wheezers, transient late wheezers, and persistent wheezers (11). Of these four groups, persistent wheezers are the children at greatest risk for the development of childhood asthma. Transient early wheezers have reduced

Table 1 Effects of Cigarette Smoking at Different Stages of the Life Cycle

Life phase (gender)	Cigarette dose	Total FEV$_1$ Reduction (mL)	FEV$_1$ Reduction (mL/yr per pack/day)
In utero (male and female)	? Intensity for 9 mos.	27.3[a]	36
Adolescence (male)	15 cigs/day for 5 yr[b]	390	104
Adolescence (female)	10 cigs/day for 5 yr[b]	340	136
Adult (male)	Variable	N/A	13[c]
Adult (female)	Variable	N/A	7[c]

[a]Adjusted for gender and maternal smoking in past year; based on 1.3% reduction and mean FEV$_1$ = 2.1 L; 1 pack/day in smoking mothers during pregnancy is assumed for relative FEV$_1$ reduction (8).
[b]Median values for cigarette smoking (9).
[c]Estimated values from Ref. 45 in Six Cities Study.

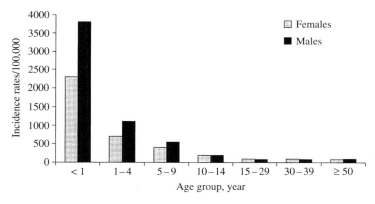

Figure 3 Annual incidence rates of asthma per 100,000 person-years, stratified by gender and age, among Rochester, MN, residents between 1964–1983. The vast majority of asthmatic subjects are diagnosed before the age of 4 years. (From Ref. 12.)

lung function at birth; this condition is strongly associated with maternal cigarette smoking. It cannot be overemphasized that over 80% of all childhood asthma is diagnosed by age 6 (12) (Fig. 3). While it has long been known that "childhood respiratory illness" is a risk factor for adult COPD, this has been though to be due, at least in part, to recall bias; i.e., individuals reporting COPD are more likely to remember early childhood respiratory illness (13). It would appear from longitudinal data in early childhood that the recall problem is of a different nature and likely has a different impact with regard to adult disease. Given the very high prevalence of early childhood wheezing and its disappearance in most individuals by the age of 6, it is clear that recall of these early childhood events in later life is likely to be poor. Even most of the 10% of children with diagnosed asthma at age 6 and "persistent wheezing" will remit at some point by early adulthood. Thus, asthma that presents as "incident" asthma in adolescence or early adulthood may simply be recrudescence of early childhood asthma and not true incident disease. A large percentage of the population will have intermediate phenotypes associated with asthma, i.e., increased airways responsiveness and allergy, and yet will be "silent" with regard to symptom (wheeze) occurrence at older ages. The importance of this "asymptomatic" airways responsiveness in population-based studies is emphasized by its high prevalence. It is clear from a large number of studies using different methodologies in different western industrialized countries that a substantial number of subjects exist with increased airways responsiveness in the asthmatic range who do not have current asthma (Table 2) (14–20). In addition, it can be shown that many of these cases have a prior history of asthma (21). Thus, airways responsiveness constitutes a susceptibility phenotype by which individuals who have this physiological trait have the potential, if they interact with relevant environmental exposures (particularly cigarette smoking, allergen exposure, and respiratory illness), to develop recurrent airflow obstruction (Fig. 4). It is hypothesized that the form of this recurrent airflow obstruction will depend on both the genetic susceptibility profile and the dose, number, and timing of environmental exposures experienced throughout life. The recurrent airflow obstruction will resemble asthma to the extent that cigarette smoking is minimal, atopy is present, and allergen exposure high, but it will begin to resemble COPD as cigarette smoking increases in dose.

IV. Lung Function Growth and Decline

As noted earlier, fixed airflow obstruction is the essence of the definition of chronic obstructive pulmonary disease. FEV_1, as a measure of lung function, tends to track consistently throughout the life of an individual. Tracking is defined as the correlation of a biological variable over time and is defined mathematically by the intraclass correlation coefficient, which is the ratio: (within-person variation)/(within-person variation between-person variation). As can be seen from Figure 5, FEV_1 tracks very consistently during growth within individuals from a very early age. In fact, the tracking correlations for FEV_1, which are on the order of 0.8–0.9 in populations, approximate the tracking correlations for height or body mass index. FEV_1

Table 2 Prevalence of Increased Airway Responsiveness in Random Population Samples of Asymptomatic Children and Adults

Ref.	Population	Criteria for positive response	% Prevalence of increased airway responsiveness	Prevalence of asymptomatic increased responsiveness	
				% of total population	% of all responsive subjects
14	East Boston, MA, random population children, young adults ($n=213$), age range 6–24	$\Delta FEV_1/FVC > 9\%$ to cold air	22	11	51
15	Australia, random population children ($n=2363$), age range 8–11	$PD_{20}FEV_1 \leq 7.8\ \mu mol$ histamine	17.9	6.7	37
16	New Zealand, random population sample ($n=766$), age 9 yr	$PD_{20}FEV_1 < 25\ mg/mL$ methacholine	22	8	30
17	Busselton, Australia, random population adults ($n=876$), mean age 49	$PD_{20}FEV_1 \leq 3.9\ \mu mol$ histamine	11	2	19
18	Netherlands, random population adults ($n=1905$), age range 14–64+	$PC_{10}FEV_1 \leq 16\ mg/mL$ histamine	24.5	14	58.5
19	Boston, MA, adult males ($n=458$), mean age 60	$PD_{20}FEV_1 \leq 50\ \mu mol$ methacholine	29.9	—	—
20	England, random population adults ($n=511$), age range 18–64	$PD_{20}FEV_1 \leq 8\ \mu mol$ histamine	14	—	—

Source: Adapted from Ref. 47.

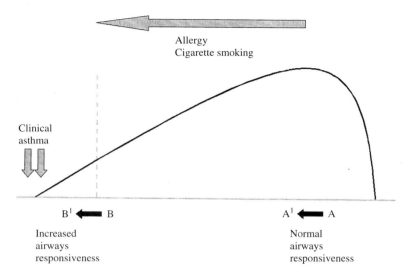

Figure 4 Schematic representation of risk for developing asthma as a function of genetic susceptibility and environmental exposures. Individuals without genetic susceptibility (A) may have some increased airways responsiveness with exposure to environmental factors such as allergic triggers and cigarette smoke (A to A^1), but they do not cross the threshold for clinical asthma. Genetically predisposed individuals (B) can cross the threshold to develop clinical asthma (B^1) with such environmental exposures.
Source: Tager IB, Hanrahan JP, Tosteson TD, Castile RB, Brown RW, Weiss ST, Speizer FE. Lung function, pre- and post-natal smoke exposure, and wheezing in the first year of life. Am Rev Respir Dis 1993;147:811–817.

follows the pattern of growth, plateau, and then decline with increasing age (Fig. 6). As shown in Figure 1, wide variability in the level of pulmonary function is present in both smoking and nonsmoking adults.

There are at least three mutually independent ways that one can reach a low level of FEV$_1$ in later adult life: one can have reduced growth, premature decline, or accelerated decline in lung function (Fig. 6). Since airways responsiveness, for a variety of physiological reasons, is strongly correlated with level of lung function (22), and since respiratory symptoms (including cough, phlegm, dyspnea, and wheezing) are also correlated with level of lung function, it stands to reason that with increased growth of FEV$_1$, there will be a decrease in respiratory symptoms and a decrease in airway responsiveness. This will contribute to as "silent" period for symptomatic disease between the ages of 15 and 35 coinciding with the plateau phase. This is because the lung has tremendous physiological

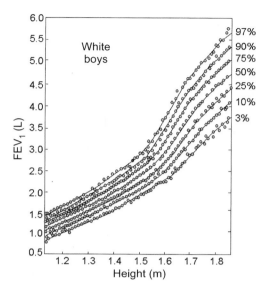

Figure 5 Tracking of FEV_1 with growth among Caucasian male children in the Six Cities Study. Tracking curves are demonstrated for individuals starting at various percentiles of FEV_1. Extremely close tracking is demonstrated—individuals typically remain on the same tracking curve during growth and development. (From Ref. 46.)

reserves, and respiratory symptoms are only modestly correlated with lung function. This silent period tends to obscure the importance of childhood events for adult disease and accentuates recall bias for these early events.

V. Factors Influencing Maximal Growth and Lung Function

Relatively little information is available concerning factors influencing maximally attained level of lung function in late adolescence and early adult life. Wang and coworkers, studying data from the Vlagtwedde/Vlaardingen population in the Netherlands, determined that the single most important factor influencing maximally attained level of lung function was the degree of airways responsiveness (23). Other factors of importance were respiratory symptoms (chronic cough, chronic phlegm, persistent wheezing, and dyspnea), cigarette smoking, and the presence of elevated numbers of eosinophils in peripheral blood. These factors were additive with regard to their effects on maximally attained level of FEV_1. The single most important

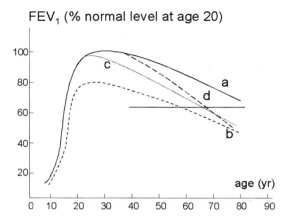

Figure 6 Hypothetical tracking curves of FEV_1 for an individual through life. The normal pattern of growth and decline in FEV_1 is shown by curve a. Significant reductions in FEV_1 can occur by: 1) normal rate of decline after a reduced maximally attained FEV_1 (curve b); 2) early initiation of FEV_1 decline following normal growth (curve c); and 3) accelerated decline in FEV_1 following normal growth (curve d). (From Ref. 44.)

respiratory symptom with regard to maximally attained FEV_1 was the occurrence of attacks of shortness of breath with wheezing. These researchers went on to investigate the influence of these factors as predictors of the development of COPD, defined as reduced FEV_1, between the ages of 36 and 55. Again, cigarette smoking, respiratory symptoms, and increased airways responsiveness were the most important predictors of subsequent fixed airflow obstruction. However, of far greater importance than of these factors was the maximally attained level of FEV_1 itself as a predictor of future level of FEV_1. These data emphasize the importance of maximal lung growth as a predictor of future adult disease.

VI. Genetics of COPD

It is generally thought that proteolytic enzymes from inflammatory cells (neutrophils and macrophages) are released into the lungs at the level of the respiratory bronchiole in response to inflammatory stimuli such as cigarette smoking (24,25). Inhibitors of these proteolytic enzymes (protease inhibitors) are responsible for controlling the inflammatory process and preventing lung tissue destruction. The most clinically important protease inhibitor of neutrophil elastase—one of the proteases hypothesized to contribute to the development of COPD—is α_1-antitrypsin (26). The α_1-antitrypsin protein is encoded by the protease inhibitor gene (PI locus on chromosome 14). More than 75 different PI alleles have been identified (27). The common M allele, which occurs with an allele frequency of $> 95\%$ in Caucasian populations, is associated with normal α_1-antitrypsin levels. The Z and null alleles are associated with severely reduced levels of α_1-antitrypsin; the S allele is associated with mildly reduced levels. Severely α_1-antitrypsin–deficient individuals (designated as PI Z), who are homozygous for the Z allele or Z null heterozygotes, often have early-onset COPD (28). The exact fraction of PI Z individuals who will develop COPD and the age of onset distribution of the disease in such individuals are unknown. With cigarette smoking, PI Z subjects tend to develop more severe pulmonary impairment at an earlier age than nonsmoking PI Z individuals. PI Z individuals do exhibit wide variability in pulmonary function impairment, even among individuals with similar smoking histories. This suggests that variability is partially explained by the interaction of smoking with PI type, but that other genes and environmental exposures are also involved.

Silverman and coworkers studied genetic and environmental factors influencing the variable development of pulmonary function impairment in α_1-antitrypsin deficiency in 52 PI Z subjects and 118 relatives (29–31). Substantial variability in pulmonary function among the PI Z subjects was noted (Fig. 7). Of particular interest in the study by Silverman and coworkers was the association of asthma, attacks of wheezing, and chest wheeziness (apart from colds) with more severe pulmonary function impairment among PI Z individuals. However, misdiagnosis of COPD as asthma in young COPD patients and similarity in respiratory symptoms in asthma and COPD are confounding factors in the assessment of the influence of asthma-related factors on the development of pulmonary function impairment in PI Z subjects. PI Z subjects with lower FEV_1 levels also reported more frequent history of pneumonia than PI Z individuals with higher levels of FEV_1, suggesting that respiratory infections may influence the development of a more severe course in PI Z subjects; however, increased risk of respiratory infections in PI Z subjects with COPD limit the interpretation of these results. There was evidence for familial aggregation of decreased lung function in the relatives of the PI Z subjects (30). Thus, unidentified genetic factors likely contribute to the development of reduced FEV_1 values in a subset of PI Z subjects.

In individuals without α_1-antitrypsin deficiency, familial aggregation of FEV_1 and of COPD within families, independent of cigarette smoking, has been reported in several studies (32–34). These data strongly support the genetic basis for the development of COPD and the potential for

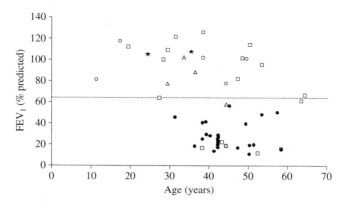

Figure 7 Effect of ascertainment bias on percent predicted FEV_1 among severely α_1-antitrypsin–deficient subjects (PI Z). Closed circles represent index PI Z subjects (individuals diagnosed with antitrypsin deficiency because they had COPD and who were the first PI Z subject identified in their family); open symbols represent nonindex subjects. Nonindex subjects were ascertained by liver disease (open circles), family studies (squares), population screening (triangles), and other pulmonary problems (stars). Marked variability in FEV_1 values is evident for the nonindex PI Z subjects. (From Ref. 29.)

gene-by-environment interaction. They also suggest the possibility that asthma and COPD, both complex diseases likely influenced by multiple genetic and environmental determinants, could share some genetic determinants.

A variety of association studies have compared the distribution of variants in genes hypothesized to be involved in the development of COPD in COPD patients and control subjects. For example, Smith and Harrison examined the distribution of variants in two exons within the microsomal epoxide hydrolase gene (35). A variant in exon 4 causes increased (or fast) enzyme activity, while a variant in exon 3 causes decreased (or slow) enzyme activity. In Scotland they studied 68 patients with a clinical diagnosis of COPD, 94 patients with pathologically proven emphysema who were undergoing lung cancer resection, and 203 blood donor controls. More homozygotes for the slow allele in exon 3 were found among the COPD subjects (19%) and the emphysema patients (22%) than among the control subjects (6%). However, a higher frequency of the fast allele was also found in the COPD group, which raises some uncertainty regarding the relationship of enzyme activity to disease pathogenesis.

Many genetic loci have been examined with the case-control association approach in COPD (36). In most cases there have been inconsistent results, with associations reported in one study which are not replicated in another study. Several factors could contribute to the inconsistent results of case-control genetic association studies in COPD. Genetic heterogeneity, or different genetic mechanisms, could contribute to difficulty in replicating associations between studies. Of course, false-positive and false-negative results could contribute to inconsistent results. In addition, case-control association studies are susceptible to supporting associations based purely on population stratification, which can result from incomplete matching between cases and controls—including differences in ethnicity and geographic origin. No association studies in COPD have been reported that used family-based controls, a study design immune to such population stratification effects. More importantly, no linkage studies have been published in COPD to identify regions of the genome which are likely to contain COPD susceptibility genes—regions in which association studies are likely to be more fruitful.

VII. Airways Responsiveness

Given the importance of childhood and early adult airways responsiveness to level of lung function, it is reasonable to hypothesize that this intermediate phenotype may relate to genetic susceptibility to the effects of cigarette smoke. Is there epidemiological and clinical data that support a relationship between increased airways responsiveness and the occurrence of respiratory symptoms and rate of decline in lung function in adult life? There are a number of reasons why FEV_1 level might be associated with increased airways responsiveness (22). There is greater central than peripheral aerosol deposition, and resistance is inversely proportional to the fourth power of the radius; thus, small changes in airway size result in large decreases in FEV_1. Peripheral resistance is much greater than central resistance in COPD. Emphysema can lead to a reduced mechanical load, thus enhancing the impact of muscular contraction on airway narrowing. At baseline, there will be an increase in bronchomotor tone, which will lower FEV_1. Finally, methodology for expressing responsiveness as a percent of baseline level of FEV_1 will also accentuate these effects (22).

For the physiological reasons given above, it was felt for a number of years that increased airways responsiveness was a consequence rather than a cause of COPD. It is clear now, from longitudinal data, that this is not the case. Xu and coworkers examined the relationship of increased airways responsiveness as a predictor of the occurrence of respiratory symptoms in adult participants in the Vlagtwedde/Vlaardingen Study (37).

Table 3 Magnitude of Effect of Increased Airway Responsiveness and Cigarette Smoking on FEV_1 Decline

	Airway responsiveness		Current smoking status	
Ref.	Mean	95% CI	Mean	95% CI
38	5.36	(0.3, 10.4)	11.6	(3.1, 19.8)
39	25.6	(− 2.6, 53.8)	2.8	(− 30.3, 35.9)
40[a]	12.5	(6.2, 18.8)	6.6[b]	(− 4.7, 17.9)
41	12.8	(1.2, 24.4)	17.2	12.54

[a]Males only.
[b]Current smokers of > 25 cigarettes/day.

They found a consistent dose-response relationship between the occurrence of chronic cough, chronic phlegm, dyspnea, persistent wheeze, and asthmatic attacks and the occurrence of increased levels of airways responsiveness to histamine. A variety of studies, summarized in Table 3, demonstrate that airways responsiveness antedates and precedes decline in lung function after controlling for baseline level of FEV_1 (38–41). In addition, the magnitude of the effects of increased airways responsiveness on decline in FEV_1 are comparable to the effects of current cigarette smoking. Variation in the size of the effects of airways responsiveness and current cigarette smoking in these studies may relate to age differences in the populations studied and to differences in the definitions of smoking status and airways responsiveness employed. Data from the Lung Health Study suggest that there may be an interaction between cigarette smoking and airways responsiveness with regard to accelerated decline in lung function (42). This interaction has not been demonstrable in population-based studies, which may not have sufficient power to demonstrate this effect.

Finally, Hospers and coworkers from Groningen, the Netherlands, demonstrated a dose-response relationship between histamine airways responsiveness and COPD mortality in the general population; increased airways responsiveness is associated with increased mortality (43). These data conclusively demonstrate that increased airways responsiveness antedates, precedes, and predicts the development of COPD symptoms, decline in lung function, susceptibility to cigarette smoke, and mortality from COPD. Thus, early life experiences with asthma, early cigarette smoke exposure, and asymptomatic airway responsiveness determine and predict the adult phenotype of chronic obstructive pulmonary disease.

VIII. Conclusions

Chronic obstructive pulmonary disease starts in utero. Childhood asthma, increased airways responsiveness, cigarette smoking exposure in early life, and largely unidentified genetic factors are important determinants of susceptibility to active cigarette smoking. Symptom remission during the plateau phase of lung function growth and decline is a function of the correlation of respiratory symptoms with lung function level. FEV_1 has a high tracking correlation and, as such, is highly predictive of disease occurrence and outcomes. However, COPD is likely a complex syndrome, composed of multiple, potentially overlapping, causes of chronic airflow obstruction. The major determinants of COPD are maximal attained level of FEV_1 airways responsiveness, and the dose and timing of cigarette smoke exposure. Further efforts of understand the genetic determinants and environmental risk factors for COPD will be required to understand this complex syndrome and to lead to improved therapy for it.

References

1. Official Statement of the American Thoracic Society: standards for the diagnosis and care of patients with chronic obstructive pulmonary disease (COPD) and asthma. Am Rev Respir Dis 1987; 136:225–244.
2. Speizer FE, Tagar IB. Epidemiology of chronic mucus hypersecretion and obstructive airways disease. Epidemiol Rev 1979; 1:124–142.
3. Gelb AF, Hogg JC, Muller NL, Schein MJ, Kuei J, Tashkin DP, Epstein JD, Kollin J, Green RH, Zamel N, Elliott WM, Hadjiaghai L. Contribution of emphysema and small airways in COPD. Chest 1996; 109:353–359.
4. Thurlbeck WM. Aspects of chronic airflow obstruction. Chest 1977; 77:341–349.
5. Benson V, Marano MA. Current estimates from the National Health Interview Survey, 1995. Vital health Stat 10 1998; 199:1–428.
6. Hoyert DL, Kochanek KD, Murphy SL. Deaths: final data for 1997. Natl Vital Stat Rep 1999; 47:1–104.
7. Burrows B, Knudson RJ, Cline MG, Lebowitz MD. Quantitative relationships between cigarette smoking and ventilatory function. Am Rev Respir Dis 1997; 115: 195–205.
8. Cunningham J, Dockery DW, Speizer FE. Maternal smoking during pregnancy as a predictor of lung function in children. Am J Epid 1994; 139:1139–1152.
9. Tager IB, Munoz Z, Rosner B, Weiss ST, Carey V, Speizer FE. Effect of cigarette smoking on the pulmonary function of children and adolescents. Am Rev Respir Dis 1985; 131:752–759.
10. Xu X, Weiss ST, Rijcken B, Schouten JP. Association of smoking and changes in smoking habits with rate of loss FEV1: a new insight into gender differences. Eur Respir J 1994; 7:1056–1061.

11. Martinez FD, Wright AL, Taussig LM, Holberg CJ, Halonen M, Morgan WJ. Asthma and wheezing in the first six years of life. N Eng J Med 1995; 332:133–138.
12. Yunginger JW, Reed CE, O'Connell EJ, Melton LJ, O'Fallon WM, Silverstein MD. A community based study of the epidemiology of asthma. Am Rev Respir Dis 1992; 146:888–894.
13. Burrows B, Taussig LM. As the twig is bent, the tree inclines. Am Rev Respir Dis 1980; 122:813–816.
14. Weiss ST, Tager IB, Weiss JW, Munoz A, Speizer FE, Ingram RH. Airways responsiveness in a population sample of adults and children. Am Rev Respir Dis 1984; 129:898–902.
15. Salome CM, Peat JK, Britton WJ, Woolcock AJ. Bronchial hyperresponsiveness in two populations of Australian schoolchildren. I. Relation of respiratory symptoms and diagnosed asthma. Clin Allergy 1997; 17:271–281.
16. Sears MR, Jones DT, Holdaway DM, Hewitt CJ, Flannery EM, Herbison PG, Silva PA. Prevalence of bronchial reactivity to inhaled methacholine in New Zealand children. Thorax 1986; 41:283–289.
17. Woolcock AJ, Peat JK, Salome CM, Yan K, Anderson SD, Schoeffel RE, McCowage G, Killalea T. Prevalence of bronchial hyperresponsiveness and asthma in a rural adult population. Thorax 1987; 42:361–368.
18. Rijcken B, Schouten JP, Weiss ST, Speizer FE, Van der Lende R. The relationship of nonspecific bronchial responsiveness to respiratory symptoms in a random population sample. Am Rev Respir Dis 1987; 136:62–68.
19. Sparrow D, O'Connor G, Colton T, Barry CL, Weiss ST. The relationship of nonspecific bronchial responsiveness to the occurrence of respiratory symptoms and decreased levels of pulmonary function. The Normative Aging Study. Am Rev Respir Dis 1987; 135:1255–1260.
20. Burney PG, Britton JR, Chinn S, Tattersfield AE, Papacosta AO, Kelson M, Anderson F, Corfield DR. Descriptive epidemiology of bronchial reactivity in an adult population: results from a community study. Thorax 1987; 42:38–44.
21. Sears MR, Burrows B, Flannery EM, Herbison GP, Hewitt CJ, Holdaway MD. Relation between airway responsiveness and serum IgE in children with asthma and apparently normal children. N Eng J Med 1991; 325:1067–1071.
22. O'Connor G, Sparrow D, Weiss ST. The role of allergy and nonspecific airway hyerresponsiveness in the pathogenesis of chronic obstructive pulmonary disease. Am Rev Respir Dis 1989; 140:225–252.
23. Wang X, Mensinga TT, Schouten JP, Rijcken B, Weiss ST. Determinants of maximally attained level of pulmonary function during the plateau phase (ages 15–35). Unpublished.
24. Janoff A. Elastases and emphysema: current assessment of the protease-antiprotease hypothesis. Am Rev Repir Dis 1985; 132:417–433.
25. Gadek JE, Parelt ER. The protease anti-protease balance within the human lung: implications for the pathogenesis of emphysema. Lung 1990; 168:552–564.
26. Travis J, Salvesen GS: Human plasma proteinase inhibitors. Ann Rev Biochem 1983; 52:655–709.

27. Brantly M, Nukiwa T, Crystal RG: Molecular basis of alpha-1 antitrypsin deficiency. Am J Med 1988; 84(suppl 6A):13–31.
28. Silverman EK, Speizer FE. Risk factors for the development of chronic obstructive pulmonary disease. Med Clin North Am 1996; 80:501–522.
29. Silverman EK, Pierce JA, Province MA, Rao DC, Campbell EJ. Variability of pulmonary function in alpha 1-antitrypsin deficiency: clinical correlates. Ann Intern Med 1989; 111:982–991.
30. Silverman EK, Province MA, Campbell EJ, Pierce JA, Rao DC. Variability of pulmonary function in alpha 1-antitrypsin deficiency: residual family resemblance beyond the effect of the Pi locus. Hum Hered 1990; 40:340–355.
31. Silverman EK, Province MA, Rao DC, et al. A family study of the variability of pulmonary function in alpha 1-antitrypsin deficiency: quantitative phenotypes. Am Rev Respir Dis 1990; 142:1015–1021.
32. Kueppers F, Miller RD, Gordon H, et al. Familial prevalence of chronic obstructive pulmonary disease in a matched pair study. Am J Med 1977; 63:336–342.
33. Larson RK, Barman ML, Kueppers F, Fudenberg HH. Genetic and environmental determinants of chronic obstructive pulmonary disease. Ann Intern Med 1970; 72:627–632.
34. Silverman EK, Chapman HA, Drazen JM, Weiss ST, Rosner B, Campbell EJ, O'Donnell WJ, Reilly JJ, Ginns L, Mentzer S, Wain J, Speizer FE. Genetic epidemiology of severe, early-onset chronic obstructive pulmonary disease. Risk to relatives for airflow obstruction and chronic bronchitis. Am J Respir Crit Care Med 1998; 157:1770–1778.
35. Smith CA, Harrison DJ. Association between polymorphism in gene for microsomal epoxide hydrolase and susceptibility to emphysema. Lancet 1997; 350:630–633.
36. Sandford AJ, Weir TD, Pare PD, Genetic risk factors for chronic obstructive pulmonary disease. Eur Respir J 1997; 10:1380–1391.
37. Xu X, Rijcken B, Schouten JP, Weiss, ST. Airways responsiveness and development and remission of chronic respiratory symptoms in adults. Lancet 1997; 350:1431–1434.
38. Frew AJ. Kennedy SM, Chan-Yeung M, Methacholine responsiveness, smoking, and atopy are risk factors for accelerated FEV1 decline in male working populations. Am Rev Respir Dis 1992; 146:878–838.
39. Tracey M, Villar A, Dow L, Coggon D, Lampe FC, Holgate ST. The influence of increased bronchial responsiveness, atopy, and serum IgE on decline in FEV1: a longitudinal study in the elderly. Am J Respir Crit Care Med 1995; 151:656–662
40. Rijcken B, Xu X, Schouten JP, Rosner B, Weiss ST. Airway hyperresponsiveness to histmaine associated with accelerated decline in FEV_1. Am J Respir Crit Care Med 1995; 151:1377–1382.
41. O'Connor GT, Sparrow D, Weiss ST. A prospective longitudinal study of methacholine airway responsiveness as predictor of pulmonary function decline: the Normative Aging Study. Am J Respir Crit Care Med 1995; 152:87–92.

42. Tashkin DP, Altose MD, Connett JE, Kanner RE, Lee WW, Wise RA, Methacholine reactivity predicts changes in lung function in smokers with early chronic obstructive lung disease: The Lung Health Study Research Group. Am J Respir Crit Care Med 1990; 153:1802–1804.
43. Hospers JJ, Postma DS, Schouten JP, Weiss ST, Rijcken B. Histamine airway hyperresponsiveness predicts mortality from COPD in a general population sample. Lancet 2000; 356(9238):1313–1317.
44. Rijcken B. Bronchial responsiveness and COPD risk: an epidemiologic study (postdoctoral dissertation), Groningen, The Netherlands.
45. Xu X, Dockery DW, Ware JH, Speizer FE, Ferris BG Jr. Effects of cigarette smoking on rate of loss of pulmonary function in adults: a longitudinal assessment. Am Rev Respir Dis 1992; 146:1345–1348.
46. Wang X, Dockery DW, Wypij D, Fay ME, Ferris BG Jr. Pulmonary function between 6 and 18 years of age. Pediatr Pulmonol 1993; 15:75–88.
47. Weiss ST, Sparrow D, eds. Airway Responsiveness and Atopy in the Development of Chronic Lung Disease. New York: Raven Press, 1989:220.

5

Risk Factors for the Progression of COPD

HUIB A. M. KERSTJENS and DIRKJE S. POSTMA

University Hospital Groningen
Groningen, The Netherlands

I. Introduction

Patients with chronic obstructive pulmonary disease (COPD) character-istically complain about chronic cough, sputum production, and dyspnea, especially on exertion. They experience frequent exacerbations and, in more advanced disease, hospitalizations. COPD typically affects middle-aged and older persons who either smoke or have a smoking history, but the disorder does not occur exclusively in smokers. The American Thoracic Society defines COPD as a disease state characterized by the presence of airflow limitation due to chronic bronchitis or emphysema (1). In many patients the disease is relentlessly progressive, with increasing loss of lung function, leading to early disability and premature death. In this chapter we will first look at the definition of the disease. We focus on its progressive nature, and especially on risk factors for accelerated decline and survival. Subsequently, risk factors for other markers of disease progression such as exacerbation and hospitalization rates and loss of quality of life will be briefly discussed.

It is useful to emphasize that in this chapter we have searched for risk factors of progression of COPD, not development of COPD. The risk factors for development of COPD are discussed in Chapter 4. At first glance one could perhaps expect the risk factors for development and progression to be similar, but they need not be. As an example, mucus hypersecretion is so closely associated with the diagnosis of COPD (especially the chronic bronchitis component) that the finding of a correlation with increased lung function decline intuitively makes sense. This correlation has—many years after Fletcher and Peto could find no relation (2)—indeed been found in a study by Vestbo and colleagues (3). However, once the diagnosis of COPD is made, once the susceptible smoker has identified himself or herself, a further relation between mucus hypersecretion and decline need not be the case and indeed has not been found.

II. Definition of Disease and Progression

In current guidelines COPD is divided into two categories: emphysema and/ or chronic obstructive bronchitis (1,4). Both condition can occur in one person at the same time, and it is still far from clear whether emphysema always passes through a stage of chronic bronchitis. There is every reason to believe that COPD indeed is not one homogeneous disease, and the current subdivision will undoubtedly be changed in the future: it has little relation to prognosis or to therapy, and it has traditionally had the problem of opposing a symptom-based definition (chronic bronchitis) to a histopathological definition (emphysema). The realization that COPD is not one homogeneous disease is important when interpreting the literature on risk factors associated with progression of disease. In other words, group selection is very relevant for the outcome of a study, and it may differ substantially between studies. This can be demonstrated by the results of a study by Kanner and colleagues in 84 patients with a label of COPD (5): "The criteria for admission into the study were the presence of chronic bronchitis and/or emphysema as defined by the American Thoracic Society (6). A diagnosis of chronic bronchitis was acceptable, as was a history of episodic wheezing suggesting a diagnosis of asthma if it accompanied clinical findings consistent with chronic bronchitis and/or emphysema." They found decline in their COPD population to be as follows: 62.5 mL/yr in emphysema, 30.5 mL/yr in bronchiectasis, 12.2 mL/yr in chronic bronchitis, 90.0 mL/yr in combined chronic bronchitis plus emphysema, and 70.8 mL in COPD plus asthma (5). In most contemporary studies, however there is no attempt to separate different clinical pictures under the umbrella term COPD.

COPD is commonly perceived to be a relentlessly progressive disease. Usually progression is defined as decline in lung function and more specifically in FEV_1. Why is progression so narrowly defined? It is clear that patients never enter the clinic complaining about their lung function. There are several reasons why pulmonologists persist in defining disease progression by FEV_1. The first is the close association between FEV_1 level and survival in COPD (2,7,8). The second is the good reproducibility of the measurement (9). Death (or survival) due to COPD could of course also be labeled as a clear endpoint in studies looking at progression of disease. What other endpoints could serve to define progression, especially endpoints with more day-to-day relevance to the patient? Patients express complaints about dyspnea, especially on exertion, chronic cough and sputum production, fatigue, and disability. Many patients will complain about high exacerbation frequencies and certainly hospitalization rates. In short, they will complain about their quality of life, though in nonstandardized terminology. Pulmonologists now have some tools for assessing quality of life (10,11), but their value in day-to-day patient care is as yet unclear.

III. Risk Factors for Lung Function Decline

A. Methodological Problems in Determining Decline

Studies vary considerably in the populations they report on, and different populations will yield different declines (12). Variable definitions of disease are employed (see above). Studies also differ substantially in the severity of disease of the population under investigation: patients from an epidemiological setting will frequently have milder disease compared to patients from outpatient settings of secondary or tertiary referral centers. Some of the studies have been retrospective in nature, with highly variable (between patients) and varying (on time) medical interventions during the observation period. In some studies the prognostic factors were measured at the end of the follow-up period (13,14), and thus the predictive nature of these studies may well be biased. An important problem of all long-term follow-up studies and certainly of such studies in COPD is the survivor effect. If the least diseased, or those showing the least progression, survive longest in series, this will bias the end results. A significant survivor effect, for instance, seems to play a role in the IPPB trial, where a lower initial FEV_1 is found to be related to a more favorable long-term slope (15). Another problem associated with defining decline is regression to the mean: patients with, by chance, a low FEV_1 at the start of a study are bound to show a more favorable decline from there on and vice versa (12).

B. Smoking Status

Smoking status is the most important factor consistently associated with a steeper decline in lung function (Table 1). This was first demonstrated in working men by Fletcher and colleagues (2), followed by many others (16). It holds true not only for the development of airways obstruction but also for further progression. There is a dose-response effect of smoking on rate of decline, the effect being greater with more cigarettes, more years, and more pack-years smoked (2,17–20). This effect has been more clearly demonstrated in epidemiological cohorts than in patients with established disease. Most studies have demonstrated the detrimental effects with respect to smoking of cigarettes, but more recent larger studies have been able to document this for cigar and pipe tobacco as well (20,21). As far as we are aware, no data are available on the influence of environmental tobacco smoke on decline in patients with established disease. There are, however, convincing data about the detrimental influence of environmental tobacco smoke in nondiseased subjects in utero (22), during infancy (23), and in

Table 1   Risk Factors for Decline in FEV_1 in Patients with Established COPD

Factor	Direction of relation	Evidence
Active smoking	neg.	+++
Passive smoking	n.d.	
Age	neg.	++
FEV_1	x	++
Airways hyperresponsiveness	neg.	+++
Bronchodilator response	?	−
Allergy	x	+
Asthmatic features	pos.	+
Body mass index	x	+
Mucus hypersecretion	n.d.	
Inflammation	neg.	+
Socioeconomic class	pos.	+
Psychological score SIP	pos.	+
Occupational dust exposure	neg.	+
Area of residence		+

pos., less decline with higher level of factor, or with factor present; neg., more decline with higher level of factor, or with factor present; x, no relation found in study/studies; ?, contradictory data; n.d., no sound data available; +++, several high-quality studies; ++, reasonable evidence; +, some evidence, or balance of evidence in given direction; −, studies available, but contradictory evidence.

adulthood (24). It is important to realize that a low FEV_1 in a patient over 45 years of age can be due to detrimental effects of smoking during any (combination) of the four periods of change in FEV_1: a smaller intrauterine growth, a decreased growth of lung function during infancy, a shortened plateau phase during early adulthood, and a steeper decline during adult life (see Fig. 1).

C. Airway Hyperresponsiveness

Airway hyperresponsiveness is not a hallmark of COPD, but nevertheless occurs frequently in patients with COPD in studies measuring the phenomenon: 64% in a study by Bahous et al. (27), 70% in a series from Ramsdale et al. (28), 46% in a study by Yan et al. (29), and finally 68% in the Lung Health Study (30). After smoking, airway hyperresponsiveness is the factor found most consistently to be related to onset of COPD as well as to progression of established disease: increased hyperresponsiveness was related to a steeper decline in lung function in some older and uncontrolled studies (13,25,26). The prognostic relevance of airway hyperresponsiveness has recently been confirmed in a study with 5773 participants with early COPD followed for 5 years in a randomized controlled trial (31). Using a random effects linear model, the slope of the methacholine dose response slope was found to be a strong predictor of change in $FEV_1\%$ predicted (Fig. 2), after controlling for baseline lung function, age, sex, baseline smoking history, and changes in smoking status. Significant interactions were found between responsiveness and smoking behavior. In the first year, participants who quit smoking showed improvement in FEV_1, whereas continuing smokers showed worsening. Between years 1 and 5, lung function declined to a greater extent in continuing smokers than in sustained quitters. For both time periods, these quitter/smoker differences increased as a function of airway responsiveness (31).

D. Baseline Lung Function

In the epidemiological setting, a lower baseline FEV_1 is predictive of accelerated subsequent decline in FEV_1. This effect has been labeled the horse racing effect: those who lead the pack will finish up front (2,32). In the clinical setting, i.e., in patients with established disease, such a negative relation has not been found in most studies (5,13,25,26). This lack of correlation of baseline FEV_1 with subsequent decline in patients with established COPD does not exclude a relation between FEV_1 and survival, which in fact exists (see below). One would not anticipate this lack of relation with decline, but it could be related to a survivor effect, as seems to be the case in the IPPB trial (15). Additionally, changes in smoking statues

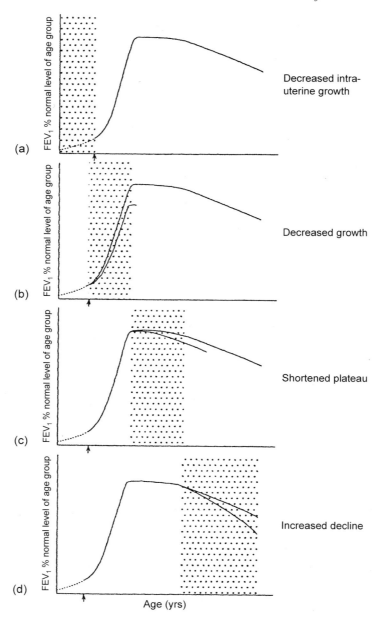

Figure 1 Phases of FEV_1 development through life cycles. (a) during pregnancy; (b) during lung function growth (0–20 yr); (c) during the plateau phase (20–40 yr); (d) during lung function decline (> 40 yr). (Modified from Ref.)

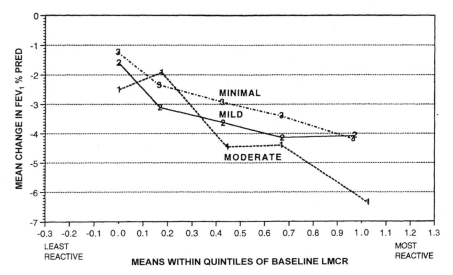

Figure 2 Mean changes in FEV$_1$ % predicted from screening to year 5 by baseline airways responsiveness. Relationships are shown separately for participants with tertiles of baseline FEV$_1$ % predicted, representing borderline and mild and moderate airway obstruction, corresponding to mean FEV$_1$ values of 85, 76, and 64% predicted, respectively. (From Ref. 31.)

during periods long enough to establish decline in FEV$_1$ with any accuracy might also obscure a relation.

E. Age

Most prediction equations for lung function for a given gender and height give linear coefficients for age. However, many authors have now demonstrated that decline accelerates with aging (33–35). Therefore, if a linear slope of, for instance, FEV$_1$ over time is used in the analysis of prognostic factors, age should come out as a significant factor for FEV$_1$ decline, which is indeed the case in the Lung Health Study (31).

F. Bronchodilator Response

Results are contradictory as to the relationship between a greater bronchodilator response and decline in FEV$_1$ in patients with COPD. Two studies from the 1970s found a negative relationship, i.e., steeper decline with a greater bronchodilator response (5,13). Three studies from the 1980s found exactly the opposite (7,15,26). Although there are clear differences in mode of expression of the bronchodilator response, possible incomplete washout of medication prior to measurement, and concomitant medication during the study, a tenable view on this issue has not yet emerged. It should be possible to merge useful data from large recently completed trials in COPD with long follow-up (Euroscop, Copenhagen, and Isolde, Lung Health Study) to obtain valuable information on prognostic factors for decline in lung function, including the bronchodilator response.

G. Allergy

Relationships have been proposed for allergy markers as prognostic factors for the development of COPD, but two studies that examined this effect in patients with established disease found no effect of positive skin tests on decline (7,25). Although higher IgE levels have been linked to less deterioration in hyperresponsiveness in COPD (36), we know of no data linking IgE levels to decline in FEV_1 in COPD. There has been one analysis from the Tucson data finding a higher rate of decline in subjects with newly diagnosed chronic bronchitis and eosinophilia (-24.5 mL/yr) compared to not having eosinophilia (-16.6 mL/yr) (37). Given the high mean FEV_1 in this study of 86 and 95% predicted in current and ex-smokers, respectively, many of these subjects did not (yet) fulfill the criteria for COPD.

H. Asthmatic Features

In at least two studies asthmatic features have been linked to a more favorable decline in FEV_1 in patient with COPD: in the Tucson data, this constituted a concomitant diagnosis of asthma (38) and in the IPPB trial wheeze (15). However, since increased hyperresponsiveness is more a hallmark of asthma than of COPD, the steeper decline in FEV_1 found with increased hyperresponsiveness would point in the opposite direction, i.e., more decline with additional asthmatic features.

I. Nutritional Status

Although weight loss has been associated with accelerated decline in FEV_1 in epidemiological series (39,40), it has not been demonstrated to be related to accelerated decline in FEV_1 in a study actually looking at the significance of nutritional status in established COPD (8).

J. Mucus Hypersecretion

The idea that mucus hypersecretion is linked to increased decline was investigated many years ago by Fletcher and colleagues, but they could not demonstrate the relation (2). The hypothesis experienced a revival with the data from Vestbo and colleagues, who found a steeper decline in subjects with mucus hyperesecretion compared to those without hypersecretion in the Copenhagen City Heart Study (3). Whether this negative relationship also applies to patients with established disease has not been investigated so far.

K. Inflammation

It is tempting to speculate that more abundant inflammation, or inflammation of a different composition in the airways or in the alveolar walls, would lead to accelerated decline in lung function. Indeed, sputum eosinophilia and sputum neutrophilia (measured at the end of the study) have been associated with a steeper decline (13,14). Since these inflammatory markers were measured at the end of the study period, it is not clear whether they were the cause or the consequence of more severe airways obstruction. Further pathophysiological data linking the inflammatory process and localization to disease progression or regression are urgently needed, but require great stamina to measure sputum or even biopsies in a large sample of patients with COPD and then to follow these patients up for a sufficiently long period.

L. Other Factors

Several other factors related to subsequent decline have been mentioned in single studies only, but most have not been confirmed by others. Examples are α_1-antitryspin level (25) or certain other phenotypes next to PiZZ such as PiMZ (41), occupational dust exposure (25), area of residence (25), socioeconomic class (5), and psychological score of the sickness impact profile (15).

IV. Effects of Intervention on Decline

Has any current intervention been proven to be effective in decreasing accelerated decline in patients with COPD? Yes, but to physicians daily struggling to help patients with advanced COPD, it is extremely clear that the list is not long, and new options are eagerly awaited (42).

A. Smoking Cessation

There should be no doubt that the single most effective intervention that can be offered to subjects with COPD is to convince and help them to quit smoking (Table 2). Earlier suggested in an uncontrolled fashion by several authors (43–45), this has recently been convincingly demonstrated in the Lung Health Study. This study included 5887 subjects with COPD that was subclinical in the sense that there was a demonstrable reduced expiratory flow but few symptoms. One third of the subjects in this randomized study continued on a usual care scheme. The other two thirds received a rather extensive smoking intervention program, including 12 smoking cessation sessions combining behavior modification and use of nicotine gum with a 5-year maintenance program to minimize relapse. The smoking intervention group was further randomized to receive either an inhaled anticholinergic agent, or a placebo. The Lung Health Study showed that successful cessation of smoking as compared to continuous smoking was associated with a significantly lower decline of FEV_1 (46). Even after 11 years the positive effects of successful smoking cessation on decline in FEV_1 persist (47). Men who quit smoking had a mean annual decline of 30.2 mL, whereas men who continued had 66.1 mL. Women who quit smoking had a mean annual decline of 21.5 mL, whereas women who continued had 54.3 mL.

Table 2 Effects of Interventions on Decline of FEV_1 in Patients with Established COPD

Intervention	Direction of relation	Evidence
Smoking cessation	pos.	+++
Long-term oxygen therapy	pos.	+
Nutritional supplementation	n.d.	
Lung transplantation	n.d.	
Lung volume reduction therapy	x	++
Rehabilitation	x	+
Mucolytics	pos.	+
Inhaled corticosteroids	x	++
β_2-Agonists	x	+
Anticholinergics	x	++
Theophyllines	n.d.	
Antibiotics	n.d.	

pos., less decline with higher level of factor, or with factor present; n.d., no sound data available; x, no relation found in study/studies; +++, several high-quality studies; ++, reasonable evidence; +, some evidence, or balance of evidence in given direction.

As expected, the difference in decline induced by being exposed to an intensive smoking cessation program or usual care was smaller than between actually stopping or continuing: over the 5-year study period, the difference in smoking cessation rates between the usual care and the intervention groups became smaller because up to 20% of patients ceased smoking in the usual care group. Nevertheless, after the first year there was still a marginally better decline in FEV_1 of 52 mL/yr with active intervention therapy as opposed to 56 mL/yr without. Although very small, this difference was statistically significant (46).

Patients who stop smoking continue to exhibit a marked inflammation in the bronchial wall, which can persist for many years after smoking has been stopped (48). It is therefore at present unclear from the pathology studies why patients who stop smoking see their decline revert back to (near) normal levels for nonsmokers.

No data are available on the effects of stopping exposure to environmental tobacco smoke. Although it would seem intuitively predictable that there will be a favorable effect on decline, it should be emphasized that side stream smoke (from the burning end of the cigarette into the environment) has constituents that are quite different from mainstream smoke.

B. Long-Term Oxygen Therapy

Several studies have examined the effects of oxygen therapy on survival in COPD (see below). In one of these studies a subgroup analysis was performed looking at effects on decline, finding a small but significant favorable effect in hypoxemic patients (49).

C. Nutritional Supplementation

There are now several studies demonstrating positive effects of nutritional supplementation on respiratory or other muscle strength (50–53). One of these also demonstrated an effect on walking distance (51). An effect on FEV_1 was not found in any of these studies, but most were too short to actually look at decline of FEV_1. The studies looking at links between specific dietary components, such as dietary *n*-3 polyunsaturated acids (54), and COPD have looked for the reduction of occurrence of COPD but not at reduction of decline in patients with established COPD.

D. Surgical Intervention

Lung transplantation has been demonstrated not to improve survival in patients with emphysema (55). Additionally, many patients with lung transplantation unfortunately after some time revert again to progressive loss of FEV_1, which is generally associated with the occurrence of bronchiolitis obliterans (56). Lung volume reduction surgery has not been shown to have an effect on decline in lung function (57).

E. Rehabilitation

Rehabilitation has been shown in a recent meta-analysis to have significant effects on health-related quality of life, especially in the domains of dyspnea and mastery (58). Additionally, it yields significant effects on exercise capacity (58). There has been one full report and one abstract of randomized controlled trials looking at the effects of a rehabilitation program on decline in FEV_1 (59,60). Both found no difference in effect on decline of a more comprehensive compared to a less intensive program. This does not preclude a positive effect on decline of a comprehensive rehabilitation program versus usual care. The latter has, however, not been tested in a clinical trial.

F. Mucolytics

In one abstract, there was a positive effect of n-acetylcysteine on decline in lung function, but only in those over 50 years old (61). In a recent systematic review of four randomized controlled trials, there seemed to be a small favorable effect on decline in FEV_1 for the group of mucolytics as a whole, but the studies were too heterogeneous for confident statements on possible effects of the mucolytics (62). Moreover, different classes of mucolytics were used. There is one large European multicenter trail, not yet published, that studied the effects of n-acetylcysteine on decline (63).

G. Other Medical Interventions

The effects of corticosteroids, bronchodilators, and antibiotics are extensively covered in separate chapters in this book, but in general have not been shown to favorably affect accelerated decline in patients with COPD (64).

V. Risk Factors Associated with Survival

A. Age and Gender

It is quite intuitive that age is related to survival in COPD (8,65,66). Age is, together with baseline FEV_1, the strongest predictor of survival in COPD (8,67) (Table 3). There has been much discussion about gender differences in

Table 3 Risk Factors for Survival in Patients with Established COPD

Factor	Direction of relation	Evidence
Active smoking	pos.	++
Passive smoking	n.d.	
Age	neg.	++
Male gender	neg.	++
FEV_1	pos.	+++
VC	pos.	++
TLC, FRC, RV/TLC	neg.	+
Airways hyperresponsiveness	x	+
Bronchodilator response	x	++
PaO_2	pos.	+++
$PaCO_2$	neg.	+++
Diffusion capacity	neg.	++
Cor pulmonale, increased PAP	neg.	++
Allergy	pos.	+
Asthmatic features	pos.	+
Body mass index	neg.	+++
Mucus hypersecretion	neg.	+
Inflammation	n.d.	
Socioeconomic class	pos.	+

pos., better survival with higher level of factor, or with factor present; neg., poorer survival with higher level of factor, or with factor present; x, no relation found in study/studies; n.d., no data available; +++, several high-quality studies; ++, reasonable evidence; +, some evidence, or balance of evidence in given direction.

mortality due to COPD. COPD used to be a male's disease, but emancipation has resulted in women catching up to male smoking habits. In older series, survival was frequently found to be worse in men than in women, but most studies did not correct for smoking habits and FEV_1 (68). In a more recent analysis, male gender was still found to be associated with poorer survival even after correction for FEV_1, age, and smoking habits (66).

B. Baseline FEV_1

The most consistent factor associated with survival in COPD next to age is baseline FEV_1. This has been shown in several older and uncontrolled studies (7,65,68–70) as well as in the IPPB trial, which followed a large group of 985 patients between 30 and 74 years of age with a clinical diagnosis of COPD comparing the effects of intermittent positive pressure

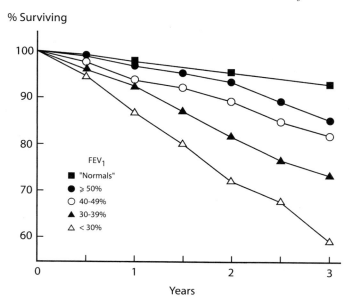

Figure 3 Survival among patients in the Intermittent Positive Pressure Breathing trial segregated according to baseline postbronchodilator FEV$_1$. (Modified from Ref. 15.)

breathing with usual care for an average follow-up of 33 months (8,71). Three-year survival ranged from 80% in patients with an FEV$_1$ over 50% predicted and decreased to under 45% in patients with an FEV$_1$ lower than 30% predicted (Fig. 3). Postbronchodilator FEV$_1$ has consistently been shown to be a better predictor of survival than prebronchodilator FEV$_1$ (8,65). FEV$_1$/VC is a very useful measure of airways obstruction and is proposed as the major parameter in determining mild COPD in the most recent guidelines of the European Respiratory Society (4). The FEV$_1$/VC, however, has been suggested to be inferior to the FEV$_1$ alone in predicting survival (65).

C. Other Lung Function Indices

Several studies have assessed other parameters of lung function in predicting survival in patients with COPD. Among these are FRC (8), TLC (8), RV/TLC (7), FVC (68), and FEV$_1$/VC (65). It is clear that many of these factors are interrelated and therefore a statistical technique looking for independent predictors of survival should be employed (7,8). Postma and colleagues compared the results of linear to multiple regression analysis looking at 5- and 10-year survival (7). In separate analyses, seven factors were significantly related to survival, including reversibility, maximal breathing capacity, and RV/TLC, but only the bronchodilator response to thiazinamium, an intramuscular anticholinergic agent, was significantly related to survival. In an additional discriminant analysis, only RV/TLC was an independent predictor of 5-year survival, next to the response to thiazinamium and the p-wave amplitude on ECG (7). The presence of frank cor pulmonale has been found by other groups as well to predict mortality in COPD (65). There has been at least one study finding pulmonary artery pressure to be related to poorer survival, more so than hypoxemia or hypercapnia (72).

In the IPPB trial, a stepwise proportional hazards model was performed. After adjusting for age and postbronchodilator FEV_1 only TLC, exercise tolerance, and resting heart rate were related to mortality (8). In the same trial, factors that may be thought of as reflecting emphysema, such as DL_{CO}, FRC, and TLC, affected survival in a relatively minor way in the multivariate model.

D. Bronchodilator Response and Airways Hyperresponsiveness

At least four studies have related a greater bronchodilator response to better survival in COPD (7,15,65,73), though the relationship has not been found invariably (74). The positive relationship became smaller in the IPPB trial after introducing postbronchodilator FEV_1 as compared to prebronchodilator FEV_1.

Given the important predictive value of increased airways hyperresponsiveness for the development of COPD and for decline in established COPD, it is important to evaluate the same effect on survival. Postma and colleagues also investigated the effect of increased histamine hyperresponsiveness but could not demonstrate a relation to 5- or 10-year survival (7).

E. Impairments in Gas Exchange

There are many studies linking lowered PaO_2 to shortened survival (68,73–79) as well as nocturnal oxygen desaturation (80). Additionally, increased $PaCO_2$ is unfavorable for survival (7,49,68,73,74,76,78,79,81). Impaired carbon monoxide diffusing capacity has also been shown by several authors to be linked to survival (65,68,76,79). These parameters are however, interrelated, and most studies did not look at independent prediction. Decreased exercise capacity has been linked to shortened survival (15,67), as has increased resting heart rate (7,8,81).

F. Smoking

The main cause of development of COPD is exposure to smoking. COPD is rare in lifetime nonsmokers and has been estimated to have an incidence of 5% in three large representative U.S. surveys from 1971 to 1984 (82). Several studies have linked continued smoking to decreased survival in COPD (7,66,68,83,84). We are unaware of any studies linking environmental tobacco smoke exposure to shortened survival in patients with established COPD.

G. Nutritional Status

The presence of malnutrition has been shown in many older studies to negatively affect survival in COPD (85–89). More recently, this notion has been reinforced with data from Gray-Donald and colleagues in a Canadian study of 348 patients followed for 3–5 years (90). They found a low body mass index and home oxygen use to be independent predictors of survival. Schols et al. performed a retrospective study including 400 patients with COPD, none of whom had received nutritional support (75). A low body mass index was a significant independent predictor of survival (Fig. 4) ($p < 0.001$). After stratification of the group into BMI quintiles, a threshold value of $25 \, \text{kg/m}^2$ was identified, below which the mortality risk was clearly increased.

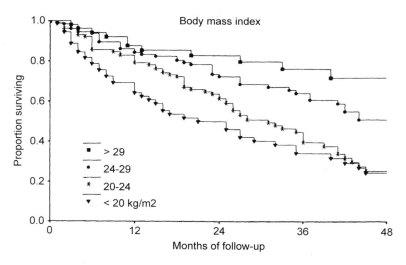

Figure 4 Kaplan-Meier plot of relation between body mass index and survival in 400 patients with COPD. (From Ref. 75.)

H. Mucus Hypersecretion and Infection

In a landmark study of London working men first published in 1976 (43), Fletcher and Peto tested the hypothesis that chronic mucus hypersecretion as marker of chronic infection would be an important prognostic factor for decline and survival. This hypothesis, later labeled the British hypothesis, was refuted by the authors themselves on the basis of a follow-up study of 792 men seen regularly over 8 years. Kanner and colleagues, however, did find a more rapid decline in patients with more frequent lower respiratory lower tract infections, which was not due to a higher incidence of these infections in those with more severe COPD as classified by FEV_1 and FEV_1/FVC (5).

More recently, the researchers joined in the Copenhagen City Heart Study generated two re-analyses of their data, looking again at the importance of mucus hypersecretion first in the general cohort (subjects with and without airways obstruction) to find an excess decline in association with chronic mucus hypersecretion (3). The analysis was not limited to a subset of subjects with airways obstruction/COPD. In an additional analysis, they looked only at the 214 cases where COPD was an underlying or contributory cause of death and who had been followed prospectively for 10–12 years (89). In 101 of these, hospital records could be obtained and the cause of death was classified as either due to pulmonary infection or not. Of subjects reporting chronic mucus hypersecretion at the initial examination, pulmonary infection was implicated in 54% of deaths, whereas this only occurred in 28% of subjects without chronic mucus hypersecretion. Controlling for covariates, especially smoking habits, chronic mucus hypersecretion was found to be a strong independent predictor of COPD-related death with pulmonary infection implicated (relative risk 3.5) but not of death without pulmonary infection (relative risk 0.9).

I. Asthmatic Features and Allergy

Burrows and coworkers in their Tucson epidemiological study looked for prognostic factors in subjects with an FEV_1 less than 65% predicted (38). The study group was divided into three subgroups, but only partial insight is given into how the three subgroups of obstructive patients were actually selected. The group selection roughly was as follows: all subjects had chronic irreversible airways obstruction, one group with and another group without an additional diagnosis of asthma, and a third group with characteristics of both. Subjects with fixed obstruction and doctor's reported asthma fared better in terms of mortality and decline of FEV_1 than the in-between group, which in turn fared better than smokers with obstruction and no asthma. Allergic patients had a better survival (38).

J. Other Factors

Some additional factors have been associated with decreased survival in patients with COPD, including which lower socioeconomic class (68).

VI. Effects of Intervention on Survival

With the current state of knowledge it is distressing to realize how little we are able to favorably influence survival in COPD. Actually, no drug to date has a documented effect on survival, although there is no retrospective cohort study suggesting an improvement with inhaled corticosteroids (91). Some other, nondrug, interventions are advantageous: smoking cessation, oxygen therapy in certain subjects, and perhaps nutritional supplementation.

A. Smoking Cessation

Smoking cessation as opposed to continued smoking in patients with established COPD results in longer survival (7,66,68,83,84) (Table 4).

Table 4 Effects of Intervention on Survival in Patients with Established COPD

Factor	Direction of relation	Evidence
Smoking cessation	pos.	+++
Long-term oxygen therapy	pos.	++
Nutritional supplementation	pos.	+
Lung transplantation	x	++
Lung volume reduction therapy	pos. and neg.	
Rehabilitation	?	−
Mucolytics	n.d.	
Inhaled corticosteroids	n.d.	
β_2-Agonists	n.d.	
Anticholinergics	n.d.	
Theophyllines	n.d.	
Antibiotics	n.d.	

pos., better survival with higher level of factor, or with factor present; neg., poorer survival with higher level of factor, or with factor present; x, no relation found in study/studies; ?, contradictory data; n.d., no data available; +++, several high-quality studies; ++, reasonable evidence; +, some evidence, or balance of evidence in given direction.

However, smoking cessation has been hard to achieve in patients with established COPD (and hence with proven increased susceptibility to the detrimental effects of cigarette smoke). One-year sustained quit rates, even after rigorous antismoking campaigns, of 25% are at the upper limit of achievable. It has been calculated that approximately 15 years of an attainable government-directed smoking reduction scenario in the Netherlands would reduce the prevalence of COPD by only 2.6% in 2010 (92). This is quite unsatisfactory, since there is a projected 41% autonomic increase in COPD in the same period in the Netherlands mainly due to aging of the population and to women catching up on smoking habits. With an extreme smoking reduction scenario, the prevalence should decrease by 8.8% again, by the year 2010. It is clear that these figures would improve considerably with longer time frames than the approximately 15 years of this projection (92). It is unfortunately the case that from a macro-economic point of view, there is no benefit to society from rigorous smoking cessation: if people stopped smoking there would be savings in health care costs, but only in the short term. Eventually, smoking cessation would lead to increased health care costs, primarily by people dying at an older age (93).

B. Long-Term Oxygen Therapy

There have been four randomized controlled trials of long-term oxygen treatment versus a control treatment. In a recent meta-analysis, these studies could not be aggregated because of too large differences in trial design and participant selection (94). There was only one double-blind trial comparing nocturnal domiciliary oxygen therapy to room air in patients with arterial desaturation at night (95). It found no difference in mortality at 3 years. Two other randomized controlled trials compared domiciliary oxygen therapy to no oxygen. The Medical Research Council Working Party study tested oxygen for at least 15 hours in 87 men and found a significant reduction in mortality of slightly more than 50% (49). The third trial, in 135 people, compared oxygen therapy for variable times versus no oxygen in people with moderate hypoxemia and found no effect on survival at 3 years (96). The length of therapy per day did not affect the analysis. Finally, 203 patients were randomized to continuous versus nocturnal domiciliary oxygen treatment in the Nocturnal Oxygen Therapy Trial Group study (78). Continuous oxygen significantly reduced mortality over 24 months (OR 0.45). In summary, it seems that domiciliary oxygen therapy has a beneficial effect on survival in patients with hypoxemia and when given for at least 15 hours per day, but the data are, we believe, as yet less convincing than often quoted.

C. Nutritional Supplementation

There have been mainly short-term controlled studies of beneficial effects of nutritional supplementation (50–52,97), thereby precluding an analysis of effects on survival. There has also recently been one post hoc analysis of a prospective study, including 203 patients with COPD who had participated in a randomized placebo-controlled trial in COPD (75). In this study, the physiological effects of nutritional therapy alone ($n = 71$) or in combination with anabolic steroid treatment ($n = 67$) after 8 weeks was studied in patients with COPD prestratified into a depleted group and a nondepleted group. Mortality was assessed as overall mortality. The Cox proportional hazards model was used to quantify the relationship between the baseline variables age, sex, spirometry, arterial blood gases, body mass index (BMI), weight gain, smoking, and subsequent overall mortality. Weight gain ($> 2\,kg/8$ weeks) in depleted and nondepleted patients with COPD, as well as increase in maximal inspiratory mouth pressure during the 8-week treatment, were significant predictors of survival.

D. Surgery

Lung transplantation does not improve survival in patients with emphysema (55). The National Emphysema Treatment Trial Group recently reported survival benefit with lung volume reduction surgery in a subgroup of patients with emphysema only (those with predominantly upper-lobe emphysema and low exercise capacity) and actually worse survival in several other subgroups (57).

E. Rehabilitation

Older reports comparing survival in a group that had received rehabilitation to a group of historical controls suggest some effect on survival. For an overview of possible effects of rehabilitation from these historical comparison studies, see the review by Hodgkin (67). Ries et al. in a more recent study evaluated 5-year follow-up in 119 patients after an 8-week comprehensive rehabilitation program followed by 1-monthly reinforcement sessions compared to an education-only program (60). They found no difference in survival between the two groups.

VII. Other Parameters of Progression of COPD

Physicians have, especially in research, focused their studies of disease progression on two parameters: survival and decline in FEV_1. These are not the parameters patients complain about when visiting their physician. Patients have complaints of cough and reduced exercise tolerance. They will mention decreased quality of life, in whatever terminology. As a marker of how well they have been doing over any recent period, patients frequently mention the number of exacerbations they have had. Together with their physician, patients will also have concerns about recent hospitalizations, certainly if these occur with increasing frequency.

A few studies have attempted to evaluate risk factors for hospitalizations for COPD. Vitacca et al. in a retrospective analysis looked 2 years back for factors predicting admission to the intensive care unit for acute COPD exacerbations (98). They found that body weight, rate of deterioration over time in FEV_1, VC, PaO_2, and $PaCO_2$ were all related to the necessity for ICU admission in patients with COPD and hypercapnic respiratory insufficiency. Vestbo and colleagues evaluated risk factors for subsequent hospitalization for COPD from an epidemiological cohort (3). They found age, active smoking, and mucus hypersecretion to be independent predictors of hospitalization (Fig. 5). Persistent chronic mucus hypersecretion was associated with an increased relative risk of 5.3 for men and 5.1 for women. After inclusion of FEV_1 in the model, these risks decreased to 2.4 for men and 1.6 for women (not significant). In a recent study, Kessler et al. found several parameters to be related to risk for subsequent hospitalization in a monovariate analysis: low body

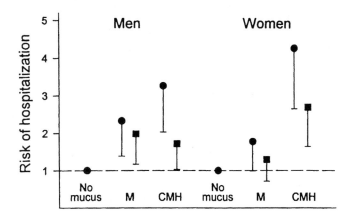

Figure 5 The association between any mucus secretion (M) and chronic mucus hypersecretion (CMH) at any of the surveys and FEV_1 decline between the two surveys adjusted for age, height, weight change, and smoking. Excess FEV_1 declines derived from multiple linear regression analyses and lower 95% confidence intervals are shown for men (left panel) and for women (right panel). (From Ref. 3.)

mass index, limited 6-minute walking test, decreased PaO_2, increased $PaCO_2$, and increased pulmonary artery pressure (99). In a multivariate model, only $PaCO_2$ and pulmonary artery pressure were independently related to hospitalization. Age and smoking habits had no relation to hospitalization.

In a recent study by Seemungal et al. there was a significant decrease in quality of life as measured by the St. George's Respiratory Questionnaire in patients with frequent exacerbations (100). Factors predictive of frequent exacerbations were daily cough, daily wheeze, daily cough and sputum, and frequent exacerbations in the previous year ($p = 0.001$). These findings demonstrate very clearly that patient quality of life is related to COPD exacerbation frequency.

VIII. Summary

COPD is commonly denoted as a relentlessly progressive disease. This notion is usually based on the progressive decline in FEV_1. Level and decline in FEV_1 are also closely related to survival: there is clearly an increased mortality from COPD, and this is rising further worldwide. Increased knowledge about risk factors for progression should lead to better understanding of the pathophysiology of COPD, as well as new therapies for a disease in which we currently have so few treatment options.

Decline in FEV_1 is related to smoking, airways hyperresponsiveness, and older age. Contrary to common belief, there are no firm data to link a lower baseline FEV_1 to decline in established COPD, whereas it is indeed linked to survival in established COPD as well as to FEV_1 decline in epidemiological cohorts. Smoking cessation is the one and only intervention with proven efficacy in reducing decline. In the subgroup of hypoxemic patients, one study suggests an effect of long-term oxygen therapy on decline. Finally, there is some evidence of a favorable effect of mucolytics on decline.

Overall mortality is above all related to level of FEV_1. Other strong predictors of decreased survival are hypoxemia, hypercapnia, and decreased body mass index. There is reasonable evidence for a negative effect of decreased diffusion capacity and cor pulmonale.

Finally being male and being older are unfavorable in regard to survival. Again, the intervention with proven efficacy is smoking cessation. In the subgroup of hypoxemic patients, there is reasonable evidence for a positive effect of long-term oxygen therapy. Lung transplantation unfortunately does not improve survival in patients with emphysema.

It is important to realize that patients complain more about decreased exercise tolerance and frequent exacerbations or hospitalizations than about low FEV_1. The link between FEV_1 and survival is relatively strong, but FEV_1 has a poor relationship with exercise tolerance. Frequent exacerbations have been proven to decrease quality of life. Future research into interventions in COPD should focus more on prevention of exacerbations and on improving the area patients complain about: reduced quality of life.

References

1. American Thoracic Society. Standards for the diagnosis and care of patients with chronic obstructive pulmonary disease. ATS statement. Am J Respir Crit Care Med 1995; 152:S77–S120.
2. Fletcher CM, Peto R, Tinker CM, Speizer FE. The Natural History of Chronic Bronchitis and Emphysema. An Eight-Year Study of Early Chronic Obstructive Lung Disease in Working Men in London. Oxford: Oxford University Press, 1976.
3. Vestbo J, Prescott E, Lange P. Copenhagen City Heart Study Group. Association of chronic mucus hypersecretion with FEV_1 decline and chronic obstructive pulmonary disease morbidity. Am J Respir Crit Care Med 1996; 153:1530–1535.
4. Siafakas NM, Vermeire P, Pride NB, Paoletti P, Gibson J, Howard P, Yernault JC, Decramer M, Higenbottam T, Postma DS, Rees J. Optimal assessment and management of chronic obstructive pulmonary disease (COPD). A consensus statement of the European Respiratory Society. Eur Respir J 1995; 8:1398–1420.
5. Kanner RE, Renzetti ADJ, Klauber MR, Smith CB, Golden CA. Variables associated with changes in spirometry in patients with obstructive lung diseases. Am J Med 1979; 67:44–50.
6. Committee on Diagnostic Standards for Nontuberculous Respiratory Diseases. Chronic bronchitis, asthma, and pulmonary emphysema. Am Rev Respir Dis 1962; 85:762–768.
7. Postma DS, Burema J, Gimeno F, May JF, Smit JM, Steenhuis EJ, et al. Prognosis in severe chronic obstructive pulmonary disease. Am Rev Respir Dis 1979; 119:357–367.
8. Anthonisen NR. Prognosis in chronic obstructive pulmonary disease: results from multicenter clinical trials. Am Rev Respir Dis 1989; 140:S95–S99.
9. Quanjer PH. Lung volumes and forced ventilatory flows: report working party standardization of lung function tests European Community for Steel and Coal. Eur Respir J 1993; 6(suppl 16):5–40.
10. Jones PW. Quality of life measurement for patients with diseases of the airways. Thorax 1991; 46:676–682.

11. Guyatt GH, Berman LB, Townsend M, Pugsley SO, Chambers LW. A measure of quality of life for clinical trials in chronic lung disease. Thorax 1987; 42: 773–778.

12. Kerstjens HAM, Brand PLP, Postma DS. Risk factors for accelerated decline among patients with chronic obstructive pulmonary disease (review). Am J Respir Crit Care Med 1996; 154:S266–S272.

13. Barter CE, Campbell AH. Relationship of constitutional factors and cigarette smoking to decrease in 1-second forced expiratory volume. Am Rev Respir Dis 1976; 113:305–314.

14. Stanescu D, Sanna A, Veriter C, Kostianev S, Calcgani PG, Fabbri LM, Maestrelli P. Airways obstruction, chronic expectoration, and rapid decline of FEV1 in smokers are associated with increased levels of sputum neutrophils. Thorax 1996; 51:267–271.

15. Anthonisen NR, Wright EC, Hodgkin JE, IPPB-Trial-Group. Prognosis in chronic obstructive pulmonary disease. Am Rev Respir Dis 1986; 133:14–20.

16. Kerstjens HAM, Rijcken B, Schouten JP, Postma DS. Decline of FEV_1 by age and smoking status: facts, figures, and fallacies (review). Thorax 1997; 52:820–827.

17. U.S. Department of Health and Human Services. A Report of the Surgeon General: The Health Consequences of Smoking—Chronic Obstructive Lung Disease. Washington, DC: U.S. Government Printing Office, 1984.

18. Burchfiel CM, Marcus EB, Curb JD, MacLean CJ, Vollmer WM, Johnson LR, et al. Effects of smoking and smoking cessation on longitudinal decline in pulmonary function. Am J Respir Crit Care Med 1995; 151:1778–1785.

19. Lange P, Groth S, Nyboe J, Mortensen J, Appleyard M, Jensen G, et al. Effects of smoking and changes in smoking habits on the decline of FEV1. Eur Respir J 1989; 2:811–816.

20. Xu X, Weiss ST, Rijcken B, Schouten JP. Smoking, changes in smoking habits, and rate of decline in FEV1: new insight into gender differences. Eur Respir J 1994; 7:1056–1061.

21. Lange P, Groth S, Nyboe J, Mortensen J, Appleyard M, Jensen G, Schnohr P. Decline of the lung function related to the type of tobacco smoked and inhalation. Thorax 1990; 45:22–26.

22. Ehrlich RI, Du Toit D, Jordaan E, Zwarenstein M, Potter P, Volmink JA, Weinberg E. Risk factors for childhood asthma and wheezing. Importance of maternal and household smoking. Am J Respir Crit Care Med 1996; 154:681–688.

23. Wang X, Wypij D, Gold DR, Speizer FE, Ware JH, Ferris BG Jr., Dockery DW. A longitudinal study of the effects of parental smoking on pulmonary function in children 6–18 years. Am J Respir Crit Care Med 1994; 149:1420–1425.

24. Xu X, Li B. Exposure-response relationship between passive smoking and adult pulmonary function. Am J Respir Crit Care Med 1995; 151:41–46.

25. Campbell AH, Barter CE, O'Connell JM, Huggins R. Factors affecting the decline of ventilatory function in chronic bronchitis. Thorax 1985; 40:741–748.

26. Postma DS, de Vries K, Koëter GH, Sluiter HJ. Independent influence of reversibility of air-flow obstruction and nonspecific hyperreactivity on the long-term course of lung function in chronic airflow obstruction. Am Rev Respir Dis 1986; 134:276–280.

27. Bahous J, Cartier A, Ouimet G, Pineau L, Malo JL. Nonallergic bronchial hyperexcitability in chronic bronchitis. Am Rev Respir Dis 1984; 129:216–220.

28. Ramsdale EH, Morris MM, Roberts RS, Hargreave FE. Bronchial responsiveness to methacholine in chronic bronchitis: relationship to airflow obstruction and cold air responsiveness. Thorax 1984; 39:912–918.

29. Yan K, Salome CM, Woolcock AJ. Prevalence and nature of bronchial hyperresponsiveness in subjects with chronic obstructive pulmonary disease. Am Rev Respir Dis 1985; 132:25–29.

30. Tashkin DP, Altose MD, Bleecker ER, Connett JE, Kanner RE, Wong-Lee W, Wise R. Lung Health Study Research Group. The Lung Health Study: airway responsiveness to inhaled methacholine in smokers with mild to moderate airflow limitation. Am Rev Respir Dis 1992; 145:301–310.

31. Tashkin DP, Altose MD, Connett JE, Kanner RE, Lee WW, Wise RA. Lung Health Study Research Group. Methacholine reactivity predicts changes in lung function over time in smokers with early chronic obstructive pulmonary disease. Am J Respir Crit Care Med 1996; 153:1802–1811.

32. Burrows B, Knudson RJ, Camilli AE, Lyle SK, Lebowitz MD. The "horse-racing effect" and predicting decline in forced expiratory volume in one second from screening spirometry. Am Rev Respir Dis 1987; 135:788–793.

33. Burrows B, Lebowitz MD, Camilli AE, Knudson RJ. Longitudinal changes in forced expiratory volume in one second in adults. Methodologic considerations and findings in healthy nonsmokers. Am Rev Respir Dis 1986; 133:974–980.

34. Glindmeyer HW, Lefante JJ, McColloster C, Jones RN, Weill H. Blue-collar normative spirometric values for Caucasian and African-American men and women aged 18 to 65. Am J Respir Crit Care Med 1995; 151:412–422.

35. Brandli O, Schindler C, Kunzli N, Keller R, Perruchoud AP, Sapaldia team. Lung function in healthy never smoking adults: reference values and lower limits of normal of a Swiss population. Thorax 1996; 51:277–283.

36. Renkema TEJ, Kerstjens HAM, Schouten JP, Vonk JM, Koëter GH, Postma DS. The importance of serum IgE for level and longitudinal change in airways hyperresponsiveness in COPD. Clin Exp Allergy 1998; 28:1210–1218.

37. Lebowitz MD, Postma DS, Burrows B. Adverse effects of eosinophilia and smoking on the natural history of newly diagnosed chronic bronchitis. Chest 1995; 108:55–61.

38. Burrows B, Bloom JW, Traver GA, Cline MG. The course and prognosis of different forms of chronic airways obstruction in a sample from the general population. N Engl J Med 1987; 317:1309–1314.

39. Wang M-L, McCabe L, Hankinson JL, Shamssain MH, Gunel E, Lapp NL, Banks DE. Longitudinal and cross-sectional analyses of lung function in steelworkers. Am J Respir Crit Care Med 1996; 153:1907–1913.

40. Chinn DJ, Cotes JE, Reed JW. Longitudinal effects of change in body mass on measurements of ventilatory capacity. Thorax 1996; 51:699–704.

41. Eriksson S, Lindell SE, Wiberg R. Effects of smoking and intermediate alpha 1-antitrypsin deficiency (PiMZ) on lung function. Eur J Respir Dis 1985; 67(4):279–285.

42. Barnes PJ, New therapies for chronic obstructive pulmonary disease. Thorax 1998; 53:137–147.

43. Fletcher CM, Peto R, Tinker CM. The natural history of chronic bronchitis and emphysema. Oxford: Oxford University Press, 1976, pp. 70–85.

44. Hughes JA, Hutchison DCS, Bellamy D, Dowd DE, Ryan KC, Hugh-Jones P. The influence of cigarette smoking and its withdrawal on the annual change of lung function in pulmonary emphysema. Q J Med 1982; 202:115–124.

45. Postma DS, Sluiter HJ. Prognosis of chronic obstructive pulmonary disease: the Dutch experience. Am Rev Respir Dis 1989; 140:S100–S105.

46. Anthonisen NR, Connett JE, Kiley JP, Altose MD, Bailey WC, Buist AS, Conway WA, Enright PL, Kanner RE, O'Hara P, Owens GR, Scanlon PD, Tashkin DP, Wise RA, Lung Health Study Research Group. Effects of smoking intervention and the use of an inhaled anticholinergic bronchodilator on the rate of decline of FEV1: the Lung Health Study. JAMA 1994; 272:1497–1505.

47. Scanlon PD, Connett JE, Waller LA, Altose MD, Bailey WC, Buist AS. Smoking cessation and lung function in mild-to-moderate chronic obstructive pulmonary disease. The Lung Health Study. Am J Respir Crit Care Med 2000; 161(2 pt 1):381–390.

48. Turato G, Di Stefano A, Maestrelli P, Mapp CE, Ruggieri MP, Roggeri A, Fabbri LM, Saetta M. Effect of smoking cessation on airway inflammation in chronic bronchitis. Am J Respir Crit Care Med 1995; 152:1262–1267.

49. Medical Research Council Working Party. Long term domiciliary oxygen therapy in chronic hypoxic cor pulmonale complicating chronic bronchitis and emphysema. Lancet 1981; i:681–686.

50. Efthimiou J, Fleming J, Gomes C, Spiro SG. The effect of supplementary oral nutrition in poorly nourished patients with chronic obstructive pulmonary disease. Am Rev Respir Dis 1988; 137(5):1075–1082.

51. Rogers RM, Donahoe M, Costantino J. Physiologic effects of oral supplemental feeding in malnourished patients with chronic obstructive pulmonary disease. A randomized control study. Am Rev Respir Dis 1992; 146(6): 1511–1517.

52. Whittaker JS, Ryan CF, Buckley PA, Road JD. The effect of refeeding on peripheral and respiratory muscle function in malnourished chronic obstructive pulmonary disease patients. Am Rev Respir Dis 1990; 142(2):283–288.

53. Schols AMWJ, Soeters PB, Mostert R, Pluymers RJ, Wouters EFM. Physiologic effects of nutritional support and anabolic steroids in patients with chronic obstructive pulmonary disease—placebocontrolled randomized trial. Am J Respir Crit Care Med 1995; 152:1268–1274.

54. Shahar E, Folsom AR, Melnick SL, Tockman MS, Comstock GW, Gennaro V, et al. Dietary n-3 polyunsaturated acids and smoking-related chronic obstructive pulmonary disease. N Engl J Med 1994; 331:228–233.

55. Hosenpud JD, Bennett LE, Keck BM, Edwards EB, Novick RJ. Effect of diagnosis on survival benefit of lung transplantation for end- stage lung disease. Lancet 1998; 351(9095):24–27.

56. Sundaresan S, Trulock EP, Mohanakumar T, Cooper JD, Patterson GA. Prevalence and outcome of bronchiolitis obliterans syndrome after lung transplantation. Washington University Lung Transplant Group. Ann Thorac Surg 1995; 60(5):1341–1346.

57. Fishman A, Martinez F, Naunheim K, Piantadosi S, Wise R, Ries A, Weinmann G, Wood DE. A randomized trial comparing lung-volume-reduction surgery with medical therapy for severe emphysema. N Engl J Med 2003; 348(21):2059–2073.

58. Lacasse Y, Wong E, Guyatt GH, King D, Cook DJ, Goldstein RS. Meta-analysis of respiratory rehabilitation in chronic obstructive pulmonary disease. Lancet 1996; 348:1115–1119.

59. Strijbos JH, Wijkstra PJ, Postma DS, Koëter GH. Five year effects of rehabilitation at different settings in patients with chronic obstructive pulmonary disease. Eur Respir J 1999; 14(suppl 30):15S–16S.

60. Ries AL, Kaplan RM, Limberg TM, Prewitt LM. Effects of pulmonary rehabilitation on physiologic and psychosocial outcomes in patients with chronic obstructive pulmonary disease. Ann Intern Med 1995; 122(11):823–832.

61. Lundbäck B, Lindström M, Andersson S, Nyström L, Rosenhall L, Stjernberg N. Possible effect of acetylscysteine on lung function. Eur Respir J 1992; 5(suppl 15):289s.

62. Poole PJ, Black PN. Mucolytic agents for chronic bronchitis. The Cochrane Library, Issue 3. Oxford: Update Software, 1999.

63. Decramer M, Dekhuijzen PN, Troosters T, van Herwaarden C, Rutten-van Molken M, van Schayck CP, Olivieri D, Lankhorst I, Ardia A. The Bronchitis Randomized On NAC Cost-Utility Study (BRONCUS): hypothesis and design. BRONCUS-trial Committee. Eur Respir J 2001; 17(3):329–336.

64. Kerstjens H, Postma D. Chronic obstructive pulmonary disease. In: Godlee F, ed. Clinical Evidence Concise Issue 9. London: BMJ Publishing Group 2003; 309–311.

65. Traver GA, Cline MG, Burrows B. Predictors of mortality in chronic obstructive pulmonary disease. Am Rev Respir Dis 1979; 119:895–902.

66. Vestbo J, Prescott E, Lange P, Schnohr P, Jensen G. Vital prognosis after hospitalization for COPD: a study of a random population sample. Respir Med 1998; 92:772–776.

67. Hodgkin JE. Prognosis in chronic obstructive pulmonary disease (review). Clin Chest Med 1990; 11:555–569.

68. Kanner RE, Renzetti ADJ, Stanish WM, Barkman HW, Klauber MR. Predictors of survival in subjects with chronic airflow limitation. Am J Med 1983; 74:249–255.

69. Peto R, Speizer FE, Cochrane AL, Moore F, Fletcher CM, Tinker CM, Higgins ITT, Gray RG, Richards SM, Gilliland J, Norman-Smith B. The relevance in adults of air-flow obstruction, but not of mucus hypersecretion, to

mortality from chronic lung disease. Results from 20 years of prospective observation. Am Rev Respir Dis 1983; 3:491–500.

70. Renzetti AD Jr., McClement JH, Litt BD. The Veterans Administration cooperative study of pulmonary function. 3. Mortality in relation to respiratory function in chronic obstructive pulmonary disease. Am J Med 1966; 41(1): 115–129.

71. The Intermittent Positive Pressure Breathing Trial Group. Intermittent positive pressure breathing therapy of chronic obstructive pulmonary disease. A clinical trial. Ann Intern Med 1983; 99:612–620.

72. Oswald-Mammosser M, Weitzenblum E, Quoix E, Moser G, Chaouat A, Charpentier C, Keesler R, Kessler R. Prognostic factors on COPD patients receiving long-term oxygen therapy: importance of pulmonary artery pressure. Chest 1995; 107:1193–1198.

73. Sahn SA, Nett LM, Petty TL. Ten-year follow-up of a comprehensive rehabilitation program for severe COPD. Chest 1980; 77(2 suppl):311–314.

74. Kawakami Y, Kishi F, Dohsaka K, Nishiura Y, Suzuki A. Reversibility of airway obstruction in relation to prognosis in chronic obstructive pulmonary disease. Chest 1988; 92:49–53.

75. Schols AMWJ, Slangen J, Volovics L, Wouters EFM. Weight loss is a reversible factor in the prognosis of chronic obstructive pulmonary disease. Am J Respir Crit Care Med 1998; 157:1791–1797.

76. Boushy SF, Thompson HK Jr., North LB, Beale AR, Snow TR. Prognosis in chronic obstructive pulmonary disease. Am Rev Respir Dis 1973; 108(6):1373–1383.

77. Mitchell RS, Webb NC, Filley GF. Chronic obstructive bronchopulmonary disease. III Factors influencing prognosis. Am Rev Respir Dis 1963; 89:878–896.

78. Nocturnal Oxygen Therapy Trial Group. Continuous or nocturnal oxygen therapy in hypoxemic chronic obstructive lung disease. A clinical trial. Ann Intern Med 1980; 93:391–398.

79. Vandenbergh E, Clement J, van de Woestijne KP. Course and prognosis of patients with advanced chronic obstructive pulmonary disease. Evaluation of functional indices. Am J Med 1973; 55:736–746.

80. Fletcher EC, Donner CF, Midgren B, Zielinski J, Levi-Valensi P, Braghiroli A, Rida Z, Miller CC. Survival in COPD patients with a daytime PaO_2 greater than 60 mm Hg with and without nocturnal oxyhemoglobin desaturation. Chest 1992; 101:649–655.

81. Burrows B, Earle RH. Course and prognosis of chronic obstructive lung disease. A prospective study of 200 patients. N Engl J Med 1969; 280:397–404.

82. Whittemore AS, Perlin SA, DiCiccio Y. Chronic obstructive pulmonary disease in lifelong nonsmokers: results from NHANES. Am J Public Health 1995; 85:702–706.

83. Hansen EF, Phanareth K, Laursen LC, Kok-Jensen A, Dirksen A. Reversible and irreversible airflow obstruction as predictor of overall mortality in asthma and chronic obstructive pulmonary disease. Am J Respir Crit Care Med 1999; 159:1267–1271.

84. Anthonisen NR, Connett JE, Enright PL, Manfreda J. Hospitalizations and mortality in the Lung Health Study. Am J Respir Crit Care Med 2002; 166(3):333–339.
85. Boushy SF, Adhikari PK, Sakamoto A, et al. Factors affecting prognosis in emphysema. Dis Chest 1964; 45:402–411.
86. Burrows B, Earle RH. Prediction of survival in patients with chronic airway obstruction. Am Rev Respir Dis 1969; 99(6):865–871.
87. Braun SR, Dixon RM, Keim NL, Luby M, Anderegg A, Shrago ES. Predictive clinical value of nutritional assessment factors in COPD. Chest 1984; 85(3): 353–357.
88. Wilson DO, Rogers RM, Wright EC, Anthonisen NR. Body weight in chronic obstructive pulmonary disease. The National Institutes of Health Intermittent Positive-Pressure Breathing Trial. Am Rev Respir Dis 1989; 139(6):1435–1438.
89. Prescott E, Lange P, Vestbo J. Chronic mucus hypersecretion in COPD and death from pulmonary infection. Eur Respir J 1995; 8:1333–1338.
90. Gray-Donald K, Gibbons L, Shapiro SH, Macklem PT, Martin JG. Nutritional status and mortality in chronic obstructive pulmonary disease. Am J Respir Crit Care Med 1996; 153(3):961–966.
91. Soriano JB, Vestbo J, Pride NB, Kiri V, Maden C, Maier WC. Survival in COPD patients after regular use of fluticasone propionate and salmeterol in general practice. Eur Respir J 2002; 20(4):819–825.
92. Rutten-van Molken MP, Postma MJ, Joore MA, Genugten ML, Leidl R, Jager JC. Current and future medical costs of asthma and chronic obstructive pulmonary disease in The Netherlands. Respir Med 1999; 93(11):779–787.
93. Barendregt JJ, Bonneux L, van der Maas PJ. The health care costs of smoking. N Engl J Med 1997; 337(15):1052–1057.
94. Crockett AJ, Moss JR, Cranston JM, Alpers JH. Domicilary oxygen in chronic obstructive pulmonary disease. The Cochrane Library, Issue 3. Oxford: Update Software, 1999.
95. Fletcher EC, Luckett RA, Goodnight-White S, Miller CC, Qian W, Costarangos-Galarza C. A double blind-trial of nocturnal supplemental oxygen for sleep desaturation in patients with chronic obstructive pulmonary disease and a daytime PaO2 above 60 mm Hg. Am Rev Respir Dis 1992; 145:1070–1076.
96. Gorecka D, Gorzelak K, Sliwinski P, Tobiasz M, Zielinski J. Effect of long-term oxygen therapy on survival in patients with chronic obstructive pulmonary disease with moderate hypoxaemia. Thorax 1997; 52:674–679.
97. Wilson DO, Rogers RM, Sanders MH, Pennock BE, Reilly JJ. Nutritional intervention in malnourished patients with emphysema. Am Rev Respir Dis 1986; 134(4):672–677.
98. Vitacca M, Foglio K, Scalvini S, Marangoni S, Quadri A, Ambrosino N. Time course of pulmonary function before admission into ICU. A two-year retrospective study of COLD patients with hypercapnia. Chest 1992; 102(6):1737–1741.

99. Kessler R, Faller M, Fourgauit G, Mennecier B, Weitzenblum E. Predictive factors of hospitalization for acute exacerbation in a series of 64 patients with chronic obstructive pulmonary disease. Am J Respir Crit Care Med 1999; 159:158–164.

100. Seemungal TA, Donaldson GC, Paul EA, Bestall JC, Jeffries DJ, Wedzicha JA. Effect of exacerbation on quality of life in patients with chronic obstructive pulmonary disease. Am J Respir Crit Care Med 1998; 157(5 pt 1):1418–1422.

6

Socioeconomic Burden of COPD

SEAN D. SULLIVAN, TODD A. LEE, and SARIKA OGALE

University of Washington
Seattle, Washington, U.S.A.

I. Introduction

The current trend in healthcare is to focus on controlling costs in an attempt to minimize the gap between individual expectations for access to medical care and the availability of societal resources to fund such care. Those in charge of financing, reimbursing, and providing healthcare aim at striking a balance between the objectives of lowering total costs of care and optimizing the health of their patients. These two objectives, however, are often in conflict with each other. Decision makers have to make choices between adoption of cost-increasing technologies that have the potential to improve health and spending in other areas that compete for the same limited resources. These decisions are complicated due to healthcare budget constraints, limited government budgets, rising prices, and an aging population. Thus, decision makers would prefer to base their choices on rational and consistent methods of evaluation designed to meet the dual objective of maximizing health given the limited budget. A common and accepted approach to comparing the relative value of healthcare interventions in creating better health outcomes is cost-effectiveness analysis.

The use of this decision making process requires an understanding of the social, functional, and economic burden of illness and the costs and outcomes associated with different interventions.

As a result of concerns about increasing healthcare costs, more sophisticated health technology assessments are being adopted that not only analyze the safety and efficacy of interventions, but also assess the impact on costs. These techniques have changed the informational requirements of decision makers, particularly in the following areas: 1) the epidemiology and burden of disease, 2) the total cost of illness, 3) the institutional and policy environment, and 4) the cost-effectiveness of health interventions.

The goal of his chapter is to review the evidence on disease burden, cost of illness, and cost-effectiveness of interventions as they relate to chronic obstructive pulmonary disease (COPD). Few studies have quantified the economic consequences of the morbidity and mortality associated with COPD, and all these studies are limited to North America and western Europe. Therefore, the information presented in this chapter is limited to treatment patterns and technologies used in developed countries. It is important to note that the review and assessment of economic evaluations is not comprehensive, but is intended to give a broad summary of the available literature and to highlight studies that follow reasonable standards for economic evaluation.

II. Economic Burden

The total economic burden of a disease is defined as the financial impact the particular condition has on society. Economic burden (or cost of illness) studies provide insight into the economic impact that COPD has on individuals, families, and the society as a whole. This approach separates the costs into direct and indirect costs associated with the disease. Direct costs are those associated with the intervention or treatment, while indirect costs are those resulting from output losses that can be attributed to the disease (loss of work or school time, decreased productivity, etc.). Economic burden studies are useful for gauging the importance of the disease and hence assist policy decisions about allocation of resources.

The total economic burden of a disease is affected both by the costs (direct and indirect) of the interventions used in the treatment of the disease as well as the prevalence of the disease in the population. Because of its high prevalence, the course of the disease, and high costs of treatment, COPD exacts a heavy social and economic toll on society. Data from North America and some European countries presented in this chapter may be instructive in understanding the relative economic burden of COPD in developed nations.

A. The United States

In the United States, the prevalence of chronic bronchitis and emphysema (the two major components of COPD) in 1996 was 16 million cases or 60.4 per 1000 persons (U.S. Census) (1). According to estimates for the year 2000 from the National Heart, Lung and Blood Institute, the annual economic burden of COPD in the United States is $30.4 billion (2). This estimate includes $14.7 billion in direct expenditures, 6.5 billion in indirect morbidity costs, and $9.2 billion in costs related to premature mortality. COPD and its attendant morbidity and mortality result in an estimated $1,900 in costs to the society per person per year—almost three times that for asthma. Table 1 displays comparable estimates of the direct and indirect costs of various lung disorders in the United States for the year 1993.

In a specific study of COPD-related illness in the Untied States, Sullivan et al. examined the National Medical Expenditure Survey in order to define the contribution of individual cost components to overall illness burden (3). These data indicated that the largest proportion of total medical expenditures was for hospitalizations and emergency department care (72.8%). Outpatient clinic and office visits accounted for 15.0% of expenditures, and prescription drug costs were responsible for 12.2%. Medical expenditures were disproportionately distributed among the sample, with a small number of patients accounting for a large proportion of expenditures. The references line in Figure 1 shows that over 70% of the total medical expenditures result from treating only 10% of COPD patients.

Table 1 Comparison of Direct and Indirect Costs of Lung Disease, 1993[a]

Condition	Total costs	Direct medical costs	Indirect, mortality	Indirect, morbidity	Total indirect
COPD	23.9	14.7	4.5	4.7	9.2
Asthma	12.6	9.8	0.9	0.9	2.8
Influenza	14.6	1.4	0.1	13.1	13.2
Pneumonia	7.8	1.7	4.6	1.5	6.1
Tuberculosis	1.1	0.7	—	—	0.4
Respiratory Cancer	25.1	5.1	17.1	2.9	20.0

[a]Costs in billions, U.S. 1993.
Source: Division of Epidemiology, National Heart, Lung and Blood Institute, 1996.

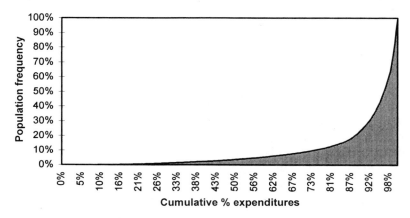

Figure 1 Distribution of medical care expenditures among respondents with COPD: 1987 National Medical Expenditure Survey, United States.
Source: National Medical Expenditure Survey, 1987.

An analysis of the Medicare insurance program for the elderly in the United States demonstrated that expenditures for beneficiaries with COPD were nearly 2.5 times higher than per capita expenditures of those without COPD ($8,482 vs. $3,511) (4). As with other serious chronic conditions, the most severely affected individuals incurred a substantial share of all costs. Nearly 50% of the total Medicare payment for COPD patients were incurred by approximately 10% of the Medicare beneficiaries with COPD, a trend similar to that seen in the analysis by Sullivan and colleagues (3,4).

Hospitalization-related costs—the largest portion of all expenditures for patients with COPD—commonly occur in the latter stages of the disease. The Sullivan et al. study estimated that per capita expenditures for inpatient hospitalizations in the COPD cohort were 2.7 times the per capita expenditures of the non-COPD cohort ($5,409 vs. $2,001). These data indicate that treatments that reduce the incidence and costs of hospitalization could substantially impact the overall healthcare costs associated with COPD.

B. The United Kingdom

Data from the United Kingdom's Office of National Statistics showed that there were 203,193 hospital admissions in Northern Ireland, Scotland, Wales, and England for COPD in 1994 (5). The average length of hospital stay among those admitted for a COPD-related diagnosis was nearly 10 days. The NHS Department of Health published data in 1996 showing that the medical cost of COPD in the United Kingdom was approximately $2,300 per person per year (6). Unlike the United States, the largest proportion (47.5%) of healthcare expenditures for COPD patients in the United Kingdom was on pharmaceutical treatments. The remaining proportions of expenditures were 24.5% for ambulatory oxygen therapy, 17.8% for hospital-based care, and 10.2% for primary care and community-based services.

A more recent analysis of the economic burden in the United Kingdom placed the cost of COPD to the NHS at £486 million in 1996 (7). Using an estimate of diagnosed prevalence of COPD in the United Kingdom of approximately 1%, the authors estimated a medical cost of $1,250 per person with COPD. Emergency and inpatient care accounted for 46.0% of all COPD-related costs. The largest fraction of costs for outpatient care was for oxygen treatments (32.1%). The remaining distribution of medical expenditures was for general practitioner consultations (4.4%) and prescription medications (17.5%). In addition, the authors estimated the indirect costs due to lost work productivity and disability, as a consequence of morbidity, and premature mortality associated with COPD. Persons with COPD had 24 million days of work loss during 1996. Non-medical economic impact amounted to an estimated £600 million for attendance at home and disability living allowance and £1.5 billion to employers for work absence and reduced productivity.

C. Sweden

Expenditures for COPD-related medical care in Sweden were estimated at 2.784 billion Swedish Kronor (SEK) in 1991 ($1 = SEK 6.05 (8)). This estimate includes 1.085 billion SEK for direct medical costs and 1.699 billion SEK for indirect costs attributable to COPD. Of the direct expenditures, the largest component was inpatient hospital care, which accounted for 47.4% (514 million SEK). Pharmaceutical expenditures totaled 137 million SEK (12.6%) and outpatient care made up the remainder of the direct costs at 434 million SEK (40.0%). Table 2 shows that, unlike the United States, the relative indirect cost of COPD in Sweden and the United Kingdom exceeded the direct medical care cost. However, the per capita total expenditures for COPD are quite similar between the three countries.

D. The Netherlands

Rutten-van Mölken and colleagues estimated present and future asthma and COPD related direct medical costs in the Netherlands (9). Using a prevalence-based cost-of-illness approach, estimates of direct medical costs for COPD and asthma in 1993 were $346 million and were expected to reach

Table 2 Four-Country Comparison of Direct and Indirect Costs of COPD[a]

Country (Ref.)	Year	Direct cost	Indirect cost	Total	Per capita[b]
United Kingdom (7)	1996	778	3,312	4,090	$65
The Netherlands (8)	1993	256	N/A	N/A	N/A[c]
Sweden (9)	1991	179	281	460	$60
United States (2)	1993	14,700	9,200	23,900	$87

[a]Costs in millions, U.S.$.
[b]Per capita valuation based on 1993 population estimates from the United Nations Population Council and expressed in 1993 US dollars.
[c]The authors did not provide estimates of indirect costs.

$555 million by 2010. The prevalence of COPD in 1993 in the Netherlands was 314,634 cases or 21 cases per 1000 persons. Annual costs per COPD patient in 1993 were estimated at $813, and the breakdown of costs for COPD showed inpatient hospitalization accounted for 57% of the total direct costs. Medication accounted for an additional 23% of medical costs. Given the prevalence of COPD and the cost per patient, the total direct costs for COPD in 1991 were $256 million. The authors did not estimate the nonmedical economic impact of COPD on the Netherlands economy. Thus, comparisons against other countries could not be undertaken.

Individuals with COPD frequently receive professional medical care services in their homes. In many European countries, national health insurance plans provide coverage for oxygen therapy, visiting nursing services, rehabilitation, and even mechanical ventilation in the home, although coverage for specific services may vary from country to country (10). These services are considered a direct medical expenditure that is part of the economic burden of COPD. No study has estimated the total social economic cost of providing these services. In 1997 government-sponsored insurance funds in the United States spent $17.7 billion on home health services, about 4% of all public expenditures on health care that year (11).

Furthermore, any estimate of direct medical expenditures for home care may underrepresent the true cost of home care to society, because it ignores the economic value of the care provided by family members to those with COPD. The value of the care provided by family members is considered a direct nonmedical expenditure for this condition. In the developing world it is likely that the economic value of family-provided care exceeds the value of care provided by health delivery systems. Thus, in terms of productivity loss, COPD may be doubly burdensome for low-income countries, since it often affects the ability and intensity of the affected individual and one or more relatives to work outside the home. Since human capital is often the most important national asset for developing countries, COPD may represent a serious threat to their economies.

The data on the economic burden of COPD are sparse, particularly outside of North America and Europe. While we can learn much from the relatively few studies on economic impact, data are needed on the use, cost, and relative distribution of medical and nonmedical resources for COPD in countries where the medical and human capital consequences of COPD are significant.

E. The Confronting COPD Survey

Confronting COPD in North America and Europe (12) was an economic analysis of data from large-scale surveys conducted in seven countries (Canada, France, Italy, the Netherlands, Spain, the United Kingdom, and the United States). Direct costs, indirect costs, overall societal costs, and cost components were compared among the seven nations. The mean direct costs per patient per year were higher in the United States ($4119) and Spain ($3196), while they were much lower in the Netherlands ($606) and France ($522). The United Kingdom and the United States reported the highest number of primary care practitioner visits, and the United States had the most specialist visits (1.51 per person in the past year), of which 0.27 per person were unscheduled. The Spanish sample exhibited the highest inpatient and emergency department admission rates. More than half of the direct costs in the United States, Canada, Italy, Spain, and United Kingdom could be assigned to inpatient hospitalizations, whereas in the Netherlands more than half of the direct costs came from prescription medications. The Netherlands also had the lowest level of hospitalization rates, indicating an inverse relationship between hospitalizations and medication use. The highest productivity loss was reported in the United States where the indirect costs amounted to $1,527 per patient. Table 3 presents the mean annual per capita direct, indirect, and societal costs of COPD in the seven nations.

III. Social Burden

Data on the societal and economic burden of COPD in developing countries have not been published in the medical or health economics literature. The economic burden of COPD may vary widely between developed and developing countries, and in some nations it may not be possible to obtain reliable data form which to gauge the cost impact of individual disease. Since mortality offers only a limited perspective on the total burden of the disease, it is necessary to find other measures of disease burden that may be more consistent and measurable across nations.

Table 3 Mean, Annual per Person Direct, Indirect, and Societal Costs of COPD in Seven Countries

Country	Direct cost	Indirect cost	Societal cost
United States	$4,119	$1,527	$5,646
Canada[a]	$1,258	$758	$2,023
United Kingdom[a]	$1,254	$1,261	$2,522
France[a]	$522	$1,064	$1,587
Italy[a]	$1,245	$47	$1,292
Spain[a]	$3,196	$296	$3,493
Netherlands[a]	$606	$405	$1,011

[a]Conversion rates for the year 2002 were used for converting European and Canadian currencies to U.S.$.
Source: Ref. 12.

In an effort to foster an independent, evidence-based approach to public health priority setting and evaluation, the World Bank initiated the Global Burden of Disease (GBD) Study in 1992 (13). The study was designed to develop internally consistent estimates of mortality from 107 major causes of death, disaggregated by age and sex, for the world split into eight geographic regions. This study was also designed to estimate the fraction of mortality and disability attributable to 10 major risk factors using a composite measure of the burden of each health problem, called the Disability-Adjusted Life Year (DALY). The DALYs for a specific condition are the sum of years lost because of premature mortality, and years of life lived with disability, adjusted for the severity of the disability.

The leading causes of DALYs lost in the world in 1990 and the numbers projected to 2020 are shown Table 4. In 1990, COPD ranked as the 12th most burdensome condition in the world with 2.1% of total DALYs lost. According to the projection from the GBD study, COPD will rank 5th in 2020 with 4.1% of total DALYs lost, behind only ischemic heart disease, major depression, traffic accidents, and cerebrovascular disease. This substantial increase in the global burden of COPD projected over the next 20 years reflects the consequences of increased tobacco use worldwide.

IV. Economic Evaluations

A. Smoking Cessation

The literature on the effectiveness of smoking cessation programs is quite extensive, and the results are strikingly similar. Investing healthcare

Table 4 Leading Causes of Disability-Adjusted Life-Years (DALY) Lost in the World: 1990 and 2020 (Projected)

Disease or injury	Rank 1990	Percent of total DALYS	Rank 2020	Percent of total DALYS
Lower respiratory infections	1	8.2	6	3.1
Diarrheal diseases	2	7.2	9	2.7
Perinatal period conditions	3	6.7	11	2.5
Unipolar major depression	4	3.7	2	5.7
Ischemic heart disease	5	3.4	1	5.9
Cerebrovascular disease	6	2.8	4	4.4
Tuberculosis	7	2.8	7	3.1
Measles	8	2.6	25	1.1
Road traffic accidents	9	2.5	3	5.1
Congenital anomalies	10	2.4	13	2.2
Malaria	11	2.3	19	1.5
COPD	*12*	*2.1*	*5*	*4.1*
Trachea, bronchus, lung cancer	33	0.6	15	1.8

Source: Murray and Lopez, Global Burden of Disease, 1996. Ref. 13.

resources in smoking cessation programs is cost effective in terms of medical costs per life year gained. A recent review of studies found that the median societal costs of various smoking cessation interventions was approximately £17,000 per life year gained (14). Cost-effectiveness studies for smoking cessation report favorable cost-effectiveness ratios for interventions such as nicotine transdermal patches, physician and other health professional counseling with and without patches, self-help and group programs, and community-based stop-smoking contests. Similarly, a comprehensive guidance document published in *Thorax* showed that smoking cessation programs produced cost-effectiveness ratios that ranged from £212 to £873 per life year gained and were thus a very good health care value for the Untied Kingdom NHS (15).

B. Home Oxygen

Supplemental home oxygen is usually the most costly component of outpatient therapy for adults with emphysema who require this therapy (16). Studies of the cost-effectiveness of alternative outpatient oxygen delivery methods in the United States and Europe suggest that oxygen concentrator devices may be cost saving compared to cylinder delivery systems (17,18).

C. Education and Pulmonary Rehabilitation

Education and pulmonary rehabilitation programs have been shown to have beneficial effects in patients with COPD (19). Education programs have been promoted as an economically attractive intervention for individuals with COPD, but the data are less clear (20,21). A Canadian study found that the incremental cost of pulmonary rehabilitation was $11,597 CDN per person. Statistically significant improvements in dyspnea, fatigue, emotional health, and mastery were observed (22).

An observational study with a small number of subjects found that patients in a pulmonary rehabilitation program utilized fewer healthcare services compared to those without rehabilitation (23). Because of study design limitations, it is unclear whether these results are generalizable to a larger, more diverse group of patients. The initial costs of the rehabilitation program may be offset if urgent care, emergency room visits, or hospitalizations are subsequently reduced.

A lingering question regarding pulmonary rehabilitation programs is whether the physiological and psychological benefits from the program fade over time. The benefits of rehabilitation programs have been observed to diminish as time from the intervention increases (16).

D. Home-Based Care

Economic studies of home care services have yielded both positive and negative results. One study of a northern Canadian native tribe found that quality of life improved and hospital days per admission fell after a home care program was instituted (24). A randomized, controlled trial in England found that substituting home care for inpatient hospital care produced no greater improvement in health outcomes while increasing costs (25,26). A recent review of home care for several conditions, including COPD, found that home care did not appear to improve health outcomes, while the cost impact was mixed (27).

E. Lung Volume–Reduction Surgery

Lung volume–reduction surgery (LVRS) has been an available option for treating disabling emphysema in developed countries, but the cost-effectiveness of this approach had not been evaluated until recently. Considerable debate has centered on the role of LVRS in treating end-stage emphysema since evidence evaluating the surgery in controlled trials was lacking. It has been estimated that widespread adoption of LVRS could cost the U.S. health economy more than $6 billion in the first several years of adoption (29). The Health Care Financing Administration has stated that Medicare will no longer provide reimbursement for LVRS until sufficient evidence exists regarding the safety and efficacy of the treatment.

A number of studies have estimated costs of LVRS in small numbers of patients. Elpern and colleagues analyzed the hospital costs associated with LVRS in 52 consecutive patients (30). Total hospital costs ranged from $11,712 to $121,829 and were significantly associated with length of stay, both in the ICU and for total length of stay in the hospital. The mean cost per hospitalization was $30,976, and the median cost was $19,771. A small number of individuals incurred extraordinary costs as a result of complications, causing the wide range in total hospital costs and the disparity between the mean and median.

Albert et al. also evaluated the hospital charges for LVRS at a single institution (31). The investigators evaluated 23 consecutive patients admitted for LVRS and found charges ranging from $20,032 to $75,561, with a median charge of $26,669. The results from this study suggest that the costs of LVRS may decrease as complication rates are reduced, and the average length of stay falls over time as caregivers gain experience with the procedure.

In a very recent randomized clinical trial, LVRS was compared with medical therapy after pulmonary rehabilitation (32). The trial showed no benefit overall, but some benefit in post hoc subgroups. Cost-effectiveness of LVRS was calculated over the duration of the trial, and the modeling was used for estimation over a 10-year follow-up period. The cost-effectiveness ratio for LVRS as compared with medical therapy during 3 years after initiation of treatment was $190,000 per quality-adjusted life-year (QALY) gained from the societal perspective ($193,000 per QALY from the health insurer perspective). At 10 years and using assumptions about sustained benefits, costs, and survival, the cost-effectiveness ratio was estimated to be $53,000 per QALY gained. Both the within trial and model-based estimates exclude a subgroup of patients that were found to be at high risk of mortality during intermediate assessments. The authors found the 10-year estimates to be unstable in their analyses but speculate that LVRS may be cost effective if the quality-of-life benefits could be maintained over time.

F. Transplantation

Lung transplantation is a costly but often effective therapy in the late stages of COPD. Studies of lifetime expenditures for lung transplantation have ranged from $110,000 to well over $200,000 (33). Unlike LVRS, the costs associated with lung transplantation remain elevated for months to years after surgery due to the high cost of complications and immunosuppression regimens.

G. Pharmacological Interventions

Sclar and colleagues analyzed the medical care expenditures of COPD patients treated with various pharmaceutical interventions (34). Their study estimated medical expenditures for prescription, physician, laboratory, and hospital services over 15 months in individuals newly diagnosed with COPD. The average adjusted cost of healthcare services for an individual over the study period ranged from $596 to $954 in 1994.

Rutten-van Mölken and associates investigated the costs and effects of adding inhaled anti-inflammatory therapy to inhaled β_2-agonists in subjects with moderately severe obstructive lung disease (35). Patients with both COPD and asthma were enrolled in the study. The addition of inhaled corticosteroids led to significant improvement in pulmonary function and symptom-free days, whereas addition of inhaled ipratropium bromide produced no clinical improvements. Analysis of the health economic endpoints showed that the average annual direct medical care cost savings associated with the use of inhaled corticosteroids were not offset by the increase in costs from the average annual price of the inhaled product. The incremental cost-effectiveness for inhaled corticosteroid was $201 per 10% improvement in FEV_1 and $5 for each symptom-free day gained. The cost-effectiveness of ipratropium was not evaluated because of the lack of clinical benefit observed in the trial. A study published recently compared fluticasone propionate (1000 µg/day) with placebo in patients with moderate to severe COPD (36). The fluticasone propionate group had fewer exacerbations overall, but the numbers of patients completely exacerbation-free over the study period were not significantly different between the two groups. The fluticasone group also had significantly greater improvements in lung function, lower symptom scores, and more successfully treated patients (FEV_1 improvement from baseline > 10%). Overall direct costs and total costs (including indirect costs) were not significantly different between the two groups, whereas nondrug direct costs were lower for the fluticasone group. The ICER per successfully treated patient was £0.25/day from the NHS perspective and −£3.39 from the societal perspective. The cost per moderate-severe exacerbation-free patient was £0.25/day from the NHS perspective. Treatment with fluticasone was thus found to be cost effective in the management of COPD in this population.

At least two studies looking at the cost-effectiveness of long-acting β_2-agonists have been published in 2003. Jones et al. conducted an economic evaluation comparing salmeterol plus usual therapy to usual therapy alone in patients with COPD (37). The salmeterol group had significantly more patients successfully treated (FEV$_1$ improvement >15%), a higher percentage of symptom-free nights and days, and more patients with a clinically significant improvement in their health status. Although the salmeterol group had higher overall costs the costs due to hospitlization, GP visits and other COPD medications were lower for this group. The ICER for salmeterol was £5.67 per additional symptom-free night, £12.33 per additional day with symptom score < 2, £4.62 per successfully treated patient, and £4.44 per day per person with significantly improved health status (SGRQ). Hogan et al. compared inhaled formoterol dry powder (12 and 24 μg BID) versus ipratropium bromide (40 μg QID) pressurized metered dose inhaler and placebo (38). In the clinical trial formoterol was found to be superior to the other arms with respect to lung function (FEV$_1$), reduced symptoms, frequency of bad days, need for rescue medications, and QOL (SGRQ). The ICER comparing ipratropium to placebo was $273 while that comparing formoterol 12 μg to ipratropium was $1,611 per additional liter of FEV$_1$. The ICER comparing formoterol 12 μg to placebo was $34.51 per QOL change score. The inclusion of information on hospitalizations from the original trial led to the ICER comparing formoterol 12 μg with ipratropium bromide to decrease from $1,611 to $892 for FEV$_1$ and from $34.51 to $28.81 for QOL, considering hospital costs to be $500/ day. This demonstrates the large impact of hospitalizations on the overall costs and results of the economic evaluation.

More recent data suggest that ipratropium alone or in combination with albuterol can reduce the cost for persons with COPD. Jurbran and colleagues performed a retrospective, chart-based cost-minimization analysis of theophylline versus ipratropium for patients with COPD (39). They found that patients treated with ipratropium had lower costs and a greater number of complication-free months compared to patients taking theophylline. Similarly, Fiedman et al. showed in a post hoc analysis of two randomized trials ($n = 1067$) that patients on a fixed combination of ipratropium and albuterol had improved pulmonary outcomes and reduced exacerbation frequency resulting in lower healthcare costs when compared to patients on albuterol alone (40). The lower healthcare costs were a direct result of fewer hospital days (46 vs. 103) and fewer patient days of changed or added antibiotics (302 vs. 429) in the group randomized to combination therapy compared to those on albuterol alone.

Another important group of pharmaceuticals is the anti-infectives used in the treatment of acute exacerbation of chronic bronchitis (AECB). In addition to antibiotic treatments, those experiencing an acute exacerbation of chronic bronchitis often require expensive inpatient care including intensive care stay and mechanical ventilation (41). Ciprofloxacin has been studied as a cost-effective alternative to usual care regimens for the treatment of AECB (42). The authors conclude that ciprofloxacin was cost effective in a subset of patients with moderate to severe chronic bronchitis who had at least four AECBs in the past year. Torrance et al. found that the use of ciprofloxacin compared to usual antibiotics in AECBs provided better outcomes but at higher costs (43). From the societal perspective, the use of ciprofloxacin increased annual cost $578 CDN compared to usual antibiotic treatment, and the incremental cost-effectiveness ratio was $18,600 per QALY gained. In a study by Halpern et al. (44), compared with clarithromycin, gemifloxacin treatment resulted in significantly more patients without a recurrence of AECB requiring antibiotic treatment (63.8% vs. 73.8%). Hospitalizations formed the largest portion of the direct costs in both study groups (46% in the gemfloxaxin group and 60% in the clarithromycin group). Gemfloxacin treatment resulted in lower costs as well as better effectiveness and hence was the dominant treatment in the cost-effectiveness study. From a review of AECB studies stated above and some additional studies, Halpern et al. (45) made some important observations and conclusions. They found that drug acquisition price is not the major cost driver in AECB treatment, but the choice of antibiotic does affect the total costs. Lower-priced (or higher-priced) medicines should not automatically be assumed to be cost effective, but the possibility of other costly consequences, such as hospitalizations, should be considered. It is clear from the literature that hospitalizations from a major portion of the costs for AECBs, as well as COPD treatment in general, and attention to minimizing these is imperative.

V. Conclusions

Because COPD is highly prevalent and can be severely disabling, medical expenditures for treating COPD can represent a substantial economic burden for societies and public and private payers worldwide. Nevertheless, very little economic information concerning COPD is available in the literature today. Economic burden-of-illness studies have only been conducted in a few developed countries. In the developing world, direct medical care costs may be less important than the impact of COPD on workplace and home productivity, yet we lack even basic information on economic burden in these countries. Another important knowledge gap is the paucity of formal economic evaluations of COPD-related prevention and treatment interventions. In an environment where resources available for medical care are limited and there are competing demands, studies that assess value for money are important. One notable highlight is smoking cessation, where economic evaluations have shown various programs to have favorable cost-effectiveness ratios. As options for treating COPD grow, more research will be needed to help guide caregivers and health budget managers regarding the most efficient and effective ways of managing this disease.

References

1. Adams PF, Hendershot GE, Marano MA. Current estimates from the National Health Interview Survey, 1996. National Center for Health Statistics. Vital Health Stat 10(200), 1999.
2. National Heart, Lung and Blood Institute. Data fact sheet: COPD. Available at: http://www.nhlbi.nih.gov/health/public/lung/other/copd_fact.htm
3. Sullivan SD, Strassels S, Smith DH. Characterization of the incidence and cost of COPD in the US. European Respiratory Society, September 1996. Stockholm, Sweden. Eur Respir J 1996; 9(suppl 23):421s.
4. Grasso ME, Weller WE, Shaffer TJ, Diette GB, Anderson GF. Capitation, managed care, and chronic obstructive pulmonary disease. Am J Respir Crit Care Med 1998; 158:133–138.
5. Office of National Statistics. Mortality Statistics (revised) 1994. England and Wales. London: HMSO, 1996.
6. NHS Executive. Burden of disease: a discussion document. Leeds: Department of Health, 1996.
7. Calverly PMA. Chronic Obstructive Pulmonary Disease: The Key Facts. London: British Lung Foundation, 1998.
8. Jacobson L, Hertzman P, Lofdahl C-G, Skoogh B-E, Lindgren B. The economic impact of asthma and COPD in Sweden 1980 and 1991. Respir Med 2000; 94(3):247–255.
9. Rutten-van Mölken MP, Postma MJ, Joore MA, Van Genugten ML, Leidl R, Jager JC. Current and future medical costs of asthma and chronic obstructive pulmonary disease in The Netherlands. Respir Med 1999; 93:779–787.
10. Fauroux B, Howard P, Muir JF. Home treatment for chronic respiratory insufficiency: the situation in Europe in 1992. The European Working Group on Home Treatment for Chronic Respiratory Insufficiency. Eur Respir J 1994; 7:1721–1726.
11. Centers for Medicare & Medicaid Services, Office of the Actuary, National Health Statistics Group, 1997.
12. Wouters EF. Economic analysis of the Confronting COPD survey: an overview of results. Respir Med 2003; 97(suppl C):S3–14.
13. The global burden of disease: a comprehensive assessment of mortality and distability from diseases, injuries and risk factors in 1990 and projected to 2020. In: Murray CJL, Lopez AD. eds. The Global Burden of Disease and Injury Series: v.1. Cambridge, MA: Harvard University Press, 1996.

14. Tengs TO, Adams ME, Pilskin JS, Safran DG, Siegel JE, Weinstein MC, Graham JD. Five hundred life saving interventions and their cost-effectiveness. Risk Analysis. 1995; 15:369–390.

15. Parrott S, Godfrey C, Raw M, West R, McNeill A. Guidance for commissioners on the cost effectiveness of smoking cessation interventions. Thorax. 1998; 53(suppl 5, pt. 2):S1–38.

16. Petty TL, O'Donohue WJ Jr. Further recommendations for prescribing, reimbursement, technology development, and research in long-term oxygen therapy. Summary of the Fourth Oxygen Consensus Conference, Washington, D.C., October 15–16, 1993. Am J Respir Crit Care Med 1994; 150:875–877.

17. Pelletier-Fleury N, Lanoe JL, Fleury B, Fardeau M. The cost of treating COPD patients with long-term oxygen therapy in a French population. Chest 1996; 110:411–416.

18. Heaney LG, McAllister D, MacMahon J. Cost minimisation analysis of provision of oxygen at home: are the *Drug Tariff* guidelines cost effective? BMJ 1999; 319:19–23.

19. Ries AL, Kaplan RM, Limberg TM, Prewitt LM. Effects of pulmonary rehabilitation on physiologic and psychological and psychosocial outcomes in patients with chronic obstructive pulmonary disease. Ann Intern Med 1995; 122:823–832.

20. Folgering H, Rooyakkers J, Herwaarden C. Education and cost/benefit ratios in pulmonary patients. Monaldi Arch Chest Dis 1994; 49:166–168.

21. Tougaard L, Krone T, Sorknaes A, Ellegaard H. Economic benefits of teaching patients with chronic obstructive pulmonary disease about their illness. The PASTMA Group. Lancet 1992; 339:1517–1520.

22. Goldstein RS, Gort EH, Guyatt GH, Feeny D. Economic analysis of respiratory rehabilitation. Chest 1997; 112:370–379.

23. Ries AL. Position paper of the American Association of Cardiovascular and Pulmonary Rehabilitation: scientific basis of pulmonary rehabilitation. J Cardiopulmo Rehabil 1990; 10:418–441.

24. Miles-Tapping C. Home care for chronic obstructive pulmonary disease: impact of the Iqaluit program. Arctic Med Res 1994; 53:163–175.

25. Shepperd S, Harwood D, Gray A, Vessey M, Morgan P. Randomised controlled trial comparing hospital at home care with inpatient hospital care. II: cost minimisation analysis. BMJ 1998; 316:1791–1796.

26. Shepperd S, Harwood D, Jenkinson C, Gray A, Vessey M, Morgan P. Randomised controlled trial comparing hospital at home care with inpatient hospital care. I: three month follow up of health outcomes. BMJ 1998; 316:1786–1791.

27. Soderstrom L, Tousignant P, Kaufman T. The health and cost effects of substituting home care for inpatient acute care: a review of the evidence. CMAJ 1999; 160:1151–1155.

28. Huizenga HF, Ramsey SD, Albert RA. Estimated growth of lung volume reduction surgery among Medicare enrollees. 1994–1996. Chest. 1998; 114(6):1583–1587.

29. Gentry C. Second Opinion. Why Medicare covers a new lung surgery for just a few patients. Wall Street Journal, June 29, 1998; Section A, p. 1.
30. Elpern EH, Behner KG, Klontz B, et al. Lung volume reduction surgery. An analysis of hospital costs. Chest 1998; 113:896–899.
31. Albert RK, Lewis S, Wood D, Benditt JO. Economic aspects of lung volume reduction surgery. Chest 1996; 110:1068–1071.
32. The national emphysema treatment trial research group. Cost-effectiveness of Lung-Volume Reduction Surgery for patients with severe emphysema. N Engl J Med 2003; 348:2092–2102.
33. Molken MP, Van Doorslaer EK, Rutten FF. Economic appraisal of asthma and COPD care: a literature review 1980–1991. Soc Sci Med 1992; 35:161–175.
34. Sclar DA, Leff RF, Skaer TL, Robison LM, Nemic NL. Ipratropium bromide in the management of chronic obstructive pulmonary disease: effect on health service expenditures. Clin. Ther 1994; 16:595–601.
35. Rutten-van Mölken MP, Van Doorslaer EK, Jansen MC, Kerstjens HA, Rutten FF. Costs and effects of inhaled corticosteroids and bronchodilators in asthma and chronic obstructive pulmonary disease. Am J Respir Crit Care Med 1995; 151:975–982.
36. Ayres JG, Price MJ, Efthimiou J. Cost-effectiveness of fluticasone propionate in the treatment of chronic obstructive pulmonary disease: a double-blind randomized, placebo-controlled trial. Respir Med 2003; 97(3):212–220.
37. Jones PW, Wilson K, Sondhi S. Cost-effectiveness of salmeterol in patients with chronic obstructive pulmonary disease: an economic evaluation. Respir Med 2003; 97(1):20–26.
38. Hogan TJ, Geddes R, Gonzalez ER. An economic assessment of inhaled formoterol dry powder versus ipratropium bromide pressurized metered dose inhaler in the treatment of chronic obstructive pulmonary disease. Clin Ther 2003; 25(1):285–297.
39. Jubran A, Gross N, Ramsdell J, Simonian R, Schuttenheim K, Sax M, Kaniecki DJ, Arnold RJ, Sonnenberg FA. Comparative cost-effectiveness analysis of theophylline and ipratropium bromide in chronic obstructive pulmonary disease. A three center study. Chest 1993; 103:78–84.
40. Friedman M, Serby CW, Manjoge SS, Wilson JD, Hilleman DE, Witek TJ Jr. Pharmacoeconomic evaluation of a combination of ipratropium plus albuterol compared with ipratropium alone and albuterol alone in COPD. Chest 1999; 115:635–641.
41. Connors AF, Dawson NV, Thomas C, Hawell FE Jr., Desbiens N, Fulkerson WJ, Kussin P, Bellamy P, Goblman L, Knaus WA. Outcomes following acute exacerbations of severe chronic obstructive lung disease. Am J Respir Crit Care Med 1996; 154:959–967.
42. Grossman R, Maukherjee J, Vaughan D, Eastwood C, Cook R, La Forge J, Lampon N. A 1-year community based health economic study of ciprofloxacin vs. usual antibiotic treatment in acute exacerbation of chronic bronchitis. Chest 1998; 113:131–141.

43. Torrance G, Walker V, Grossman R, Mukherjee J, Vaughan D, La Forge J, Lampron N. Economic evaluation of ciprofloxacin compared with usual antibacterial care for the treatment of acute exacerbations of chronic bronchitis in patients followed for 1 year. Pharmacoeconomics 1999; 16:499–520.
44. Halpern M, Palmer C, Zodet M, Kirsch J. Cost-effectiveness of gemifloxacin: results from the GLOBE study. Am J Health-Syst Pharm 2002; 59:1357–1365.
45. Halpern M, Higashi M, Bakst A, Schmier J. The economic impact of acute exacerbations of chronic bronchitis in the United States and Canada: a literature review. J Managed Care Pharm 2003; 9(4):353–359.

7

Pathology of COPD

JAMES C. HOGG

St. Paul's Hospital
Vancouver, British Columbia, Canada

The cigarette smoking habit is the single most important risk factor for developing COPD. This habit produces lung inflammation in all smokers (1), and this inflammatory process underlies the pathogenesis of the chronic bronchitis (2), airways obstruction (3,4), emphysematous destruction (5), and the early vascular lesions associated with pulmonary hypertension in COPD (6–8). However, there is not a tight correlation between the total accumulated dose of smoking and disease, and large series of cases such as that shown in Figure 1 have established that smoking accounts for only a small percentage of the variance in the decline in lung function. This suggests that other factors must add to the risk of smoking, and epidemiological studies have identified age, gender, environmental pollution, occupation, socioeconomic status, birth weight, recurrent infections, allergy, and genetic constitution as factors that independently increase the risk of developing COPD (9). The purpose of this chapter is to review the pathology of the lung lesions that contribute to the natural history of COPD and the changes that occur during acute exacerbations that periodically complicate this condition.

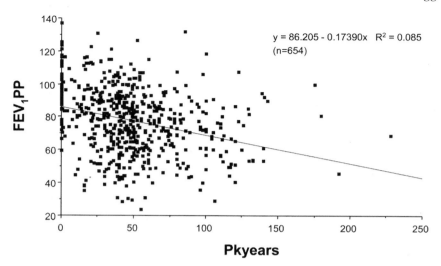

Figure 1 FEV_1 versus smoking history in a large series of patients that required lung resection for tumor. Although there is a statistically significant relationship between FEV_1 decline and smoking history, the r^2 value is low, indicating that it only accounts for a small % of the variance in the decline of FEV_1. Therefore, factors other than smoking must account for the fact that only a minority of smokers develops severe airways obstruction.

I. Chronic Bronchitis

Chronic bronchitis is defined by the symptoms of cough and sputum production, and these symptoms can occur alone or in combination with airways obstruction, emphysema and pulmonary hypertension, and right heart failure (10). Material that penetrates into the lower airway is normally cleared up by the mucociliary escalator and swallowed without producing either cough or sputum. The inflammatory response underlying the pathogenesis of cough and sputum production is located in the mucosa, gland, and gland ducts of the larger cartilaginous airway (3), where it produces an exudate of fluid and cells that interferes with normal mucociliary clearance and increases the amount of material that must be cleared. This exudate is formed by the effects of inflammatory mediators on the microvessels of the bronchial circulation that allow protein to leak out of vessels and promote the migration of inflammatory cells out of the vessels into the interstitial space and lumen of the bronchi. Small amounts of mucus are added to this exudate by mucus-secreting cells in the surface epithelium and the epithelial glands (Fig. 2). Reid introduced the measurement of the

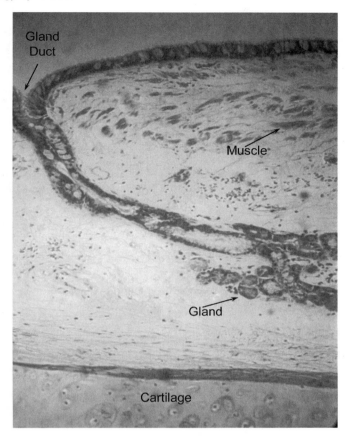

Figure 2 Low power photomicrograph of a normal bronchus showing the opening of the gland duct into the lumen and duct leading to the submucosal gland. The bronchial muscle and cartilage are clearly labeled.

size of the mucus glands as a pathological yardstick for the symptoms of chronic bronchitis (11), and other investigators have used a variety of techniques to examine airway gland size. Ryder et al. (12) showed a clear difference in bronchial mucus gland size between smokers and nonsmokers in a large series of cases, and Thurlbeck and Angus (13) reported an overlap in gland size between groups with and without chronic bronchitis. These data suggest that smoking tends to increase gland size and that chronic bronchitis can be present with or without mucus gland enlargement. When there is an increase in gland size, it is associated with an increase in cell mass within the gland and a shift from serous to mucus cells with production of

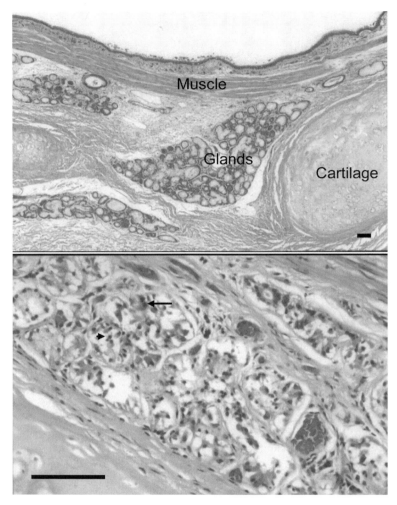

Figure 3 Chronic bronchitis is associated with an inflammatory process that involves the mucosa, gland ducts, and glands of the bronchi that are between 2 and 4 mm in internal diameter.

several types of glyoproteins (14,15). Several of the genes involved in mucus production by these cells have now been identified, and factors that control their expression in both health and disease are under active investigation.

Mullen et al. (Fig. 3) showed that chronic bronchitis was associated with inflammation of the airway mucosal surface, the submucosal glands, and gland ducts, particularly in the smaller bronchi between 2 and 4 mm in diameter (2). The nature of the cells present in the inflammatory process have been investigated in biopsy studies which show that the CD8 + lymphocytes are present in excess numbers in smokers with chronic bronchitis (16,17). This increase in CD8 + cells suggests the presence of a population of cytotoxic T lymphocytes that might be searching out cells containing intracellular parasites such as viruses. Elliott et al. (18) reported that cells in the epithelium, glands, and gland ducts of human airways are latently infected with adenovirus and express a viral protein capable of amplifying the cigarette smoke–induced inflammatory process. Although the mechanisms responsible for the amplification of smoke–induced bronchial inflammation in patients with chronic bronchial inflammation in patients with chronic bronchitis are only partially understood, has become clear that this inflammatory process is responsible for the exudate in the airway lumen, the changes in the epithelium and epithelial glands, the stimulation of the extracellular matrix that increases the smooth muscle and connective tissue in the airway wall (19), and the degenerative changes in the airway cartilage that occurs in chronic bronchitis (20,21). These structural changes all contribute to a long-term deterioration in the function of the cartilaginous conducting airways, particularly those that involve the mucosa and glands to make the airways easier to infect.

II. Airways Obstruction

The smaller conducting airways that include bronchi and bronchioles less than 2 mm in diameter are the site of airway obstruction in COPD (2,22). In the normal lung, the total cross-sectional area of the airways increases rapidly as the gas-exchanging surface is approached (23), and direct measurements of airways resistance in canines (24) established that the small peripheral airways < 2 mm in diameter offer very little resistance to airflow. Similar measurements in human lungs (2) confirmed that the resistance of airways < 2 mm in internal diameter make up a small percentage of total airways resistance in the normal lung (Fig. 4) but account for the majority of the increase in airways resistance in disease (Fig. 5). Although some have argued (22) that a larger proportion of the total resistance should be attributed to peripheral airways in the normal lung, there is agreement that the peripheral airways are the major site of increased airway resistance in COPD (2,22).

The pathological changes proposed to increase peripheral airways resistance in fully developed COPD include a reduction in the support these small airways receive from alveolar walls attached to their outer walls through the surrounding connection tissue sheath (25,26), and structural

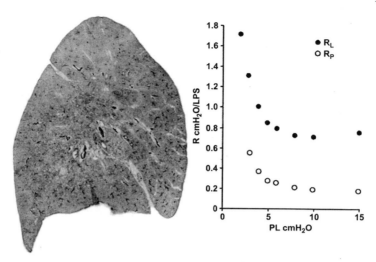

Figure 4 Gross photograph of paper-mounted whole lung section of a normal lung. The data on the right were obtained from this lung using a retrograde catheter technique (right). Total airways resistance (R_L) and the component of this resistance attributed to the peripheral airways < 2 mm in diameter. These data show that in the normal lung, the resistance of the peripheral airways (R_P) make up a relatively small percentage of the total airways resistance (R_L). (From Ref. 3.)

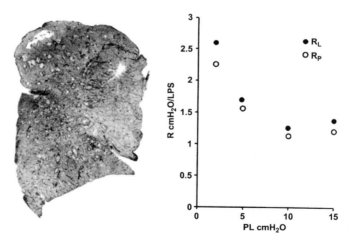

Figure 5 Paper-mounted section of a lung from a patient with mild centrilobular emphysema. Total lower airways resistance (R_L) and peripheral airways resistance (R_P) were measured using the technique described in Ref. 3. R_L has approximately doubled (compared to normal in Fig. 4), and the majority of this increase is due to a large increase in peripheral airways resistance.

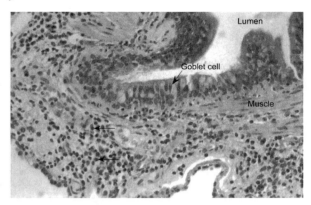

Figure 6 Bronchiole from a case of severe COPD. The airway wall of this peripheral airway has been thickened by a chronic inflammatory process that contains large numbers of mononuclear cells. There has also been an increase in the number of goblet cells in the epithelial lining of the airway surface.

narrowing of the airway lumen produced by the inflammatory process (2,4,27). The histological appearance of peripheral airways in cases of COPD with high resistance (Fig. 6) shows that the chronic inflammatory process is present in these airways and that this process thickens the airway wall and narrows its lumen. Matsuba and Thurlbeck (27) showed that the peripheral airways were disproportionately narrow in patients with COPD, and a systematic analysis of peripheral airways resistance has suggested that this airway narrowing made a greater contribution to the increase in airways resistance than a reduction in the alveolar support produced by emphysematous destruction of the alveolar walls (3).

III. Emphysema

A. Terminology

The terms used to describe the pathology of emphysema are based on the anatomy of the normal lung. Miller (28) defined the secondary lobule as the part of the lung surrounded by connective tissue septae (Fig. 7A) and the acinus as the portion of the lung parenchyma supplied by a single terminal bronchiole (Fig. 8). As each secondary lobule contains several terminal bronchioles, it follows that each lobule contains several acini. Miller also introduced the term "primary lobule" to describe an alveolar duct and the collection of alveolar sacs that it supplies, but this term has fallen out of usage.

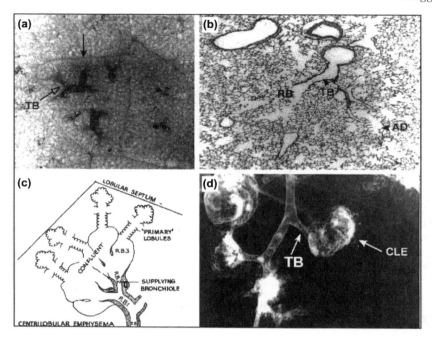

Figure 7 (a) Normal lung photographed from the pleural surface after a postmortem bronchogram was performed. The connective tissue outlining the secondary lobule is clearly seen (solid arrow), and a terminal bronchiole (TB) indicated by a clear arrow supplies a single acinus. (b) Photomicrograph of an acinus showing a terminal bronchiole (TB), respiratory bronchiole (RB), and alveolar ducts (AD). Their structure is represented by the fine spray of contrast at the end of the terminal bronchiole shown in the bronchogram in (A). (c) Diagram of the lesion in centrilobular emphysema showing the dilation and destruction of the respiratory bronchioles. (From Ref. 32.) (d) Postmortem bronchogram showing a centrilobular emphysematous lesion (CLE) outlined by bronchographic material.

B. Centrilobular/Centriacinar Emphysema

Figure 7 shows examples of the centriolobular form of emphysema that results from dilatation and destruction of the respiratory bronchioles. This form of emphysema was briefly described by Gough in 1952 (29), by McLean in Australia in 1956 (30), and in a more detailed report by Leopold and Gough in 1957 (31). Dunnill (32) suggested that centriacinar emphysema was a better term than centrilobular because the disease is located in the acinus and not all of the acini in a lobule need be affected. However, as individual centriacinar lesions frequently coalesce, the term centrilobular

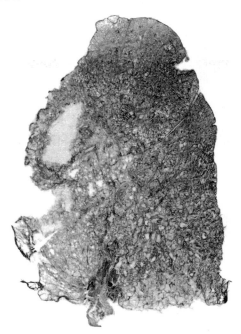

Figure 8 Paper-mounted whole lung section from patients with severe panacinar emphysema, which is predominant in the lower lobes. Thurlbeck has shown that this lower lobe predominance is obvious in advanced cases such as this but does not reach statistical significance in less advanced disease.

emphysema has become firmly entrenched in the literature. This form of emphysema affects the upper regions of the lung more commonly than the lower (33–35). Heppleston and Leopold (36,37) emphasized that the parent airways supplying the centriacinar lesions were often narrowed due to an inflammatory reaction that was peribronchiolar in location and involved both a polymorphonuclear and mononuclear leukocyte infiltration. They also showed that the fragmented strands of tissue within the lesions are inflamed. They seperated a lesion they had first described in coalworkers (37) from the centrilobular form and referred it as focal emphysema. This lesion also involved the respiratory bronchioles, was less destructive than the centrilobular form, contained large quantities of pigment, and was supplied by airways that were neither inflamed nor stenosed (36). Wyatt (38) challenged the view that there was any difference between focal and centrilobular emphysema, and Thurlbeck (39) thought that they might be distinguished when the disease was mild. Dunnill's (32) view was that the separation of focal from centrilobular emphysema was based largely on semantic arguments that add little to our understanding of either the mechanism of the lung destruction or its functional consequences. The two conditions probably have a similar origin, with focal emphysema being more widely distributed and less severe than the classic centrilobular form.

C. Panacinar/Panlobular Emphysema

Panacinar emphysema refers to dilatation and destruction throughout the acinus that results in uniform destruction of the entire lobule when all of the acini in it are involved. Wyatt et al. (40) provided a detailed account of this lesion in 1962, although it had been described under different names by earlier investigators. Thurlbeck (35) showed that the mildest form of this disease is difficult to discern unless the slices of fixed inflated lung are impregnated with barium sulfate and examined under water using low magnification. In some cases the disease is clearly more severe in the lower lobe (Fig. 8), but Thurlbeck believed this only becomes statistically significant in advanced cases. The association between α_1-antitrypsin deficiency (α1P1) and severe emphysema was first described by Laurell and Eriksson (41). The high incidence of severe emphysema in some families and reports of severe panacinar emphysema in young subjects with normal levels of α_1-antitrypsin suggest that other genetic deficiencies make persons more susceptible to the development of emphysema (43,44). Indeed, the wide variation in the prevalence of emphysema in the face of similar heavy cigarette smoking histories has caught the imagination of the geneticists and led to an active search for susceptibility genes.

D. Distal Acinar Emphysema

The terms distal acinar, mantle, and paraseptal emphysema are used to describe lesions that occur in the periphery of the lobule. This type of lesion is commonly found along the lobular septae, particularly in the subpleural region. The lesion can occur in isolation, where it has been associated with spontaneous pneumothorax in young adults and bullous lung disease in older individuals. However, isolated distal acinar destruction if often found in association with other forms of emphysema (32).

E. Miscellaneous Forms of Emphysema

There are several forms of emphysema, which will be only briefly described here because they are only marginally relevant to the pathology of adult COPD. The emphysema that forms around scars lacks any special distribution in the lobule and is referred to as irregular emphysema. Bullous disease of the lung arising from the paraseptal form of emphysema discussed earlier can occur in isolation, and if the cysts become large enough they may interfere with lung function. Surgical removal of these large isolated lesions can have a very positive effect. Unilateral emphysema, or McLeod's syndrome, has been described following severe infections with measles and adenovirus infection that produced severe bronchiolitis in the affected lung. Congenital lobar emphysema is a developmental abnormality affecting newborn children that has been fully discussed elsewhere (32).

F. Summary of Terminology

The terminology used to describe emphysema has been helpful, but the precise nature of these descriptions becomes unhelpful in severely diseased lungs. Although it is possible to find cases of pure centrilobular emphysema and pure panacinar emphysema, it is much more common to see both forms of the disease in the same lung in advanced cases. When an entire lobule has been destroyed and the destruction of many lobules has coalesced into large lesions, the value of terms such as panacinar and centrilobular as precise descriptors is reduced.

IV. Pulmonary Hypertension

In contrast to people with normal lungs, persons with minimal COPD elevate their pulmonary vascular pressures during exercise (6). This increase in vascular pressure is the result of a rise in intrathoracic pressure caused by an increase in the time required to empty the lung during expiration (6). However, as this rise in intrathoracic pressure affects both pulmonary artery and pulmonary venous pressures, the elevation in driving pressure, i.e., $P_A - P_V$, remains appropriate for the increase in cardiac output, and there is no increase in pulmonary vascular resistance. As the resistance to lung emptying increases with the progression of COPD, alveolar pressure begins to rise above intrathoracic pressure when breathing rates increase during exercise. This shifts portions of the lung from Zone III conditions where the driving pressure is $P_A - P_V$ to Zone II conditions where the driving pressure is $P_{PA} - P_{ALV}$ and there is an elevation in pulmonary vascular resistance that results in a greater increase in pulmonary arterial pressure.

Wright et al. (6) have shown that the minor changes in pulmonary hemodynamics that occur in minimal to moderate COPD produce structural changes in the vessel wall that include thickening of the intimal and adventitial layers without a change in the media (Table 1). These early changes appear to be associated with abnormalities in the ventilation perfusion (V/Q) ratio and with inflammatory changes involving the vessel wall (7,8). These structural changes progress with hypertrophy of the

Table 1 Comparison of Nonsmokers and Smokers with Minimal and Moderate Emphysema[a]

		Smokers with COPD	
	Nonsmokers	Minimal emphysema	Moderate emphysema
Sex (M/F)	0/3	7/0	6/0
Age (yr)	60 ± 2	59 ± 4	62 ± 2
Smoking history (pack-years)	0	65 ± 1	63 ± 9
PO_2 (mm Hg)	—	71 ± 3	79 ± 6
TLC (% pred)	97 ± 5	119 ± 3	113 ± 7
VC (% pred)	98 ± 3	103 ± 5	95 ± 5
FRC (% pred)	93 ± 10	133 ± 5	125 ± 7
RV (% pred)	95 ± 9	146 ± 6	134 ± 9
$FEV_1/FVC \times 100$	88 ± 3	63 ± 4	68 ± 4
FEF_{25-75} (% pred)	119 ± 9	43 ± 8	48 ± 7
DL_{CO} (% pred)	115 ± 19	87 ± 11	58 ± 5[b]
K, (% pred)	—	112 ± 5	154 ± 4
Emphysema grade	0	7 ± 2	28 ± 7
Total airway score	97 ± 37	140 ± 17	222 ± 23
Inflammation score	13 ± 5	28 ± 10	31 ± 6
Ppa (mmHg)			
Rest room air		17 ± 3	13 ± 1
Exercise room air		27 ± 4	34 ± 3
Rest oxygen		17 ± 3	15 ± 1
Exercise oxygen		27 ± 4	27 ± 3
Ppaw (mmHg)			
Rest room air		9 ± 2	5 ± 1
Exercise room air		15 ± 4	16 ± 2
Rest oxygen		10 ± 2	5 ± 1
Exercise oxygen		13 ± 3	10 ± 2[c]
Cardiac index (1/min/m)			
Rest room air		2.7 ± 3	3.2 ± 0.4
Exercise room air		5.3 ± 0.5	6.7 ± 1.6
Rest oxygen		2.8 ± 0.2	3.4 ± 0.5
Exercise oxygen		5.9 ± 0.9	6.3 ± 1.2
Pulmonary vascular resistance (dynes/cm^{-5}/s^{-1})			
Rest room air		146 ± 56	142 ± 30
Exercise room air		111 ± 32	182 ± 53
Rest oxygen		117 ± 34	160 ± 31
Exercise oxygen		112 ± 26	161 ± 39

Table 1 Continued

	Nonsmokers	Smokers with COPD	
		Minimal emphysema	Moderate emphysema
Vessel morphology			
% intima	14 ± 0.6	18 ± 0.5^d	21 ± 0.6^e
% media	17 ± 0.6	18 ± 0.4	19 ± 0.5
% adventitia	69 ± 1	64 ± 0.7	60 ± 0.8^d
Area of vessel wall (mm^2)	0.12 ± 0.02	0.26 ± 0.02^d	0.34 ± 0.02^e

[a]Values are mean $\pm$ SE.
[b]Compared with minimal emphysema group, $p < 0.05$.
[c]Compared with exercise room air, $p < 0.01$.
[d]Compared with control (nonsmoking group), $p < 0.05$.
[e]Compared with control (nonsmoking group), $p < 0.01$.

smooth muscle layer and the changes in the extracellular matrix of the wall that lead to scarring and a permanent reduction in the vessel lumen (44,45). The V/Q mismatch produces hypoxia, which stimulates the vascular smooth muscle to shorten, and this acts in series with the thickening in the vessel wall to further reduce the vascular lumen. In the end stage of the disease, emphysematous destruction of the capillary bed also contributes to pulmonary arterial hypertension by increasing the pressures required to perfuse the pulmonary vascular bed, but the relationship between emphysema and right ventricular hypertrophy is not a simple one (46,47). The onset of right heart failure leads to systemic venous dilation and peripheral venous stasis, which initiates venous thrombosis and predisposes to embolization into the pulmonary circulation, which further increases the load on the right heart.

V. Acute Exacerbations of COPD

The natural history of COPD is complicated by acute exacerbations that can result in death, an acceleration of the downhill course of the developing COPD with more frequent hospital admissions, and an increase in the likelihood of a poor outcome (48). In a large series of 1016 adult patients admitted for exacerbations, 51% had lung infections, 26% had heart failure, 12% had a variety of other disorders that included pulmonary embolism and pneumothorax, and in 30% no cause for the acute deterioration was found. This study clearly showed that of the problems that were not directly attributable to the underlying disease, the most frequent was a super-imposed infection.

Body surfaces such as the upper airways and oropharynx are permanently infected with a large number of organisms that make up their natural flora. These organisms exist in a symbiotic relationship with the host without producing harmful effects. Disease is the result of tissue damage produced by organisms capable of invading the natural tissue barriers and resisting the cellular and humoral defence mechanisms of the host. The lower respiratory tract of the normal lung is sterile and almost always becomes infected from a source above the larynx. Aspiration is common even in healthy people, especially during sleep, but their adverse effects are readily managed by the host-defense mechanisms of the lower airways. As these natural defense mechanisms are compromised in COPD, it is easier for pathogens to overcome the host defenses, damage airway and parenchymal tissue, and induce an inflammatory and/or immune response that results in disease.

The pathology of acute exacerbations of COPD is difficult to study because tissue obtained at autopsy or by biopsy reflects the underlying pathology as well as the acute insult. Examination of the lower respiratory tract during acute viral infection (49–53) shows diffuse reddening and swelling of the larynx, trachea, and bronchi. Light microscopic examination of the tissue shows evidence of ciliary damage and desquamation of the epithelium, frequently exposing a thickened and sometimes hyalinized basement membrane. There is also evidence of submucosal edema with vascular congestion and infiltration of neutrophils and mononuclear cells. Later in the course of the disease, reparative and destructive processes may be present simultaneously with complete resolution of the epithelial necrosis occurring over a period of weeks to months. In experimental models of viral infection, this inflammatory process can persist long after the virus has stopped replicating, and there is excellent evidence that much of this pathology is produced by an immune response of the virus and not by the damage the virus does to the host tissue (54).

Saetta et al. (55) performed an important study on patients with exacerbations of COPD that were for the most part much milder than those described in Connors's series (48). They performed bronchoscopy and biopsied the lower airways of 11 patients during acute exacerbations and compared the results to a separate group of 12 patients who were stable at the time of biopsy. The most interesting finding was a 30-fold increase in the number of eosinophils during exacerbation with a smaller but still significant increase in the number of neutrophils, T lymphocytes, and VLA-1–positive and TNFα-positive cells. No attempt was made to determine if infection was responsible for the exacerbations, and it is difficult to assess if these findings are relevant to the exacerbations seen in patients with more severe COPD (48). It does, however, point the way to the type of study that will be required to come to grips with this problem of understanding the pathozenesis of these accute episodes.

Population-based studies suggest that persons with chronic lung disease experience more acute lower respiratory symptoms than healthy controls and that these symptoms are associated with serological responses to influenza type A and B, RSV, parainfluenza 1, 2, and 3, and coronaviruses (57). Other studies (58) suggest that rhinovirus might be added to this list, but most of the misery produced by this group of viruses may be limited to the upper respiratory tract. Acute viral infections of the upper airways predispose to aspiration, which exposes the lower airways to infection by bacteria. The increased risk of aspiration of a mucoid exudate loaded with bacteria from the upper airways during an infection of the upper airways accounts for the introduction of organisms such as *Streptococcus pneumoniae Staphylococcus aureus*, and *Haemophilus influenzae* into the lower respiratory tract.

The positive effects of antibiotic treatment on some acute exacerbations of COPD reflects the fact that a proportion of these events are precipitated by bacterial infection (59) and the response of some exacerbations to steroids could reflect their influence on the inflammatory and immunopathological response to the viruses (60).

VI. Summary

The precise mechanisms responsible for the excess inflammation and accelerated decline in lung function experienced by the susceptible smoker remain to be determined. However, the data suggest that the inflammatory process must be amplified in this susceptible minority of smokers to produce chronic bronchitis, fixed airways obstruction, and emphysematous lung destruction.

The cigarette smoke–induced inflammatory process that underlies the pathogenesis of the disease in the large airways is based in the mucosa, gland ducts, and glands of intermediate-sized bronchi, where it produces an exudate of plasma, inflammatory cells, and mucus in the airway lumen. Attempts to clear this exudate by cough and expectoration result in the symptoms of chronic bronchitis. Fixed airways obstruction is caused by inflammation of the smaller bronchi and bronchioles less than 2 mm in internal diameter. This inflammatory process thickens the wall, narrows the lumen, and destroys the parenchymal support of these small airways.

As the resistance of the peripheral airways is normally low, the effects of the inflammatory process must reach an advanced stage before total airway resistance is increased. Emphysematous destruction of the lung surface has been attributed to a functional imbalance between the proteolytic enzymes and their inhibitors in the cigarette smoke–induced inflammatory exudate involving gas exchanging surface of the lung, but the precise identification of both enzyme and inhibitor is a subject of continued investigation.

This combination of airway and parenchymal disease slows the rate of emptying of the lung, which causes intrathoracic pressure to rise during expiration first during exercise and then at rest. The rise in intrathoracic pressure increases both arterial and venous pressures without changing vascular resistance. When lung emptying becomes further compromised and alveolar pressures rise above intrathoracic pressure during exercise, there is a shift in lung blood flow from Zone III to Zone II conditions and an increase in vascular resistance. The relatively minor changes in pulmonary vascular hemodynamics that occur in mild COPD result in changes in the intima and adventitia of the small pulmonary blood vessels. Progression of the disease further compromises the pulmonary vessels resulting in muscular hypertrophy, reorganization of the extracellular matrix, a thickening of the vessel wall, and a narrowing of its lumen. These changes permanently elevate vascular resistance, which is further increased by the effect of hypoxia on the pulmonary vascular smooth muscle. The progressive destruction of the lung by emphysema reduces the capillary bed and further increases the pressure required to perfuse the pulmonary circulation. This cascade of events leads to right heart failure and systemic venous stasis, which precipitates venous thrombosis and pulmonary embolism to further compromise the pulmonary circulation.

The natural history of COPD is complicated by acute exacerbations that often require hospital admission and treatment with antibiotics, bronchodilators, oxygen, assisted ventilation, and systemic steroids. These exacerbations are precipitated both by the effects of the underlying disease and by a predisposition to infection with a wide range of viruses and bacteria that target lung tissue. Although it is difficult to separate the pathology of these acute events from that of the underlying disease, studies attempting to demonstrate these acute changes are beginning to appear.

References

1. Niewoehner DE, Kleinerman J, Reisst DB. Pathologic changes in the peripheral airways of young cigarette smokers. N Engl J Med 1974; 291:755–758.

2. Mullen JBM, Wright JL, Wiggs B, Pare PD, Hogg JC. Reassessment of inflammation in the airways of chronic bronchitis. Br Med J 1985; 291:1235–1239.

3. Hogg JC, Macklem PT, Thurlbeck WM. Site and nature of airways obstruction in chronic obstructive lung disease. N Engl J Med 1968; 278:1355–1360.

4. Cosio M, Ghezzo M, Hogg JC, et al. The relation between structural changes in small airways and pulmonary function tests. N Engl J Med 1978; 298:1277–1281.

5. Janoff A. Biochemical links between cigarette smoking and pulmonary emphysema. J Appl Physiol 1983; 55:285–293.

6. Wright JL, Lawson L, Pare PD, Hooper RO, Peretz DI, Nelems JM, Schultzer M, Hogg JC. The structure and function of the pulmonary vasculature in mild chronic obstructive pulmonary disease. Am Rev Respir Dis 1983; 128:702–707.

7. Barbera JA, Riverola A, Roca J, Ramirez J, Wagner PD, Ros D, Wiggs BR, Rodriguez-Roisin R. Pulmonary vascular abnormalities and ventilation-perfusion relationships in mild chronic obstructive pulmonary disease. Am J Respir Crit Care Med 1994; 149:423–429.

8. Peinado VI, Barbera JA, Abate P, Ramirez J, Roca J, Santos S, Rodriguez-Roisin R. Inflammatory reaction in pulmonary muscular arteries of patients with mild chronic obstructive pulmonary disease. Am J Respir Crit Care Med 1999; 159:1605–1611.

9. Pride NB, Burrows B. Development of impaired lung function: natural history and risk factors. In: Calverly P. and Pride N. eds. Chronic Obstructive Lung Disease. London: Chapman and Hall Medicla, 1995; 69–91.

10. Ciba guest symposium report: terminology, definitions and classifications of chronic pulmonary emphysema and related conditions. Thorax 1959; 14: 286–299.

11. Reid L. Measurement of the bronchial mucous gland layer: a diagnostic yardstick in chronic bronchitis. Thorax 1960; 15:132–141.

12. Ryder RC, Dunnill MS, Anderson JA. A quantitative study of the bronchial mucus gland volume, emphysema and smoking in a necropsy population. J Pathol 1971; 104:59–71.

13. Thurlbeck WM, Angus GE. The distribution curve for chronic bronchitis. Thorax 1964; 19:436–442.

14. Lamb D, Reid L. Mitotic rates, goblet cell increase and histochemical changes in mucus in rat bronchial epithelium during exposure to sulphur dioxide. J Path Bacteriol 1968; 96:97–111.

15. Lamb D, Reid L. Goblet cell increase in rat bronchial epithelium after exposure to cigarette and cigar tobacco smoke. Br Med J 1969; 1:33–35.

16. O'Shaughnessy TC, Ansari TW, Barnes NC, Jeffery PK. Inflammation in bronchial biopsies of subjects with chronic bronchitis: inverse relationship of CD-8+ T lymphocytes with FEV1. Am J Respir Crit Care Med 1997; 155:382–387.

17. Saetta M, Di Stefano A, Maestrelli P, et al. Activated T-lymphocytes and macrophages in bronchial mucosa of subjects with chronic bronchitis. Am Rev Respir Dis 1993; 147:301–306.

18. Elliott WM, Hayashi S, Hogg JC. Immunodetection of adenoviral E1A proteins in human lung tissue. Am J Respir Cell Mol Biol 1995; 12:642–648.

19. Dunnill MS, Massarella GR, Anderson JA. A comparision of the quantitative anatomy of the bronchi in normal subjects in status asthmaticus, in chronic bronchitis, and in emphysema. Thorax 1969; 24:176–179.

20. Thurlbeck WM, Pun R, Toth J, Fraser RG. Bronchial cartilage in chronic obstructive lung disease. Am Rev Respir Dis 1974; 109:73–80.

21. Haraguichi M, Shemura S, Shirata K. Morphologic analysis of bronchial cartilage in chronic obstructive pulmonary disease and bronchial asthma. Am J Respir Crit Care Med 1999; 159:1005–1013.

22. van Braband T, Cauberghs M, Verbeken E, Moerman P, Lauweryns JM, van de Woestijne KP. J Appl Physiol Respir Environ Exercise Physiol 1983; 55:1733–1742.

23. Weibel ER. Morphometry of the Human Lung. New York: Academic Press, 1963.

24. Macklem PT, Mead J. Resistance of central and peripheral airways measured by the retrograde catheter. J Appl Physiol 1967; 22:395–401.

25. Dayman H. Mechanics of airflow in health and emphysema. J Clin Invest 1951; 3031:1175–1190.

26. Butler J, Caro C, Alkaler R, Dubois AB. Physiological factors affecting airway resistance in normal subjects and in patients with obstructive airways disease. J Clin Invest 1960; 39:584–591.

27. Matsuba K, Thurlbeck WM. The number and dimensions of small airways in emphysematous lungs. Am J Pathol 1972; 67:265–275.

28. Miller WS. The Lung. 3rd ed. 1943, Charles C Thomas, Springfield, IL: pp 191–193.

29. Gough J. Discussion on the diagnosis of pulmonary emphysema. Proc Royal Soc Med 1952; 45:576–577.

30. McLean KH. Macroscopic anatomy of pulmonary emphysema. Aust Ann Med 1956; 5:73–88.

31. Leopold JG, Gough J. The centrilobular form of hypertrophic emphysema and its relation to chronic bronchitis. Thorax 1957; 12:219–235.

32. Dunnill MS. Emphysema. Pulmonary Pathology. Churchill-Livingstone Edinburgh 1982:81–112.

33. Heard BE. Further observations on the pathology of pulmonary emphysema in chronic bronchitis. Thorax 1959; 14:58–70.

34. Snider GL, Brody JS, Doctor L. Subclinical pulmonary emphysema. Incidence and anatomic patterns. Am Rev Respir Dis 1962; 85:66–83.

35. Thurlbeck WM. The incidence of pulmonary emphysema with observations on the relative incidence and spatial distribution of various types of emphysema. Am Rev Respir Dis 1963; 87:206–215.

36. Heppleston AG, Leopold JG. Chronic pulmonary emphysema: anatomy and pathogenesis. Am J Med 1953; 31:279–291.
37. Heppleston AG, Leopold JG. The pathologic anatomy of simple pneumoconiosis in coal workers. J Pathol Bacteriol 1953; 66:235–246.
38. Wyatt JP. Macrosection and injection studies of emphysema. Am Rev Respir Dis 1959; 80:94–103.
39. Thurlbeck WM. Chronic Airflow Obstruction in Lung Disease. Philadelphia: WB Saunders, 1976.
40. Wyatt JP, Fischer VW, Sweet HC. Panlobular emphysema: anatomy and pathodynamics. Dis Chest 1962; 41:239–259.
41. Laurell CB, Eriksson S. The electrophoretic alpha, globulin pattern of serum in alpha$_1$ antitrypsin deficiency. Scand J Clin Lab Invest 1963; 15:132–140.
42. Schleusener A, Talamo RC, Pare JAP, Thurlbeck WM. Familial emphysema. Am Rev Respir Dis 1968; 98:692–696.
43. Martelli NA, Goldman E, Roncoroni AJ. Lower zone emphysema in young patients without alpha-1 antitrypsin deficiency. Thorax 1974; 29:237–244.
44. Hale KA, Niewoehner DE, Cosio MG. Morphologic changes in the muscular pulmonary arteries: relationship to cigarette smoking, airway disease and emphysema. Am Rev Respir Dis 1980; 122:273–278.
45. Heath D, Edwards JE. The pathology of hypertensive pulmonary vascular disease. Circulation 1958; 18:533–547.
46. Hicken P, Brewer D, Heath D. The relation between the weight of the right ventricle of the heart and the internal surface area and number of alveoli in the human lung in emphysema. J Path Bacteriol 1966; 92:529–546.
47. Hicken P, Brewer D, Heath D. The relation between the weight of the right ventricle and the percentage of abnormal air space in the lung in emphysema. J Pathol Bacteriol 1966; 92:519–528.
48. Connors AF Jr., Dawson NV, Thomas C, Harrell FE Jr., Desbiens N Fulkerson WJ, Kussin P, Bellamy P, Goldman L, Knaus WA. Ostructive lung disease. Am J Respir Crit Care Med 1996; 154:959–967.
49. Hers JF. Disturbances of the ciliated epithelium due to influenza virus. Am Rev Respir Dis 1966; 93:162–172.
50. Hers JF, Masurel N, Mulder J. Bacteriology and histopathology of the respiratory tract and lungs in fatal Asian influenza. Lancet 1958; II: 1141–1143.
51. Hers JF, Mulder J. Broad aspects of the pathology and pathogenesis of human influenza. Am Rev Respir Dis 1961; 83(suppl): 64–67, 84–97.
52. Martin CM, Cunin CM, Gottlieb LS, Barnes MW, Liu C, Finland M. Asian influenza A in Boston, 1957–1958. Arch Intern Med 1959; 103:516–531.
53. Walsh JJ, Dietlein LF, Low FN, Burch GE, Mogabgab WJ. Bronchotracheal response in human influenza. Arch Intern Med 1961; 108:376–388.
54. Vitalis TZ, Keicho N, Itabashi S, Hayashi S, Hogg JC. A model of latent adenovirus 5 infection in the guinea pig (*Cavia procellus*). Am J Respir Cell Mol Biol 1996; 14:225–231.

55. Saetta M, Di Stefano A, Maestrelli P, Turato G, Ruggieri MP, Roggeri A, Calcagni P, Mapp CE, Ciaccia A, Labbri LM. Airway eosinophilia in chronic bronchitis during exacerbations.

56. Monto AS, Higgins MW, Ross HW. The Tecumseh study of respiratory illness. VIII. Acute infection in chronic respiratory disease and comparison groups. Am Rev Respir Dis 1975; 111:27–36.

57. Wiselka MJ, Kent J, Cookson JB, Nicholson KG. Impact of respiratory virus infection in patients with chronic chest disease. Epidemiol Infec 1993; 111:337–346.

58. Smith CB, Golden CA, Kanner RE, Renzetta AD. Association of viral and myocplasmal pneumonia infections with acute respiratory illness in patients with chronic obstructive pulmonary disease. Am Rev Respir Dis 1980; 121: 225–232.

59. Anthonisen NR, Manfreda J, Warren CP, Hershfield ES, Harding GK, Nelson NA. Antibiotic therapy in exacerbations of COPD. Ann Interin Med 1987; 106:196–204.

60. Niewoehner DE, Erbland ML, Deupree RH, Collins D, Gross NJ, Light RW, Anderson P, Morgan NA. Effect of systemic glucocorticoids on exacerbations of chronic obstructive pulmonary disease.

8

Inflammatory Mechanisms

R. A. STOCKLEY

Queen Elizabeth Medical Center
Edgbaston, Birmingham, England

I. Introduction

Inflammation is a complex process involving cellular, protein, and biochemical mediators. Side effects include tissue damage, which in the lung can lead to many of the clinical and pathological features of patients with chronic obstruction pulmonary disease (COPD). In recent years there has been an increase in the literature on inflammation in COPD, although at present this is somewhat confusing as research tries to bridge the gap between basic mechanisms and clinical observation. Part of the problem relates to the use of the term COPD itself, which is a group of conditions defined on the basis of predominantly fixed airflow limitation. This airflow limitation may relate to problems in the large airways, occlusion of small airways, and dynamic airways collapse as a result of loss of connective tissue (often a feature of emphysema). There is now extensive literature involving studies of tissue biopsies of the large and small airways, bronchial and bronchoalveolar lavage, sputum and sputum induction.

Generally all of these approaches indicate that inflammation is a feature of the lung in patients with COPD. This includes an increase in the number of lymphocytes in the tissues (1), and an increase in mast cells, neutrophils, and sometimes eosinophils in the airway (2). However, the role of these cells remains somewhat confusing since their numbers, activation, and pathogenic role will depend on the site being sampled, the presence of disease, current smoking or pollution exposure, treatment, bacterial colonization, and the presence or absence of exacerbations. This chapter breaks down the mechanisms by considering two regions of the lung: first, the alveolar region and peripheral airways with respect to the development of emphysema, and second, the larger airways with relevance to bronchial disease. In reality, this separation may be only anatomical since patients often have pathological changes throughout the lung and it is possible that the same inflammatory processes produce different pathological changes depending on the site at which they take place. Nevertheless, until further work leads to clarification of this issue, it remains most appropriate to consider the pathological processes that lead to emphysema and those that lead to bronchial disease separately.

II. Emphysema

Emphysema is defined pathologically and it is generally accepted that the destruction of lung connective tissue, and in particular lung elastin, is central to its development. Animal models have demonstrated that instillation of enzymes only with the ability to destroy elastin are capable of producing emphysematous changes in the lungs. In addition, factors that influence elastin turnover and repair (3,4) have also been shown to amplify the pathological changes that develop.

So far three enzymes that are likely to be relevant in humans have been demonstrated to produce emphysema in experimental animals. These include the neutrophil serine proteinases, neutrophil elastase (5) and proteinase 3 (6), and the cysteine proteinase cathepsin B (7). Most data have been centered on the role of neutrophil elastase largely for historical reasons, and the importance of the other two enzymes remains to be determined. Neutrophil elastase is preformed during neutrophil maturation in the bone marrow and is released on activation of the mature cell as the azurophil granules undergo exocytosis and the enzyme diffuses outwards. In addition, some enzyme becomes associated with the cell membrane, where it retains its enzymatic activity (8).

Neutrophil elastase has been identified in the interstitium of pathological specimens obtained from patients with emphysema. Studies have shown that the amount of emphysema relates directly to the amount of neutrophil elastase present, suggesting an effect and cause (9). It should be noted that although neutrophil elastase is classically associated with a neutrophil, it is also present in some monocytes (10). Studies have indicated that a subset of these cells that respond to chemoattractants and are therefore likely to migrate into the tissues are also a source of the enzyme (10). Activation of this subpopulation of monocytes results in the complete release of elastase, which may be critical in cell migration (see later).

Neutrophils and macrophages are increased in number in the lungs of cigarette smokers. In addition, pathological studies have indicated that the number of neutrophils relates to the degree of emphysema (see Chap. 7). Furthermore, studies in smokers who have developed subclinical emphysema show an increase in elastase in bronchoalveolar lavage fluid compared to nonsmokers or smokers who have not developed emphysema (11). The elastase was inactive, being present in inhibitory complex with α_1-antitrypsin, but reflects the amount that had been released. The fact that the elastase was inactive does not negate a role in the development of emphysema since the important and critical processes take place in the lung interstitium where the connective tissue is present and not in the airway where the enzyme is harvested.

A. The Interstitium

Lung connective tissue forms a tight matrix, which includes fibrillary elastin. Animal models have shown that elastase leads to destruction of lung elastin, which subsequently reaccumulates but is associated with the development of emphysematous change (12). Thus, destruction of the fibrillary form of the elastin in the interstitium by free elastase activity is likely to be central to the development of emphysema in humans.

A migrating neutrophil has to traverse the interstitial space between the endothelial cell layer of the blood vessel to the epithelial layer of the airway. In order to penetrate the tight matrix the neutrophil has to "punch" a hole, and studies have shown that elastase is important in connective tissue degradation when neutrophils are activated by a chemoattractant (13). Indeed, studies with the connective tissue fibronectin have shown that when neutrophils adhere tightly to the substrate, it is digested by neutrophil elastase even in the presence of supernormal concentrations of effective proteinase inhibitors such as α_1-antitrypsin (14). This indicates that in close cell substrate contact, there is an area of obligate proteolysis that relates to the concentration of elastase being released. Studies have indicated that the amount of elastase in the azurophil granule would result in a concentration in the immediate vicinity of a released granule being some 2 orders of magnitude above the physiological concentration of the naturally occurring inhibitors. Thus, it would not be possible to prevent an activated neutrophil from destroying connective tissue with which it is in close contact. Indeed, the degree of damage is even worse when the inhibitor concentration is low as in α_1-antitrypsin deficiency. Studies have indicated that such subjects have critically low levels, resulting in a greatly amplified degree of tissue destruction (see Chap. 19). However, the ability of neutrophils to digest connective tissue is also increased when the proteinase inhibitor has a reduced association rate constant for elastase. Studies with α_1-antitrypsin of the PIZ phenotype have indicated that it is also less effective at controlling this process than α_1-antitrypsin of the PIM phenotype (15). This influence of association rate constant may also be important in determining the degree of damage, since α_1-antitrypsin recovered from the lungs of smokers has shown a similar reduction in association rate constant (16).

Alpha$_1$-antitrypsin undoubtedly protects the tissues from destruction, as does the other major inhibitor in the lung, secretory leukoproteinase inhibitor. Thus, these two inhibitors will serve to minimize the degree of tissue destruction that occurs. However as indicated above, it is not possible to control this completely. Therefore destruction of lung elastin is likely (in most patients) to reflect the degree of neutrophil traffic, and the more cells that migrate and the more activated they are, the greater the degree of destruction and the more emphysematous change that will develop. This process will be amplified in subjects with α_1-antitrypsin deficiency even without a change in the nature or number of migrating neutrophils (Fig. 1).

B. Mechanisms of Cell Migration

As indicated above, migration of inflammatory cells through connective tissue by necessity initiates some damage. Early studies have indicated that the number of cells harvested by bronchoalveolar lavage is increased in smokers (17). In addition, patients with early emphysema also have an increase in inflammatory cells, particularly neutrophils in the peripheral airways (11). However, the mechanisms involved in cell recruitment are only partly understood. Cigarette smoke is a major etiological factor in the development of emphysema, and studies have shown that cigarette smoke is capable of stimulating epithelial cells to produce the chemokine interleukin (IL)-8 (18). This protein is a major neutrophil chemoattractant and may thus be central to the recruitment of neutrophils into the peripheral airways. Mechanisms by which cigarette smoke initiates this change are largely unknown, although recent studies have indicated that oxidants can also activate epithelial cells to release IL-8 (19), and cigarette smoke is known to be a major source of oxidants. However IL-8 is also released by macrophages, and these cells are present in large numbers in the peripheral airways of patients who smoke (20).

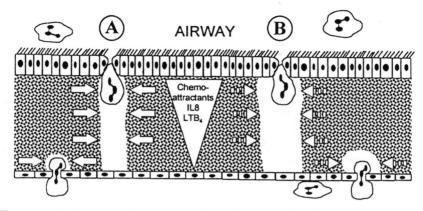

Figure 1 Diagrammatic representation of connective tissue destruction by migrating neutrophils. (A) A neutrophil migrates through the interstitium of a subject with normal proteinase inhibitors in response to airway chemoattractants. The area of surrounding tissue degradation is tightly restricted by the antiproteinases. (B) A similar migrating neutrophil in the presence of subjects with a deficiency of proteinase inhibitors such as α_1-antitrypsin leads to a much greater area of connective tissue destruction.

The role of IL-8 in the pathogenesis of emphysema has received little attention. However, McCrae and colleagues (21) measured IL-8 in lavage samples obtained from healthy smokers and nonsmokers. In general, they found that the IL-8 levels were not increased except in a small subgroup of healthy smokers. They demonstrated that these samples also had increased neutrophil chemotactic activity and hypothesized that this could be the susceptible population of smokers who eventually develop severe airflow obstruction. Clearly these findings would be consistent with our understanding of the cellular basis of the development of emphysema, and over many years increased neutrophil recruitment in response to IL-8 in this small subgroup would lead to excessive damage to interstitial elastin and potentially the progressive development of emphysema.

At present there is little information to determine why a small subgroup should have an excessive IL-8 response to smoking, either directly or indirectly. However, recent work by Hogg and colleagues has suggested that latent viral infections may play a role (22), and epithelial cells transfected by adenovirus do show increased cytokine response (23). Nevertheless, several other factors known to be present in the lung, including tumor necrosis factor (TNF) α, IL-1 β, bacterial endotoxin, and steroid therapy, may all have an effect on IL-8 production by epithelial cells.

Finally, recent data by Tanino and colleagues (24) have shown that IL-8 concentrations are increased in lung lavage fluids from patients with subclinical emphysema, suggesting that it may be an early feature of disease leading to neutrophil accumulation and tissue destruction resulting in the emphysema. Clearly regulation of this major neutrophil chemoattractant is worthy of further study and may provide further insight into the pathogenesis of airflow obstruction that develops in only a subpopulation of subjects.

The role of other chemoattractants is even less clear. Leukotriene B_4 (LTB4) is a potent neutrophil chemoattractant found in the lung. Studies in patients with α_1-antitrypsin deficiency have implicated LTB4 as being the major mediator of the excessive neutrophil recruitment seen in these subjects (25). Lavage studies indicated not only that the LTB4 concentrations were increased in α_1-antitrypsin deficient subjects, but also that the macrophage was likely to be the source perhaps stimulated by neutrophil elastase (see Chap. 19). Whether LTB4 plays a role in neutrophil recruitment to the peripheral airways of non-α_1-antitrypsin–deficient subjects remains uncertain, although it may play an important role in the major airways (see later).

Other chemotactic factors may be of importance in determining neutrophil influx at the alveolar level. For instance, nicotine itself is a chemoattractant (26), and studies have shown that α_1-antitrypsin elastase complexes can also recruit neutrophils (27), and damage to α_1-antitrypsin by oxidants can also change this protein into a chemoattractant (28). Finally, there may be other chemoattractants present including GROα and MIP1α, although in general the role of these additional factors has yet to be explored in detail (29).

C. Increased Cellular Response

A further mechanism that would result in increased neutrophil recruitment to the airways of susceptible smokers would be an enhanced cellular response. For instance, β-endorphin has been shown to prime neutrophils, resulting in an increase in a subsequent chemotactic response (30). Indeed, studies have shown that neutrophils from patients who have established emphysema do show an increased chemotactic response, and this probably relates to an overexpression of chemoattractant receptors (31). In addition, the destructive potential of the cells can vary from subject to subject, and data have shown that neutrophils from patients with established emphysema have an increased capacity to digest connective tissue (32). Whether this indicates a small degree of initial activation by a factor or factors unknown is currently uncertain, but stimulation of these cells leads to a further increase in their capacity to digest connective tissue, and this remains higher than for neutrophils from controlled matched subjects (32). The implication of these findings, therefore, is that even if the chemoattractants being released in the lungs of smokers is normal, the peripheral neutrophils of those who have emphysema are both recruited in greater numbers and cause a greater degree of connective tissue destruction as they are recruited compared to smoking subjects who do not have emphysema. Again, further studies of the exact mechanisms involved are indicated.

D. Adhesion Molecules

Adhesion molecules on neutrophils and their counterreceptors on epithelial cells are necessary for cell adherence and migration. Studies of these receptors and their function in COPD have been few and far between. Immunohistology has shown that E selectin is upregulated on vascular endothelium in patients with chronic obstructive bronchitis (33). Noguera and colleagues have shown increased expression of CD11/CD18 on neutrophils in stable COPD but lower concentrations of the soluble component of its endothelial counter receptor ICAM1 (34). The exact implications of these findings have yet to be determined but suggest neutrophil activation/priming as a preliminary step to increased adhesion and migration. The reduced soluble ICAM1 was thought to reflect endothelial dysfunction, which may impair the process.

Although most studies have concentrated on the role of the neutrophil in emphysema, it is well known that macrophage numbers are also increased in smokers. The source of these macrophages is unknown, but in general it is believed that most are derived from circulating monocytes. Studies have shown that these circulating cells are a heterogeneous population, and a small proportion of the cells show an ability to respond to chemotactic agents (10). This subgroup is phenotypically distinct and contains neutrophil elastase. As the cells are activated and adhere, they release the elastase, and this may play a role in their migration from the circulation to the airways. Whether this population of cells is different in smokers who develop emphysema is unknown.

E. Role of Other Enzymes

For historical reasons, and indeed observational ones, neutrophil elastase has long been considered the major mediator of tissue destruction leading to emphysema. However in animal studies, proteinase 3 has been shown to produce emphysematous lesions (6), and it could therefore play a role in human disease. The proteinase 3 gene is located close to the neutrophil elastase gene on chromosome 19 (35). These two enzymes are co-expressed during cell differentiation and packaged into the same azurophil granule. Both enzymes would be released simultaneously, and arguments that apply to neutrophil elastase and the role of cell migration could be directly applicable to proteinase 3.

The only other enzyme that has been shown directly to produce emphysematous lesions in animal models is cathepsin B (7). This cysteine proteinase is produced by alveolar macrophages and is also present in epithelial cells. Control and activity of this enzyme in the lung is largely unknown, but in secretions in the absence of inflammation, cathepsin B seems to be present largely as a pro-enzyme. In the present of inflammation, the enzyme becomes active, and it is believed that one mechanism leading to this activation is cleavage of the pro-enzyme by neutrophil elastase (36). Thus if cathepsin B plays a key role in the development of emphysema in humans, it may be indirectly by activation of the pro-enzyme following release of neutrophil elastase. Again, further studies are required to determine the role of this enzyme, its source, and the role of inflammation.

More recently, studies using gene knockout and gene transfection technologies have suggested that a further elastase from the macrophage (37) or even enzymes with collagenolytic activity (38) may play a role in emphysema development. If so, the inflammatory cells expressing these enzymes and their recruitment and activation will be of importance in understanding the pathogenic processes involved.

At present there is little evidence to support the role of these other enzymes in humans. Lavage samples have shown that collagenolytic enzymes are present in bronchoalveolar lavage samples from patients with emphysema (39), raising the options of cause or effect. These studies, however, have shown no difference between current or ex-smokers with emphysema. Since epidemiological studies have indicated that smoking cessation leads to a significant reduction in the physiological progression of the disease, the studies with collagenase would indicate that it is an effect of emphysema rather than a direct cause, since its activity should be lower in ex-smokers. Of importance in this argument, it should be noted that in the same studies neutrophil elastase in the lavage samples was decreased in emphysematous patients who had ceased to smoke, providing more evidence for the role this enzyme in development of disease.

However, recent studies have investigated the role of matrix metallo-proteinase 9 (MMP9) and the tissue inhibitor or metalloproteinase 1 (TIMP1), which also inhibits MMP9. This enzyme is predominantly produced by macrophages and has the ability in vitro to digest lung matrix proteins, including elastin. Alveolar macrophages are found in increased numbers in the peripheral airways of smokers and patients with emphysema. Betsuyaku and colleagues found increased amounts of MMP in the lungs of patients with subclinical emphysema (40), although macrophages were not thought to be the source.

On the other hand, studies in healthy smokers showed no increase in MMP9 in lavage but indicated that the macrophages harvested at the same time produced more of the enzyme (41). This effect is even greater in macrophages from COPD patients (42), although the concentration of MMP in lavage from these patients and whether they had emphysema was not documented. Clearly further studies are indicated to determine whether this in vitro observation has implications for the pathogenesis of emphysema.

III. Bronchial Disease

Bronchial disease is also a feature of patients with COPD. This area of the lung is much more accessible to study, and assessment expectorated sputum or induced sputum can give a guide to inflammation within the large airways. For these reasons there has been a rapidly increasing literature confirming the presence of inflammatory cells and inflammatory mediators. Keatings et al. have demonstrated an increase in the proportion of neutrophils in healthy smokers, but a greater increase in subjects who had COPD (43). In addition, this increase in COPD was related to the severity of airflow obstruction. These observations were compatible with neutrophil recruitment in response to IL-8 since a slight increase in concentration was found in the smokers, but a much greater increase in those with COPD. Finally, the authors also assessed TNFα and found a major increase of this pro-inflammatory cytokine in COPD. The study suggested a major role for the neutropil in the airway, but in particular a greater effect in smokers who had airflow obstruction compared to those who did not, suggesting a cause and effect.

The neutrophil, and in particular neutrophil elastase, has been implicated in the pathology of airways disease. Patients with COPD have evidence of epithelial damage with squamous cell metaplasia, and mucous gland hyperplasia is often present with excess mucus production. These factors influence mucociliary clearance, which is reduced in COPD, and finally there is evidence of increased airways leakage with transudation of serum proteins into the airway secretions. All these changes can be induced by neutrophil elastase, both in vitro and in vivo (44), suggesting that this enzyme can also be a key mediator of airways disease. In addition, studies with neutrophil cathepsin G (5) and cathepsin B (45) have shown that both enzymes can also induce bronchial disease. Since cathepsin G is also present in the azurophil granule of the neutrophil together with neutrophil elastase, they will be released simultaneously and their effects will depend upon neutrophil recruitment, as has been argued earlier. For cathepsin B to have an effect it would need to be activated by neutrophil elastase (see above), and thus even if this enzyme is an important mediator of bronchial disease, neutrophilic infiltration may be central to the process.

Bronchial biopsies from patients with COPD have in some instances been supportive of this general concept, whereas in others the data seem to contradict a central role for the neutrophil. For instance, in the study by Turato et al. macrophage numbers were increased in subjects with chronic bronchitis, as was the expression of the adhesion molecules E selectin and ICAM 1 (46). In this study there was no obvious difference between current or ex-smokers and the neutrophils were not increased in subjects who had bronchitis compared to healthy controls. Di Stefano and colleagues (47) found increased number of T lymphocytes in subjects with bronchitis and airflow limitation and an inverse correlation between the number of lymphocytes and FEV_1. In addition, the number of macrophages was also increased in subjects with chronic bronchitis and airflow obstruction, whereas the number of neutrophils was not influenced by the FEV_1. On the other hand, a study by Saetta and colleagues in 1997 found that smokers with symptoms of chronic bronchitis had increased numbers of neutrophils as well as macrophages in the bronchial glands compared to asymptomatic smokers (48). In addition, subjects also had increased numbers of neutrophils in the epithelium.

Studies of bronchial secretions, either spontaneous sputum or induced sputum, have been somewhat more consistent (43,49,50). In general, all such studies shown an increase in the number of neutrophils in the airways in COPD, which suggests that compartmentalization is an important phenomenon in the interpretation of biopsy specimens. The neutrophil is a short-lived cell that migrates rapidly from the circulation into the airway. The time spent in the interstitium would be short, and hence identification of these cells in biopsies would be difficult even in the presence of a continuous stream of migrating cells. On the other hand, lymphocytic cells and macrophages are much longer lived and are much more likely to be found in the interstitial spaces.

Recruitment of neutrophils in bronchial disease has largely been attributed to the local production of IL-8. Clearly this is consistent with the function of IL-8, and in some studies IL-8 has been said to be the only chemoattractant of importance (51). Undoubtedly IL-8 has been shown to relate to the number of neutrophils in the secretion either directly (52) or indirectly by assessing the neutrophil product myeloperoxidase (53). Such correlations have been used to support the role of IL-8 in neutrophil recruitment, but it should be noted that the neutrophil itself is a source of

IL-8 and such correlations may in part be measuring only the neutrophils and their activation.

TNFα can initiate IL-8 production by epithelial cells, and studies in COPD have indicated that TNFα concentration is increased in the airways (43). In addition, bacterial products such as endotoxin can also stimulate epithelial cells to release a variety of pro-inflammatory cytokines including TNFα, IL-6, and IL-8 (54). Thus, there is good in vitro evidence to indicate mechanisms whereby IL-8 may drive neutrophil recruitment. However, once in the airway, activation of the neutrophils can lead to further release of IL-8 (55) as well as leukotriene B$_4$ (56). Both of these chemoattractants released from the neutrophils may amplify the inflammatory process leading to further neutrophil recruitment. Indeed, studies of airway secretions have indicated that a significant proportion of the chemotactic activity is due to LTB4 as well as IL-8 (57), and in COPD LTB4 may be more important especially in α_1-antitrypsin deficiency (58). It should be noted that even these two chemoattractants do not account for all the chemotactic activity of the secretions, suggesting that other chemoattractants are present. The role that each of these plays in the neutrophilic influx into the airways will require specific intervention studies.

IV. Factors That Influence Airways Inflammation

Interpreting data related to airways inflammation in patients with COPD depends on careful considerations of all the factors that may influence the process. Clearly of major importance is the definition of COPD and the physiological and radiological abnormalities that are associated with this generic diagnosis. Furthermore, it is of importance to note that bronchial disease may be anatomically distinct from alveolar disease, and thus inflammation at one site may not be characteristic of inflammation at the other. In addition, there may be many local factors that influence the degree of inflammation as well as its nature.

A. Smoking

Smoking is a major factor in the pathogenesis of COPD, and many patients have ceased to smoke because of their disease. In the early study of Keatings et al., smoking itself induced a degree of airways inflammation, whereas in COPD it was much greater (43). Biopsy reports have not shown much difference between smokers and ex-smokers, but this does not seem to be consistent with the beneficial effect of smoking cessation on disease progression. It is possible that secretion sampling from the airway does not reflect the pathological processes that lead to the reduction in FEV$_1$.

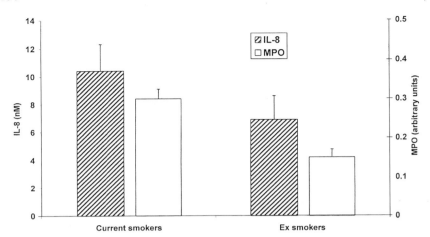

Figure 2 The mean sputum IL-8 concentration is shown for current ($n = 22$) and ex-smokers ($n = 20$) with COPD. In addition, the myeloperoxidase concentration in the samples is also shown in arbitrary units (open histograms).

It is equally possible that the differences between smokers and ex-smokers may be subtle, making it difficult to separate the physiological from the pathological response. Recent data from our own group have shown that ex-smokers matched for treatment and airflow obstruction have slight but significant differences in the concentrations on IL-8 and myeloperoxidase in the airway secretions compared to current smokers (see Fig. 2). Such an observation would be consistent with the inflammatory effect of cigarette smoke and a role of neutrophils recruited to the airway.

B. Chemoattractants

As intimated above, the majority of studies have considered IL-8 to have a major role in neutrophil recruitment in the airways. Indeed, strong correlations between IL-8 and neutrophils or myeloperoxidase (53) would support such a concept. However, in studying a wide range of airways inflammation, it is clear that the relationship between IL-8 and neutrophil recruitment is not a simple linear one (see Fig. 3). The data suggest that there may be a threshold between the IL-8 concentration and the degree of neutrophilic influx, thus influencing the severity of inflammation. A similar threshold does not seem to occur between LTB4 and myeloperoxidase (57), which suggests that this might be an early chemoattractant and IL-8 a late chemoattractant causing additional cell recruitment.

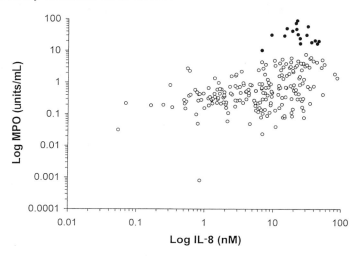

Figure 3 Graph showing the relationship between IL-8 and the concentration of myeloperoxidase for samples of patients with varying degrees of bronchial inflammation. Note that the relationship appears curvilinear, suggesting a threshold above which excess neutrophil accumulation occurs in response to very little extra change in IL-8.

C. Steroids

Corticosteroids are generally accepted to be anti-inflammatory. Many if not most patients with COPD are currently being treated with inhaled and occasionally oral corticosteroids. Certainly studies in vitro would suggest that steroids might have a beneficial effect on the release of chemoattractants such as IL-8 by airways cells (59). However, there is currently some controversy concerning whether steroids influence airways inflammation in vivo. Some authors have failed to show any effects of inhaled corticosteroids on airway inflammation (60). On the other hand, previous studies using oral steroids have shown clear effects (61), and inhaled studies have shown subtle but significant effects (62). In addition, airway neutrophilia has been shown to be reduced in patients on inhaled steroids (63) and in a long-term study of inhaled corticosteroids in COPD the number of exacerbations has been shown to be influenced by treatment (64). Recently we have shown that the pro-inflammatory response to nebulized hypotonic saline can be abrogated in patients receiving inhaled corticosteroids, but not in those receiving no such therapy (see Fig. 4). Thus, on balance it appears that corticosteroids have a beneficial effect, but it is possible that in some patients other factors such as continued smoking or bacterial colonization (see below) may offset

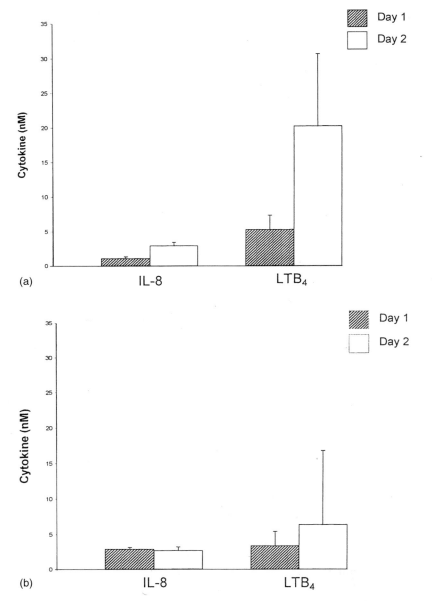

Figure 4 The average concentrations of IL-8 (closed histograms) and LTB4 (open histograms) are shown for patients on the first and second day of sputum induction with nebulized saline. (a) Data for subjects not receiving inhaled corticosteroids on a regular basis. (b) Subjects on continuous treatment with inhaled corticosteroids.

the beneficial effects of corticosteroid therapy. However, these observations have to be reconciled with the failure of several trials to show an influence of inhaled corticosteroids on the decline of lung function (65–67). These studies suggest that either the patients are resistant to corticosteroid therapy, the treatment does not alter the relevant inflammatory process, or (more likely) the inhaled therapy does not reach the critical site (small airways, alveoli, and interstitium) where the disease processes causing airflow obstruction are continuing. Nevertheless, a further study has suggested that inhaled steroids reduce mortality in COPD (68), suggesting that this defined endpoint is related to inflammation. Further carefully designed studies with appropriate end points are necessary to resolve the uncertainty.

D. Bacteria

Approximately 30–40% of patients with COPD and sputum production are colonized by bacteria (69). Studies have shown that bacterial products can potentially influence airways inflammation by the release of pro-inflammatory cytokines from epithelial cells (54). Bacterial colonization may be facilitated by defective mucociliary clearance in COPD, but usually this state is no more symptomatic than in patients who are not colonized. However, recent data indicate that the size of the microbial colonizing load is critical in determining airways inflammation (70). When the bacterial load is small, there seems to be no effect, whereas when the load exceeds 10^6 colony-forming units (CFU)/mL, airways inflammation increases and is associated with further neutrophil recruitment (see Fig. 5). Thus, careful quantitative microbiology is imperative when assessing airways inflammation in COPD. The role of inflammation generated by neutrophils in response to bacterial colonization on lung function decline is worthy of further study. Recent data have indicated that exacerbations of COPD (that are often bacterial) do relate to decline in lung function (71), at least supporting this concept.

E. Alpha$_1$-Antitrypsin Deficiency

Alpha$_1$-antitrypsin has conventionally been thought to be an inhibitor with a key role in the lung interstitium and alveolar region, whereas secretory leukoproteinase inhibitor is thought to be more important in the major airways, protecting them from elastase-induced damage. Recent data from our own group indicate that airways inflammation is increased in patients with α_1-antitrypsin deficiency when matched with nondeficient subjects for smoking history, the degree of airflow obstruction, treatment, and, most importantly, the airway bacterial load (see Fig. 6). These data would suggest that α_1-antitrypsin has a major role in the protection and modulation of airways inflammation (72). These data again suggest a key role for

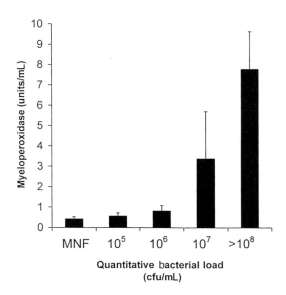

Figure 5 Releationship between sputum myeloperoxidase concentration and bacterial colonizing load. Histograms are the mean and standard error, and the size of the microbial load is indicated on the horizontal axis.

neutrophil elastase, which is avidly inhibited by α_1-antitrypsin, as a mediator of airways inflammation and the pathogenesis of bronchial disease. Augmentation therapy with intravenous α_1-antitrypsin has been shown to reduce the elastase activity and the airway concentration of LTB4 (73), which is the major neutrophil chemoattractant in the airways of these patients (58).

F. Exacerbations

Exacerbations of COPD would be expected to alter airways inflammation. However, exacerbations are poorly defined and dependent on a change in the patient's symptomatology. Thus, an exacerbation may not necessarily reflect a change in airways inflammation. Studies have shown that corticosteroids (74) and antibiotics (75) influence exacerbations in a proportion of the patients, suggesting that inflammation and bacterial infection play a role in some of the episodes. Studies have indicated increased neutrophil recruitment (76), increased oxidant burden (77), and a change in airways inflammation (78) during such episodes. However, the degree of change may reflect the severity of the exacerbation. For instance,

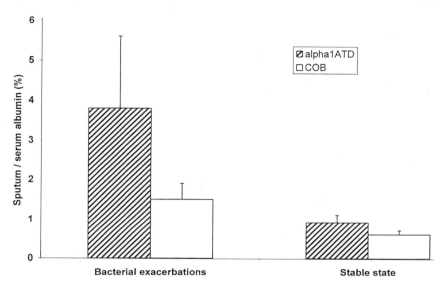

Figure 6 The degree of serum protein transudation is shown as the mean sputum-to-serum albumin ratio $\pm$ SE lines. Data are for patients with α_1-antitrypsin deficiency (hatched histograms) and patients with a similar degree of airflow obstruction but no α_1-antitrypsin deficiency (open histograms). Results are shown for patients presenting with a bacterial exacerbation of their disease as well as in the stable clinical state. (Data derived from Ref. 59.)

patients hospitalized with clear bacterial exacerbations have a much greater inflammatory response than those who are managed as outpatients (see Fig. 7). Furthermore, the number of exacerbations influences lung function decline (see above), suggesting that the associated inflammation plays a role.

The presence of bronchial disease is clearly associated with airways inflammation. Whereas the etiology may be diverse, studies have indicated that the presence of chronic bronchitis is related to progression of COPD (79). Undoubtedly smoking, bacterial colonization, and exacerbations will influence this inflammatory process as well as morbidity and mortality, and further studies are required to determine the pathological changes that influence airflow obstruction and the key mechanisms responsible.

V. Role of the Eosinophil

Classically COPD has been considered to be a neutrophil-dependent condition. However, recent studies have suggested that the eosinophil may

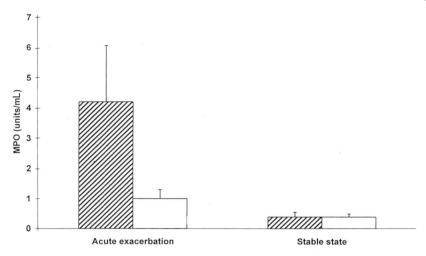

Figure 7 Myeloperoxidase concentration of sputum samples obtained for patients with acute exacerbation of COPD and in a stable clinical state. The hatched histograms indicate patients who were admitted to the hospital with an acute bacterial exacerbation, and the open histograms are results from patients who underwent treatment as outpatients.

also play a role. In support of this is the observation that some patients have increased numbers of eosinophils in induced sputum (80). Furthermore, in exacerbations of COPD eosinophil numbers have been shown to rise. The interpretation of these data is complex. First, COPD is a generic term that may cover a variety of conditions, and there is an overlap with asthma, which is more classically associated with the eosinophil. Thus, the eosinophil data may indicate a subset of patients with COPD who have a different etiology, pathogenic process, and response to treatment. Indeed, recent studies have indicated that the present of sputum eosinophilia is a good indicator of subsequent physiological response to steroid therapy (81). In addition, many patients with COPD have clearly demonstrable reversibility of airflow obstruction, and studies indicate that this is related to sputum eosinophilia (82). Finally, it should be noted that eosinophils (if primed) can migrate in response to IL-8 (83). It is possible that the numbers of eosinophils seen in the airways of some patients with COPD may reflect a secondary response to IL-8 as part of the neutrophilic inflammation rather than a specific eosinophilic response. The increase in eosinophils from exacerbations of COPD (although significant) is the same or somewhat less than the neutrophilic response in the same patients (84). Clearly further studies are necessary to determine whether the eosinophil has a major role in COPD or whether it represents a true distinct subset of patients.

In conclusion inflammation is a constant feature of COPD and is thought to play a crucial role in the pathogenic processes. However, at present the data being collected are being interpreted without careful consideration of the site of the pathology, treatment, microbial colonization, or the patient phenotype. Better definitions of the subgroups and appreciation of the anatomical region being sampled and its relationship to physiological and pathological change is mandatory.

References

1. Saetta M, Baraldo S, Corbino L, Turato G, Braccioni F, Rea F, Cavallesco G, Tropeano G, Mapp CE, Maestrelli P, Ciaccia A, Fabbri LM. CD8 + ve cells in the lungs of smokers with chronic obstructive pulmonary disease. Am J Respir Crit Care Med 1999; 160:711–717.
2. Pesci A, Balbi B, Majori M, Cacciani G, Bertacco S, Alciato P, Donner CF. Inflammatory cells and mediators in bronchial lavage of patients with chronic obstructive pulmonary disease. Eur Respir J 1998; 12:380–386.
3. Kuhn C, Starcher BC. The effect of Lathyrogens on the evolution of elastase induced emphysema. Am Rev Respir Dis 1980; 122:453–460.
4. O'Dell BL, Kilburn KH, Mackenzie WN, Thurston RJ. The lung of the copper deficient rat. Am J Pathol 1978; 91:413–432.
5. Lucey EC, Stone PJ, Breuer R, Christensen PG, Calore JD, Catanese A, Franz-Blau C, Snider GL. Effect of combined human neutrophil cathepsin G and elastase on induction of secretory cell metaplasia and emphysema in hamsters with in vitro observations on elastolysis by these enzymes. Am Rev Respir Dis 1985; 132:362–366.
6. Kao RC, Wehner NG, Skubitz KM, Gray BH, Hoidal JR. Proteinase 3—a distinct human polymorphonuclear leukocyte proteinase that produced emphysema in hamsters. J Clin Invest 1988; 82:1963–1973.
7. Lesser M, Padilla ML, Cordozo C. Induction of emphysema in hamsters by intratracheal installation of cathepsin B. Am Rev Respir Dis 1992; 145:661–668.
8. Owen CA, Campbell MA, Sannes PL, Boukedes SS, Campbell EJ. Cell-surface-bound elastase and cathepsin G in human neutrophils. A novel non-oxidative mechanism by which neutrophils focus and preserve catalytic activity of serine proteinases. J Cell Biol 1995; 131:775–789.
9. Damiano VV, Tsang A, Kucich U, et al. Immunolocalization of elastase in human emphysematous lungs. J Clin Invest 1986; 78:482–493.
10. Owen CA, Campbell MA, Boukedes SS, Stockley RA, Campbell EJ. A discrete subpopulation of human monocytes expresses a neutrophil-like proinflammatory (P) phenotype. Am J Physiol 1994; 267 (6 pt 1):L775–785.

11. Yoshiola A, Betsuyaku T, Nishimura M, Miyamoto K, Kondo T, Kawakami Y. Excessive neutrophil elastase in bronchoalveolar lavage fluid in subclinical emphysema. Am J Respir Crit Care Med 1995; 152:2127–2132.

12. Kuhn C, Slodkowska J, Smith T, Starcher B. The tissue response to exogenous elastase. Bul Europ Physiopath Resp 1980; 16:127–137.

13. Sibille Y, Lwebuga-Mukasa JS, Polomski L, Merrill WW, Ingbar DH, Gee JBL. An in-vitro model for polymorphonuclear-leukocyte-induced injury to extra cellular matrix. Am Rev Respir Dis 1986; 134:134–140.

14. Campbell EJ, Senior RM, McDonald JA, Cox DW. Proteolysis by neutrophils. Relative importance of cell-substrate contact and oxidative inactivation of proteinase inhibitors in vitro. J Clin Invest 1982; 70:845–852.

15. Ogushi F, Fells GA, Hubbard RC, Straus SD, Crystal RG. Z-type α1 antitrypsin is less competent that M1 type anitrypsin as an inhibitor of neutrophil elastase. J Clin Invest 1987; 80:1366–1374.

16. Ogushi F, Hubbard RC, Vogelmeier C, Fells GA, Crystal RG. Risk Factors for emphysema. Cigarette smoking is associated with a reduction in the association rate constant of lung α1-antitrypsin for neutrophil elastase. J Clin Invest 1991; 87:1060–1065.

17. Hunninghake GW, Crystal RG. Cigarette smoking and lung destruction: accumulation of neutrophils in the lungs of cigarette smokers. Am Rev Respir Dis 1983; 128:833–838.

18. Tadashi M, Romberger DJ, Thompson AB, Robbins RA, Heires A, Rennard SI. Cigarette smoke induces interleukin 8 release from human bronchial epithelial cells. Am J Respir Crit Care Med 1997; 155:1770–1776.

19. Nishikawa M, Kakemizu N, Ito T, Kudo M, Kaneko T, Suzuki M, Udaka N, Ikeda H, Okubo T. Superoxide mediates cigarette smoke-induced infiltration of neutrophils into the airways through nuclear factor-kB activation and IL-8 mRNA expression in guinea pigs in vivo. Am J Respir Cell Mol Biol; 1999:189–198.

20. Harris JO, Swenson EW, Johnson JE. Human alveolar macrophages: comparison of phagocytic ability, glucose utilization and ultrastructure in smokers and non-smokers. J Clin Invest 1970; 49:2086–2096.

21. McCrea KA, Ensor JE, Nall K, Blicker ER, Hasday JD. Altered cytokine regulation in the lungs of cigarette smokers. Am J Respir Crit Care Med 1994; 150:696–703.

22. Matsuse T, Heashi S, Kuwano K, Keunecke H, Jefferies WA, Hogg JC. Latent adenoviral infection in the pathogenesis of chronic airways obstruction. Am Rev Respir Dis 1992; 146:177–184.

23. Keicho N, Elliott WM, Hogg JC, Heashi S. Adenovirus E1A regulates IL-8 expression induced by endotoxin in pulmonary epithelial cells. Am J Physiol (Lung Cell Mol Physiol) 1997; 16:L1046–L1052.

24. Tanino M, Betsuyaku T, Takeyabu K, et al. Increased levels of interleukin-8 in BAL fluid from smokers susceptible to pulmonary emphysema. Thorax 2002; 57:405–411.

25. Hubbard RC, Fells G, Gadek J, Pacholok S, Humes J, Crystal RG. Neutrophil accumulation in the lung in alph-1-antitrypsin deficiency; spontaneous release of leukotriene B4 by alveolar macrophages. J Clin Invest 1991; 88:891–897.

26. Totti N, McCusker KT, Campbell EJ, Griffin GL, Senior RM. Nicotine is chemotactic for neutrophils and enhances neutrophil responsiveness to chemotactic peptides. Science 1984; 223:169–171.

27. Banda MJ, Rice AG, Griffin GL, Senior RM. The inhibitory complex of human alpha-1 proteinase inhibitor and human leukocyte elastase is a neutrophil chemoattractant. J Exp Med 1988; 167:1608–1617.

28. Stockley RA, Shaw J, Afford SC, Morrison HM, Burnett D. Effect of alpha-1-proteinase inhibitor on neutrophil chemotaxis. Am J Respir Cell Mol Biol 1990; 2:163–170.

29. Traves TL, Culpitt SV, Russell REK, Barnes PJ, Donnelly LE. Increased levels of the chemokines GROα and MCP-1 in sputum samples from patients with COPD. Thorax 2002; 57:590–595.

30. Pasnik J, Tchorzewski H, Baj Z, Luciak M, Tchorzewski M. Priming effect of met-enkephalin and β-endorphin on chemiluminescence, chemotaxis and CD11b molecule expression on human neutrophils in vitro. Immunol Lett 1999; 67:77–83.

31. Stockley RA, Grant RA, Llewellyn-Jones CG, Hill SL, Burnett D. Neutrophil formyl peptide receptors: relationship to peptide induced responses and emphysema. Am J Respir Crit Care Med 1994; 149:464–468.

32. Burnett D, Chamba A, Hill SL, Stockley RA. Neutrophils from subjects with chronic obstructive lung disease show enhanced chemotaxis and extracellular proteolysis. Lancet 1987; 8567:1043–1046.

33. Di Stefano A, Maestrelli P, Roggeri A, Turato G, Calabro S, Potena A, Mapp CE, Ciaccia A, Covalev L, Fabbri LM, Saetta M. Up-regulation of adhesion molecules in the bronchial mucosa of subjects with chronic obstruction bronchitis. Am J Respir Crit Care Med 1994; 149:803–810.

34. Noguera A, Busquets X, Souleda J, Villaverde M, MacNee W, Agusti AGN. Expression of adhesion molecules and G proteins in circulating neutrophils in chronic obstructive pulmonary disease. Am J Respir Crit Care Med 1998; 158:1664–1668.

35. Heusel JW, Hanson RD, Silverman GA, Ley TJ. Structure and expression of a cluster of human haematopoietic serine proteinase genes found on chromosone 14q11.2. J Biol Chem 1991; 266:6152–6158.

36. Buttle DJ, Abrahamson M, Burnett D, Mort JS, Barrett AJ, Dando PM, Hill SL. Human sputum cathepsin B degrades proteoglycan, is inhibited by alpha-2-macroglobulin and is modulated by neutrophil elastase cleavage of cathepsin B precursor and cystatic C. Biochemistry 1991; 276:325–331.

37. Hautamaki RD, Kobayashi DK, Senior RM, Shapiro SD. Requirement for macrophage elastase for cigarette smoke-induced emphysema in mice. Science 1997; 277:2002–2004.

38. D'Armiento J, Dalal SS, Okaela Y, Berg RA, Chada K. Collagenase expression in the lungs of transgenic mice causes pulmonary emphysema. Cell 1992; 71:955–961.

39. Finlay GA, Russell KJ, McMahon KJ, Darcy EM, Masterton JB, Fitzgerald MX, O'Connor CM. Elevated levels of matrix metalloproteinases in broncho-alveolar lavage fluid in emphysematous patients. Thorax 1997; 52:502–506.

40. Betsuyaku T, Nishimura M, Tukeyabu K, Tanino M, Venge P, Xu S, Kawakami Y. Neutrophil granule proteins in bronchoalveolar lavage fluids from subjects with subclinical emphysema. Am J Respir Crit Care Med 1999; 159:985–1991.

41. Lim S, Roche N, Oliver B, Mattos W, Barnes PJ, Fan Chung K. Balance of matrix metalloprotease-9 and tissue inhibitor of metalloprotease-1 from alveolar macrophages in cigarette smokers. Regulation by interleukin-10. Am J Respir Crit Care Med 2000; 162:1355–1360.

42. Russell REK, Culpitt SV, DeMatos C, Donnelly L, Smith M, Wiggins J, Barnes PJ. Release and activity of matrix metalloproteinase-9 and tissue inhibitor of metalloproteinase-1 by alveolar macrophages from patients with chronic obstructive pulmonary disease. Am J Respir Cell Mol Biol 2002; 26:602–609.

43. Keatings VM, Collins PD, Scott DM, Barnes PJ. Differences in interleukin-8 and tumour necrosis factor-alpha in induced sputum from patients with chronic obstructive pulmonary disease or asthma. Am J Respir Crit Care Med 1996; 153:530–534.

44. Stockley RA. Obstructive airway disease: proteases/anti-proteases: pathogenesis and role in therapy. Clin Pulm Med 1998; 5:203–210.

45. Cordozo C, Padilla ML, Choi H-SH, Lesser M. Goblet cell hyperplasia in large intra-pulmonary airways after intra-tracheal injection of cathepsin B into hamsters. Am Rev Respir Dis 1992; 145:675–679.

46. Turato G, Di Stefano A, Maestrelli P, Mapp CE, Ruggieri MP, Roggeri A, Fabbri LM, Saetta M. Effect of smoking cessation on airway inflammation in chronic bronchitis. Am J Respir Crit Care Med 1995; 152(4 pt 1):1262–1272.

47. Di Stefano A, Turato G, Maestrelli P, Mapp CE, Ruggieri MP, Roggeri A, Boschetto P, Fabbri LM, Saetta M. Airflow limitation in chronic bronchitis is associated with T-lymphocyte and macrophage infiltration of the bronchial mucosa. Am J Respir Crit Care Med 1996: 153(2):629–632.

48. Saetta M, Turato G, Facchini FM, Corbino L, Lucchini RE, Casoni G, Maestrelli P, Mapp CE, Ciaccia A, Fabbri LM. Inflammatory cells in the bronchial glands of smokers with chronic bronchitis. Am J Respir Crit Care Med 1997: 156(5):1633–1639.

49. Peleman RA, Rytila PH, Kips JC, Joos GF, Pauwells RA. The cellular composition of induced sputum in chronic obstructive pulmonary disease. Eur Respir J 1999; 13:839–843.

50. Hoshi H, Ohno I, Honma M, Tanno Y, Yamauchi K, Tamura G, Shirato K. IL-5, IL-8 and GM-CSF immunostaining of sputum cells in bronchial asthma and chronic bronchitis. Clin Exp Allergy 1995; 25(8):720–728.

51. Richman-Eisenstat JB, Jorens PG, Hebert CA, Ueki I, Nadel JA. Interleukin-8: an important chemoattractant in sputum of patients with chronic inflammatory airway diseases. Am J Physiol 1993; 264:L413–L418.

52. Riise GC, Ahlstedt S, Larsson S, Enander I, Jones I, Larsson P, et al. Bronchial inflammation in chronic bronchitis assessed by measurement of cell products in bronchial lavage fluid. Thorax 1995; 50(4):360–365.

53. Yamamoto C, Yoneda T, Yoshikawa M, Fu A, Tokuyama T, Tsukaguchi K, Narita N. Airway inflammation in COPD assessed by sputum levels of interleukin-8. Chest 1997; 112(2):505–510.

54. Khair OA, Devalier JL, Abdilaziz MM, Sapsford RJ, Davis RJ. The effect of haemophilus influenzae endotoxin on synthesis of IL-6, IL-8, TNF-α and expression of ICAM-1 in cultured human bronchial epithelial cells. Eur Respir J 1994; 7:2109–2116.

55. Takahashi GW, Andrews DF, Lilly MB, Singer JW, Alderson MR. Effect of granulocyte-macrophage colony-stimulating factor and interleukin-3 on interleukin-8 production by human neutrophils and monocytes. Blood 1993; 81:357–364.

56. Ford-Hutchinson AW, Bray MA, Doig MW, Shipley ME, Smith MJ. Leukotriene B4—a potent chemokinetic and aggregating substance released form polymorphonuclear leukocytes. Nature (London) 1980; 286:264–265.

57. Hill A, Bayley D, Stockley R. The inter-relationship of sputum inflammatory markers in patients with chronic bronchitis. Am J Respir Crit Care Med 1999; 160:893–898.

58. Woolhouse IS, Bayley DL, Stockley RA. Sputum chemotactic activity in chronic obstructive pulmonary disease: effect of α_1-antitrypsin deficiency and the role of leukotriene B_4 and interleukin 8. Thorax 2002; 57:709–714.

59. Mukaida N, Morita M, Ishikawa Y, Rice N, Okamoto S, Kasahara T, Matsushima K. Novel mechanism with glucocorticoid-mediated gene expression. Nuclear factor-κ as a target for glucocorticoid-mediated interleukin 8 gene repression. J Biol Chem 1994; 269:13289–13295.

60. Keatings VM, Jatakanon A, Worsdell YM, Barnes PJ. Effect of inhaled and oral glucocorticoids on inflammatory indices in asthma and COPD. Am J Respir Crit Care Med 197; 155:545–548.

61. Wiggins J, Elliot JA, Stevenson RD, Stockley RA. Effect of corticosteroids on sputum solphase protease inhibitors in chronic obstructive pulmonary disease. Thorax 1982; 37:652–656.

62. Llewellyn-Jones CG, Harris TAJ, Stockley RA. Effect of fluticasone proprionate on sputum of patients with chronic bronchitis and emphysema. Am J Respir Crit Care Med 1996; 153:616–621.

63. Confalonieri M, Mainardi E, Della Porta R, Bernorio S, Gandola L, Beghe B, Spanevella A. Inhaled corticosteroids reduce neutrophilic bronchial

inflammation in patients with chronic obstructive pulmonary disease. Thorax 1998; 53(7):583–585.

64. Paggiaro PL, Dahle R, Bachran I, Frith L, Hollingworth K, Efthimiou J. Multi-center randomised placebo—control trial of inhaled fluticasone proprionate in patients with chronic obstructive pulmonary disease. Lancet 1998; 351:773–780.

65. Burge PS, Calverley PMA, Jones PW, Spencer SA, Anderson JA, Maslen TK. Randomised, double blind, placebo controlled study of fluticasone propionate in patients with moderate to severe chronic obstructive pulmonary disease; the ISOLDE trial. BMJ 2000; 320:1297–1303.

66. Lung Health Study Research Group. Effects of inhaled triamcinolone on the decline in pulmonary function in chronic obstructive pulmonary disease. NEJM 2000; 343:1902–1909.

67. Pauwels RA, Lofdahl C, Laitinen LA, Schouten JP, Postma DS, Pride NB, Ohlssan S. Long-term treatment with inhaled budesonide in persons with mild chronic obstructive pulmonary disease who continue smoking. NEJM 1999; 340:1948–1953.

68. Sin DD, Tu JV. Inhaled corticosteroids and the risk of mortality and readmission in elderly patients with chronic obstructive pulmonary disease. Am J Respir Crit Care Med 2001; 164:580–584.

69. Monso E, Ruiz J, Tosell A, Manterola J, Fiz J, Morera J, Ausina V. Bacterial infection in chronic obstruction pulmonary disease. A study of stable and exacerbated outpatients using the protected specimen brush. Am J Respir Crit Care Med 1995; 152:1316–1320.

70. Hill AT, Campbell EJ, Hill SL, Bayley DL, Stockley RA. Association between airway bacterial load and markers of airway inflammation in patients with stable chronic bronchitis. Am J Med 2000; 109:288–295.

71. Dowson LJ, Guest PJ, Stockley RA. Longitudinal changes in physiological, radiological and health status measurements in α_1-antitrypsin deficiency and factors associated with decline. Am J Respir Crit Care Med 2001; 164:1805–1809.

72. Hill AT, Campbell EJ, Bayley DL, Hill SL, Stockley RA. Evidence for excessive bronchial inflammation during an acute exacerbation of COPD in patients with alpha-1 antitrypsin deficiency (PiZ). Am J Respir Crit Care Med 1999. 160:1968–1975.

73. Stockley RA, Bayley DL, Unsal I, Dowson L. The effect of augmentation therapy on bronchial inflammation in α1-antitrypsin deficiency. Am J Respir Crit Care Med (2002); 165:1494–1498.

74. Thompson WH, Neilson CP, Carvalho P, Charan NB, Crowley JJ. Controlled trial of oral prednisolone in out patients with acute COPD exacerbation. Am J Respir Crit Care Med 1996; 154:407–512.

75. Anthonisen NR, Manfreda J, Waren CPW, Hevohfield ES, Harding GK, Nelson NA. Antibiotic therapy in exacerbations of chronic obstructive pulmonary disease. Ann Intern Med 1987; 106:196–204.

76. Maestrelli P, Saetta M, Di Stefano A, Calcagni PG, Turato G, Ruggieri MP, Roggeri A, Mapp CE, Fabbri LM. Comparison of leukocyte counts in sputum bronchial biopsies and bronchoalveolar lavage. Am J Respir Crit Care Med 1995; 152:1926–1931.

77. DeKhuijzen PNR, Aben KKH, Dekker I, Aarts LPHJ, Weidlers PLML, van Herwaarden CLA, Bast A. Increased exhalation of hydrogen peroxide in patients with stable and unstable chronic obstructive pulmonary disease. Am J Respir Crit Care Med 1996; 154:813–816.

78. Stockley, RA, Burnett D. Alpha 1 antitrypsin and leukocyte elastase in infected and non-infected sputum. Am Rev Respir Dis 1979; 120:1081–1086.

79. Vestbo J, Prescott E, Lange P. Association of mucus hypersecretion with FEV1 decline and chronic obstructive pulmonary disease morbidity. Am J Respir Crit Care Med 1996; 153:1530–1535.

80. Gibson PG, Woolley KL, Carty K, Murree-Allen K, Saltos N. Induced sputum eosinophil cationic protein (ECP). Measurement in asthma and chronic obstructive airways disease. Clin Exp Allergy 1998; 28:1081–1088.

81. Pizzichini E, Pizzichini MM, Gibson P, Parameswaran K, Gleich GJ, Berman L, Dolovich J, Hargreave FE. Sputum eosinophilia predicts benefit from Prednisone in smokers with chronic obstructive bronchitis. Am J Respir Crit Care Med 1998; 158(5 pt 1):1511–1517.

82. Brightling CE, Monteiro W, Ward R, Parker D, Morgan MD, Wardlaw AJ, Pavord ID. Sputum eosinophilia and short-term response to prednisolone in chronic obstructive pulmonary disease: a randomized controlled trial. Lancet 2000; 356:1480–1485.

83. Brandolini L, Sergi R, Caselli G, Baraschi D, Locati M, Sozzanl S, Bertini R. Interleukin-1 beta and interleukin-8-stimulated chemotaxis and elastase release in human neutrophils via its type 1 receptor. Eur Cytokine Netw 1997; 8:173–178.

84. Saetta M, Di Stefano A, Maestrelli P, Turato G, Ruggieri MP, Roggeri A, Calcagni P, Map CE, Ciaccia A, Fabbri LM. Airway eosinophilia in chronic bronchitis during exacerbations. Am J Respir Crit Care Med 1994; 150:1646–1652.

9

Defective Repair in COPD: The American Hypothesis

STEPHEN RENNARD

University of Nebraska Medical Center
Omaha, Nebraska, U.S.A.

I. Introduction

Chronic obstructive pulmonary disease (COPD) refers to a heterogeneous collection of disorders that share a common physiological abnormality: limitation of expiratory airflow (1,2). Rigorous definition of COPD has been difficult, in part because it represents a collection of disorders that are themselves heterogeneous. In general, many disorders including cystic fibrosis, bronchiectasis, and localized airway lesions are excluded from the definition of COPD. Current usage includes both chronic bronchitis and emphysema within the definition of COPD, recognizing that either condition may be present without clinically significant airflow limitation. Asthma is also characterized by airflow limitation, but, in contrast to COPD, where airflow limitation may be partially reversible, in asthma airflow limitation is largely reversible either spontaneously or with treatment. Recent evidence, however, suggests that asthma per se may be associated with progressive irreversible loss of expiratory airflow (3,4). This has led to semantic and nosological difficulties. The currently accepted best definition of COPD, adopted by the Global Initiative for Chronic

Table 1 Geographic Hypotheses for COPD Pathogenesis

Hypothesis	Proponent[a]	Lung site	Mechanism
Dutch	Orie (7,8)	Airways	Reactivity
British	Fletcher et al. (11)	Airways	Infection/mucus
"Swedish"	Laurell and Eriksson (229)	Alveoli	Proteolytic destruction
"American"	Liebow (23)	Alveoli	Defective repair

[a]Many investigators contributed to the development of these ideas.

Obstructive Pulmonary Disease (GOLD) is: "COPD is a disease state characterized by airflow limitation that is not fully reversible. The airflow limitation is both progressive and associated with an abnormal inflammatory response of the lungs to noxious particles and gases" (5).

Several anatomical lesions can contribute to airflow limitation in COPD (6). In the airways, smooth muscle contraction, edema of the airway wall, the presence of secretions within the airway lumen, and peribronchiolar fibrosis with airway narrowing can all limit airflow. The loss of alveolar wall that characterizes emphysema leads both to loss of lung elastic recoil and loss of the radial attachments that help maintain small airway patency. Several hypotheses have been proposed to account for the development of these lesions and subsequent physiologic abnormalities (Table 1). While these have been regarded historically as competing hypotheses, current thinking suggests they are not exclusive and that the consequences of multiple mechanisms can account for the heterogeneity that characterizes COPD.

II. Historical Background

In the 1960s, two hypotheses were proposed to account for airflow limitation due to airways disease. One concept, which became known as the Dutch hypothesis, suggested that airways hyperreactivity, the physiological hallmark of asthma, could lead directly to airway alterations associated with more or less fixed airflow limitation (7,8). Epidemiological studies demonstrating that airways reactivity is a risk factor for accelerated loss of lung function in COPD in smokers (9) and that individuals with clinical asthma are at risk for accelerated loss of expiratory airflow (3,4) support this hypothesis. Some patients with asthma, moreover, appear to progress to the development of COPD (10).

A competing hypothesis, the British hypothesis, suggested that chronic bronchial infection was associated with mucus hypersecretion, which, in turn, led to inflammation, airway damage, and the fixed airflow limitation characteristic of COPD. The early studies of Fletcher et al. (11) suggested that mucus hypersecretion was not a risk factor for the development of fixed airflow limitation, and the British hypothesis was generally disregarded. More recent studies, however, provide evidence supporting the concept that mucus hypersecretion is a risk factor for the development of airflow limitation in COPD (12). Exacerbations with increased cough and mucus production may also be associated with increased loss of airflow (13). Importantly, the British and Dutch hypotheses are not exclusive. It seems likely that both may be correct and that different individuals may have either of them to different degrees.

Although not referred to by geographic origin, much of the thinking regarding the pathogenesis of emphysema derives from the studies of the Swedish investigators Laurell and Eriksson in the 1960s. These investigators defined the association of congenital α_1 protease inhibitor deficiency with emphysema leading to the protease antiprotease hypothesis (14,15). In the context of this review, could be called the Swedish hypothesis. The concept that proteolytic activity in excess of antiproteolytic defense mechanisms leads to tissue destruction has been greatly studied. Experimental and human studies support the concept, which has also been substantially expanded (16–19). Enzymes in addition to neutrophil elastase and inhibitors in addition to α_1 protease inhibitor are now believed to also play roles. In addition, destructive mechanisms in addition to proteolysis, including both oxidant injury (20) and possibly toxic peptides (21), have also been suggested to contribute to tissue damage. Interaction among these mechanisms, moreover, provides for amplification of destructive processes. By causing tissue destruction and emphysema, these processes lead to loss of lung elastic recoil and, therefore, to expiratory airflow limitation (6). A series of recent studies, moreover, have provided evidence that proteases and oxidants likely also contribute to the development of airways disease (22).

Another hypothesis was proposed at about the same time by the American pathologist Liebow to account for the development of emphysema (23). He noted that the alveolar capillaries are a major structural component of the alveolar wall. Loss of capillaries, he suggested, should result in loss of alveolar wall and the development of emphysema. Expanding this concept of tissue maintenance in balance with tissue turnover or destruction leads to the so-called American hypothesis: that defective repair contributes to the development of COPD (24). Importantly, defective repair is not exclusive of any of the other hypotheses, but rather, repair likely interacts with tissue destruction, infection, and reactivity. The current chapter will provide an overview of the evidence relating to repair in lung as it relates to COPD pathogenesis.

III. Airway Repair

Repair of the lungs was first evaluated and has been best studied in the airways. In the 1950s, Wilhelm demonstrated that mechanical injury of the rat trachea is followed by an orderly series of repair events that can restore epithelial integrity (Fig. 1) (25). These investigations have been confirmed and extended by several investigators (26–29), and the molecular and cellular events that contribute to repair are being defined.

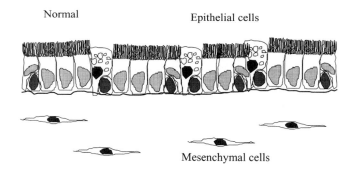

Figure 1 Schematic representation of events following injury in the airway. It is likely that similar events transpire in the alveolar structures. See text for details. (a) Normal epithelium. Only the epithelial cells and mesenchymal cells are shown. Vessels, nerves, and migratory and resident inflammatory cells also present. (b) Fifteen minutes following wounding. After injury, leakage of plasma proteins results in the formation of a provisional matrix. Cells on the margin of the wound are activated to migrate into the wound. Cells present in the wound likely release mediators. (c) Six hours after wounding. Epithelial cells have migrated into the wound and have altered their differentiated phenotype. The cells become flattened and reestablish epithelial integrity. (d) Twenty-four hours after wounding. Marked proliferation occurs in the epithelial cell in the original defect. (e) Seventy-two hours after wounding. Proliferation and accumulation of mesenchymal cells occurs. The epithelial cells have ceased replication and are beginning to differentiate. (f) Six weeks after injury. Epithelial differentiation has resulted in normal epithelial cell populations. The subjacent mesenchymal cell accumulation has also resolved. Normal structure has been restored.

A. Epithelial Repair

Under normal conditions, the epithelial and mesenchymal cells within the airway are relatively stable. A very small percentage of mostly basal cells appear to be dividing and presumably account for normal epithelial cell turnover (30). In response to injury, however, a rapid response ensues.

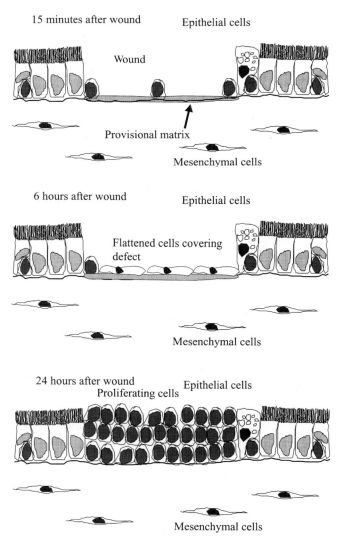

Figure 1 Continued.

72 hours after wound   Epithelial cells

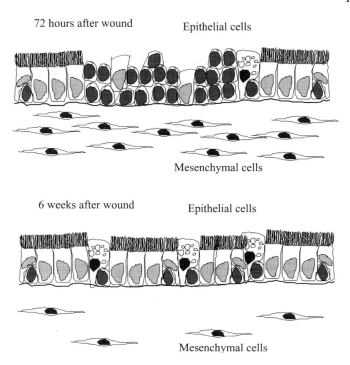

Mesenchymal cells

6 weeks after wound   Epithelial cells

Mesenchymal cells

Figure 1 Continued.

Within minutes following mechanical injury, for example, plasma leakage results in the development of a provisional matrix (29,31). Epithelial cells adjacent to a wound begin to migrate within minutes and alter their phenotypes so that within hours an epithelial barrier comprised of markedly flattened cells can be restored (27,32,33). Epithelial cells that accumulate within an area of mechanical injury rapidly proliferate (27,33), and a large percentage of the cells may be dividing 24 hours following injury. Within several days, however, proliferation ceases, and the epithelial cells that have accumulated in the area of injury begin to differentiate. Over a course of days to weeks, these cells can reassume a normal pseudostratified columnar appearance and can reform the epithelium with a normal distribution of goblet and ciliated cells.

The cells that accumulate early in the injury process express cytokeratin 14, a cytoskeletal protein characteristic of basal cells, and this marker persists through the early phases of the developmental process (28). In contrast, histochemical markers including cytokeratin 18 that are characteristic of columnar cells become present only later in the repair process. This led Shimizu and colleagues to suggest that basal cells may be the precursor cells responding to airway injury (28). In this context, repair may be distinct from airway development as, at least in some species, basal cells are present within the airway only at a relatively late stage during development (34,35). In addition, basal cells are prominent in the proximal airways but become progressively more rare in the more distal airways (36,37). The presence of basal cell markers in regenerating cells could, alternatively, represent a marker of dedifferentiation rather than reflect cell of origin. In addition, a progenitor cell that could contribute to both normal tissue maintenance and to repair following injury has been identified within gland ducts (38). The precursor cells that mediate repair in the airway, therefore, remain incompletely defined. Finally, which cell types play a role in the distal airways remains to be fully delineated, although Clara cells have been suggested to play a role (39,40).

B. Mediators of Repair

A number of in vitro and in vivo studies have begun to suggest candidate mediators that may regulate repair processes in the airway. The first step, migration of epithelial cells into a wounded area, has been evaluated in several in vitro systems. Using primary isolates of bovine bronchial epithelial cells, Shoji et al. demonstrated migration in response to chemotactic stimuli using the blindwell Boyden chamber technique in which cells migrate through holes in a membrane (41). Insulin-like growth factor-1 (IGF-1) (41), fibronectin (42), and fragments of extracellular matrix (43) are also capable of driving epithelial cell chemotaxis. It is likely that the cells present in the wound can also contribute to the production of factors regulating repair. In this context, transforming growth factor (TGF)-β is a multifunctional cytokine believed to play an important role in tissue repair in multiple tissues (44,45). TGF-β is produced by airway epithelial cells (46,47) and, among its other actions, is capable of stimulating these cells to produce the glycoprotein fibronectin (48,49). Fibronectin, in turn, is a macromolecule that mediates a number of interactions between cells and extracellular matrix (50). With regard to airway repair following injury, fibronectin is a potent chemoattractant for airway epithelial cells (42). Interestingly, airway epithelial cell-derived fibronectin is a much more potent chemoattractant than is plasma fibronectin, suggesting that fibro-nectin could function in this capacity even in the presence of fibronectin derived from plasma leakage (42). However, it is unlikely that de novo production of fibronectin or polypeptide growth factors accounts for the initial chemotaxis of epithelial cells. These responses are observed within minutes, time frames generally regarded as too short for the induction of new gene expression or even protein production from preformed message. These mediators could, of course, play important roles in subsequent waves of cell migration.

Formation of eicosinoids or release of preformed mediators could contribute to rapid increases in epithelial cell movement (51). In this context, peptides derived from nerves and from neuroendocrine cells can increase in vitro epithelial cell migration (52). Moreover, the initial phase is slowed as repair proceeds following neuropeptide blockade, suggesting a role for neuropeptides in early repair events (53). Serum is also a potent chemotactic stimulus (42). Thus, it is also possible that the leakage of plasma, in addition to generating a provisional matrix (54), also generates chemotactic factors that contribute to epithelial cell recruitment.

Several investigators have utilized an in vitro wound-repair technique in which cells are removed from a small area of a culture dish and the ability of cells to migrate into and fill the resulting defect can be assessed (55,56). With this technique, Zahm (55) and Kim (57) have demonstrated that epidermal growth factor (EGF) can augment epithelial-cell-mediated wound closure. The EGF receptor is present in the normal airway epithelium and is upregulated in the injured epithelium in asthma. Inhibition of EGF receptor signaling blocks in vitro wound closure mediated by a human airway epithelial cell line (58). Interestingly, there is an associated increase in TGF-β production (see below). Taken together, these data suggest a key role for EGF in augmenting epithelial repair. Other mediators may play similar roles. Tumor necrosis factor (TNF)-α (59) and hepatocyte growth factor (HGF) (60), members of the EGF family that signal through a family of closely related receptors, as well as keratinocyte growth factor (KGF) (61) and prostaglandin E (PGE) (51) have all been demonstrated to accelerate epithelial cell migration in similar assay systems.

C. Matrix and Proteases

Epithelial cell migration occurs over a surface, and the composition of the matrix likely has important effects. Epithelial cells, for example, migrate more rapidly over interstitial collagen-coated surfaces than they do over basement membrane collagen (62). Extracellular matrix, moreover, has a complex structure, and partial proteolytic cleavage, which may occur during injury, can expose novel binding sites for cell surface integrins that may affect both chemotaxis and differentiation (63). While the importance of such processes for in vivo repair remains undefined, epithelial cells migrate more rapidly across protease-treated extracellular matrix (62). In addition, inhibition of matrix metalloproteinases (MMPs) with nonselective inhibitors inhibits epithelial repair in in vitro explants of human tracheas. Matrilysin (MMP-7) may be particularly important in this regard. It is expressed in normal airway epithelium, and its expression increases during repair in an in vitro model (64). Several MMPs are expressed by epithelial cells in skin wounds, including MMP-1, MMP-3, MMP-9, and MMP-10, but MMP-7 was the only MMP among those tested prominent in human airway epithelial cells. Similarly, the MMP-7 knockout mouse has markedly deficient epithelial repair, further supporting a role for MMP-7 in epithelial repair in the airway.

Expression of MMP-3, MMP-9, and MMP-2 has been noted to be increased in other in vitro models of airway epithelial injury (65). The expression of these enzymes correlates with migratory ability (65,66). Moreover, exogenous MMP-9 increases migration. In contrast, exogenous MMP-2 inhibits migration (67). The MMPs are generally released as inactive precursors that are activated by a variety of mechanisms, including proteolytic cleavage. In this context, induction of uPA (urine-type plasminogen activator) at the leading edge of a wound has been reported (68). Since uPA can activate MMP-9 and blockade uPA of activity decreases migration, this suggests a model in which uPA activation leads to MMP-9 activation, which in turn facilitates epithelial cell migration. Undoubtedly many other interactions among the many proteases likely present following injury could also play roles. It also seems likely that the proteases involved will vary with the nature of the injury, the stage of repair, and, possibly, with species. Regulation of protease expression in airway epithelial cells, therefore, is likely to be a key feature of repair. Conversely, abnormal regulation of proteases may be a key feature in pathological processes.

Early after mechanical wounding of the rat trachea, migrating cells are observed as individual cells streaming away from the wounded edge (69). A different pattern of migration is observed in many of the in vitro wound closure assays noted above, where the epithelial cells commonly migrate as a sheet in which cells at the leading edge are attached both to each other and to their neighbors (55,59). The cytokine HGF, sometimes termed scatter factor, induces epithelial cell detachment from their neighbors and migration as individual cells (70), and it can increase the rate of closure of wounds in vitro (60). HGF also can have important effects in alveolar repair following bleomycin injury. Whether it plays a role in airway repair following mechanical injury or in COPD, however, remains to be established.

Epithelial cells can interact with extracellular matrix through several receptors. In vitro, antibodies to α 2, α 3, and α 6 integrins blocked wound closure on type IV collagen but not on laminin. In contrast, antibodies to β1 integrin blocked closure on all surfaces tested (71). This suggests that several integrins interacting with multiple substrates may play roles. Following wounding in one study, epithelial cells at the edge of a mechanical wound expressed V, β5, and β6 integrins. These integrins are not highly expressed in normal epithelium (72), and their induction has been suggested to alter the function of cells in a wound. αVβ6 integrin, for example, can activate TGF-β by inducing a conformational change in the latent TGF-β molecule (73). TGF-β, in turn, is believed to mediate many repair responses. A number of controversies and questions remain regarding integrin expression by epithelial cells in wound repair. Herard et al., for example, reported increased epithelial cell expression of $\alpha_5\beta_1$ integrin and fibronectin, but no change in expression of αV, α2, or α3 integrin (74). Experimental differences may account for these differences between investigators in injury-induced integrin expression. Nevertheless, it is clear that airway epithelial cells can express several integrins and that their expression can be modulated in the face of injury. It is likely, therefore, that migrating cells can utilize a different repertoire of receptors than do cells present in the normal airway.

The phenotypic changes observed in epithelial cells participating in the wound repair response are accompanied by changes in the gene expression. Alterations in cell surface expression of specific isoforms of CD44, for example, have been described that may also play a role in regulating the process of migration (75). Alterations in cell surface receptor expression may also contribute to the susceptibility of the repairing epithelium to pathogens. Some bacteria adhere to epithelial cells through fibronectin, and increased fibronectin expression on airway epithelial cells has been suggested to increase bacterial adherence and to predispose to airway colonization (76). Increases in epithelial cell expression of ICAM-1 can result from cytokines likely present following wounding (77). This could increase the ability of inflammatory cells to bind to the airway epithelium and therefore susceptibility of the airway epithelium to collateral damage during an inflammatory response (78).

D. Proliferation and Differentiation

Following recruitment, epithelial cells proliferate and then redifferentiate, potentially restoring epithelial architecture. It is likely that many regulatory factors control epithelial cell proliferation and differentiation during repair. Fibroblasts (79), epithelial cells (37,80,81), and mononuclear phagocytes (82) can produce epithelial cell growth factors. A number of potential epithelial cell growth factors have been identified (37,83). Some, including IGF-1 (84), EGF (80), HGF (81), and fibronectin (85), can stimulate epithelial cell recruitment as well as epithelial cell proliferation.

Epithelial cells have an endogenous capacity to differentiate. In vitro cultures of epithelial cells maintained on a filter in growth-supporting medium proliferate and form a layer of cells several cells thick (86). Proliferation, however, spontaneously stops. If such cultures are transferred to an air/liquid interface, differentiation will "spontaneously" take place with the formation of both ciliated cells and mucin-expressing cells resembling goblet cells. Thus, epithelial cells themselves can produce the mediators that regulate proliferation and can undergo complex differentiation into several cells types without an external source of mediators. However, exogenous mediators also can regulate differentiation. Activation of the EGF receptor by both ligand- and non-ligand-mediated mechanisms is a potent inducer of mucin gene expression (87–89). Oxidants generated by inflammatory cells can activate the EGF receptor (90). It is likely, therefore, that the inflammatory response present in the airways in COPD can modify repair responses by altering differentiation signals. Inasmuch as inflammation is chronically present in COPD, such mechanisms could lead to the altered epithelial differentiation that is characteristically present. Other factors can also play roles. A study evaluating ozone injury in rats suggested that capsaicin ablation of lung sensory C fibers resulted in impaired repair processes in the small airways. These results suggest that neuropeptides may contribute to epithelial repair following injury (91).

E. Mesenchymal Cells

Mesenchymal cells are also recruited and activated during repair following injury. Following mechanical injury of the airway, mesenchymal cells accumulate beneath the injured area in a wave of recruitment and proliferation, which follows by a few days that of the epithelial cells (69). Many of the same mediators that drive epithelial cell recruitment and proliferation, such as TGF-β, fibronectin, and EGF, are also potent stimuli for fibroblast recruitment and proliferation, suggesting that epithelial and mesenchymal responses may be linked. In addition, just as fibroblasts can stimulate epithelial cells (79), epithelial cells are potential sources of factors, including fibronectin (92), IGF-1 (93), endothelin (94), and PDGF (95), which can stimulate fibroblasts. TGF-β is also a potent stimulator of fibroblast fibronectin production, and fibronectin is a potent fibroblast chemoattractant (92,96–98). These mediators could, therefore, account for the recruitment of mesenchymal cells into the vicinity of an injured area as well. The mutual interactions between epithelial cells and fibroblasts resemble those essential for normal lung morphogenesis (99). This has led to the concept that many of the interactions that regulate development are, to some extent, recapitulated during repair following injury (100). Finally, other structural cells present in the airway, including chondrocytes (101), can also release mediators that can regulate repair.

The role that mesenchymal cells play in normal repair remains to be established. However, it is clear that overabundant recruitment and accumulation of mesenchymal cells and their products can result in fibrosis. Peribronchiolar fibrosis together with the contraction that characterizes fibrotic tissues likely accounts for the airway narrowing and airflow limitation in many patients with COPD (6). Several mechanisms could account for excessive accumulation of fibrotic tissue during the repair process. These could include: (1) excessive or prolonged production of pro-fibrotic mediators; (2) the presence of an overabundance of cells responding to pro-fibrotic mediators; (3) an increased sensitivity of potential target cells; (4) ineffective signals leading to termination of pro-fibrotic responses; and (5) ineffective resolution of the mesenchymal cell fibrotic response. While current evidence for these various mechanisms in the airways is limited, some sometimes controversial evidence exists in support for all. Immuno-histochemical studies of the airways have investigated TGF-β expression in the airways of individuals with chronic bronchitis compared to individuals with asthma and normal subjects. Vignola and colleagues (102), using an antibody that recognizes TGF-β isoforms 1, 2, and 3, found increased staining in the epithelium of patients with COPD. Using a cDNA probe specific for TGF-β1, increased gene expression was demonstrated in parallel with the immunohistochemical findings. In contrast, Aubert et al. (103) found no differences using antibodies and cDNA probes specific for TGF-β1. While there were methodological differences between the studies, the issue of whether TGF-β levels are increased in airways disease remains unresolved. TGF-β, moreover, is regulated not only by control of its production, but also by its activation. It is likely that several pathways may activate TGF-β in vivo.

Fibronectin, as noted above, may be produced in response to TGF-β and can also participate in repair responses. Consistently, fibronectin is present in higher concentration in the bronchoalveolar lavage samples of individuals with chronic bronchitis (104). Endothelin I (105,104) and neuropeptides (107,108) have also been reported in COPD and may increase with exacerbations (109,110). These agents are known to have stimulatory activity on fibroblasts and may, therefore, contribute to the development of airways dysfunction (111–114). These observations provide some support for the increased and/or prolonged production of pro-fibrotic mediators in chronic bronchitis.

The airways of individuals with chronic bronchitis are characterized by an increased population of mesenchymal cell (102). While data from the airways are limited, fibroblasts isolated from a variety of other tissues are heterogeneous, and those associated with the formation of fibrosis generally are more sensitive to pro-fibrotic stimuli and produce greater quantities of extracellular matrix macromolecules (115–118). This suggests that altered distribution of fibroblast subpopulations as well as well as increased numbers of fibroblasts may contribute to the formation of fibrosis. Interestingly, fibroblasts with different phenotypes may be differentially responsive to chemotactic stimuli such as fibronectin (119), thus providing a mechanism to change the distribution of mesenchymal cells within the airway in response to injury.

While the signals that lead to initiation of fibrotic responses are partially defined, fewer data exist regarding the mediators responsible for terminating fibrotic responses. Several mediators that can inhibit "pro-fibrotic" responses have been described (120–122). It is likely that defects in inhibitory processes could contribute to fibrosis in the airways. Resolution of fibrotic responses has been definitively documented in a number of tissues, including the lung. In the airways, for example, the intraluminal fibrosis that is characteristic of bronchiolitis obliterans can resolve completely, at least in some settings (123–125). The cellular processes that drive this resolution, including the degradation and removal of extracellular matrix and the apoptosis and removal of accumulated mesenchymal cells, remain to be defined. Inadequate resolution, however, may well account for the persistence of intraluminal fibrosis in some conditions such as rheumatoid arthritis.

Epithelial cells, as noted above, can produce a variety of factors that can drive fibrotic responses (47,92,126,127). Production of these factors, moreover, can be modulated by external stimuli. In this regard, bacterial endotoxin is capable of stimulating epithelial cells to release increased activity, which can drive fibroblast mediated contraction of extracellular matrices (47). This contractile process may be the mechanism by which scars contract. Within the airway, circumferential contraction likely accounts for the narrowing that leads directly to fixed airflow limitation (128,129). The production of factors that stimulate contractile activity in response to endotoxin could be one mechanism by which chronic bacterial infection of the airways may lead to fixed airflow limitation.

F. Vasculature

Proliferation of blood vessels is a characteristic feature of granulation tissue. Increased microvasculature has been described in asthma (130,131) and, although less well studied, probably in chronic bronchitis (132,133), and likely contributes to airflow limitation by making the airways more susceptible to edema. In addition, alteration of vascular endothelial cell adhesion molecule expression may predispose the airways to inflammation (131). The airway vasculature is part of the systemic circulation, but whether airway vessels respond similarly to other systemic vessels is undetermined.

IV. Alveolar Repair

The alveolar epithelial response to injury likely resembles that of the airway epithelium in many respects. Different experimental methods have been used to evaluate alveolar injury and repair, however. The alveoli are not readily accessible to mechanical injury, so much of the understanding of alveolar response to injury comes from chemical toxins, particularly bleomycin. This injury model, however, has been used primarily to model the development of pulmonary fibrosis. Interestingly, in α_1 protease inhibitor-deficient mice, bleomycin injury leads to the development of emphysema (134), supporting the concept that injury may lead to varying pathology depending on subsequent events. In vitro culture systems have also been used to model alveolar responses, but alveolar type I cells are not routinely cultured and type II-like cells are relatively difficult to culture. As a result, cell lines, particularly the A549 alveolar carcinoma-derived cell line, which resembles alveolar type II cells, have been used extensively. Similar to airway epithelial cells, both HGF and KGF promote epithelial cell recruitment and proliferation following injury (135,136). After bleomycin injury, both are present (137) and may mitigate the severity of injury. Following bleomycin injury, HGF induces the expression of uPA (138) and reduces the severity of fibrosis as indicated by collagen deposition (138). Similarly, KGF reduces the severity of allogeneic injury in a bone marrow transplantation model (139). Other cytokines also contribute to alveolar epithelial repair. IL-1, for example, increases alveolar cell migration perhaps indirectly by stimulating TNF-α and EGF (140).

A. Vasculature

Damage of alveoli also affects the vasculature. Loss of pulmonary capillary bed is a defining feature of emphysema. That inadequate maintenance of the pulmonary vascular bed could be a primary cause of emphysema was originally suggested by Liebow (23). Since that time, understanding of vascular cell biology has advanced considerably. Vascular endothelial growth factor (VEGF) is a mediator thought to be crucial for both the development and maintenance of pulmonary vessels. It is a growth factor for endothelial cells, and in its absence endothelial cells can undergo apoptosis (141). Liebow's concept that vasculopathy can contribute to the development of emphysema and that VEGF deficiency may play a role in this process has been supported by recent studies by Kasahara and colleagues. In a rat model, blockade of VEGF signaling induces endothelial cell apoptosis and leads to the formation of emphysema (142). Interestingly, blockade of apoptosis with an inhibitor of caspase prevents the development of emphysema. Consistently, in human lungs, both increased apoptosis of endothelial cells as well as epithelial cells and decreased expression of VEGF and one of the VEGF receptors has been described (143). Genetic variations in VEGF metabolism may account for the varying susceptibility to develop COPD. For example, the suggestion that different VEGF splice variants are expressed during normal events and following repair (144) provides one mechanism for incomplete restoration of normal architecture following some injuries. However, another study found no relationship between the presence of a common polymorphism associated with low VEGF levels and emphysema (145).

B. Emphysema

Emphysema is characterized by destruction of alveolar walls with a loss of lung elastic recoil. In this context, much of the elastic recoil of the lung is accounted for by elastic fibers. It has been, therefore, of great interest that enzymes with elastolytic activity are capable of inducing emphysema (146). Elastin is an extraordinarily stable macromolecule and, under normal circumstances, may be stable throughout the lifetime of an adult individual. For example, Shapiro and colleagues used two methods to estimate the lifetime of elastin in adults (147). Taking advantage of the fact that only levo-aspartic acid is incorporated into macromolecules but that aspartic acid undergoes a very slow epimerization, the relative presence of the dextro form of aspartic acid was measured in elastin samples obtained from lungs at autopsy. A very slow and gradual accumulation of d-aspartic acid was noted which appeared to be linear throughout the lifetime of individuals, increasing from approximately 10% at age 20 to 15% at age 80. A second method, taking advantage of the increase in environmental $[^{14}C]$ associated with nuclear weapons testing provided confirmatory data. With this method, the percentage of $[^{14}C]$ in elastin within the lungs corresponded to the environmental $[^{14}C]$ levels during lung development and was independent of age. These results suggest that elastin is deposited within the lung during development and growth and then remains throughout an individual's lifetime.

These results, however, do not preclude a role for abnormal repair processes in the development of emphysema. First, turnover of a small percentage of lung elastin may not have been observed with the methods used by Shapiro and colleagues. More importantly, both in vitro and in vivo studies suggest that elastin fibers can undergo repair following injury. In this context, Stone and colleagues demonstrated that elastin fibers partially degraded and rendered soluble by elastase exposure can be repolymerized and rendered insoluble through the action of cellular repair mechanisms (148). Similarly, morphological disruption of elastin fibers caused by elastase exposure in vitro can be reversed in cell culture (148,149). These observations suggest that repair of elastin fibers can be mediated not only by the de novo synthesis of new tropoelastin monomers, but also by the "salvage" of partially damaged extracellular elastin as well.

The concept that repair plays a role in the development of emphysema is also supported by animal model studies. In this context, induction of emphysema with elastase can result in an initial decrease in elastin content (146). Elastin synthesis, however, is stimulated by elastase exposure, and after an initial decrease, elastin concentrations can return to near-normal levels (150,151). Other macromolecules may be similarly affected. In this regard, collagen synthesis is also stimulated by elastase exposure (152). Moreover, several studies suggest that collagen concentrations within the lung may increase with mild emphysema (153–155) and there may be focal collagen accumulations (156). Presumably this could represent part of an attempt at tissue repair following injury. Whether the accumulation of such fibrotic material compromises lung function remains to be determined.

The normal lung is characterized by the presence of numerous alveolar pores (157). While these pores may provide for collateral ventilation between alveoli (158), in many cases these pores are likely covered by surfactant (159). The physiological significance of these structures, therefore, remains controversial. The observation that pore size increases with age (159) and with the development of emphysema has suggested that these structures may represent the earliest lesions of emphysema (160–163). The mechanisms by which pores may be repaired remain to be defined. Type II alveolar epithelial cells, however, can be observed at the margins of pores (164). The fact that these cells are believed to be both the precursor of all alveolar epithelial cells (165) and the major cells responsible for both routine metabolic activity and repair within the alveoli is suggestive that repair of pores can take place (166).

The concept that repair of emphysema can occur in vivo was established by Massaro and Massaro. In rats following elastase-induced emphysema, retinoic acid is capable of inducing new alveolar wall formation (167), although lung function is not restored completely. Retinoic acid is thought to be a key mediator signaling alveolarization during development (168). The degree to which alveolar repair following experimental emphysema recapitulates developmental events is unestablished.

C. Defective Repair and Emphysema

Several lines of evidence suggest that defects in repair mechanisms can contribute to the formation of emphysema. In this regard, blocking the activity of lysyloxidase by the administration of either the inhibitor β-amino proprionitrile or penicillamine exacerbates the formation of elastase-induced emphysema (169). Rendering animals copper deficient can also block lysyloxidase activity as copper is a required cofactor, and this deficiency can also lead to emphysema in rats (170) and pigs (171).

Starvation is also associated with both the development and worsening of emphysema. Human studies in the Warsaw ghetto suggest that starvation per se may lead to development of emphysema in humans (172). Animal studies support a role for starvation in altering lung structure both in developing (173–175) and adult animals (162,176). Starvation, moreover, can significantly exacerbate the emphysema induced by elastase exposure (177). In mice, mechanisms leading to starvation-associated loss of alveolar wall may be activated within hours of calorie restriction. Lymphocyte elaboration of granzyme A and B may play a role in this process (178).

Severe emphysema is often associated with significant weight loss. Interestingly, undernourished individuals with COPD are much more likely to have significant emphysema, as manifest by reduction in diffusion capacity, than are individuals with similar degrees of airflow associated with normal or excessive body weight (179). Weight loss in COPD, moreover, is generally regarded as a poor prognostic factor (180,181). Increased work of breathing consequent to the physiological abnormalities characterizing COPD has been suggested as one explanation for the weight loss in COPD (182). The weight loss, however, may be associated with a generalized catabolic, or at least non-anabolic, state. This could lead to ineffective repair mechanisms and could be associated with worsening emphysema.

It is also possible that the weight loss per se could be associated with the inflammatory processes associated with COPD. In this context, while controversial (183,184), elevated levels of circulating TNF-α have been reported in individuals with COPD (185) and, in particular, with associated weight loss (186). Similarly, monocytes isolated from individuals with COPD and associated weight loss have been reported to have increased production of TNF in response to standard stimuli (187). Increased levels of TNF-α have been reported in the induced sputum (188) and airway wall (189) of patients with COPD. In the airways, TNF-α is thought to be an early step leading to amplification of inflammatory response by driving the production of other mediators such as interleukin (IL)-8. Circulating TNF-α could contribute to weight loss, as TNF-α is generally regarded as a cachectic factor. Interestingly, administration of TNF interperitoneally has been associated with the development of emphysema (190). In this regard, TNF-α is generally an inhibitor of fibroblast pro-fibrotic responses (121,191,192). It is possible, therefore, that, among its other actions, TNF-α may contribute to the development of emphysema by inhibiting repair response.

D. Cigarette Smoke

The most important risk factor for the development of COPD is cigarette smoke. Smoke can affect the lungs in many ways, increasing inflammation and compromising antioxidant and antiprotease protective mechanisms. Smoke can also adversely affect repair mechanisms. Inflammation induced by cigarette smoke could lead to the production of cytokines such as TNF-α that could affect repair as described above. In addition, similar to the insults described above, cigarette smoke can inhibit the activity of lysyl-oxidase (193). Consistent with this, cigarette smoke exposure in amounts insufficient to cause emphysema has been associated with inhibition of elastin biosynthesis and accumulation in the first week following elastase exposure (194) and has been reported to lead to worsening of emphysema over a 6-month interval following exposure in animal models (195).

Cigarette smoke can also directly affect the cells that participate in repair. In this context, cigarette smoke inhibits fibroblast chemotaxis, proliferation (196), matrix production, and contraction of extracellular collagenous gels (197). Smoke similarly inhibits airways epithelial chemotaxis and proliferation (198,199). Cigarette smoke inhibits VEGF expression in an in vitro culture system (200). Moreover, oxidant injury contributes to the apoptosis and emphysema that develops following VEGF blockade, suggesting that smoke may exacerbate this mechanism as well (201).

E. Other Agents

Other agents associated with emphysema may also compromise repair processes. Cadmium exposure has been associated with the development of emphysema (202,203). Interestingly, the role of inflammation in cadmium-associated emphysema has not been well established. Cadmium, however, like cigarette smoke, is capable of inhibiting fibroblast responses including proliferation (204), matrix molecule production (204,205), and contraction of three-dimensional collagen gels (206). Cadmium, therefore, may also contribute to the development of emphysema, at least in part, by inhibiting repair responses. Cadmium may be related to smokers' emphysema, as increased cadmium levels have been noted in smokers and are associated with increased risk of COPD (207).

Taken together, these observations suggest that smoke may contribute to the development of emphysema, not only by initiating inflammatory responses leading to tissue destruction, but also by compromising repair responses which may serve to mitigate damage.

V. Overview of the American Hypothesis

A. Normal, Defective, and Excessive Repair

The studies reviewed above support the concept that the lung is a dynamic organ in which tissue turnover is required for the maintenance of normal structure and increased repair can take place following injury. If such repair processes are adequate, tissue structure and function can be maintained in the face of injurious insults. However, defective repair could contribute to the development of the anatomical lesions that contribute to airflow limitation in COPD.

Of the lesions contributing to fixed airflow limitation, two are believed to be most important. Tissue destruction with loss of lung elastic recoil is the major mechanism by which emphysema causes airflow limitation (6). This lesion is frequently of paramount importance, particularly in severe disease, as evidenced by autopsy studies (208,209). In patients with milder disease, however, bronchiolar narrowing associated with peribronchiolar fibrosis plays a prominent role (128,129,208–210). This suggests the possibility that individuals with COPD may have several distinct anatomical processes. It is possible, therefore, that one process may account for the physiological abnormalities at one time during the course of a patient's illness, while a different process may supervene at a later time.

This also raises a interesting paradox: how can inadequate repair, such as develops in emphysema, be caused by the same factors and be present together with excessive repair, such as airway fibrosis. This may depend on subtle differences at different tissue sites. In this context, normal repair may be a fine balance between fibrosis and tissue loss. As noted above, bleomycin is widely used to induce pulmonary fibrosis, but causes emphysema in α_1-deficient mice (134). That this balance can be modified is also supported by the observations that KGF (139) and HGF (138) can mitigate lung damage and that prostaglandin E, which generally inhibits mesenchymal cells in repair (120,211–213), stimulates epithelial cells (51). This concept is further supported by the observation of Smad3-deficient mice. These animals have defective TGF-β-induced signaling, a process thought to contribute to the development of fibrosis. But, although the lung has not been studied, have accelerated epithelial repair in the skin (214). Interestingly, cigarette smoke can inhibit repair processes in both epithelial cells and fibroblasts. In the latter, however, the effects of smoke are density dependent. At high cell densities, cigarette smoke can lead to activation of latent TGF-β and thus could also be profibrotic under some conditions (215).

B.   Cells, Involved in Repair

The relationships among differentiated cells in the lung, committed progenitor cells, and multipotent stem cells is undefined. However, pluripotential stem cells are present in the lung and can, under experimental conditions, be induced to form nonpulmonary tissues such as the formed elements of blood (216). Precursor cells capable of differentiation have been described in the ducts of airway glands (38) and in defined sites in small airways (217,218). The cells present in the normal airway are also capable of undergoing both proliferation and differentiation. In the airways, both basal cells (219) and columnar cells (220) have been suggested to have precursor functions. In the small airways, Clara cells (40), and in the alveoli, type II cells (165,221), are thought to serve this function. Circulating stem cells can also be recruited into the lung (222–225) and have been reported to contribute to alveolar and airway epithelial cells as well as to endothelial cells and tissue mesenchymal cells. Recruitment of donor cells into lung parenchyma has been reported in humans following bone marrow transplantation (226). Interestingly, although not uniformly observed, type I cells derived from circulating stem cells have been reported in the absence of stem cell-derived type II cells (225,227), calling into question the precursor-progeny relationship between these cell types. Ortiz et al. noted that transplantation of stem cells could alter the response to bleomycin (228). That several sources of cells may participate in repair following injury in the lung raises some interesting possibilities. Specifically, repair mediated by locally recruited precursor cells may have very different pathophysiological consequences than repair mediated by stem cells recruited from the circulation or other sites.

C.   Potential for Therapeutic Intervention

The concept that disrupted repair contributes to the development of airflow limitation suggests several potential therapeutic approaches. Stimulation of epithelial repair may be able to restore function following injurious insults. Similarly, stimulation of alveolar wall formation could slow or even reverse the development of emphysema. Conversely, inhibition of repair mechanisms may prevent the development of peribronchial fibrosis. As the molecular and cellular mechanisms that underlie repair and remodeling become better defined, potential targets for intervention will be identified.

The successful development of such therapies will require maintaining the balance between excessive and inadequate repair, either of which could have adverse consequences. The development of such therapies, however, would have great utility to slow or reverse the progressive natural history of COPD.

References

1. Celli BR, Snider GL, Heffner J, Tiep B, Ziment I, Make B, Braman S, Olsen G, Phillips Y. Standards for the diagnosis and care of patients with chronic obstructive pulmonary disease. Am J Respir Crit Care Med 1995; 152:S77–S120.
2. Siafakas, NM, Vermeire P, Pride NB, Paoletti P, Gibson J, Howard P, Yernault JC, Decramer M, Higenbottam T, Postma DS, Rees J. Optimal assessment and management of chronic obstructive pulmonary disease (COPD). Eur Respir J 1995; 8:1398–1420.
3. Peat JK, Woolcock AJ, Cullen K. Rate of decline of lung function in subjects with asthma. Eur J Respir Dis 1987; 70:171–179.
4. Lange P, Parner J, Vestbo J, Schnor P, Jensen G. A 15-year follow-up study of ventilatory function in adults with asthma. N Engl J Med 1998; 339:1194–1200.
5. Global Strategy for the Diagnosis, Management, and Prevention of Chronic Obstructive Pulmonary Disease. 2003,
6. Niewoehner DE. Anatomic and pathophysiological correlations in COPD. In: Baum GL et al. eds. Textbook of Pulmonary Diseases. Philadelphia: Lippincott-Raven, 1998: 823–842.
7. Orie NG, Sluiter HJ, DeVries K, Tammeling GJ, Witkop J. The host factor in bronchitis. In: Orie NGM, Sluiter HJ, eds. Bronchitis, An International Symposium. Assen, Netherlands, 1961: 43–59.
8. Burrows B. Airways obstructive disease: pathogenetic mechanisms and natural histories of the disorders. Med Clin North Am 1990; 74:547–560.
9. Tashkin DP, Altose MD, Connett JE, Kanner RE, Lee WW, Wise RA. Methacholine reactivity predicts changes in lung function over time in smokers with early chronic obstructive pulmonary disease. Am J Respir Crit Care Med 1996; 153:1802–1811.
10. Ulrik CS, Backer V. Nonreversible airflow obstruction in life-long nonsmokers with moderate to severe asthma. Eur Respir J 1999; 14:892–6.
11. Fletcher C, Peto R, Tinker C, Speizer FE. The Natural History of Chronic Bronchitis and Emphysema. New York: Oxford University Press, 1976: 1–272.
12. Vestbo J, Prescott E, Lange P. Association of chronic mucus hypersecretion with FEV_1 decline and chronic obstructive pulmonary disease morbidity. Am J Respir Crit Care Med 1996; 153:1530–1535.
13. Donaldson GC, Seemungal TAR, Bhowmik A, Wedzicha JA. Relationship between exacerbation frequency and lung function decline in chronic obstructive pulmonary disease. Thorax 2002; 57:847–852.

14. Paupe J. Immunotherapy with an oral bacterial extract (OM-85 BV) for upper respiratory infections. Respiration 1991; 58:150–154.
15. Martin RJ, Pak J, Moore EG. Overnight theophylline concentrations and effects on sleep and lung function in chronic obstructive pulmonary disease. Am Rev Respir Dis 1992; 145:540–544.
16. McElvaney NG, Crystal RG. Proteases and lung injury. In: Crystal RG, West JB, eds. The Lung: Scientific Foundations. Philadelphia: Lippincott-Raven, 1997: 2205–2218.
17. McElvaney NG, Crystal RG. Antiproteases and lung defense. In: Crystal RG, et al., eds. The Lung: Scientific Foundations. Philadelphia: Lippincott-Raven, 1997: 2219–2235.
18. Lucey EC, Stone PJ, Snider GL. Consequences of proteolytic injury. In: Crystal RG, et al., eds. The Lung: Scientific Foundations. Philadelphia: Lippincott-Raven, 1997; 2237–2250.
19. Hautamaki, RD, Kobayashi DK, Senior RM, Shapiro SD. Requirement for macrophage elastase for cigarette smoke-induced emphysema in mice. Science 1997; 277:2002–2004.
20. Rahman I, MacNee W. Role of oxidants/antioxidants in smoking induced lung disease. Free Radic Biol Med 1996; 21:669–681.
21. Brassart B, Randoux A, Hornebeck W, Emonard H. Regulation of matrix metalloproteinase-2 (gelatinase A, MMP-2), membrane type matrix metallo-proteinase-1 (MT1-MMP) and tissue inhibitor of metalloproteinases-2 (TIMP-2) expression by elastin derived peptides in human HT-1080 fibrosarcoma cell line. Clin Exp Metastasis 1998; 16:489–500.
22. Nadel JA. Role of neutrophil elastase in hypersecretion during COPD exacerbations, and proposed therapies. Chest 2000; 117:386S–389S.
23. Liebow AA. Pulmonary emphysema with special reference to vascular changes. Am Rev Respir Dis 1959; 80:67–93.
24. Rennard SI. COPD: overview of definitions, epidemiology and factors influencing its development. Chest 1998; 113:235S–241S.
25. Wilhelm DL. Regeneration of tracheal epithelium. J Pathol Bacteriol 1953; 55:543–550.
26. Lane BP, Gordon R. Regeneration of rat tracheal epithelium after mechanical injury. Exp Biol Med 1974; 145:1139–1144.
27. Keenan KP, Combs JW, McDowell EM. Regeneration of hamster tracheal epithelium after mechanical injury. Virchows Arch 1982; 41:193–214.
28. Shimizu T, Nishihara M, Kawaguchi S, Sakakura Y. Expression of phenotypic markers during regeneration of rat tracheal epithelium following mechanical injury. Am J Respir Cell Mol Biol 1994; 11:85–94.
29. Erjefalt JS, Persson CG. Airway epithelial repair: breathtakingly quick and multipotentially pathogenic. Thorax 1997; 52:1010–1012.
30. Boers JE. Composition and Proliferation of Normal Human Tracheobronchial Mucosa. Maastricht: Masstricht Universitaire Pers, 1997: 134.
31. Persson CGA, Erjefalt JS, Andersson M, Greiff L, Svensson C. Extravasation, lamina propria flooding ande lumenal entry of bulk plasma

exudate in mucosal defence, inflammation and repair. Pulm Pharmacol 1996; 9:129–139.

32. Lane BP, Gordon R. Regeneration of rat tracheal epithelium after mechanical injury. Proc Soc Exp Biol Med 1974; 145:1139–1144.

33. Erjefalt J. Airway Epithelial Shedding: Morphological and Functional Aspects In Vivo. Lund, Sweden, 1996.

34. McDowell EM, Newkirk C, Coleman B. Development of hamster tracheal epithelium: I. A quantitative morphologic study in the fetus. Anat Rec 1985; 213:429–447.

35. Plopper CG, Alley JL, Weir AJ. Differentiation of tracheal epithelium during fetal lung maturation in the rhesus monkey *Macaca mulatta*. Am J Anat 1986; 175:59–71.

36. Plopper CG, Mariassy AT, Wilson DW, Alley JL, Nishio SJ, Nettesheim P. Comparison of nonciliated tracheal epithelial cells in six mammalian species: ultrastructure and population densities. Exp Lung Res 1983; 5:281–294.

37. Robbins RA, Rennard SI. Biology of airway epithelial cells. In: Crystal RG, et al. (eds) The Lung: Scientific Foundations Second Edition, Philadelphia: Lippincott-Raven, 1997: 445–457.

38. Borthwick DW, Shahbazian M, Krantz QT, Dorin JR, Randell SH. Evidence for stem-cell niches in the tracheal epithelium. Am J Respir Cell Mol Biol 2001; 24:662–670.

39. Brody AR, Hook GER, Cameron GS, Jetten AM, Butterick CJ, Nettesheim P. The differentiation capacity of Clara cells isolated from the lungs of rabbits. Lab Invest 1987; 57:219.

40. Hook GER, Brody AR, Cameron GS, Jetten AM, Gilmore LB, Nettesheim P. Repopulation of denuded tracheas by Clara cells isolated from the lungs of rabbits. Exp Lung Res 1987; 12:311–329.

41. Shoji S, Ertl RF, Linder J, Koizumi S, Duckworth WC, Rennard SI. Bronchial epithelial cells respond to insulin and insulin-like growth factor-I as a chemoattractant. Am J Respir Cell Mol Biol 1990; 2:53–557.

42. Shoji S, Ertl RF, Linder J, Romberger DJ, Rennard SI. Bronchial epithelial cells produce chemotactic activity for bronchial epithelial cells: possible role for fibronectin in airway repair. Am Rev Respir Dis 1990; 141:218–225.

43. Rickard KA, Taylor J, Rennard SI, Spurzem JR. Migration of bovine bronchial epithelial cells to extracellular matrix components. Am J Respir Cell Mol Biol 1993; 8:63–68.

44. Roberts AB, Sporn MB, Assoian RK, Smith JM, Roche NS, Wakefield LM, Heine UI, Liotta LA, Falanga V, Kehrl JH, Fauci AS. Transforming growth factor type beta: rapid induction of fibrosis and angiogenesis in vivo and stimulation of collagen formation in vitro. Proc Natl Acad Sci USA 1986; 83:4167–4171.

45. Roberts AB. Molecular and cell biology of TGF-beta. Miner Electrolyte Metab 1998 24:111–119.

46. Sacco O, Romberger D, Rizzino A, Beckmann J, Rennard SI, Spurzem JR. Spontaneous production of transforming growth factor beta 2 by primary

culture of bronchial epithelial cells: effects on cell behavior in vitro. J Clin Invest 1992; 90:1379–1385.

47. Mio T, Liu X, Adachi Y, Striz I, Skold CM, Romberger DJ, Spurzem JR, Illig MG, Ertl R, Rennard SI. Human bronchial epithelial cells modulate collagen gel contraction by fibroblasts. Am J Phys 1998; 274:L119–L126.

48. Romberger DJ, Beckmann JD, Claassen L, Ertl RF, Rennard SI. Modulation of fibronectin production of bovine bronchial epithelial cells by transforming growth factor-beta. Am J Respir Cell Mol Biol 1992; 7:149–155.

49. Wang A, Cohen DS, Palmer E, Sheppard D. Polarized regulation of fibronectin secretion and alternative splicing by transforming growth factor. J Biol Chem 1991; 266:15558–15560.

50. Ruoslahti E. Fibronectin and its receptors. Annu Rev Biochem 1988; 57:375–413.

51. Savla U, Appel HJ, Sporn PH, Waters CM. Prostaglandin E(2) regulates wound closure in airway epithelium. Am J Physiol Lung Cell Mol Physiol 2001; 280:L421–431.

52. Kim JS, McKinnis VS, White SR. Migration of guinea pig airway epithelial cells in response to bombesin analogues. Am J Respir Cell Mol Biol 1997; 16:259–266.

53. Kim JS, McKinnis VS, Adams K, White SR. Proliferation and repair of guinea pig tracheal epithelium after neuropeptide depletion and injury in vivo. Am J Physiol 1997; 273:L1235–1241.

54. Erjefalt JS, Erjefalt I, Sundler F, Persson CGA. Microcirculation-derived factors in airway epithelial repair in vivo. Microvasc Res 1994; 48:161–178.

55. Zahm JM, Chevillard M, Puchelle E. Wound repair of human surface respiratory epithelium. Am J Respir Cell Mol Biol 1991; 5:242–248.

56. Herard AL, Zahm JM, Pierrot D, Hinnrasky J, Fuchey C, Puchelle E. Epithelial barrier integrity during in vitro wound repair of the airway epithelium. Am J Respir Cell Mol Biol 1996; 15:624–632.

57. Kim JS, McKinnis VS, Nawrocki A, White SR. Stimulation of migration and wound repair of guinea-pig airway epithelial cells in response to epidermal growth factor. Am J Respir Cell Mol Biol 1998; 18:66–74.

58. Puddicombe SM, Polosa R, Richter A, Krishna MT, Howarth PH, Holgate ST, Davies DE. Involvement of the epidermal growth factor receptor in epithelial repair in asthma. FASEB J 2000; 14:1362–1374.

59. Ito H, Rennard SI, Spurzem JR. Mononuclear cell conditioned medium enhances bronchial epithelial cell migration but inhibits attachment to fibronectin. J Lab Clin Med 1996; 127:494–503.

60. Zahm JM, Debordeaux C, Raby B, Klossek JM, Bonnet N, Puchelle E. Motogenic effect of recombinant HGF on airway epithelial cells during the in vitro wound repair of the respiratory epithelium. J Cell Physiol 2000; 185:447–453.

61. Waters CM, Savla U. Keratinocyte growth factor accelerates wound closure in airway epithelium during cyclic mechanical strain. J Cell Physiol 1999; 181:424–432.

62. Rickard KA, Taylor J, Spurzem JR, Rennard SI. Extracellular matrix and bronchial epithelial cell migration. Chest 1992; 01:17S–18S.
63. Yokosaki Y, Matsuura N, Sasaki T, Murakami I, Schneider H, Higashiyama S, Saitoh Y, Yamakido M, Taooka Y, Sheppard D. The integrin alpha(9)beta(1) binds to a novel recognition sequence (SVVYGLR) in the thrombin-cleaved amino-terminal fragment of osteopontin. J Biol Chem 1999; 274:36328–36334.
64. Dunsmore SE, Saarialho-Kere UK, Roby JD, Wilson CL, Matrisian LM, Welgus HG, Parks WC. Matrilysin expression and function in airway epithelium. J Clin Invest 1998; 102:1321–1331.
65. Buissson AC, Gilles C, Polette M, Zahm JM, Birembaut P, Tournier JM. Wound repair-induced expression of a stromelysins is associated with the acquisition of a mesenchymal phenotype in human respiratory epithelial cells. Lab Invest 1996; 74:658–669.
66. Legrand C, Gilles C, Zahm JM, Polette M, Buisson AC, Kaplan H, Birembaut P, Tournier JM. Airway epithelial cell migration dynamics. MMP-9 role in cell-extracellular matrix remodeling. J Cell Biol 1999; 146:517–529.
67. de Bentzmann S, Polette M, Zahm JM, Hinnrasky J, Kileztky C, Bajolet O, Klossek JM, Filloux A, Lazdunski A, Puchelle E. *Pseudomonas aeruginosa* virulence factors delay airway epithelial wound repair by altering the actin cytoskeleton and inducing overactivation of epithelial matrix metalloproteinase-2. Lab Invest 2000; 80:209–219.
68. Legrand C, Polette M, Tournier JM, de Bentzmann S, Huet E, Monteau M, Birembaut P. uPA/plasmin system-mediated MMP-9 activation is implicated in bronchial epithelial cell migration. Exp Cell Res 2001; 264:326–363.
69. Erjefalt JS, Erjefalt I, Sundler F, Persson GA. In vivo restitution of airway epithelium. Cell Tissue Res 1995; 281:305–316.
70. Stoker M. Effect of scatter factor on motility of epithelial cells and fibroblasts. J Cell Physiol 1989; 139:565–569.
71. White SR, Dorscheid DR, Rabe KF, Wojcik KR, Hamann KJ. Role of very late adhesion integrins in mediating repair of human airway epithelial cell monolayers after mechanical injury. Am J Respir Cell Mol Biol 1999; 20:787–796.
72. Pilewski JM, Latoche JD, Arcasoy SM, Albelda SM. Expression of integrin cell adhesion receptors during human airway epithelial repair in vivo. Am J Physiol 1997; 273:L256–263.
73. Munger JS, Huang X, Kawakatsu H, Griffiths MJ, Dalton SL, Wu J, et al. The integrin alpha $\alpha v \beta 6$ binds and activates latent TGF beta 1: a mechanism for regulating pulmonary inflammation and fibrosis. Cell 1999; 96:319–328.
74. Herard AL, Pierrot D, Hinnrasky J, Kaplan H, Sheppard D, Puchelle E, Zahm JM. Fibronectin and its alpha 5 beta 1-integrin receptor are involved in the wound-repair process of airway epithelium. Am J Physiol 196; 21:L726–L733.

75. Leir SH, Baker JE, Holgate ST, Lackie PM. Increased CD44 expression in human bronchial epithelial repair after damage or plating at low cell densities. Am J Physiol Lung Cell Mol Physiol 2000; 278:L1129–L1137.

76. de Bentzmann S, Roger P, Puchelle E. *Pseudomonas aeruginosa* adherence to remodelling respiratory epithelium. Eur Respir J 1996; 9:2145–2150.

77. Striz I, Mio T., Adachi Y, Heires P, Robbins RA, Spurzem JR, Illig MJ, Romberger DJ, Rennard SI. IL-4 induces ICAM-1 expression in human bronchial epithelial cells and potentiates TNF-α. Am J Physiol 1999; 277:L58–L64.

78. DeRose V, Robbins RA, Snider RM, Spurzem JR, Thiele GM, Rennard SI, Rubinstein I. Substance P increases neutrophil adhesion to bronchial epithelial cells. J Immunol 1994; 152:1339–1346.

79. Shoji S, Rickard KA, Takizawa H, Ertl RF, Linder J, Rennard SI. Lung fibroblasts produce growth stimulatory activity for bronchial epithelial cells. Am Rev Respir Dis 1990; 141:433–439.

80. Tsao MS, Zhu H, Viallet J. Autocrine growth loop of the epidermal growth factor receptor in normal and immortalized human bronchial epithelial cells. Exp Cell Res 1996; 223:268–273.

81. Tsao MS, Zhu H, Giaid A, Viallet J, Nakamura T, Park M. Hepatocyte growth factor/scatter factor is an autocrine factor for human normal bronchial epithelial and lung carcinoma cells. Cell Growth Differ 1993; 4:571–579.

82. Takizawa H, Beckmann J, Shoji S, Classen LR, Ertl RF, Linder J, Rennard SI. Pulmonary macrophages can stimulate cell growth of bovine bronchial epithelial cells. Am J Respir Cell Mol Biol 1990; 2:245–255.

83. Jetten AM, Vollberg TM, Nervi C, George MD. Positive and negative regulation of proliferation and differentiation in tracheobronchial epithelial cells. Am Rev Respir Dis 1990; 142:S36–S39.

84. Oyamada H, Kayaba H, Kamada Y, Kuwasaki T, Yamada Y, Kobayashi Y, Cui C, Honda K, Saito N, Chihara J. An optimal condition of bronchial cell proliferation stimulated by insulin-like growth factor-I. Int Arch Allergy Immunol 2000; 122(suppl 1):59–62.

85. Aoshiba K, Rennard SI, S. JR. Fibronectin supports bronchial epithelial cell adhesion and survival in the absence of growth factors. Am J Phys 1997; 273:L684–693.

86. Whitcutt MJ, Adler KB, Wu R. A biphasic chamber system for maintaining polarity of differentiation of cultured respiratory tract epithelial cells. In Vitro Cell Dev Biol 1988; 24:420.

87. Takeyama K, Dabbagh K, Lee HM, Agusti C, Lausier JA, Ueki IF, Grattan KM, Nadel JA. Epidermal growth factor system regulates mucin production in airways. Proc Natl Acad Sci USA 1999; 96:3081–3086.

88. Guzman K, Randell SH, Nettesheim P. Epidermal growth factor regulates expression of the mucous phenotype of rat tracheal epithelial cells. Biochem Biophys Res Commun 1995; 217:412–418.

89. Hill AT, Bayley D, Stockley RA. The interrelationship of sputum inflammatory markers in patients with chronic bronchitis. Am J Respir Crit Care Med 1999; 160:893–889.

90. Takeyama K, Dabbagh K, Jeong Shim J, Dao-Pick T, Ueki IF, Nadel JA. Oxidative stress causes mucin synthesis via transactivation of epidermal growth factor receptor: role of neutrophils. J Immunol 2000; 164:1546–1552.

91. Vesely KR, Hyde DM, Stovall MY, Harkema JR, Green JF, Schelegle ES. Capsaicin-sensitive C-fiber-mediated protective responses in ozone inhalation in rats. J Appl Physiol 1999; 86:951–962.

92. Shoji S, Rickard KA, Ertl RF, Robbins RA, Linder J, Rennard SI. Bronchial epithelial cells produce lung fibroblast chemotactic factor: fibronectin. Am J Respir Cell Mol Biol 1989; 1:13–20.

93. Harrison NK, Dawes KE, Kwon OJ, Barnes PJ, Laurent GJ, Chung KF. Effects of neuropeptides on human lung fibroblast proliferation and chemotaxis. Am J Physiol 1995; 268:L278–L283.

94. Endo T, Uchida Y, Matsumoto H, Suzuki N, Nomura A, Hirata F, Hasegawa S. Regulation of endothelin-1 synthesis in cultured guinea pig airway epithelial cells by various cytokines. Biochem Biophys Res Commun 1992; 14:1594–1599.

95. Shimizu S, Gabazza EC, Hayashi T, Ido M, Adachi Y, Suzuki K. Thrombin stimulates the expression of PDGF in lung epithelial cells. Am J Physiol Lung Cell Mol Physiol 2000:L503–510.

96. Varga J, Rosenbloom J, Jimenez SA. Transforming growth factor beta (TGF beta) causes a persistent increase in steady-state amounts of type I and III collagen and fibronectin mRNAs in normal human dermal fibroblasts. J Biochem 1987; 247:597–604.

97. Postlethwaite AE, Keski-Oja J, Balian G, Kang AH. Induction of fibroblast chemotaxis by fibronectin: Localization of the chemotactic region to a 140,000 molecular weight non-gelatin binding fragment. J Exp Med 1980; 153:494–499.

98. Gauss-Muller E, Kleinman HK, Martin GR, Schiffmann E. Role of attachment factors and attractants in fibroblast chemotaxis. J Lab Clin Med 1980; 96:1071–1080.

99. Cardoso WV. Molecular regulation of lung development. Annu Rev Physiol 2001; 63:471–494.

100. Holgate ST, Davies DE, Lackie PM, Wilson SJ, Puddicombe SM, Lordan JL. Epithelial-mesenchymal interactions in the pathogenesis of asthma. J Allergy Clin Immunol 2000; 104:193–204.

101. Hicks W Jr, Sigurdson L, Gabalski E, Hard R, Hall L, 3rd, Gardella J, Powers C, Kumar N, Lwebuga-Mukasa J. Does cartilage down-regulate growth factor expression in tracheal epithelium? Arch Otolaryngol Head Neck Surg 1999; 125:1239–1243.

102. Vignola, AM, Chanez P, Chiappara G, Merendino A, Pace E, Rizzo A, la-Rocca AM, Bellia V, Bonsignore G, Bousquet J. Transforming growth

factor-beta expression in mucosal biopsies in asthama and chronic bronchitis. Am J Respir Crit Care Med 1997; 156:591–599.

103. Aubert J-D, Dalal BI, Bai TR, Roberts CR, Hayashi S, Hogg JC. Transforming growth factor beta-1 gene expression in human airways. Thorax 1994; 49:225–232.

104. Romberger D, Daughton D, Claassen L, Ertl R, Ghafouri M, Robbins RA, Von Essen SG, Thompson AB, Rennard SI. Increased fibronectin in bronchial lavage fluid of chronic bronchitis. Am Rev Respir Dis 1992; 145:A761.

105. Sofia M, Mormile M, Faraone S, Carratu P, Alifano M, Di Benedetto G, Carratu L. Increased 24-hour endothelin-1 urinary excretion in patients with chronic obstructive pulmonary disease. Respiration 1994; 61:263–268.

106. Chalmers GW, Macleod KJ, Sriram S, Thomson LJ, McSharry C, Stack BH, Thomson NC. Sputum endothelin-1 is increased in cystic fibrosis and chronic obstructive pulmonary disease. Eur Respir J 1999; 13:1288–1292.

107. Tomaki M, Ichinose M, Miura M, Hirayama Y, Yamauchi H, Nakajima N, Shirato K. Elevated substance P content in induced sputum from patients with asthma and patients with chronic bronchitis. Am J Respir Crit Care Med 1995; 151:613–617.

108. Chanez P, Springall D, Vignola AM, Moradoghi-Hattvani A, Polak JM, Godard P, Bousquet J. Bronchial mucosal immunoreactivity of sensory neuropeptides in severe airway diseases. Am J Respir Crit Care Med 1998; 158:985–990.

109. Sofia M, Maniscalco M. Endothelin in acute exacerbations of COPD. Thorax 2001; 56:819.

110. Polzin A, Pletz M, Erbes R, Raffenberg M, Mauch H, Wagner S, Arndt G, Lode H. Procalcitonin as a diagnostic tool in lower respiratory tract infections and tuberculosis. Eur Respir J 2003; 21:939–943.

111. Takuwa N, Takuwa Y, Yanagisawa M, Yamashita K, Masaki T. A novel vasoactive peptide endothelin stimulates mitogenesis through inositol lipid turnover in Swiss 3T3 fibroblasts. J Biol Chem 1989; 264:7856–7861.

112. Peacock AJ, Shock A, Gray AJ, Reeves JT, Chmabers R, Laurent GJ. The effect of endothelin-1 on the growth and chemotaxis of fibroblasts. Eur Respir J 1990; 3:336S.

113. Ziche M, Morbidelli L, Pacini M, Dolara P, Maggi CA. NK1-receptors mediate the proliferative response of human fibroblasts to tachykinins. Br J Pharmacol 1990; 100:11–14.

114. Kahler CM, Herold M, Wiedermann CJ. Substance P: a competence factor for human fibroblast proliferation that induces the release of growth-regulatory arachidonic acid metabolites. J Cell Physiol 1993; 156:579–587.

115. Philpps RP, Borrello MA, Blieden TM. Fibroblast heterogeneity in the periodontium and other tissues. J Periodont Res 1997; 32:159–165.

116. Torry DJ, Richards CD, Podor TJ, Gauldie J. Anchorage-independent colony growth of pulmonary fibroblasts derived from fibrotic human lung tissue. J Clin Invest 1994; 93:1525–1532.

117. Botstein GR, Sherer GK, Leroy EC. Fibroblast selection in scleroderma. Arthritis Rheum 1982; 25:189–195.
118. Torry DJ, Richards CD, Podor TJ, Gauldie J. Modulation of the anchorage-independent phynotype of human lung fibroblasts obtained from fibrotic tissue following culture with retinoid and corticosteriod. Exp Lung Res 1996; 22:231–244.
119. Kawamoto M, Matsunami T, Ertl RF, Fukuda Y, Ogawa M, Spurzem JR, Yamanaka N, Rennard SI. Selective migration of α-smooth muscle actin-positive myofibroblasts toward fibronectin in the Boyden's blindwell chamber. Clin Sci 1997; 93:355–362.
120. Bitterman PB, Wewers MD, Rennard SI, Adelberg S, Crystal RG. Modulation of alveolar macrophage-driven fibroblast proliferation by alternative macrophage mediators. J Clin Invest 1986; 77:700–708.
121. Diaz A, Munoz E, Johnston R, Korn JH, Jimenez SA. Regulation of human lung fibroblast alpha 1 procollagen gene expression by tumor necrosis factor alpha, interleukin-1 beta, and prostaglandin E2. J Biol Chem 1993; 268:10364–10371.
122. Sempowski GD, Derdak S, Phipps RP. Interleukin-4 and interferon-gamma discordantly regulate collagen biosynthesis by functionally distinct lung fibroblast subsets. J Cell Physiol 1996; 167:290–296.
123. Epler GR, Colby T, McLoud TC, Carrington CB, Gaensler EA. Bronchiolitis obliterans organizing pneumonia. N Engl J Med 1985; 312:152–158.
124. Costabel U, Guzman J, Teschler H. Bronchiolitis obliterans with organizing pneumonia: outcome. Thorax 1995; 50:S59–S64.
125. King TE. Bronchiolitis. In: Schwarz MI, King TE, eds. Interstitial Lung Disease. St. Louis, MO, Mosby-Year Book, 1993:463–495.
126. Kawamoto M, Romberger DJ, Nakamura Y, Tate L, Ertl RF, Spurzem JR, Rennard SI. Modulation of fibroblast type I collagen and fibronectin production by bovine bronchial epithelial cells. Am J Respir Cell Mol Biol 1995; 12:425–433.
127. Nakamura Y, Tate L, Ertl RF, Kawamoto M, Mio T, Adachi Y, et al. Bronchial epithelial cells regulate fibroblast proliferation. Am J Physiol 1995; 269:L377–L387.
128. Matsuba K, Wright JL, Wiggs BR, Pare PD, Hogg JC. The changes in airways structure associated with reduced forced expiratory volume in one second. Eur Respir J 1989; 2:834–839.
129. Kuwano K, Bosken CH, Pare PD, Bai TR, Wiggs BR, Hogg JC. Small airways dimensions in asthma and in chronic obstructive pulmonary disease. Am Rev Respir Dis 1993; 148:1220–1225.
130. Salvato G. Quantitative and morphological analysis of the vascular bed in bronchial biopsy specimens from asthmatic and non-asthmatic subjects. Thorax 2001; 56:902–906.
131. Vrugt B, Wilson S, Bron A, Holgate ST, Djukanovic R, Aalbers R. Bronchial angiogenesis in severe glucocorticoid-dependent asthma. Eur Respir J 2000; 15:1014–1021.

132. Hogg JC. Chronic obstructive pulmonary disease: an overview of pathology and pathogenesis. Novartis Found Symp 2001; 234:4–26.
133. McDonald DM. Angiogenesis and remodeling of airway vasculature in chronic inflammation. Am J Respir Crit Care Med 2001; 164:S39–45.
134. Cavarra E, Martorana PA, Bartalesi B, Fineschi S, Gambelli F, Lucattelli M, Ortiz L, Lungarella G. Genetic deficiency of alpha1-PI in mice influences lung responses to bleomycin. Eur Respir J 2001; 17:474–480.
135. Michelson PH, Tigue M, Panos RJ, Sporn PH. Keratinocyte growth factor stimulates bronchial epithelial cell proliferation in vitro and in vivo. Am J Physiol 1999; 277:L737–742.
136. Ohmichi H, Matsumoto K, Nakamura T. In vivo mitogenic action of HGF on lung epithelial cells: pulmotrophic role in lung regeneration. Am J Physiol 1996; 270:L1031–1039.
137. Adamson IYR, Bakowska J. Relationship of keratinocyte growth factor and hepatocyte growth factor levels in rat lung lavage fluid to epithelial cell regeneration after bleomycin. Am J Pathol 1999; 155:949–954.
138. Dohi M, Hasegawa T, Yamamoto K, Marshall BC. Hepatocyte growth factor attenuates collagen accumulation in a murine model of pulmonary fibrosis. Am J Respir Crit Care Med 2000; 162:2302–2307.
139. Panoskaltsis-Mortari A, Taylor PA, Rubin JS, Uren A, Welniak LA, Murphy WJ, Farrell CL, Lacey DL, Blazar BR. Keratinocyte growth factor facilitates alloengraftment and ameliorates graft-versus-host disease in mice by a mechanism independent of repair of conditioning-induced tissue injury. Blood 2000; 96:4350–4356.
140. Geiser T, Jarreau PH, Atabai K, Matthay MA. Interleukin-1β augments in vitro alveolar epithelial repair. Am J Physiol Lung Cell Mol Physiol 2000; 279:L1184–L1190.
141. Neufeld G, Cohen T, Gengrinovitch S, Poltorak Z. Vascular endothelial growth factor (VEGF) and its receptors. FASEB J 1999; 13:9–22.
142. Kasahara Y, Tuder RM, Taraseviciene-Stewart L, Le Cras TD, Abman S, Hirth PK, Waltenberger J, Voelkel NF. Inhibition of VEGF receptors causes lung cell apoptosis and emphysema. J Clin Invest 2000; 106:1311–1319.
143. Kasahara Y, Tuder RM, Cool CD, Lynch DA, Flores SC, Voelkel NF. Endothelial cell death and decreased expression of vascular endothelial growth factor and vascular endothelial growth factor receptor 2 in emphysema. Am J Respir Crit Care Med 2001; 163:737–744.
144. Watkins RH, D'Angio CT, Ryan RM, Patel A, Maniscalco WM. Differential expression of VEGF mRNA splice variants in newborn and adult hyperoxic lung injury. Am J Physiol Lung Cell Mol Physiol 1999; 276:L858–L867.
145. Sakao S, Tatsumi K, Hashimoto T, Igari H, Shino Y, Shirasawa H, Kuriyama T. Vascular endothelial growth factor and the risk of smoking-related COPD Chest 2003; 124:323–327.
146. Snider G, Lucey E, Stone P. Animal models of emphysema. Am Rev Respir Dis 1986; 133:149–169.

147. Shapiro SD, Endicott SK, Province MA, Pierce JA, Campbell EJ. Marked longevity of human lung parenchymal elastic fibers deduced from prevalence of D-aspartate and nuclear weapons-related radiocarbon. J Clin Invest 1991; 87:1828–1834.

148. Stone PJ, Morris SM, Thomas KM, Schuhwerk K, Mitchelson A. Repair of elastase-digested elastic fibers in acellular matrices by replating with neonatal rat-lung lipid interstitial fibroblasts or other elastogenic cell types. Am J Respir Cell Mol Biol 1997; 17:289–301.

149. Morris SM, Thomas KM, Rich CB, Stone PJ. Degradation and repair of elastic fibers in rat lung interstitial fibroblast cultures. Anat Rec 1998; 250:397–407.

150. Senior RM, Tegner H, Kuhn C, Ohlsson K, Starcher BC, Pierce JA. The induction of pulmonary emphysema with human leukocyte elastase. Am Rev Respir Dis 1977; 116:469–475.

151. Karlinsky JB, Fredette J, Davidovits G. The balance of lung connective tissue elements in elastase-induced emphysema. J Lab Clin Med 1983; 102:151–162.

152. Kuhn C, Yu SY, Chraplyvy M. The induction of emphysema with elastase: II. Changes in connective tissue. Lab Invest 1976; 34:372–380.

153. Cardoso WV, Sekhon HS, Hyde DM, Thurlbeck WM. Collagen and elastin in human pulmonary emphysema. Am Rev Respir Dis 1993; 147:975–981.

154. Pierce JA, Hocott JB, Ebert RV. The collagen ad elastin content of the lung in emphysema. Ann Intern Med 1961; 55:210–221.

155. Lang MR, Fiaux GW, Gillooly M, Stewart JA, Hulmes DJS, Lamb D. Collagen content of alveolar wall tissue in emphysematous and non-emphysematous lungs. Thorax 1994; 49:319–326.

156. Vlahovic G, Russell ML, Mercer RR, Crapo JD. Cellular and connective tissue changes in alveolar septal walls in emphysema. Am J Respir Crit Care Med 1999; 160:2086–2092.

157. Kawakami M, Takizawa T. Distribution of pores within alveoli in the human lung. J Appl Physiol 1987; 63:1866–1870.

158. Menkes H, Traystman R, Terry P. Collateral ventilation. Fed Proc 1979; 38:22–26.

159. Gillett NA, Gerlach RF, Muggenburg BA, Harkema JR, Griffith WC, Mauderly JL. Relationship between collateral flow resistance and alveolar pores in the aging beagle dog. Exp Lung Res 1989; 15:709–719.

160. Port CD, Ketels KV, Coffin DL, Kane P. A comparative study of experimental and spontaneous emphysema. J Toxicol Environ Health 1977; 2:589–604.

161. Takaro T, Gaddy LR, Parra S. Thin alveolar epithelial partitions across connective tissue gaps in the alveolar wall of the human lung: ultrastructural observations. Am Rev Respir Dis 1982; 126:326–331.

162. Sahebjami H, Wirman JA. Emphysema-like changes in the lungs of starved rats. Am Rev Respir Dis 1981; 124:619–624.

163. Parra SC, Gaddy LR, Takaro T. Early ultrastructural changes in papain-induced experimental emphysema. Lab Invest 1980; 42:277–289.

164. Mazzone RW, Kornblau S. Size of pores of Kohn: influence of trans-pulmonary and vascular pressures. J Appl Physiol 1981; 51:739–745.
165. Adamson IYR, Bowden DH. Derivation of Type 1 epithelium from Type 2 cells in the developing rat lung. Lab Invest 1975; 32:736.
166. Mason RJ, Shannon JM. Alveolar type II cells. In: Crystal RG, West JB eds. The Lung: Scientific Foundations, 2nd ed. Philadelphia: Lippincott-Raven, 1997, 543–555.
167. Massaro G, Massaro D. Retinoic acid treatment abrogates elastase-induced pulmonary emphysema in rats. Nat Med 1997; 3:675–677.
168. Massaro GD, Massaro D. Postnatal treatment with retinoic acid increases the number of pulmonary alveoli in rats. Am J Physiol 1996; 270:L305–L310.
169. Kuhn C, Starcher BC. The effect of lathyrogens on the evolution of elastase-induced emphysema. Am Rev Respir Dis 1980; 122:453–460.
170. O'Dell BL, Kilburn KH, McKenzie WN, Thurston RJ. The lung of the copper-deficient rat. A model for developmental pulmonary emphysema. Am J Pathol 1978; 91:413–432.
171. Soskel NT, Watanabe S, Hammond E, Sandberg LB, Renzetti AD, Crapo JD. A copper-deficient, zinc-supplemented diet produces emphysema in pigs. Am Rev Respir Dis 1982; 126:316–325.
172. Stein J, Fenigstein H. Anatomie pathologique de la maladie de famine. In: Apfelbaum E, ed. Maladie de Famine. American Joint Distribution Committee (1946), 21–27.
173. Das RM. The effects of intermittent starvation on lung development in suckling rats. Am J Pathol 1984; 117:326–332.
174. Lechner AJ, Winston DC, Bauman JE. Lung mechanics, cellularity, and surfactant after prenatal starvation in guinea pigs. J Appl. Physiol 1986; 60:1610–1614.
175. Sahebjami H, Domino M. Effects of repeated cycles of starvation and refeeding on lungs of growing rats. J Appl Physiol 1992; 73:2349–2354.
176. Karlinsky JB, Goldstein RH, Ojserkis B, Snider GL. Lung mechanics and connective tissue levels in starvation-induced emphysema in hamsters. Am J Physiol 1986; 251:R282–R288.
177. Sahebjami H, Vassallo CL. Influence of starvation on enzyme-induced emphysema. J Appl Physiol 1980; 48:284–288.
178. Massaro D, Massaro GD, Baras A, Hoffman EP, Clerch LB. Calorie-related rapid onset of alveolar loss, regeneration, and changes in mouse lung gene expression. Am J Physiol Lung Cell Mol Physiol 2003;
179. Sahebjami H, Doers JT, Render ML, Bond TL. Anthropometric and pulmonary function test profiles of outpatients with stable chronic obstructive pulmonary disease. Am J Med 1993; 94:469–474.
180. Wilson DO, Rogers RM, Hoffman RM. Nutrition and chronic lung disease. Am Rev Repir Dis 1985; 132:1347–1365.
181. Schols AM, Slangen J, Vovovics L, Wouters EF. Weight loss is a reversible factor in the prognosis of chronic obstructive pulmonary disease. Am J Respir Crit Care Med 1998; 157:1791–1797.

182. Donahoe M, Rogers RM, Wilson DO, et al. Oxygen consumption of the respiratory muscles in normal and in malnourished patients with chronic obstructive pulmonary disease. Am Rev Respir Dis 1989; 140:385–391.
183. Schols AMWJ, Buurman WA, Staal-van den Brekel AJ, Dentener MA, Wouters EFM. Evidence for a relation between metabolic derangements and increased levels of inflammatory mediators in a subgroup of patients with chronic obstructive pulmonary disease. Thorax 1996; 51:819–824.
184. Keman S, Wilemse B, Tollerud DJ, Guevarra L, Schins RP, Borm PJ. Blood interleukin-8 production is increased in chemical workers with bronchitic symptoms. Am J Indust Med 1997; 32:670–673.
185. Yasuda N, Gotoh K, Minatoguchi S, Asano K, Nishigake K, Nomura M, et al. An increase of soluble fas, an inhibitor of apoptosis, associated with progession of COPD. Respir Med 1998; 92:993–999.
186. Di Francia M, Barbier D, Mege JL, Orehek J. Tumor necrosis factor-alpha levels and weight loss in chronic obstructive pulmonary disease. Am J Respir Crit Care Med 1994; 150:1453–5.
187. ****#11057:
188. Keatings VM, Collins PD, Scott DM, Barnes PJ. Differences in interleukin-8 and tumor necrosis factor-α in induced sputum from patients with chronic obstructive pulmonary disease or asthma. Am J Respir Crit Care Med 1996; 153:530–534.
189. Mueller R, Chanez P, Campbell AM, Bousquet J, Heusser C, Bullock GR. Different cytokine patterns in bronchial biopsies in asthma and chronic bronchitis. Respir Med 1996; 90:79–85.
190. Sulkowska M, Sulkowski S, Terlikowski S, Nowak HF. Tumor necrosis factor-alpha induces emphysema-like pulmonary tissue rebuilding. Changes in type II alveolar epithelial cells. Pol J Pathol 1997; 48:179–188.
191. Mauviel A, Heino J, Kahari V-M, Hartmann D-J, Loyau G, Pujol J-P, Vuorio E. Comparative effects of interleukin-1 and tumor necrosis factor-alpha on collagen production and corresponding procollagen mRNA levels in human dermal fibroblasts. J Invest Dermatol 1991; 96:243–249.
192. Rapala KT, Vaha-Kreula MO, Heino JJ, Vuorio EI, Laato MK. Tumor necrosis factor alpha inhibits collagen synthesis in human and rat tissue fibroblasts. Experentia 1996; 52:70–74.
193. Laurent P, Janoff A, Kagan HM. Cigarette smoke blocks cross-linking of elastin in vitro. Am Rev Respir Dis 1983; 127:189–192.
194. Osman M. Cigarette smoke impairs elastin resynthesis in lungs of hamsters with elastase-induced emphysema. Am Rev Respir Dis 1985; 132:640–643.
195. White RR, Coggins CRE. Effects of cigarette smoke on elastase-induced emphysema. Am Rev Respir Dis 1982; 125:S214.
196. Nakamura Y, Romberger DJ, Tate L, Ertl RF, Kawamoto M, Adachi Y, Mio T, Sisson JH, Spurzem JR, Rennard SI. Cigarette smoke inhibits lung fibroblast proliferation and chemotaxis. Am J Respir Crit Care Med 1995; 151:1497–1503.

197. Carnevali S, Nakamura Y, Mio T, Liu X, Takigawa K, Romberger DJ, Spurzem JR, Rennard SI. Cigarette smoke extract inhibits fibroblast-mediated collagen gel contraction. Am J Physiol Lung Cell Mol Physiol 1998; 274:L591–L598.

198. Cantral DE, Sisson JH, Veys T, Rennard SI, Spurzem JR. Effects of cigarette smoke extract on bovine bronchial epithelial cell attachment and migration. Am J Physiol 1995; 268:L723–L728.

199. Wang H, Liu X, Umino R, Skold CM, Zhu Y, Kohyama T, Spurzem JR, Romberger DJ, Rennard SI. Cigarette smoke inhibits human bronchial epithelial cell repair processes. Am J Respir Cell Mol Biol 2001; 25:772–779.

200. Tuder RM, Wood K, Taraseviciene L, Flores SC, Voekel NF. Cigarette smoke extract decreases the expression of vascular endothelial growth factor by cultured cells and triggers apoptosis of pulmonary endothelial cells. Chest 2000; 117:241S–242S.

201. Tuder RM, Zhen L, Cho CY, Taraseviciene-Stewart L, Kasahara Y, Salvemini D, Voelkel NF, Flores SC. Oxidative stress and apoptosis interact and cause emphysema due to vascular endothelial growth factor receptor blockade. Am J Respir Cell Mol Biol 2003; 29:88–97.

202. Lane RE, Campbell ACP. Fatal emphysema in two men making a copper cadmium alloy. Br J Ind Med 1954; 11:118–122.

203. Driscoll KE, Hassenbein DG, Howard BW, Isfort RJ, Cody D, Tindah MH. Cloning, expression and functional characterization of rat MIP-2: a neutrophil chemoattractant and epithelial cell mitogen. J Leukoc Biol 1995; 58:359–364.

204. Chambers RC, McAnulty RJ, Shock A, Campa JS, Tyalor AJN, Laurent GJ. Cadmium selectively inhibits fibroblast procollagen production and proliferation. Am J Physiol 1994; 267:L300–L308.

205. Chambers RC, Laurent GJ, Westergren-Thorsson G. Cadmium inhibits proteoglycan and procollagen production by cultured human lung fibroblasts. Am J Respir Cell Mol Biol 1998; 19:498–506.

206. Liu XD, Umino T, Zhu YK, Wang HJ, Spurzem JR, Romberger DJ, Rennard SI. A study on the effect of cadmium on human lung fibroblasts. Chest 2000; 117:247S.

207. Mannino DM. Personal communication.

208. Mitchell RS, Stanford RE, Johnson JM, Silvers GW, Dart G, George MS. The morphologic features of the bronchi, brochioles and alveoli in chronic airway obstruction: a clinicopathologic study. Am Rev Respir Dis 1976; 114:137–145.

209. Nagai A, West WW, Thurlbeck WM. The national institutes of health intermittent positive-pressure breathing trial: pathology studies II. Correlation between morphologic findings, clinical findings, and evidence of expiratory airflow obstruction. Am Rev Respir Dis 1985; 132:946–953.

210. Nagai A, West WW, Paul JL. The national institutes of health intermittent positive pressure breathing trial: pathology studies. Am Rev Respir Dis 1985; 132:937–945.

211. Mio T, Adachi Y, Romberger DJ, Spurzem JR, Ertl RF, Carnevali S, Rennard SI. Human bronchial epithelial cells modulate collagen gel contraction by fibroblasts. Am J Respir Crit Care Med 1995; 151:A561.

212. Kohyama T, Ertl RF, Valenti V, Spurzem J, Kawamoto M, Nakamura Y, Veys T, Allegra L, Romberger D, Rennard SI. Prostaglandin E$_2$ inhibits fibroblast chemotaxis. Am J Physiol 2001; 281:L1257–L1263.

213. Fine A., Goldstein RH. The effect of PGE2 on the activation of quiescent lung fibroblasts. Prostaglandins 1987; 33:903–913.

214. Ashcroft GS, Yang X, Glick AB, Weinstein M, Letterio JL, Mizel DE, Anzano M, Greenwell-Wild T, Wahl SM, Deng C, Roberts AB. Mice lacking Smad3 show accelerated wound healing and an impaired local inflammatory response. Nat Cell Biol 1999; 1:260–266.

215. Wang H, Liu X, Umino T, Kohyama T, Zhu YK, Wen FQ, Spurzem JR, Romberger DJ, Kim HJ, Rennard SI. Effect of cigarette smoke on fibroblast-mediated gel contraction is dependent on cell density. Am J Physiol Lung Cell Mol Physiol 2003; 284:L205–213.

216. Abe S, Lauby G, Boyer C, Manouilova L, Rennard SI, Sharp JG. Lung cells transplanted to irradiated recipients generate lymphohematopoietic progeny. Am J Respir Cell Mol Biol 2003.

217. Giangreco A, Reynolds SD, Stripp BR. Terminal bronchioles harbor a unique airway stem cell population that localizes to the bronchoalveolar duct junction. Am J Pathol 2002; 161:173–182.

218. Hong KU, Reynolds SD, Giangreco A, Hurley CM, Stripp BR. Clara cell secretory protein-expressing cells of the airway neuroepithelial body micro-environment include a label-retaining subset and are critical for epithelial renewal after progenitor cell depletion. Am J Respir Cell Mol Biol 2001; 24:671–681.

219. Inayama Y, Hook GER, Brody AR, Cameron GS, Jetten AM, Gilmore LB, Gray T, Nettesheim P. The differentiation potential of tracheal basal cells. Lab Invest 1988; 58:706.

220. Johnson NF, Hubbs AF. Epithelial progenitor cells in the rat trachea. Am J Respir Cell Mol Biol 1990; 3:579–585.

221. Otto WR. Lung epithelial stem cells. J Pathol 2002; 197:527–535.

222. Krause DS, Theise ND, Collector MI, Henegariu O, Hwang S, Gardner R, Neutzel S, Sharkis SJ. Multi-organ, multi-lineage engraftment by a single bone marrow-derived stem cell. Cell 2001; 105:369–377.

223. Theise ND, Henegariu O, Grove J, Jagirdar J, Kao PN, Crawford JM, Badve S, Saxena R, Krause DS. Radiation pneumonitis in mice: a severe injury model for pneumocyte engraftment from bone marrow. Exp Hematol 2002; 30:1333–1338.

224. Devine SM, Cobbs C, Jennings M, Bartholomew A, Hoffman R. Mesenchymal stem cells distribute to a wide range of tissues following systemic infusion into nonhuman primates. Blood 2003; 101:2999–3001.

225. Abe S, Lauby G, Boyer C, Rennard SI, Sharp JG. Transplanted bone marrow and bone marrow side population (SP) cells contribute progeny to the lung and liver in irradiated mice. Cytotherapy. In Press.

226. Suratt BT, Cool CD, Serls AE, Chen L, Varella-Garcia M, Shpall EJ, Brown KK, Worthen GS. Human pulmonary chimerism following hematopoietic stem cell transplantation. Am J Respir Crit Care Med 2003. In Press.

227. Kotton DN, Ma BY, Cardoso WV, Sanderson EA, Summer RS, Williams MC, Fine A. Bone marrow-derived cells as progenitors of lung alveolar epithelium. Development 2001; 128:5181–5188.

228. Ortiz LA, Gambelli F, McBride C, Gaupp D, Baddoo M, Kaminski N, Phinney DG. Mesenchymal stem cell engraftment in lung is enhanced in response to bleomycin exposure and ameliorates its fibrotic effects. Proc Natl Acad Sci USA 2003; 100:8407–8411.

229. Laurell CB, Eriksson S. The electrophoretic alpha 1-globulin pattern of serum in alpha 1-antitrypsin deficiency. Scand J Clin Lab Invest 1963; 15:132–140.

10

Proteinases in COPD

STEVEN D. SHAPIRO

Harvard Medical School
and Brigham and Women's Hospital
Boston, Masachusetts, U.S.A.

I. The Pathogenesis of Emphysema

Pulmonary emphysema is a major component of the morbidity and mortality of chronic obstructive pulmonary disease (COPD), a condition that is estimated to afflict in excess of 24 million persons and has become the fourth leading cause of death in the United States. However, major increases in cigarette smoking are occurring in many underdeveloped countries, particularly China. Cigarette-related diseases will become the leading cause of death worldwide within a decade (1). COPD alone is expected to account for 1.5 million deaths per year in China within the next half century (2). Despite increasing knowledge regarding the mechanisms of COPD, there has been limited translation into pharmacotherapy for COPD. This chapter will explore the role of proteinases in the pathogenesis of emphysema. Strategies to inhibit lung destruction could halt the progression of airspace enlargement and airflow obstruction in COPD.

II. Proteinase-Antiproteinase Hypothesis

Emphysema is defined as enlargement of the peripheral airspaces of the lung, including respiratory bronchioles, alveolar ducts, and alveoli, accompanied by destruction of the walls of these structures (3). In 1963, Laurell and Eriksson reported an association of chronic airflow obstruction and emphysema with a deficiency of serum α_1-antitrypsin (α_1-AT) (4), and in 1964, Gross and associates described the first reproducible model of emphysema in experimental animals by injecting the lungs with the plant protease papain (5). Together, these two observations formed the basis for the proteinase-antiproteinase hypothesis of emphysema that has been the prevailing concept of the pathogenesis of emphysema ever since.

The pathogenesis of garden-variety emphysema associated with cigarette smoking can be dissected into four interrelated events (Fig. 1). 1) Chronic exposure to cigarette smoke may lead to inflammatory cell

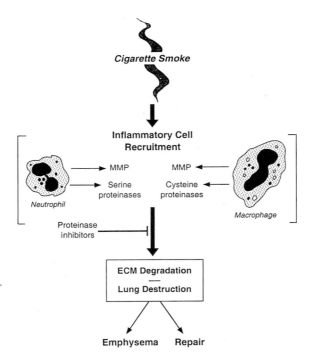

Figure 1 Emphysema results when chronic exposure to cigarette smoke leads to inflammatory cell recruitment release of elastolytic proteinases in excess of inhibitors and ineffective repair of alveoli and elastic.

recruitment within the terminal airspaces of the lung. 2) These inflammatory cells release elastolytic proteinases in excess of inhibitors in local micro-environments, causing damage to the extracellular matrix (ECM) of the lung. 3) Structural cells of the lung are killed either in response to lost matrix or as a primary event. 4) Ineffective repair of alveoli and elastic fibers and perhaps other extracellular matrix components results in airspace enlargement that defines pulmonary emphysema.

III. Inflammatory Cell Proteinases

A variety of techniques have been used to determine the burden of inflammatory cells in lungs of patients with COPD. Induced sputum measures inflammation in large airways, bronchoalveolar lavage (BAL) determines content of nonfixed inflammatory cells in the lower airspace, and (immuno)histochemical techniques assay lung tissue cells in fixed sections. These techniques are complementary but allow only a "snapshot" in time of a dynamic process and cannot determine causation. Nevertheless, what has emerged is that neutrophils are the predominant upper airway inflammatory cell, while macrophages are the most abundant host defense cell in the lower airspace (6). CD8+ and CD4+ T cells are also found in significant numbers throughout the lung. The role of eosinophils, mast cells, and other cell types remains intriguing.

Few neutrophils are present in the lungs of nonsmokers. Cigarette smoking leads to neutrophil retention in the pulmonary microcirculation and deposition in the lung parenchyma. This is apparently achieved by increasing adhesiveness of neutrophils and pulmonary microvascular endothelium, and possibly by increasing neutrophil stiffness so that they do not deform enough to allow pulmonary capillary transit. The neutrophil soon becomes quite deformable as it "slithers" through the cellular and ECM barriers into the lung parenchyma (7). In addition to a 5- to 10-fold increased number of neutrophils in lavage fluids from smokers compared to nonsmokers, Hogg and colleagues have been able to quantify large numbers of neutrophils and other inflammatory cells in samples from patients with end-stage emphysema undergoing volume-reduction surgery (see Chap. 7). Saetta found neutrophils in particular associated with airway wall mucous glands.

The fact that neutrophil serine proteinases have a pH optimum of about 7.4 suggests that these enzymes could damage lung tissue if liberated from the neutrophil. Also, the fact that activated neutrophils can concentrate active neutrophil elastase and cathepsin G on their plasma surface (8) may help explain how these enzymes can function in the extracellular environment despite large excesses of α_1-AT and other inhibitors. Apart from digesting lung elastin and other types of extracellular matrix, neutrophil proteinases may participate in the regulation of the inflammatory response via the stimulation or activation of cytokines. For example, neutrophil elastase in bronchial fluid from cystic fibrosis patients induces interleukin (IL)-8 transcription in airway epithelial cells in culture, and the cathepsin G:α_1-antichymotrypsin complex promotes transcription of IL-6 (9). Neutrophil elastase (NE) is also a potent secretagogue, contributing to mucus production in COPD. NE proteolytic activity is required for upregulation of Muc 5a, which acts via stabilization Muc 5a mRNA (10).

Neutrophils readily release secondary and tertiary granule components including the elastolytic metalloproteinase, gelatinase B (MMP-9), upon activation. Whether primary granule components that contain the more destructive serine proteinases are released in vivo is less clear. However, since the half-life of the neutrophil is less than a day following release form the bone marrow, destructive enzymes could be released from apoptotic neutrophils if not cleared by tissue macrophages. Thus, interaction between macrophages and neutrophils may be critically important in maintaining the structural integrity in the lung.

Neutrophil serine proteinases are characterized by conserved His, Asp, and Ser residues that form a charge relay system that functions by transfer of electrons form the carboxyl group of Asp to the oxygen of Ser which then becomes a powerful nucleophile able to attack the carbonyl carbon atom of the peptide bond of the substrate. All of these enzymes are synthesized as pre-proenzymes in the endoplasmic reticulum and processed by cleavage of the signal peptide (pre-) and removal of a dipeptide (pro-) by dipeptidylpeptidase I, and stored in granules as active packaged proteins. Distinct subsets of serine proteinases are expressed in a lineage-restricted manner in immune and inflammatory cells. Serine proteinases are also expressed in a developmentally specific manner. For example, neutrophil elastase, proteinase 3, and cathepsin G are major components of primary or azurophil granules that are formed during a very specific stage during the development of myeloid cells.

Neutrophil elastase has activity against a broad range of extracellular matrix proteins, including elastin. Following the discovery of α_1-AT deficiency and the capacity of NE to cause emphysema in experimental animals, NE has been considered to be of primary importance in the pathogenesis of pulmonary emphysema. Further evidence supporting involvement of NE in this disease process includes (11,12): 1) the presence of NE and neutrophils in the lung tissue and BAL of patients with emphysema in some (but not all) studies, 2) smoking leads to an acute increase in a specific peptide released by NE action on fibrinogen, and 3) cigarette smoke can oxidize a methionine residue in the reactive center of α_1-AT, inactivating α_1-AT and thus altering the NE:α_1-AT balance (see below). Whether this inactivation occurs in vivo is uncertain. Proteinase 3 (PR3) is roughly 40% as potent as NE against elastin. PR3 has been shown to cause emphysema in experimental animals (13). This molecule has been identified as the autoantigen target of cytoplasmic-staining anti-PMN autoantibody in Wegener's granulomatosis. Cathepsin G (CG) is stored in neutrophil primary granules and to a lesser degree in mast cells and a subset of peripheral blood monocytes. CG is a chymotryptic serine proteinase with the capacity to degrade ECM components. CG has 20% the elastolytic capacity of HNE. CG may facilitate neutrophil penetration of epithelial and endothelial barriers by increasing their permeability.

Neutrophils contain two matrix metalloproteinases (MMPs), gelatinase B (MMP-9) and neutrophil collagenase (MMP-8). In the neutrophil these MMPs are stored in large quantities within specific granules. Neutrophil collagenase can degrade interstitial collagens, but not elastin. MMP-9, expressed by many cell types, is active against a number of substrates, including denatured collagens (gelatins), basement membrane components, and elastin.

Peripheral blood monocytes resemble neutrophils in that they contain serine proteinases NE and CG in peroxidase-positive granules that are similar to the azurophil granules of neutrophils. These proteinases are synthesized by monocyte precursors in the bone marrow and can be rapidly released by the circulating cell, perhaps for transvascular migration. As monocytes differentiate into macrophages in tissues, they lose their armamentarium of serine proteinases and acquire the capacity to synthesize and secrete metalloproteinases. Expression of serine proteinases is limited to a subset of proinflammatory monocytes ($\sim 15\%$ of total), which appear to be those capable of tissue penetration (14).

Alveolar macrophages are the most abundant defense cells in the lung, both under normal conditions and particularly during states of chronic inflammation. Alveolar macrophages are prominent in the respiratory bronchioles of cigarette smokers where emphysematous changes are first manifest. Because they are capable of producing factors that both promote destruction of extracellular matrix and protect against matrix destruction, it is apparent that the macrophage may have a complex role in the pathogenesis of emphysema (15). Alveolar macrophages have the capacity to degrade elastin by means of several different proteolytic enzymes, and use of gene targeting has demonstrated a direct role for their involvement in animal models of emphysema (discussed below).

Cysteine (thiol) proteinases (16) represent a large, diverse group of plant and animal enzymes with amino acid homology at the active site only. Human alveolar macrophages produce the lysosomasl thiol proteinases cathepsins B, H, L, and S. These enzymes share similar sizes of 24–32 kDa and high-mannose side chains (typical of proteins targeted for lysosomal accumulation). Cathepsins B and H have little endopeptidase activity and may function to activate other proteins similar to a distant relative—interleukin converting enzyme. Cathepsin C or dipeptidyl peptidase I has limited extracellular matrix-degrading activity but is required for activation of nearly all matrix-degrading serine proteinase pro-enzymes to their active form. Cathepsins L and S have large active pockets with relatively indiscriminate substrate specificities that include elastin and other matrix components. These enzymes have an acidic pH optima, but cathepsin S retains $\sim 25\%$ of its elastolytic capacity at neutral pH (making it approximately equal to NE). Cathepsin K is a potent elastase predominantly expressed in osteoclasts but also by macrophages in the vasculature and perhaps other tissues. Thus, these enzymes clearly have the capacity to cause lung destruction when targeted to the cell surface or extracellular space, particularly in acidic microenvironments.

Matrix metalloproteinases (17,18) comprise a family of 23 human matrix-degrading enzymes believed to be essential for normal development and physiological tissue remodeling and repair. Abnormal expression of metalloproteinases has been implicated in many destructive processes, including tumor cell invasion and angiogenesis, arthritis, atherosclerosis, arterial aneurysms, and pulmonary emphysema. MMPs are secreted as inactive proenzymes, which are activated at the cell membrane surface or within the extracellular space by proteolytic cleavage of the N-terminal domain. Catalytic activity is dependent on coordination of a zinc ion at the active site and is specifically inhibited by members of another gene family, the tissue inhibitors of matrix metalloproteinases (TIMPs). Four TIMPs have been described. Optimal activity of MMPs is around pH 7.4. MMP family members share about 40–50% identity at the amino acid level, and they possess common structural domains. Domains include a pro-enzyme domain that maintains the enzyme in its latent form, an active domain that coordinates binding of the catalytic zinc molecule, and (except for matrilysin) a C-terminal domain involved in substrate, cell, and TIMP binding. The gelatinases A and B (MMP-2 and MMP-9, respectively) have an additional fibronectin-like domain, which mediates their high binding affinity to gelatins and elastin. MMP-9 has one more domain with homology to type V collagen. Membrane-type MMPs (MT–MMPs) have an additional membrane-spanning domain.

Individual members of the MMP family can be loosely divided into groups based on their matrix-degrading capacity. As a whole, they are able to cleave all extracellular matrix components. The collagenases (MMP-1, -8, and -13) have the unique capacity to cleave native triple helical interstitial collagens. MMP-1 has a small active-site pocket and a restricted substrate specificity. MMP-8 and MMP-13 are able to cleave other ECM components, but not elastin. There are two gelatinases of 72 kDa (gelatinase A, MMP-2) and 92 kDa (gelatinase, MMP-9), which differ in their cellular origin and regulation, but share the capacity to degrade gelatins (denatured collagens), type IV collagen, elastin and other matrix proteins. Stromelysins (MMP-3, -10) have a broad spectrum of susceptible substrates, including most basement membrane components. MMP-11 is termed but has little homology to the other stromelysins, and human MMP-11 has a mutation in humans, making it a poor proteinase. Matrilysin (MMP-7), the smallest MMP (28 kDa as a proenzyme) has the broad substrate specificity of stromelysin, plus it has some elastase activity. While a potent and potentially destructive enzyme, gene targeting of MMP-7 has also demonstrated a physiological role for this MMP in tracheal wound repair (Dunsmore et al., 1998) and activation of defensins (19). Macrophage elastase (MMP-12) also has a potent broad substrate specificity, which includes elastin. MMP-12 is required for cigarette smoke-induced emphysema in mice, as described below. MT-MMPs are located at the cell surface, and at least one MT-MMP, MT1-MMP, activates MMP-2. MT-MMPs also appear to directly degrade ECM proteins, but their catalytic capacities are not well defined at present. MMPs are active against a variety of proteins besides the extracellular matrix. For example, MMPs cleave and activate latent TNF-α, thereby regulating inflammation, they cleave plasminogen, generating the antiangiogenic fragment, angiostatin (20), and they cleave TEP1 augmenting tissue thrombosis (21). MMPs (22), particularly MMP-12 (23), degrade and inactivate α_1-AT, thus indirectly enhancing the activity of NE. Thus, MMPs play both direct and indirect roles in the matrix destruction associated with emphysema and may indirectly influence cytokine release and angiogenesis that could influence the development and progression of COPD.

Alveolar macrophages produce several MMPs, including significant amounts of MMP-12, MMP-9, and smaller amounts of MMP-3 and MMP-7. Human macrophages have the capacity to produce MMP-1, an enzyme not present in rodents. MT1-MMP (MMP-14) also appears to be a macrophage product. Expression of these MMPs is highly regulated, and under quiescent conditions, such as in normal mature lung tissue, MMPs are essentially not expressed. They are induced and their production and activity are carefully controlled during normal repair and remodeling processes.

Table 1 Elastases Present in the Lung

Elastase	Porteinase class	Cell of origin	Molecular mass[a] (kDa)	Other matrix substrates	Elastolytic capacity at pH 7.5 (%)
Neutrophil elastase	Serine	Neutrophil (monocyte)	27–31	bm components[b]	100
Proteinase 3	Serine	Neutrophil (monocyte)	28–34	bm components[b]	40
Cathepsin G	Serine	Neutrophil (monocyte) (mast cells)	27–32	bm components[b]	20
MMP-9	Matrix metalloproteinase	Neutrophil, macrophage, endothelial cell	92–95	Denatured collagens, types IV, V, and VII collagen	30
MMP-12	Matrix metalloproteinase	Macrophage	54	bm components[b]	35
Cathepsin L	Cysteine	Macrophage	29	(Inactive at pH 7.5)	0[c]
Cathepsin S	Cysteine	Macrophage CD4 T cell	28	(Unknown)	80

[a]Denotes (pre)proenzyme forms.
[b]bm components include fibronectin, laminin, entactin, vitronectin, and type IV collage (nonhelical domains).
[c]These enzymes are significantly more potent than neutrophil elastase at pH 5.5.
Parentheses denote minor cellular sources.
Source: Adapted from Ref. 47.

With chronic inflammation, regulation of MMPs can go awry, and MMPs can be produced in excess and at inappropriate sites. Alveolar macrophages cultured from patients with COPD expressed MMP-1 and MMP-9, while macrophages from subjects without COPD did not express these enzymes (24). In this study, MMP-12 appeared to be induced in cigarette smokers with and without COPD. As discussed below, overexpression of MMP-1 in the lungs of transgenic mice led to enlarged airspaces characteristic of emphysema.

Many cells in the lung have the capacity to produce MMPs. Eosinophils produce significant amounts of MMP-9. T lymphocytes produce MMP-2, MMP-3, and MMP-9. Using gene-targeted mice, it was shown that contact hypersensitivity is dependent upon T-cell MMP activity. Stromelysin-1 (MMP-3) was required for sensitization, whereas gelatinase B (MMP-9) was required for timely resolution of the reaction to antigenic challenge.

Various resident lung cells can produce MMPs, including fibroblasts, which are a potential prominent source of MMP-1, -2, and -3, and the MT-MMPs. Type II alveolar epithelial cells produce MMP-7 in addition to other MMPs. Endothelial cells also produce a variety of MMPs such as MMP-1 and MMP-9. Considering the variety of lung cells capable of producing MMPs, it seems plausible that MMPs could participate in the lung destruction resulting in emphysema.

IV. Proteinase Inhibitors

A. Proteinase Inhibitors in Plasma

Human plasma contains at least six proteins that function as proteinase inhibitors (Table 2). Together they make up about 10% of the total plasma proteins. At a concentration of 150–350 mg/dL, α_1-AT has the highest concentration of the plasma inhibitors. α_1-AT belongs to a family of serine proteinase inhibitors called the serpins. Serpins have considerable sequence homology, particularly around their reactive sites. They are important for homeostasis, since they exert some control over such major proteolytic cascades as the complement system and coagulation. Another major inhibitor is α_2-macroglobulin, a large protein usually restricted to the bloodstream because of its mass, 725,000 kDa. α_2-Macroglobulin inhibits proteinases of several classes by entrapping proteinases following cleavage of susceptible regions of the molecule.

The clearest example of the association of proteinase-antiproteinase imbalance and emphysema occurs with inherited deficiency of α_1-AT. α_1-AT is a glycoprotein of 52 kDa synthesized primarily by the liver, consisting of a single polypeptide chain of 394 amino acids. Proteolytic inhibition of

Table 2 Proteinase Inhibitors Present in the Lung

Proteinase inhibitor	Molecular mass (kDa)	Cell origin	Proteinases inhibited
α_1-AT[a]	52	Hepatocyte (Macrophage)	Neutrophil serine proteinases (especially NE)
SLPI	12	Large airway epithelial cells Type II pneumocytes	Neutrophil serine proteinases[b] (except NE)
Elafin	12	Large airway epithelial cells	Neutrophil serine proteinases
α_2-Macroglobulin	725,000	Hepatocytes Lung fibroblasts (Macrophages)	Serine proteinases, MMPs, cysteine proteinases
TIMPs	21–27.5	Macrophages Lung parenchymal resident cells	MMPs
Cystatin C	13	Bronchial epithelial cells (Macrophages)	Cysteine proteinases

Parentheses denote minor cellular sources.
[a]α_1-AT has greater affinity for NE than PR3 and CG.
[b]SLPI does not inhibit NE.
Source: Adapted from Ref. 47.

NE and other serine proteinases by α_1-AT involves cleavage of the strained reactive open center of α_1-AT between methionine[358] and serine[359], resulting in an altered, relaxed α_1-AT conformation in complex with the proteinase. Formation of the complex renders the proteinase inactive, and because the complex is quite stable, inactivation is essentially permanent. The association and inhibition of α_1-AT with NE is much faster than with other serine proteinases, including trypsin, yet the name α_1-antitrypsin is used for historical reasons.

Several α_1-AT phenotypes are associated with very low serum concentrations of α_1-AT and emphysema. Of these, the Pi Z phenotype is by far the most common, accounting for more than 95% of such individuals. The small remainder consists of individuals with Pi SZ, Pi null-null, or Pi null-Z phenotypes. Pi Z individuals have about 15% of the normal serum concentration of α_1-AT. The abnormality leading to the Pi Z phenotype is a point mutation involving a single nucleotide at codon 342 that results in coding for lysine instead of glutamic acid. This amino acid substitution changes the charge attraction between the amino acids at positions 342 and 290 present in the normal form of α_1-AT and prevents the formation of a fold in the molecule. With this change in tertiary structure, the molecule is susceptible to aggregation of α_1-AT in the endoplasmic reticulum that impedes secretion of the protein from the hepatocyte. In addition, its rate of association with NE is significantly slower than the association rate of normal α_1-AT with NE (25). The prevalence of the Pi Z phenotype in the United States is about 1 in 3000 people. The Z allele is rare in Asians and African Americans.

Most Pi Z individuals eventually become symptomatic with COPD, but there is considerable variation, and some individuals reach advanced age with minimal symptoms. In a group of Pi Z subjects and their families, Silverman and colleagues (26) confirmed the wide variability in pulmonary function among Pi Z subjects and found evidence for familial factors that segregated with deterioration in pulmonary function. This striking variability in COPD between Pi Z individuals is a vivid illustration of how little is known about the mechanistic basis for COPD. Smoking has a marked effect on the age at which shortness of breath appears. On average, Pi Z smokers have symptoms by age 40, about 15 years earlier than Pi Z nonsmokers.

B. Tissue-Derived Inhibitors

Low molecular weight serine proteinase inhibitors are abundant in airway fluid and hence thought to represent the primary defense against proteinase-mediated airway damage. Secretory leukoprotease inhibitor (SLPI) is a 12 kDa protein produced by mucus-secreting and epithelial cells in the airway as well as type 2 pneumocytes. SLPI inhibits NE and CG and many other serine proteinases, but not PR3. Elafin, also produced by airway secretory and epithelial cells, is released as a 12 kDa precurser, which is processed to a 6 kDa form that specifically inhibits NE and PR3. These inhibitors are able to inhibit NE bound to substrate, giving them an added dimension that α_1-AT lacks.

Airway mucus contains several other substances that partially inhibit NE including polyanionic molecules such as mucins, other glycosaminoglycans, and fatty acids. DNA, released from inflammatory leukocytes, binds to SLPI, greatly enhancing its rate of association with NE. The relative contribution of each of these molecules to proteinase inhibition is unknown.

Tissue inhibitors of metalloproteinases comprise a family of proteins (four to date) with molecular masses ranging between 21 (TIMP-2, nonglycosylated) and 27.5 (TIMP-1, glycosylated) (41). Each TIMP inhibits MMPs via tight, noncovalent binding with 1:1 stoichiometry. TIMP-1 binds to the C-terminal domain of MMPs, but how this leads to inhibition of catalysis is unknown. Those MMPs that lack the C-terminal domain, including MMP-7 and the fully processed form of MMP-12, are still susceptible to TIMP inhibition, although with a lower Ki. TIMP-2 is secreted complexed to MMP-2 in fibroblasts. A significant body of work has uncovered complex mechanisms whereby TIMP-2 not only inhibits MMP-2, but is also involved in docking pro-MMP-2 to the cell surface, where the enzyme is activated by MT1-MMP. TIMP-3 is expressed predominantly by epithelial cells and binds to extracellular matrix.

TIMPs are secreted from many cell types and are abundant in tissues. Alveolar macrophages secrete both a variety of metalloproteinases as well as TIMP-1 and TIMP-2. Endotoxin induces synthesis of macrophage MMPs and TIMP-1, but inhibits TIMP-2 production (27). Other cytokines, such as interferon-γ(IFNγ), inhibit MMP-1 and MMP-3 expression in macrophages with little effect on TIMP-1 (28). Thus, depending on the inflammatory stimulus, MMPs and TIMPs may be coordinately regulated, perhaps to limit tissue injury during normal remodeling associated with inflammation, or regulation may be discoordinate, potentially leading to tissue injury.

Cystatins represent families of cysteine proteinase inhibitors, some of which are strictly intracellular, while others, such as cystatin C, possess a signal peptide and are secreted by a variety of cells into the extracellular fluid. Cystatin C, comprised of a single nonglycosylated 120-amino-acid peptide chain (13 kDa), forms reversible 1:1 complexes with enzymes in competition with substrates. Cystatin C is the most ubiquitous cystatin, found in all human tissues and body fluids tested, providing general protection against tissue destruction by intracellular cathepsin enzymes leaking from dying cells. It is also a product of alveolar macrophages.

V. Use of Animal Models to Determine the Role of Proteinases in Emphysema

Animal models were critical in the development of the elastase-antielastase hypothesis and continue to play a critical role in deciphering the pathogenesis of emphysema. Genetic manipulation in mice, particularly when combined with a model of long-term cigarette smoke exposure, has and will help define the contribution of several proteinases to the development of emphysema (Fig. 2).

A. Elastase- and Chemical-Induced Emphysema

Since Gross's initial experiments, investigators have instilled a variety of proteinases into the lungs of many small and large animals. A common feature is that administration of elastolytic enzymes including pancreatic elastase, neutrophil elastase, and proteinase 3 results in airspace enlargement (13,29–31). Pancreatic elastase produces the most consistent and

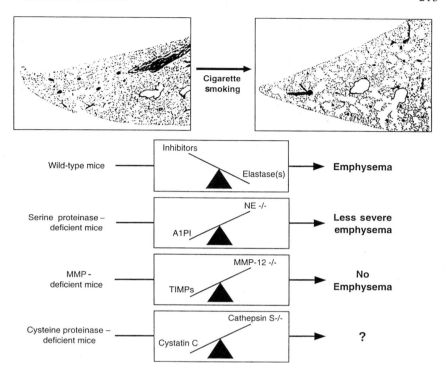

Figure 2 Murine model of cigarette-induced emphysema and potential application to elastase-deficient mice. Low-power magnification (40 ×) of heamatoxylin and eosin stained lung sections obtained from a wild-type C57BL/6 (nonsmoking) control mouse (left) and a mouse exposed to cigarette smoke for 6 months (right). Note enlarged lung volumes (both inflated 25 cm H_2O) and enlarged alveolar spaces characteristic of emphysema in smoke-exposed mouse. The elastase-antielastase hypothesis would predict that lung destuction in wild-type mice was secondary to a shift in the balance favoring unopposed elastase activity (depicted by scale). This model is being applied to gene-targeted mice lacking individual serine (such as neutrophil elastase, NE), metallo- (such as macrophage elastase, MMP-12), and cysteine (such as cathepsin S) proteinases.

impressive airspace enlargement. Instillation of nonelastolytic enzymes such as bacterial collagenase do not cause emphysema. Overexpression of proteinases by either simple intratracheal instillation or more modern transgenic methods can determine whether an enzyme has the capacity to cause emphysema (when applied to mature, full developed lungs). However, these models cannot identify which proteinases are involved in the pathogenesis of emphysema associated with cigarette smoking, nor can they be used to decipher events upstream of proteinase release. Moreover, cigarette smoke exposure may cause a variety of other abnormalities not observed with simple overexpression of a proteinase. Nevertheless, the elastase model continues to have utility due to its relative simplicity and the fact that it allows for first-order approximation for study of downstream event, particularly alveolar repair. For example, elastase instillation has recently been used to demonstrate that retinoic acid has the capacity to promote alveolarization and lung repair in adult male rats (32). In addition, although instillation of elastase causes immediate airspace enlargement, there is an ensuing inflammatory response and further lung destruction from endogenous proteinases. Whether chemotactic mechanisms and participating proteinases are similar to COPD is unclear but of interest.

B. Cigarette Smoke-Induced Emphysema

The chemicals and irritants used in experimental animal to induce inflammation and emphysema include lipopolysaccharide (LPS), cadmium chloride, nitrogen dioxide, inorganic dusts, and ozone. Results from these models have been reviewed elsewhere (33). These models have contributed to our knowledge of lung injury, but none have replicated exposure to cigarette smoke as a model for authentic COPD.

Several animal species have been exposed to cigarette smoke over the years, including dogs, rabbits, guinea pigs, and rodents (33). Recent focus has been on the mouse since it provides unique opportunities for genetic manipulation. Other advantages of the mouse include extensive knowledge of mouse biology, abundant mouse cDNA probes and antibodies, rapid breeding, large litter sizes, small size (advantage for dosing expensive pharmaceutical agents, a disadvantage for surgical (models), and relatively cheap housing. Exposure of mice to long-term cigarette smoke, using smoking chambers similar to those described in the past for other species, results in a variety of changes in lung structure. The mouse upper airway differs from humans in that submucosal glands are sparse and restricted to the trachea. Similar to humans, mice have ciliated epithelial cells that are altered in response to cigarette smoke. Epithelial cells lose their cilia and columnar shape and undergo metaplasia. Mice have less airway branching before terminating in acinar units. Also, unlike humans, the mouse lower airspace lacks respiratory bronchioles and the alveolar to airspace dimensions are significantly less in the mouse than observed in other species, including rats. Overall, the mouse alveolar space is very similar to that of humans, and following exposure to cigarette smoke, inflammatory cell recruitment and airspace enlargement closely mimics the human response (34).

The main strength of mouse models is the ability to develop genetic gain of function and loss of function models. Overexpression of proteinases in transgenic mice was used by DiArmento and colleagues (35), who found that a human collagenase-1 (MMP-1) transgene driven by the haptoglobin reporter unexpectedly resulted in lung-specific expression in severel independent founder lines. These mice developed enlarged airspaces characteristic of emphysema. This was the first demonstration that an MMP could directly cause emphysema. Also, since MMP-1 is inactive against mature elastin, this result suggested that collagen degradation was sufficient to cause emphysema. This study raises the important concept that collagen turnover is involved in emphysema. Clearly there is loss of collagen from destroyed alveoli, but there is also excess collagen accumulation in the small airways (Wright, 1995). Thus, collagen turnover in emphysema is likely important but complicated.

As discussed above, overexpression has limited ability to decipher disease pathogenesis. Gene targeting or targeted mutagenesis by homologous recombination in embryonic stem cells has allowed investigators to generate strains of mice that lack individual proteins, providing specific loss of function models. Combination of gene targeting with the cigarette smoke exposure model provides an opportunity to perform highly controlled experiments that differ with respect to expression of a single protein in mammals. Strains of mice deficient in individual candidate proteinases can be compared to determine their contribution to the development emphysema in response to cigarette smoke.

Macrophage elastase (MMP-12), nearly undetectable in normal macrophages, is expressed in human alveolar macrophages of cigarette smokers and in patients with emphysema, but not normal lung tissue. Application of wild-type (MMP-12+/+) mice to long-term cigarette smoke exposure led to inflammatory cell recruitment followed by alveolar space enlargement similar to the pathological defect in humans. However, mice deficient in macrophage elastase (MMP-12−/−) were protected from development of emphysema despite long-term smoke exposure (34). Surprisingly, MMP-12−/− mice also failed to recruit monocytes into their lungs in response to cigarette smoke. Because MMP-12 and most other MMPs are only expressed upon differentiation of monocytes to macrophages, it appeared unlikely that monocytes require MMP-12 for transvascular migration.

The working hypothesis is that cigarette smoke induces constitutive macrophages, which are present in lungs of MMP-12−/− mice, to produce MMP-12, which in turn cleaves elastin, thereby generating fragments chemotactic for monocytes. This positive feedback loop perpetuates macrophage accumulation and lung destruction. The concept that proteolytically generated elastin fragments mediate monocyte chemotaxis is not original. Independent studies by Senior and colleagues (36,37) as well as Hunninghake and colleagues (38) from the early 1980s demonstrated that elastase-generated elastin fragments were chemotactic for monocytes and fibroblasts. Gene targeting is merely reinforcing this as a major in vivo mechanism of macrophage accumulation in a chronic inflammatory condition. Whether human emphysema is also dependent on this single MMP is of course uncertain. At the very least, this study demonstrates a critical role of macrophages in the development of emphysema and unmasks a proteinase-dependent mechanism of inflammatory cell recruitment that may have broader biological implications.

Subsequently, several other genetically engineered mice have confirmed the capacity of MMPs/MMP-12 to cause airspace enlargement. Inducible, lung-specific transgenic mice expressing either: 1) the Th2 cytokine IL-13 (39); 2) the Th1 cytokine IFNγ (40), induce expression of MMP-12, MMP-9, and cysteine proteinases with subsequent airspace enlargement; 3) SP-D$-/-$ mice demonstrate macrophage activation MMP production and consequent emphysema (41); 4) $\alpha_v\beta6-/-$ mice develop macrophage recruitment, MMP-12 activation airspace enlargement with age (42). Emphysema is abrogated upon crossing $\alpha_v\beta6-/-$ with MMP-12$-/-$ mice or crossing $\alpha_v\beta6-/-$ with TGF-β. Since $\alpha_v\beta6$ activates TGFβ and TGF-β is known to inhibit MMP-12, this study shows that in the absence of TGF-β there is induction of MMP-12 and emphysema. However, too much TGF-β might cause fibrosis, hence a delicate balance of TGF-β appears to be critical.

NE-deficient mice have also been generated by gene targeting. These mice have demonstrated a role for NE in killing bacteria (21,43). Multiple mechanisms of NE-mediated bacterial killing have subsequently been identified, including proteolytic degradation of Omp proteins on the outer wall of gram-negative bacteria (21), degradation of bacterial toxins (44), and activation of cathelicidins (45). NE$-/-$ mice have also been applied to cigarette smoke exposure, and NE$-/-$ smoke-exposed mice were significantly protected from the development of emphysema (46).

How can there be significant protection in mice deficient in both MMP-12 and NE? A clue has come from a mouse model of bullous pemphigoid. In this model, intradermal injection of antibodies against hemidesmosomes results in neutrophil recruitment and blister formation. Blisters do not form in either MMP-9$-/-$ or NE$-/-$ mice. Further studies demonstrate that MMP-9 degrades α_1-AT, allowing NE to degrade hemidesmosomes/tight junctions and cause blisters (Liu et al., 2000). Application of MMP-9$-/-$ mice to cigarette smoke failed to demonstrate a role for MMP-9 in the development of emphysema (S. D. Shapiro, and R. M. Senior, unpublished). In this model, there is evidence that MMP-12 degrades α_1-AT, promoting NE-mediated lung destruction, and NE degrades TIMP-1. As opposed to the neutrophil predominant bullous pemphigoid model, the cigarette smoke-exposed lung is a macrophage-MMP-12-rich environment. Under these conditions, MMP-12, which is most efficient at degrading α_1-AT, plays a prominent role in degrading the large amounts of α_1-AT present in the lung. Of note, MMP-12 might influence acute neutrophil accumulation via TNF shedding (47).

VI. Summary

Although the proteinase-antiproteinase hypothesis has remained intact for 35 years, many fundamental questions related to the hypothesis are still unanswered. Inflammatory cells are the presumed source of injurious proteinases, but specifically which cells are responsible is debated. In addition, structural cells of the lung also have the capacity to produce proteinases and might contribute to proteolytic injury. What are the signals that initiate and perpetuate inflammation in the lungs during the development of emphysema? Which enzymes are involved in lung destruction, and how do they make contact with the lung extracellular matrix and maintain their catalytic activity in the presence of an abundance of proteinase inhibitors? With respect to the extracellular matrix, which ECM molecules are degraded and not appropriately repaired, and what is the role of fibrosis or excessive matrix production in emphysema?

Use of animal models combined with in vitro studies is allowing investigators to address some of these important questions in a highly controlled manner in complex organisms. The usefulness of animal models for COPD depend upon similar molecular mechanisms between species. As we learn more about similarities and differences between mice and men, and as the entire genomes are cloned and protein function determined, then we will be in an increasingly strong position to unravel the complex pathogenetic mechanisms of COPD. This knowledge should then lead to specific therapy to eliminate the pathology associated with this disease. Hopefully, in the future we can thwart cigarette smoking itself, eliminating COPD as we know it, and apply knowledge gained from this research to other inflammatory lung diseases.

References

1. Bartecchi C, MacKenzie T, Schrier R. The human costs of tobacco use. N Engl J Med 330 1994; 907–912, 975–980.
2. Peto, R, Chen, Z, Boreham, J. Tobacco—the growing epidemic. Nat Med 1999; 5:15–17.

3. Standards for the diagnosis and care of patients with chronic obstructive pulmonary disease. Am J Respir Crit Care Med 1995; 152:S77–S121.

4. Laurell CB, Erickson S. The electrophoretic alpha-globulin pattern of serum in alpha-antitrypsin deficiency. Scand J Clin Invest 1963; 15:132–140.

5. Gross P, Pfitzer E, Tolker E, Babyak M, Kaschak M. Experimental emphysema: its production with papain in normal and silicotic rats. Arch Environ Health 1965; 11:50–58.

6. Merchant RK, Schwartz DA, Helmers RA, Dayton CS, Hunninghake GW. Bronchoalveolar lavage cellularity. Am Rev Respir Dis 1992; 146:448–453.

7. Doerschuk C. Neutrophil rheology and transit through capillaries and venules. Am J Respir Crit Care Med 1999; 159:1693–1695.

8. Owen C, Campbell M, Sannes P, Boukedes S, Campbell E. Cell surface-bound elastase and cathepsin G on human neutrophils: a novel, non-oxidative mechanism by which neutrophils focus and preserve catalytic activity of serine proteinases. J Cell Biol 1995; 13:775–789.

9. Kurdowska AaJT. Acute phase protein stimulation by alpha-1-antichymotrypsin: cathepsin G complexes. Evidence for the involvement of IL-6. J Biol Chem 1990; 265:21023–21026.

10. Voynow J, Young L, Wang Y, Horger T, Rose M, Fischer B. Neutrophil elastase increases MUC5AC mRNA and protein expression in respiratory epithelial cells. Am J Physiol 1999; 276:L835–843.

11. Janoff A. State of the art. Elastases and emphysema. Am Rev Respir Dis 1985; 132:417–433.

12. Snider GL. Emphysema: the first two centuries—and beyond, Part 1. Am Rev Respir Dis 1992a; 146:1334–1344.

13. Kao RC, Wehner NG, Skubitz KM, Gray BH, Hoidal JR. Proteinase 3. A distinct human polymorphonuclear leukocyte proteinase that produces emphysema in hamsters. J Clin Invest 1988; 82:1693.

14. Campbell EJ, Cury JD, Shapiro SD, Goldberg GI, Welgus HG. Neutral proteinases of human mononuclear phagocytes—cellular-differentiation markedly alters cell phenotype for serine proteinases, metalloproteinases, and tissue inhibitor of metalloproteinases. J Immunol 1991; 146:1286–1293.

15. Shapiro S. The macrophage in COPD. Am J Respir Crit Care Med 1999.

16. Chapman HAJ, Munger JS, Shi G-P. The role of thiol proteases in tissue injury and remodeling. Am J Respir Crit Care Med 1994; 150:S155–160.

17. Parks WC, Mecham RP. Matrix Metalloproteinases—Comprehensive and Up to Date Reviews on Many Aspects of MMP Biology and Chemistry (1998). Academic Press.

18. Shapiro SD. Biological consequences of extracellular matrix cleavage by matrix metalloproteinases. Curr Opin Cell Biol 1998; 10:602–608.

19. Wilson C, Ouellette A, Satchell D, Ayabe T, Lopez-Boado Y, Stratman J, Hultgren S, Matrisian L, Parks W. Regulation of intestinal alpha-defensin activation by the metalloproteinase matrilysin in innate host defense. Science 1999; 286.

20. Cornelius LA, Nehring L, Klein, B, Pierce R, Bolinski M, Welgus HG, Shapiro SD. Generation of angiostatin by matrix metalloproteinases: effects on neovascularization. J Immunol (1998). In Press

21. Belaaouaj A, Li A, Wun T, Welgus H, Shapiro S. Matrix metalloproteinases cleave tissue factor protein inhibitor: effects on coagulation. J Biol Chem 2000; 275:27123–27128.

22. Sires UI, Murphy G, Welgus HG, Senior RM. Matrilysin is much more efficient than other metalloproteinases in the proteolytic inactivation of alpha-1-antitrypsin. Biophys Biochem Res Comm 1994; 204:613–620.

23. Gronski TJ, Martin R, Kobayashi, DK, Walsh BC, Holman MC, Van Wart HE, Shapiro SD. Hydrolysis of a broad spectrum of extracellular matrix proteins by human macrophage elastase. J Biol Chem 1997; 272: 12189–12194.

24. Finlay GA, O'Driscoll LR, Russell KJ, D'Arcy EM, Masterson, JB, Fitzgerald MX, O'Connor CM. Matrix metalloproteinase expression and production by alveolar macrophages in emphysema. Am J Respir Crit Care Med 1997; 156:240–247.

25. Lomas DA, Evans DL, Stone SR, Chang W-SW, Carre RW. Effect of the Z mutation on the physical and inhibitory properties of alpha-1-antitrypsin. Biochem 1993; 32:500–508.

26. Silverman E, Pierce J, Province M, Rao D, Campbell E. Variability of pulmonary function in alpha-1-antitrypsin deficiency: clinical correlates. Ann Int Med 1989; 111:982–991.

27. Shapiro SD, Kobayashi DK, Welgus HG. Identification of TIMP-2 in human alveolar macrophages: regulation is opposite metalloproteinases and TIMP-1. J Biol Chem 1992; 267: 13890–13894.

28. Janoff A, Sloan B, Weinbaum G, Damiano V, Sandhaus RA, Elias J, Kimbel P. Experimental emphysema induced with purified human neutrophil elastase: tissue localization of the instilled protease. Am Rev Respir Dis 1977; 115: 461.

29. Shapiro SD, Campbell EJ, Kobayashi DK, Welgus HG. Immune modulation of metalloproteinase production in human macrophages: selective pretranslation suppression of interstitial collagenase and stromelysin biosynthesis by gamma interferon. J Clin Invest 1990; 86:1204–1210.

30. Senior RM, Tegner H, Kuhn C, Ohlsson K, Starcher BC, Pierce JA. The induction of pulmonary emphysema induced with human leukocyte elastase. Am Rev Respir Dis 1977; 116, 469.

31. Snider G, Lucey EC, Christiansen TG, Stone PJ, Calore JD, Catanes A, Franzbau, C. Emphysema and bronchial secretory cell metaplasia induced in hamsters by human neutrophil products. Am Rev Respir Dis 1984; 129:155–160.

32. Massaro GD, Massaro D. Retinoic acid treatment abrogates elastase-induced pulmonary empysema in rats. Nat Med June, 1997; 675–677.

33. Snider GL, Lucey EC, Stone PJ. Animal models of emphysema. Am Rev Respir Dis 1986; 133:149–169.

34. Hautamaki RD, Kobayashi DK, Senior RM, Shapiro SD. Macrophage elastase is required for cigarette smoke-induced emphysema in mice. Science 1997; 277:2002–2004.

35. D'Armiento J, Dalal SS, Okada Y, Berg RA, Chada K. Collagenase expression in the lungs of transgenic mice causes pulmonary emphysema. Cell 1992; 71:955–961.

36. Senior RM, Griffin GL, Mecham RP. Chemotactic activity of elastin-derived peptides. J Clin Invest 1980; 66: 859–862.

37. Senior RM, Griffin GL, Mecham RP, Wrenn DS, Prasad KU, Urry DW. Val-Gly-Val-Ala-Pro-Gly, a repeating peptide in elastin, is chemotactic for fibroblasts and monocytes. J Cell Biol 1984; 99: 870–874.

38. Hunninghake GW, Davidson JM, Rernnard S, Szapiel S, Gadek JE, RG C. Elastin fragments attract macrophage precursors to diseased sites in pulmonary emphysema. Science 1981; 212:925–927.

39. Zheng T, Zhu Z, Wang Z, Homer R, Ma B, Riese R, Chapman Jr, H, Shapiro S., and JA E. Inducible targetting of IL-13 to the adult lung causes matrix metalloproteinase- and cathepsin-dependent emphysema. J Clin Invest 2000; 106:1081–1093.

40. Wang Z, Zheng T, Zhu Z, Homer R, Riese R, Chapman HJ, Shapiro S, Elias J. Interferon g induction of pulmonary emphysema in the adult murine lung. J Exp Med 2000; 192:1587–1599.

41. Wert SE, Yoshida M, LeVine AM, Ikegami M, Jones T, Ross GF, Fisher JH, Korfhagen TR, and Whitsett JA. Increased metalloproteinase activity, oxidant production, and emphysema in surfactant protein D gene-inactivated mice. Proc Natl Acad Sci USA 2000; 97:5972–5977.

42. Morris D, Huang X, Kaminski N, Wang Y, Shapiro S, Dolganov G, Glick A, Sheppard D. Loss of intergrin-mediated TGFb activation causes MMP-12 dependent pulmonary emphysema. Nature 2003; 422: 169–173.

43. Tkalcevic J, Novelli M, Phylactides M, Iredale J, Segal A, J R. Impaired immunity and enhanced resistance to endotoxin in the absence of neutrophil elastase and cathepsin G. Immunity 2000; 12:201–210.

44. Weinrauch Y, Drujan D, Shapiro S, Weiss J, Zychlinsky A. Neutrophil elastase targets virulence factors of enterobaceria. Nature 2002; 417: 91–94.

45. Cole AM, Shi J, Ceccarelli A, Kim YH, Park A, Ganz T. Inhibition of neutrophil elastase prevents cathelicidin activation and impairs clearance of bacteria from wounds. Blood 2001; 97: 297–304.

46. Shapiro S, Goldstein N, Kobayashi D, Kelley D, Houghton A, Belaaouaj A. Neutrophil elastase contributes to cigarette smoke-induced emphysema in mice (2003). Am J Pathol. In press.

47. Churg A, Wang R, Tai H, Wang X, Xie C, Dai J, Shapiro S, Wright J. Macrophage metalloelastase mediates acute cigarette smoke-induced inflammation via TNF-alpha release. Am J Pulum Crit Care Med 2003; 167: 1083–1089.

48. Senior RM, Shapiro S. Chronic obstructive pulmonary disease: epidemiology, pathophysiology and pathogenesis. In: Fishman's Pulmonary Diseases and Disorders. 3rd ed. New York: McGraw-Hill, 1997:659–681.

49. Dunsmore S E, Saarialho-Kere UK, Roby JD, Wilson CL, Matrisian LM, Welgus HG, Parks WC. Matrilysin expression and function in airway epithelium. J Clin Invest 1998; 102:1321–1331.

50. Snider G. Emphysema: the first two centuries—and beyond, Part 2. Am Rev Respir Dis 1992b; 146:1615–1622.

11

Oxidative Stress and COPD

WILLIAM MACNEE and IRFAN RAHMAN

University of Edinburg
Edinburg, Scotland

I. Summary

A number of studies have shown an increased oxidant burden and consequently increased makers of oxidative stress in the airspaces, breath, blood, and urine of smokers and patients with chronic obstructive pulmonary disease (COPD). The presence of oxidative stress has important consequences for the pathogenesis of COPD. These include oxidative inactivation of antiproteinases, airspace epithelial injury, increased sequestration of neutrophils in the pulmonary microvasculature, and gene expression of pro-inflammatory mediators. Oxidative stress may thus have a role in enhancing the inflammation, which occurs in smokers and patients with COPD, through the activation of redox-sensitive transcriptions factors such as NF-κB and AP-1, which regulate the genes for pro-inflammatory mediators as well as protective antioxidant gene expression.

The sources of the increased oxidative stress in patients with COPD derive from the increased burden of oxidants present in cigarette smoke and from the increased amounts of reactive oxygen species (ROS) released from leukocytes, both in the airspaces and in the blood. Antioxidant depletion or deficiency in antioxidants may contribute to oxidative stress. The development of airflow limitation is related to dietary deficiency of antioxidants, and hence dietary supplementation may be a beneficial therapeutic intervention in this condition. Antioxidants that have good bioavailability or molecules that have antioxidant enzyme activity may be therapies that not only protect against the direct injurious effects of oxidants, but may fundamentally alter the inflammatory events that play an important role in the pathogenesis of COPD.

II. Oxidants/Antioxidants

Biological systems are continuously exposed to oxidants generated endogenously either by metabolic reactions (e.g., for mitochondrial electron transport during respiration, released from phagocytes) or exogenously (e.g., air pollutants or cigarette smoke). The tissues are protected against this oxidative challenge by well-developed enzymatic and nonenzymatic antioxidant defense systems (1).

Oxidative stress occurs when the balance between oxidants and antioxidants shifts in favor of oxidants (2). This results from either an excess of oxidants and/or a depletion of antioxidants. Oxidative stress is thought to play an important role in the pathogenesis of a number of lung diseases (3), not only through its potential to produce direct injurious effects, but also by involvement in the molecular mechanisms that control lung inflammation. The impact of the injurious and inflammatory effects of oxidative stress, particularly those resulting from the generation of exogenous oxidants, may be particularly important in the lungs because of the enormous surface area of the airspace epithelium and its exposure to higher concentrations of oxygen than other tissues.

Chronic obstructive pulmonary disease is a slowly progressive condition characterized by airflow limitation, which is largely irreversible (4,5). A smoking history of at least 20 pack-years is usual, reflecting the fact that smoking is the main etiological factor in this condition, far outweighing any other risk factor. The pathogenesis of COPD is therefore strongly linked to the effects of cigarette smoke (6). Although nearly 90% of all patients with COPD are smokers (7), for as yet unknown and probably complex reasons only a proportion (15–20%) of smokers develop clinically apparent COPD. The fact that cigarette smoke contains 10^{17} molecules per puff (8), together with evidence of increased oxidative stress in smokers and in patients with COPD (9), has led to the proposal that an oxidant/antioxidant imbalance occurs in COPD, which is important in the pathogenesis of this condition (9,10). This chapter will review the evidence for the role of oxidative stress in the pathogenesis of COPD and the mechanisms, responses, and consequences of oxidative stress in this condition.

A. Oxidants/Free Radicals in Cigarette Smoke

Cigarette smoke is a complex mixture of over 5000 chemical compounds, of which free radicals and other oxidants are present in high concentrations (8,11). Cigarette smoke can be divided into two phases—tar and gas—which are traditionally separated by a Cambridge glass–fiber filter, which traps 99% of particles of $> 0.1 \mu m$ (8). Free radicals are present in both the tar and the gas phases of cigarette smoke. The gas phase of cigarette smoke contains approximately 10^{15} radicals per puff, primarily of the alkyl and peroxyl types. Nitric oxide (NO) is another oxidant present in cigarette smoke in concentrations of 500–1000 ppm (11). Nitric oxide reacts quickly with the superoxide anion $(O_2^{\cdot-})$ to form highly reactive peroxynitrite $(ONOO^-)$ and with peroxyl radicals to give alkyl peroxynitrites (ROONO).

The tar phase of cigarette smoke contains a high concentration of radicals, which are more stable and can be directly observable by electron spin resonance (10^{17} spins/g). Examples are the semiquinone radical, which can reduce oxygen to produce the superoxide anion $(O_2^{\cdot-})$, the hydroxyl radical ($\cdot$OH), and hydrogen peroxide (H_2O_2) (11). The tar phase is also an effective metal chelator and can bind iron to produce tar-semiquinone + tar-Fe^{2+}, which can generate H_2O_2 continuously (12,13). The gas phase of cigarette smoke contains organic carbon and oxygen centered radicals, which have short lifetimes, typically < 1 second. However, reactions occur that can prolong the effect of inhaled radicals. An examples is the slow oxidation of NO present in cigarette smoke to produce reactive nitrogen species (RNS) such as nitrogen dioxide, which can react with unsaturated compounds, such as isoprene in cigarette smoke to form carbon-centered organic radicals. These radicals react rapidly with oxygen to form peroxyl radicals, which are converted to alkoyxyl radicals by reaction with NO, resulting in more nitrogen dioxide, which can reenter the reaction (11). Gas-phase cigarette smoke also contains high concentrations of olefins and dienes.

The lung epithelial lining fluid (ELF) and mucus, which have antioxidant properties (14), are the first line of defense in the lungs against inhaled oxidants, quenching the short-lived free radicals in the gas phase of cigarette smoke. However, cigarette smoke condensate, which forms in the epithelial lining fluid, may continue to produce reactive oxygen species (ROS) for a considerable time. Cigarette smokers deposit up to 20 mg of tar per cigarette smoked, or as much as 1 g per day. Tar contains over 5000 different organic compounds, from which the water-soluble components, such as aldehydes, catechol, and hydroquinone, are extracted into the epithelial lining fluid (11). Polyphenols, such as catechols, are not free radicals, but solutions of polyphenols undergo autoxidation and polymerize to form substances that are oxidants (15). Aged polyphenols also have some reducing properties. For example, solutions of catachol and hydroqinones, in concentrations that are similar to those in cigarette smoke condensate, mobilize ferric ions from ferritin (16).

Quinone (Q)/hydroquinone (QH_2)/semiquinone($QH^{\cdot}$) in the tar phase are present in equilibrium:

$$Q + QH_2 \rightarrow 2H^+ + Q^{\cdot-}$$

Aqueous extracts of cigarette tar contain the quinone radical ($Q^{\cdot-}$), which can reduce oxygen to form the superoxide anion ($O_2^{\cdot-}$), which may dismutate to form hydrogen peroxide (H_2O_2):

$$Q^{\cdot-} + O_2 \rightarrow Q + O_2^{\cdot-}$$

$$2O_2^{\cdot-} + 2H^+ \rightarrow O_2 + H_2O_2$$

Furthermore, since both cigarette tar and lung epithelial lining fluid contain metal ions, such as iron, Fenton chemistry will result in the production of hydroxyl radical ($HO^{\cdot}$), which is a very reactive and potent oxidant.

B. Cell-Derived Oxidants

Inflammation is a characteristic feature in the lungs of smokers (17–19). Recent bronchial biopsy studies have clearly demonstrated the presence of increased number of leukocytes in the airway and distal airspace walls in smokers who develop COPD (17).

The increase in the oxidative burden produced directly by inhaling cigarette smoke is therefore further enhanced in smokers' lungs by the release of oxygen radicals from inflammatory leukocytes, both neutrophils and macrophages, which are known to migrate in increased numbers into the lungs of cigarette smokers, compared with nonsmokers (20). Moreover, the lungs of smokers with airway obstruction have more neutrophils than smokers without airway obstruction (21).

Alveolar macrophages obtained by bronchoalveolar lavage from the lungs of smokers are more activated compared with those obtained from nonsmokers (22,23). One manifestation of this is the release of increased amounts of ROS such as $O_2^{\cdot-}$ and H_2O_2 (24–27). Exposure to cigarette smoke in vitro has also been shown to increase the oxidative metabolism of alveolar macrophages (28). Subpopulations of alveolar macrophages with a higher density appear to be more prevalent in the lungs of smokers and are responsible for the increased expression of the adhesion molecule CD11/CD18 and for the increased $O_2^{\cdot-}$ production that occurs in smokers, macrophages (29).

In studies in both stable (19) and mild exacerbations of bronchitis (30), eosinophils have been shown to be prominent in the airway walls. Broncoalveolar lavage (BAL) from patients with COPD has also been shown to contain increased levels of eosinophilic cationic protein. Furthermore, peripheral blood eosinophilia is also considered to be a risk factor for the development of airway obstruction in patients with chronic bronchitis and is an adverse prognositc sign (31,32). Eosinophils produce more $O_2^{\cdot-}$ than neutrophils, which in turn generate more than macrophages. Although generally true, this does depend somewhat on the stimulus (33).

Superoxide anion and H_2O_2 can be generated by the xanthine/xanthine oxidase (XO) reaction. XO activity has been shown to be increased in cell-free bronchoalveolar lavage fluid from COPD patients, compared with normal subjects, and this was associated with increased $O_2^{\cdot-}$ and uric acid production (34). Preliminary studies also show increased XO activity in the lungs in animal models of cigarette smoke exposure (35), supporting the concept that an increased oxidative burden occurs during smoking.

Several transition metal salts react with H_2O_2 to for OH. In this regard most attention in vivo for the generation of OH has been paid to iron (36). Iron is a critical element in many oxidative reactions (Fig. 1). Free iron in the ferrous form catalyzes the Fenton reaction and the superoxide-driven Haber-Weiss reaction, which generate the hydroxyl radical, a free radical that is extremely damaging to all tissues, particularly to cell membranes, producing lipid peroxidation. In addition to their cytotoxic properties (37), lipid peroxides are increasingly recognized as being important in signal transduction for a number of important events in the inflammatory response. The generation of oxidants in epithelial lining fluid may therefore be further enhanced by the presence of increased amounts of free iron in the airspaces in smokers (38). This is relevant to COPD since the intracellular iron content of alveolar macrophages is increased in cigarette smokers and is increased further in those who develop chronic bronchitis, compared with nonsmokers (39). In addition, macrophages obtained from smokers release more free iron in vitro than those from nonsmokers (40).

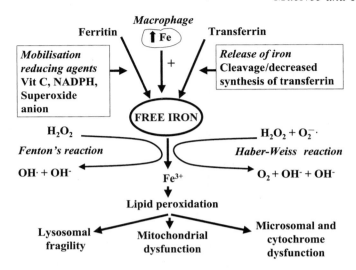

Figure 1   Sources of free iron in the lungs and associated oxidative reactions.

Lung epithelial cells are another source of ROS. Type II alveolar epithelial cells have been shown to release both H_2O_2 and O_2^- in similar quantities to alveolar macrophages (41). Indeed, the release of ROS from type II cells is able, in the presence of myeloperoxidase, to inactivate α_1-antitrypsin in vitro (41).

ROS and RNS can also be generated intracellularly from several sources such as mitochondrial respiration, the NADPH oxidase system, xanthine/xanthine oxidase, and, in the case of RNS, from arginine, by the action of nitric oxide synthetase (42) (Fig. 2). Depending on the relative amounts of ROS and RNS, particularly the amounts of O_2^- and NO, which are almost invariably produced simultaneously at sites of inflammation, these can react together to produce the powerful oxidant peroxynitrite (ONOO$^-$). Since this reaction occurs at a nearly diffusion-limited rate, it is though that NO can outcompete superoxide dismutase (SOD) for reaction who $O_2^{\cdot-}$ and thus ONOO$^-$ will be generated (43):

$$O_2^{\cdot-} - +NO^\cdot \to ONOO^-$$

The generation of peroxynitrite is thought to prolong the action of NO and to be responsible for most of the adverse effects of excess generation of NO (44). Peroxynitrite is directly toxic to cells (45,46) or may decompose to

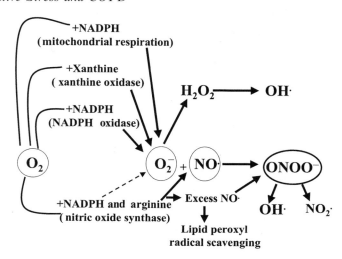

Figure 2   Sources of intracellular reactive oxygen species: O_2^- = superoxide anion; NO = nitric oxide; H_2O_2 = hydrogen peroxide; OH• = hydroxyl radical; NO_2 = nitrogen dioxide; ONOO$^-$ = peroxynitrite.

produce the hydroxyl radical:

$$ONOO^- + H^+ \rightarrow OH^\cdot + NO_2^\cdot$$

Studies have shown that in response to tumor necrosis factor-α (TNFα) and lipopolysaccharide (LPS), which are relevant stimuli for the inflammatory response in COPD, airway epithelial cells can concurrently produce increased amounts of intracellular ROS and RNS (47). This intracellular production of oxidants and the subsequent changes in intracellular redox status are important in the molecular events controlling the expression of genes for inflammatory mediators (see below).

Lipid peroxidation following the reaction of free radicals with polyunsaturated fatty acid (PuFA) side chains in membranes or lipoproteins is a further reaction that can result in cell damage and has even greater importance in this respect since it is self-perpetuating process that continues as a chain reaction (37) (Fig. 3). The presence of lipid peroxides may also have a role in the signaling events in the molecular mechanisms involved in the lung inflammation in COPD (see below).

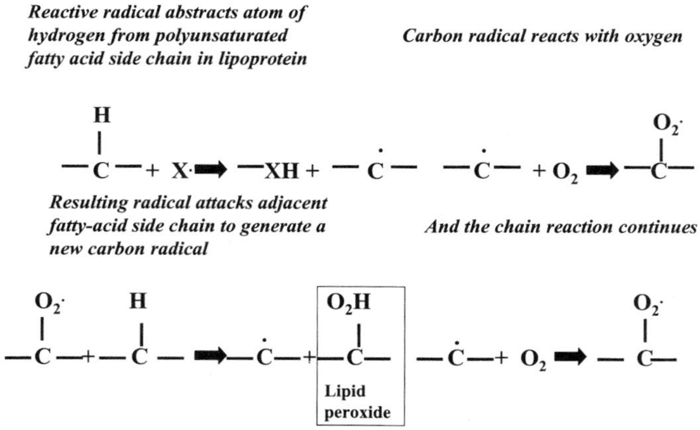

Reactive radical abstracts atom of hydrogen from polyunsaturated fatty acid side chain in lipoprotein   *Carbon radical reacts with oxygen*

$$-\overset{\overset{\textstyle H}{|}}{C}- + \; X\cdot \Rightarrow \; -XH + \; -\overset{\cdot}{C}- \qquad -\overset{\cdot}{C}- + O_2 \Rightarrow -\overset{\overset{\textstyle O_2\cdot}{|}}{C}-$$

Resulting radical attacks adjacent fatty-acid side chain to generate a new carbon radical   *And the chain reaction continues*

$$-\overset{\overset{\textstyle O_2\cdot}{|}}{C}- + \; -\overset{\overset{\textstyle H}{|}}{C}- \; \Rightarrow -\overset{\cdot}{C}- + \boxed{\begin{array}{c}-\overset{\overset{\textstyle O_2H}{|}}{C}-\\[4pt]\text{Lipid}\\\text{peroxide}\end{array}} \quad -\overset{\cdot}{C}- + \; O_2 \Rightarrow -\overset{\overset{\textstyle O_2\cdot}{|}}{C}-$$

Figure 3 Reactions producing lipid peroxidation.

III. Evidence of Oxidative Stress in Smokers and Patients with COPD

The evidence for the presence of increased oxidative stress in smokers and patients with COPD is now overwhelming (10,48,49). The only direct method to measure excessive free radical activity is by electron spin resonance using spin traps, which cannot be applied to the study of tissues at present. Most studies have therefore relied on indirect measurements of free radical activity in biological fluids. Although these markers suggest the occurrence of oxidative stress, they do not prove that it is involved in the pathogenesis of the condition.

There are now numerous studies using different techniques which have shown that increased markers of oxidative stress are present in the epithelial lining fluid, in the breath, in the urine and in the blood in cigarette smokers and in patients with COPD.

A. Evidence of Local Oxidative Stress in the Lungs

1. Antioxidants in Lung Lining Fluid

The ELF forms the interface between the airspace epithelium and the external environment and therefore forms a critical defense mechanism against inhaled oxidants or those produced by cells in the airspaces (50). An antioxidant is defined as a substance that, when present at low concentrations, compared to those of an oxidizable substrate, significantly delays or inhibits oxidation of that substrate (51). Antioxidant species in ELF

Table 1 Antioxidant Constituents of Epithelial Lining Fluid

Antioxidant	Plasma (μM)	ELF (μM)
Ascorbic acid	40	100
Glutathione	1.5	100
Uric acid	300	90
Albumin-SH	500	70
α-Tocopherol	25	2.5
β-Carotene	0.4	—

comprise low molecular weight antioxidants, metal-binding proteins, antioxidant enzymes, sacrificial reactive proteins, and unsaturated lipids (Table 1). The concentrations of non-enzymatic antioxidants vary in ELF. Some are concentrated in ELF compared to plasma, such as glutathione and ascorbate, which may indicate their relative importance (52–55). The major antioxidants in ELF include mucin, reduced glutathione, uric acid, protein (largely albumin), ceruloplasmin, and ascorbic acid (50,56).

Mucin is a glycoprotein with a core that is rich in serine and threonine, to which carbohydrates and cysteine residues (sulfhydryls) are attached. The antioxidant properties of mucus derive from the abundance of sulfhydryl and disulfide moieties in its structure (57), which would effectively scavenge oxidants such as the hydroxyl radical ($^{\bullet}$OH) (58) and would also be expected to scavenge $OCL^-/HOCL$ (59). Mucin also has metal-binding properties (60) and hence is an important antioxidant in the airways. Oxidant-generating systems, such as xanthine/xanthine oxidase, have been shown to cause the release of mucus from airway epithelial cells (61). Relevant to COPD, animal models of elastase-induced emphysema also show features of airways disease with goblet cell hyperplasia (62). In addition, neutrophil elastase is known to be a potent secretagogue for mucous glands, and therefore both oxidants and elastase may contribute to the hypermucus secretion in chronic bronchitis (63). Toxic inhalants such as cigarette smoke increase the secretion of mucins, which therefore represents a major protective mechanism in the bronchial tree.

There is limited information on the respiratory epithelial antioxidant defenses in smokers, and less for patients with COPD. Several studies have shown that glutathione (GSH) is elevated in BAL fluid (BALF) in chronic smokers (64–66).

However, the twofold increase in BALF GSH in chronic smokers may not be sufficient to deal with the excessive oxidant burden during acute smoking when acute depletion of GSH may occur (67). Rahman and colleagues (68,69) studied the acute effects of cigarette smoke condensate

(CSC) on GSH metabolism in a human alveolar epithelial cell line in vitro and in rat lungs in vivo after intratracheal CSC instillation. They found a dose and time-dependent depletion of intracellular GSH concomitant with the formation of GSH conjugates. Similar results were shown in animal lungs in vivo (68,69). Furthermore, the activities of glutathione redox system enzymes, such as glutathione peroxidase and glucose 6-phosphate dehydrogenase, transiently decreased in alveolar epithelial cells and in rat lungs after CSC exposure, possibly as a result of the action of highly electrophilic free radicals on the active site of these enzymes.

Several studies have suggested that GSH homeostasis may play a central role in the maintenance of the integrity of the lung airspace epithelial barrier. Decreasing the levels of GSH in epithelial cells leads to loss of barrier function and increased permeability (68,70). Pacht and coworkers (71) demonstrated reduced levels of vitamin E in the BAL fluid of smokers compared with nonsmokers, whereas Bui and colleagues (72) found a marginal increase in vitamin C in BALF of smokers compared to nonsmokers. Similarly, alveolar macrophages from smokers have both increased levels of ascorbic acid and augmented uptake of ascorbate (73). Increased activity of antioxidant enzymes (superoxide dismutase and catalase) in alveolar macrophages from young smokers has also been reported (74). However, Kondo et al. (75) found that increased superoxide generation by alveolar macrophages in elderly smokers was associated with decreased antioxidant enzyme activities when compared with nonsmokers. The activities of CuZnSOD, glutathione-S-transferase, and glutathione peroxidase (GP) are all decreased in alveolar macrophages from elderly smokers. However, this reduced activity was not associated with decreased gene expression, but was due to modification at the posttranslational level (75).

There appears to be no consistent change in antioxidant defenses in ELF in smokers. The apparent inconsistencies between these studies in the levels of the different antioxidants in ELF and alveolar macrophages may be due to differences in the smoking histories of chronic smokers, particularly the time of the last cigarette in relation to the sampling of and BALF, which is rarely reported in these studies.

The activities of Superoxide dismutase (SOD) and GP have been shown to be higher in the lungs of rats exposed to cigarette smoke (76). McCusker and Hoidal (74) have also demonstrated enhanced antioxidant enzyme activities in alveolar macrophages in hamsters following cigarette smoke exposure, which resulted in reduced mortality when the animals were subsequently exposed to > 95% oxygen. They speculated that alveolar macrophages undergo an adaptive response to chronic oxidant exposure that may ameliorate potential damage to lung cells from further oxidant

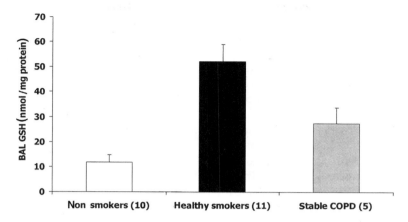

Figure 4 Levels of glutathione (GSH) in bronchoalveolar lavage (BAL) in stable and exacerbated COPD patients.

stress. The mechanisms for the induction of antioxidant enzymes in erythrocytes (77), alveolar macrophages (74), and lungs (76) by cigarette smoke exposure are currently unknown. However, it is likely to be due to the induction of antioxidant genes (see below).

In mild COPD recent studies have shown increased levels of the important antioxidant glutathione, but not to the levels that occur in chronic cigarette smokers (Fig. 4). However, there is a marked depletion of glutathione in ELF in exacerbations of COPD (78).

2. Surrogate Markers of Oxidative Stress in the Lungs

Direct measurements of oxidative stress are difficult since free radicals are highly reactive and thus short-lived. An alternative has been to measure markers of the effects of radicals on lung biomolecules, such as lipid, protein, or DNA, or to measure the stress responses to an increased oxidant burden.

There are now a number of surrogate markers of oxidative stress in the lungs which have been measured in smokers and patients with COPD. Many of these markers have been measured non-invasively in breath or breath condensate or in induced or spontaneously produced sputum. Hydrogen peroxide, measured in exhaled breath, is a direct measurement of oxidant burden in the airspaces. Smokers and patients with COPD have higher levels of exhaled H_2O_2 than normal non-smokers (79,80), and levels are even higher during exacerbations of COPD (81). The source of the increased

H_2O_2 is unknown but may in part derive from increased release of $O_2^{\cdot-}$ from alveolar macrophages in smokers (81). However, smoking in one study did not appear to influence the levels of exhaled H_2O_2 (79). The levels of exhaled H_2O_2 in this study correlated with the degree of airflow obstruction as measured by the FEV_1. However, the variability of the measurement of exhaled H_2O_2 has led to concerns over its reproducibility as a marker of oxidative stress.

Nitric oxide has been used as a marker of airway inflammation and indirectly as a measure of oxidative stress. There have been reports of increased levels of NO in exhaled breath in patients with COPD, but not to the high levels reported in asthmatics (82,83), although one study failed to confirm this result (84). Smoking increases NO levels in breath (85), and the reaction of NO with $O_2^{\cdot-}$ limits the usefulness of this marker in COPD, except perhaps to differentiate from asthma. Another defense mechanism against oxidative stress is the induction of the stress-responsive protein heme oxygenase-1 (HO-1) (86). HO-1 catalyzes the initial rate-limiting step in the oxidative degradation of heme to bilirubin. (HO-1) catalyzes the breakdown of heme to biliverdin, which is then converted by biliverdin reductase to bilirubin, which has antioxidant properties. The reaction of HO-1 with heme releases iron and carbon monoxide, which can be measured in exhaled breath and has been shown, in preliminary studies, to be elevated in patients with COPD (87). Isoprostanes are products of nonenzymatic lipid peroxidation and have therefore been used as markers of oxidative stress (88). The isoprostanes are free radical–catalyzed isomers of arachadinic acid and are stable lipid peroxidation products that circulate in plasma and are excreted in the urine (89,90). Isoprostane F2α has been shown to be elevated in cigarette smokers and can be reduced by antioxidant vitamin supplimentation (91). Urinary levels of isoprostane F2α-3 have been shown to be elevated in patients with COPD compared with control subjects (Fig. 5) and are even more elevated during exacerbations of COPD (92). Preliminary data also indicate that isoprostane F2α is elevated in exhaled breath in patients with COPD (93). Indirect measurements of lipid peroxidation products, such as thiobarbituric acid–reactive substances, have also been shown to be elevated in breath condensate in patients with stable COPD (94).

3. Evidence of Oxidative Stress in Lung Tissue

There is much evidence, from the studies described above, demonstrating the presence of oxidative stress locally in the lungs, as measured by increased levels of numerous surrogate markers of oxidative stress. However, the presence of markers of oxidative stress by no means confirm a role for

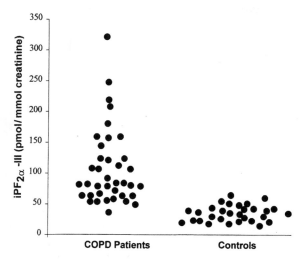

Figure 5 Urinary isoprostane $F_{2\alpha}$ (iPF$_{2\alpha}$-III) in patients with COPD and control subjects. (From Ref. 92.)

oxidative stress in the pathogenesis of COPD. Support for this link would come from the demonstration of reaction of RoS with target lung molecules and the presence of these oxidatively modified molecules in increased amounts in the lungs of smokers, particularly those who develop COPD. Increased products of lipid peroxidation have been found in the lungs of cigarette smokers, and the levels relate to the length of the smoking history (95). Furthermore, smoking-associated mitocondrial DNA mutations have been demonstrated in lungs of smokers (95), and neutrophils have been shown to cause oxidative DNA damage in alveolar epithelial cells in vitro (96). 4-Hydroxy-2-nonenal (HNE) is an aldehyde lipid peroxidation product of arachidonic acid (97). It is highly reactive and has been shown to enter cells from adducts with proteins and activate MAPKinase signaling pathways (97). It also acts as a chemoattractant for neutrophils. Recent data have shown increased expression of HNE-modified protein levels in airway and alveolar epithelial and endothelial cells in the lungs of patients with COPD compared with subjects with the same smoking history but no airways obstruction (97). This finding is important since it indicates not only the presence of increased levels of this lipid peroxidation product, but that HNE modifies proteins in lung cells to a greater extent in patients with COPD (Fig. 6). The levels of HNE adducts in alveolar and airway epithelium were shown to be inversely related to the degree of airway obstruction as measured by the FEV$_1$, suggesting a role for HNE in this

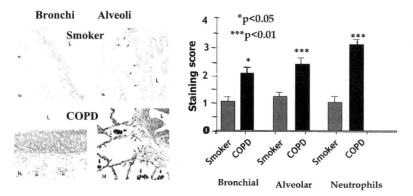

Figure 6 Photographs from immunostaining for NE in lung tissue from subjects with and without COPD: (a) non-COPD, bronchial; (b) non-COPD, alveolar; (c) COPD, bronchial; (d) COPD, alveolar. Thin arrows point to pneumocyte types I and II. Thick arrows indicate alveolar macrophages. L = airway lumen; BV = blood vessel. Note the intensely stained neutrophils in the blood vessels in (Original magnification × 200) $^*p < 0.05$; $^{***}p < 0.01$.

pathogenesis of COPD. Thus, evidence is accumulating that oxidative stress can induce reactions with target molecules in lung tissue from patients with COPD.

B. Evidence of Systemic Oxidative Stress

There has been interest recently in the concept that COPD produces not only local lung, but systemic manifestations (98). This relates not only to the systemic effects of hypoxaemia as reflected in peripheral muscle function, but also the concept that local lung inflammation may have systemic effects, such as the weight loss, which occurs in some patients and is a predictor of reduced survival (99).

One manifestation of a systemic effect is the presence of markers of oxidative stress in the blood in patients with COPD. This may be reflected as an increased sequestration of neutrophils in the pulmonary microcirculation during smoking and during exacerbations of COPD, which, as described below, may be an oxidant-mediated event (48,100,101).

Rahman and colleagues (102,103) demonstrated increased production of superoxide anion from peripheral blood neutrophils obtained from patients during acute exacerbations of COPD, which returned to normal when the patients were restudied when clinically stable. Other studies have shown that circulating neutrophils from patients with COPD show upregulation of their surface adhesion molecules, which may also be an oxidant-mediated effect (104). Activation may be even more pronounced in neutrophils that are sequestered in the pulmonary microcirculation in smokers and in patients with COPD, since neutrophils that are sequestered in the pulmonary microcirculation in animal models of lung inflammation release more ROS than circulating neutrophils (105). Thus, neutrophils, which are sequestered in the pulmonary microcirculation, may be a source of oxidative stress and may have a role in inducing endothelial adhesion molecule expression in COPD (see below).

Polyunsaturated fats and fatty acids in cell membranes are a major target of free radical attack, resulting in lipid peroxidation, a process that may continue as a chain reaction to generate peroxides and aldehydes (Fig. 3). Products of lipid peroxidation reactions can be measured in body fluids as thiobarbituric acid reactive substances (TBARS). The levels of TBARS in plasma or in BAL fluid are significantly increased in healthy smokers and patients with acute exacerbation of COPD, compared with healthy nonsmokers (24,102). However, there is a problem with the specificity of a thiobarbituric acid–malondialehyde assay as a measure of lipid peroxidation, since this assay does not directly measure the lipid peroxidation reaction. Other studies have measured the levels of conjugated dienes of linoleic acid, a secondary product of lipid peroxidation, and have shown that the levels in plasma were elevated in chronic smokers (106). In addition, elevated circulating levels of F_2-isoprostane, which is a more direct measurement of lipid peroxidation, have been found in smokers (107). Other studies have shown increased levels of fluorescent products of lipid peroxidation in smokers (108).

Lipid peroxidation products produced by oxidative stress may also activate signaling mechanisms in the inflammatory response in the airways. HNE has been shown to enter cells and activate transcription factors such as activator protein 1 (AP-1) through pathways involving MAP kinases. These events are important stress responses, which may upregulate protective antioxidant genes (109). However, HNE inhibits NF-κB activation, suggesting that a specific signaling pathway is involved in this mechanism (110). HNE may also travel between cells and become attached to plasma proteins, with the result that it may trigger effects distant from the site of the initial oxidative stress. This may be an important mechanism for the systemic effects of oxidative stress in patients with COPD. Changes in the antioxidant capacity of the blood were measured in one study as a marker of systemic oxidative stress in smokers and patients with acute exacerbations of COPD (102). Rahman and coworkers (102) found that the plasma antioxidant capacity was significantly decreased in smokers 1 hour after

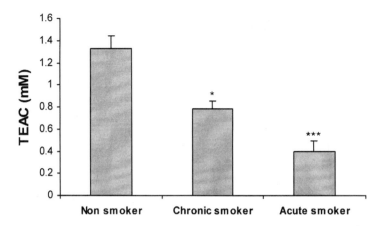

Figure 7 Plasma antioxidant capacity measured as Trolox equivalent antioxidant capacity (TEAC) in healthy nonsmokers in healthy chronic smokers who have not smoked for 12 hours and smokers who smoked 2 cigarettes 1 hour prior to measurement (acute smoker) $^*p < 0.05$ and $^{***}p < 0.001$ compared with nonsmokers. (From Ref. 102.)

smoking and in patients during acute exacerbations of COPD when compared with plasma from age-matched nonsmoking controls. The decrease in plasma antioxidant capacity in smokers may be due to a profound depletion of plasma protein sulfhydryls, as shown following cigarette smoke exposure in vitro (111). The decrease in antioxidant capacity in smokers occurred transiently during smoking and resolved rapidly after smoking cessation (Fig. 7). In exacerbations of COPD, however, the decrease in antioxidant capacity remained low for several days after the onset of the exacerbation, tending to return toward normal values at the time of recovery from the exacerbation (103) (Fig. 8). The depletion of antioxidant capacity could be explained in part by the increased release of ROS from peripheral blood neutrophils, as shown by a significant negative correlation between neutrophil superoxide anion release and plasma antioxidant capacity (102). Thus, there is clear evidence that oxidants in cigarette smoke, in vitro or in vivo, markedly decrease plasma antioxidants both in vitro and in vivo (112). Depletion of plasma antioxidants will reduce the protection against cigarette smoke–induced plasma membrane peroxidation.

Studies showing depletion of total antioxidant capacity in smokers are supported by earlier studies of measurements of the major plasma antioxidants in smokers (113–119). These studies show depletion of ascorbic

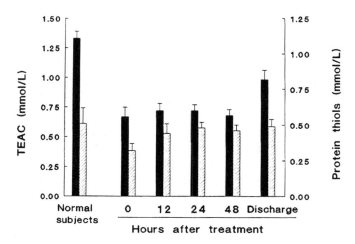

Figure 8 Time course of changes in plasma antioxidant capacity measured by Trolox equivalent antioxidant capacity (TEAC) (solid columns) and protein thiols (open columns) in normal subjects and patients during exacerbations of COPD. $p < 0.05$ for all time points during exacerbations compared with normal subjects. (From Ref. 103.)

acid, vitamin E, β-carotene, and selenium in the serum of chronic smokers (115–120). Moreover, decreased vitamin E and vitamin C levels were measured in leukocytes from smokers (121–123). However, circulating red blood cells from cigarette smokers contain increased levels of SOD and catalase, despite similar acitivity of glutathione peroxidase, and are better able to protect endothelial cells from the effects of H_2O_2 when compared with cells from nonsmokers (77).

Plasma ascorbate appears to be a particularly important antioxidant in the plasma because the gas phase of cigarette smoke induces lipid peroxidation in plasma in vitro that is decreased by ascorbate (111). Inhalation of NO from cigarette smoke as well as NO and superoxide anion released by activated phagocytes react to form peroxynitrite, which has been shown to decrease plasma antioxidant capacity by rapid oxidation of ascorbic acid, uric acid, and plasma sulfhydryls (124).

Evidence of NO/peroxynitrite activity in plasma has been demonstrated in cigarette smokers (125). Nitration of tyrosine residues or proteins in plasma leads to the production of 3-nitrotyrosine (125). Petruzzelli and colleagues (125) reported the presence of higher levels of 3-nitrotyrosine in plasma in smokers than in a group of nonsmokers. They also confirmed the presence of low levels of plasma antioxidant capacity in smokers, which were negatively correlated with the levels of 3-nitrotyrosine (125).

IV. Oxidative Stress and Airspace Epithelial Injury

The airspace epithelial surface of the lungs is particularly vulnerable to the effects of oxidative stress produced by cigarette smoke by virtue of its direct contact with the environment. At least three processes may be responsible for oxidant injury to the respiratory tract epithelial cells from cigarette smoke: (a) a direct toxic interaction of constituents of cigarette smoke (including free radicals) which have penetrated the protective antioxidant shield of the ELF; (b) damage to the cells by toxic reactive products generated by interaction between cigarette smoke and ELFs; and (c) reactions occurring subsequent to activation of inflammatory-immune processes initiated by the first two processes (50,58).

Direct oxidative damage to components of the lung matrix (such as elastin and collagen) can result from oxidants in cigarette smoke (127). Elastin synthesis and repair can also be impaired by cigarette smoke (128), which can augment proteolytic damage to matrix components and thus enhance the development of emphysema.

Injury to the epithelium may be an important early event in inflammation produced by cigarette smoke and results in an increase in airspace epithelial permeability (129). Lannan and colleagues (130) demonstrated the injurious effect of both the whole and vapor phases of cigarette smoke on human alveolar epithelial cell monolayers, as shown by increased epithelial cell detachment, decreased cell adherence, and increased cell lysis. These effects were in part oxidant-mediated since they were partially prevented by the antioxidant GSH in concentrations (500 μM) present in the epithelial lining fluid. Extra- and intracellular glutathione appears to be critical to the maintenance of epithelial integrity following exposure to cigarette smoke. Studies by Li et al. (67,70) and Rahman et al. (68) demonstrated that the increased epithelial permeability of epithelial cell monolayers in vitro and in rat lungs in vivo following exposure to cigarette smoke condensate was associated with profound changes in the antioxidant glutathione. Concentrations of GSH were considerably decreased, concomitant with a decrease in the activities of the enzymes involved in the GSH redox cycle such such as glutathione peroxidase and glucose-6-phosphate dehydrogenase by cigarette smoke exposure. Furthermore, depletion of lung GSH alone by treatment with the glutathione synthesis inhibitor buthionine sulfoximine induces increased airspace epithelial permeability both in vitro and in vivo (68,70,131).

Similar to these in vitro and animal studies, human studies have shown increased epithelial permeability in chronic smokers compared with nonsmokers, as measured by increased ^{99m}technetium-diethylenetriamine-pentacetate (^{99m}Tc-DTPA) lung clearance, with a further increase in ^{99m}Tc-DTPA clearance following acute smoking (64). Thus, cigarette smoke has a detrimental effect on alveolar epithelial cell function, which is, in part, oxidant-mediated, since antioxidants provide protection against this injurious event.

V. Oxidative Stress and Neutrophil Sequestration and Migration in the Lungs

The recruitment of neutrophils to the airspaces is initiated by the sequestration of these cells in the lung microcirculation (132). Sequestration occurs under normal circumstances in the pulmonary capillary bed and results from the size differential between neutrophils (average diameter $7 \mu M$) and pulmonary capillary segments (average diameter $5 \mu M$). Thus, a proportion of the circulating neutrophils have to deform in order to negotiate the smaller capillary segments (132). Studies using a variety of techniques, including radiolabeled or fluorescently labeled neutrophils, have supported the idea that the lungs contain a large pool of noncirculating neutrophils, which are either retained or slowly moving within the pulmonary microcirculation. Radiolabeled neutrophil studies in healthy subjects indicate that a proportion of neutrophils are normally delayed in the pulmonary circulation, compared to radiolabeled erythrocytes (100). In normal subjects there is a correlation between neutrophil deformability measured in vitro and the subsequent sequestration of these cells in the pulmonary microcirculation following their reinjection—the less deformable the cells, the greater the sequestration of these cells occurs in the pulmonary circulation (133). This provides a mechanism for the creation of a pool of sequestered or noncirculating cells in the pulmonary microcirculation, without the need to invoke margination of neutrophils in the post capillary venules, which is the mechanism by which a noncirculating pool of cells is present in the systemic circulation (134). Sequestration of neutrophils in the pulmonary capillaries allows time for the neutrophils to interact with the pulmonary capillary endothelium, resulting in their adherence to the endothelium and thereafter their transmigration across the alveolar capillary membrane to the interstitium and airspaces of the lungs in response to inflammation or infection.

Any condition leading to a decrease in neutrophil deformability will potentially increase neutrophil sequestration in the lungs. Cell activation is associated with decreased neutrophil deformability and occurs due to the assembly of the cytoskeleton, in particular the polymerization of microfilaments (F-actin), resulting in cell stiffening. Neutrophils can be activated while in transit in the pulmonary microcirculation by a number of mediators, including cytokines released from resident lung cells, alveolar macrophages, and epithelial and endothelial cells. Inhaled oxidants such as those contained in cigarette smoke and other air pollutants could influence the transit of cells in the pulmonary capillary bed. Studies in humans using radiolabeled neutrophils and red cells show a transient increase in neutrophil sequestration in the lungs during smoking (100), which returns to normal upon cessation of smoking. Using an in vitro positive pressure cell filtration technique, cells exposed to cigarette smoke in vitro decrease their deformability (135). A similar decrease in deformability can be demonstrated in vivo for neutrophils from the blood of subjects who are actively smoking (Fig. 9) (136). Since each puff of cigarette smoke contains 10^7 oxidant molecules/puff, it has been suggested that the effect of cigarette smoke on neutrophil deformability is oxidant-mediated. Support for this hypothesis comes from in vitro studies, which show that the decreased neutrophil deformability induced by cigarette smoke exposure is abolished by antioxidants, such as glutathione (135). There is also evidence that

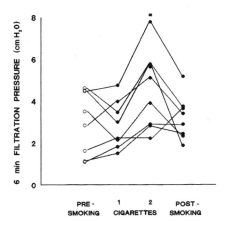

Figure 9 The pressures developed by the immediate filtration of arterial blood sampled presmoking (open circles) after one and two cigarettes and 10 minutes postsmoking (closed circles). An increase in the 6-minute filtration pressure (P_a) was observed in all eight subjects after two cigarettes. Multiple ANOVA showed a significant effect of cigarettes ($p < 0.05$) (%COHb: presmoking, $4.1 \pm 1.8\%$; two cigarettes, $5.6 \pm 2.2\%$; postsmoking, $6.0 \pm 2.0\%$). (From Ref. 136.)

oxidative stress may reach the circulation during cigarette smoking, which could result in a decrease in the deformability of neutrophils, increasing their sequestration in the pulmonary microcirculation (136). Oxidants appear to affect neutrophil deformability by altering the cytoskeleton as a result of polymerisation of actin (135).

Recent studies have also shown that cigarette smoke causes the release of neutrophils from the bone marrow and that these neutrophils may have decreased deformability and may thus preferentially sequester in the pulmonary microcirculation (137). The mechanism of this release of bone marrow neutrophils is as yet unclear, but oxidants may have a role. Thus, cigarette smoking increases neutrophil sequestration in the pulmonary microcirculation, at least in part, by decreasing neutrophil deformability.

Once sequestered, components of cigarette smoke can alter neutrophil adhesion to endothelium by upregulating CD18 integrins (138,139), which is known to upregulate the NADPH oxidase–H_2O_2-generating system (140). Inhalation of cigarette smoke by hamsters increases neutrophil adhesion to the endothelium of both arterioles and venules (138). This increased neutrophil adhesion is thought to be mediated by superoxide anion derived from cigarette smoke, since it was inhibited by pretreatment with CuZnSOD (138). Neutrophils sequestered in the pulmonary circulation of the rabbit following cigarette smoke inhalation also show increased expression of CD18 integrins (139). Changes in intracellular glutathione redox status in endothelial cells have been shown to alter the neutrophil chemotactic and other metabolic functions, such that depletion of glutathione enhanced neutrophil endothelial adhesion, an effect that was blocked by increasing intracellular glutathione with N-acetylcysteine (141). The mechanism of this change in neutrophil adhesion involves the expression of intracellular adhesion molecule-1 and E-selectin involving the activation of the transcription factor nuclear factor kappa B (NF-κB). Glutathione has been shown to be depleted in lungs exposed acutely to cigarette smoke (64,67,68,70), and therefore changes in endothelial cell glutathione may be involved in the adhesion and subsequent migration of neutrophils into the airspaces in cigarette smokers.

Increased expression of adhesion molecules on neutrophils and endothelial cells in smoke-exposed animals may result from the secondary inflammatory effects of smoking, through the release of cytokines, since direct smoke exposure in vitro does not produce increased expression of neutrophil adhesion molecules or enhance functional adherence (142). Thus, several mechanisms involving oxidants cause neutrophil sequestration in the pulmonary microcirculation in smokers. Oxidant-mediated mechanisms may also result in the increased sequestration of neutrophils, which occurs in the pulmonary microcirculation during exacerbations of COPD (101,103).

Neutrophils sequestered in the pulmonary microcirculation will subsequently respond to chemotactic components in cigarette smoke and become more adhesive to pulmonary vascular endothelial cells in preparation for migration into the airspaces. Nicotine itself is chemotactic (143). Smoke exposure in humans results in increased levels of chemotactic factors in the airspaces (144). Studies in animal models of smoke exposure (145) have shown increased neutrophil sequestration in the pulmonary microcirculation, associated with upregulation of adhesion molecules on the surface of these cells (146). Activation of neutrophils sequestered in the pulmonary microvasculature could also induce the release of reactive oxygen intermediates and proteases within the microenvironment with limited access for free radical scavengers and antiproteases. Thus, destruction of the alveolar wall, as occurs in emphysema, could result from a proteolytic or oxidant insult from the intravascular space without the need for the neutrophils to migrate into the airspaces (146).

VI. Oxidative Stress and Protease/Antiprotease Imbalance

The development of a proteinase/antiproteinase imbalance in the lungs is a central hypothesis in the pathogenesis of emphysema in smokers. This theory was developed from studies of early-onset emphysema in α_1-antitrypsin (α_1-AT)–deficient subjects. In the case of smokers with normal levels of α_1-AT, the elastase burden may be increased as a result of increased recruitment of leukocytes to the lungs, and there may be a functional deficiency of α_1-AT due to oxidative inactivation of α_1-AT in the lungs.

A large body of literature has been published in an attempt to prove the protease/antiprotease theory of the pathogenesis of emphysema. It is clear that an imbalance between an increased elastase burden in the lungs and a functional deficiency of α_1-At due to its inactivation by oxidants is an oversimplification, not least because other proteinases and other antiproteinases are likely to have a role. Early studies showed that the function of α_1-AT in bronchoalveolar lavage was decreased by around 40% in smokers, compared with nonsmokers (147). This functional α_1-AT deficiency is thought to be due to inactivation of the α_1-AT by oxidation of the methionine residue at its active site (148,149) by oxidants in cigarette smoke. Secretory leukoprotease inhibitor (SLPI), another major inhibitor of neutrophil elastase (NE), can also be inactivated by oxidants (150,151).

In vitro studies have also showed loss of α_1-AT–inhibitory capacity when treated with oxidants (152), including cigarette smoke (153). In addition, oxidation of the methionine residue in α_1-AT was confirmed in the lungs of healthy smokers (154). These studies supported the concept of inactivation of α_1-AT by oxidation of the active site of the protein. Other studies showed that macrophases from the lungs of smokers release increased amounts of ROS which could also inactivate α_1-AT in vitro (149). However, most of the α_1-AT in cigarette smokers remains active and is therefore still capable of protecting against the increased protease burden. There is also conflicting data on whether α_1-AT function lavage is altered in cigarette smokers (155), which may be due to technical differences between the studies that may have affected α_1-AT function. In addition the original observation that oxidation of $\alpha_{1\_}1$-AT occurs in bronchoalveolar lavage in smokers has not been confirmed (156).

The acute effects of cigarette smoking on the functional activity of α_1-AT in bronchoalveolar lavage fluid has also been studied and show a transient, but nonsignficant fall in the antiprotease activity of bronchoalveolar lavage fluid one hour after smoking (157). Thus, studies assessing the function of α_1-AT in either chronic or acute cigarette smoking have failed to produce a clear picture. A further hypothesis has been developed to explain these conflicting data and has invoked a contributory role for other antiproteases, such as antileukoprotease, or by observing more subtle changes, e.g., a decrease in the association rate constant of α_1-AT for neutrophil elastase, which may contribute to elastin degradation (158).

VII. Other Mechanisms Involving Oxidants Related to the Pathogenesis of COPD

The majority of the information available on the pathogenesis of COPD relates to the development of emphysema. COPD also includes the other conditions of chronic bronchitis and small airways disease. It is presumed that the mechanisms that initiate inflammation and the effects of proteolytic and oxidant-induced damage are also relevant to these conditions, although much less information is available.

The airways of smokers contain more goblet cells than do those of nonsmokers, and goblet cell activation results in mucus hypersecretion, the defining feature of chronic bronchitis. Cigarette smoke has been shown to activate epithelial growth factor (EGF) receptors by tyrosine phosphorylation (159), resulting in the induction of mucin (mucin 5ac) gene expression and synthesis in epithelial cells in vitro and the lungs in vivo (160). Apoptosis or programmed cell death of leukocytes is an important mechanism in the resolution of inflammation. However, structural lung cells may also undergo apoptosis. Hydrogen peroxide can induce apoptosis in airway epithelial cells (161). Recent evidence from both in vitro and in vivo studies in animals and in humans have shown that apoptosis occurs in smoke-exposed macrophages (162).

The marked decrease in intracellular glutathione that occurs upon exposure of cells to cigarette smoke exposure may have a role in the regulation of apoptosis (163). Recently a hypothesis has been developed that pulmonary capillary endothelial cell apoptosis, induced by cigarette smoking, may be an early event in the process that leads to alveolar wall destruction and emphysema. Studies have shown in vitro that cigarette smoke exposure triggers apoptosis (164) and that pulmonary vascular endothelial cell apoptosis induced by cigarette smoking may be an early event in the process that leads to alveolar wall destruction, a central feature of emphysema (165). Signaling pathways involving of AP-1 and NF-κB and the downregulation of the vascular endothelial growth factor receptor KDR (VEGF-KDR) have been proposed as part of the mechanism (166). Oxidants are thought to be involved since the apoptosis in lung cells associated with emphysematous lesions is also associated with increased markers of oxidative stress, specifically increased expression of the lipid peroxidation product HNE (167). Moreover, lung cell apoptosis induced by downregulation of the VEGF-KDR can be prevented by antioxidants (167).

VIII. Relationship Between Oxidative Stress and the Development of Airways Obstruction

The neutrophil appears to be a critical cell in the pathogenesis of COPD. Previous epidemiological studies have shown a relationship between circulating neutrophil numbers and the FEV_1 (168). Moreover, a relationship has also been shown between the change in peripheral blood neutrophil count and the change in airflow limitation over time (169). Another study has shown that a relationship between peripheral blood neutrophil luminol enhanced chemiluminescence, as a measure of the release of ROS and measurements of airflow limitation in young cigarette smokers (170). Even passive cigarette smoking has been associated with increased peripheral blood leukocyte counts and enhanced release of oxygen radicals (171). Oxidative stress, measured as lipid peroxidation products in plasma, has also been shown to correlate inversely with the % predicted FEV_1 in a population study (172).

In the general population there is an association between dietary intake of antioxidant vitamins and lung function. Britton and coworkers (173), in a population of 2633 subjects, showed an association between dietary intake of the antioxidant vitamin E and lung function, supporting the hypothesis that this antioxidant may have a role in protecting against the development of COPD. Another study has suggested that antioxidant levels in the diet could be a possible explanation for differences in COPD mortality in different populations (174). Dietary polyunsaturated fatty acids may protect cigarette smokers against the development of COPD (175,176). These studies support the concept that dietary antioxidant supplementation may be a possible therapy to prevent the development of COPD. Such intervention studies have been difficult to carry out (177), but there is at least some evidence to suggest that antioxidant vitamin supplementation reduces oxidant stress in smokers, measured as a decrease in Pentane levels in breath as an indication of lipid peroxides in the airways (178).

IX. Oxidative Stress and Muscle Dysfunction

Part of the systemic effects in COPD is the loss of muscle mass and dysfunction of peripheral skeletal muscles. Mechanisms underlying muscle dysfunction in COPD are not well understood. Skeletal muscles generate ROS at rest, which increases during contractile activity. It is known that oxidative stress occurs in skeletal muscles during skeletal muscle fatigue and sepsis-induced muscle dysfunction (179). The proposed mechanism for this may relate to hypoxia, impaired mitochondrial metabolism, and increased cytochrome c oxidase activity in skeletal muscles and patients with COPD (180). The levels of glutamate (a precursor of the antioxidant glutathione) are reduced in patients with severe COPD, associated with increased muscle glycolytic metabolism (181).

Associated with the lower levels of glutamate, GSH levels are also decreased. These findings suggest that an oxidant/antioxidant imbalance is involved in skeletal muscle dysfunction in patient with COPD. A causal relationship between abnormally low muscle redox potential at rest and the alterations of glutamate metabolism observed in patients with emphysema has been suggested (182), since the decreased muscle redox capacity in COPD is thought to result from a reduced ability to synthesize GSH during endurance training in patients with COPD (179). It has been suggested that oxidative stress may play a central role in mediating the muscle mass wasting in patients with COPD.

X. Oxidative Stress and Gene Expression

A. Pro-inflammatory Genes

Evidence from a large number of studies indicates that COPD is associated with airway and airspace inflammation, as shown in recent bronchial biopsy studies (18) and by the presence of markers of inflammation including interleukin (IL)-8 and tumor necrosis factor-alpha (TNFα), which are elevated in the sputum of patients with COPD (183).

Many inflammatory mediator genes, such as those for the cytokines IL-8 and TNFα and nitric oxide, are regulated by transcription factors, such as nuclear factor kappa B (NF-κB). NF-κB is present in the cytosol in an inactive form linked to its inhibitory protein IκB. Many stimuli, including cytokines and oxidants, activate NF-κB, resulting in ubiquination, cleaving of IκB from NF-κB, and the destruction of IκB in the proteosome (184). These critical events in the inflammatory response are redox sensitive. Studies in vitro show that treatment of macrophages and alveolar and bronchial epithelial cells with oxidants stimulates the release of inflammatory mediators such as IL-8, IL-1, and nitric oxide, associated with increased expression of the mRNA for the genes for these inflammatory mediators and increased nuclear binding and activation of NF-κB (185,186). In addition, a stimulus that is relevant to exacerbations of COPD, such as particulate air pollution, which has oxidant properties, also activates NF-κB in alveolar epithelial cells (187).

Thiol antioxidants such as *N*-acetylcysteine and Nacystelin, which are potential therapies in COPD, have been shown in in vitro experiments to block the release of these inflammatory mediators from epithelial cells and macrophages, by a mechanism involving increasing intracellular glutathione and decreasing NF-κB activation (185,187). The intracellular glutathione redox status, which is affected by cigarette smoke, plays a critical role in the regulation of transcription factors such as NF-κB and AP-1 (187–190).

There may also be an interaction between oxidants and tumor necrosis factor, which are both relevant mediators in COPD, producing synergistic activation of NF-κB, suggesting that anti-inflammatory and antioxidant therapies may be required together in order to prevent the activation of NF-κB in the lung inflammation that occurs in COPD (191).

B. Antioxidant Genes

An important effect of oxidative stress in the lungs is the upregulation of protective antioxidant genes. The antioxidant glutathione is concentrated in epithelial lining fluid compared with plasma (50) and has an important protective role, together with its redox enzymes in the airspaces and intracellularly in epithelial cells. Human studies have shown elevated levels of glutathione in epithelial lining fluid in chronic cigarette smokers compared with nonsmokers (56). However, this increase is not present immediately after acute cigarette smoking (24).

The discrepancy between glutathione levels in epithelial lining fluid in chronic and acute cigarette smokers has been investigated in animal models and in vitro using cultured epithelial cells (67,70,192). Exposure of airspace epithelial cells to cigarette smoke condensate in vitro produces an initial decrease in intracellular GSH with a rebound increase after 12 hours (193). This effect in vitro is mimicked by a similar change in glutathione in rat lungs in vivo following intratracheal instillation of cigarette smoke condensate (192). The initial fall in lung and intracellular glutathione after treatment with cigarette smoke condensate was associated with a decrease in the activity of gamma-glutamylcysteine synthetase (γGCS); the rate-limiting enzyme for glutathione synthesis, with recovery of the activity by 24 hours (192,193). The increased level of glutathione following cigarette smoke condensate exposure has been shown to be due to transcriptional upregulation of the gene for GSH synthesis, γGCS, by components within cigarette smoke (193,194) (Fig. 10). The mechanism by which cigarette smoke causes the upregulation of γGCS involves redox-sensitive transcription factors. Using both a gel mobility shift assay and a reporter system in which the promoter region of the γGCS gene was transfected into airway epithelial cells, cigarette smoke can be shown to activate the transcription factor activator protein-1 (AP-1) (195,196). Deletion experiments and site-directed mutagenesis in the reporter assay has shown that the proximal AP-1 site on the γGCS gene promoter region is critical for the regulation of γGCS gene expression in response to various oxidants, including cigarette smoke (196). Thus, oxidative stress, including that produced by cigarette smoking, causes upregulation of the gene involved in the synthesis of glutathione as a proective mechanism against oxidative stress. These events are likely to account for the increased level of glutathione seen in the epithelial lining fluid in chronic cigarette smokers (24). However, the injurious effects of cigarette smoke may occur repeatedly during and immediately after cigarette smoking when the lung the depleted of antioxidants, including glutathione (24).

The cytokine tumor necrosis factor (TNF), which is present as part of the airway inflammation in COPD (183), also decreases intracellular glutathione levels initially in epithelial cells by a mechanism involving the generation of intracellular oxidative stress, which is followed after 24 hours by a rebound increase in intracellular glutathione as a result of AP-1 activation and increased γGCS mRNA expression (196). Corticosteroids have been used as anti-inflammatory agents in COPD, but there is still

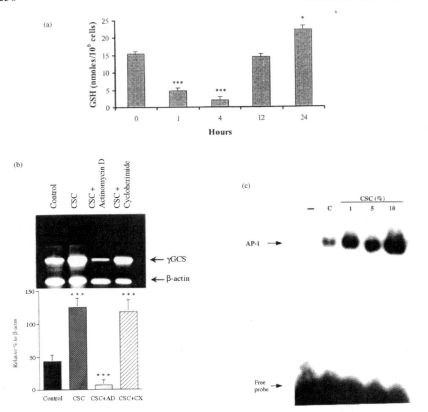

Figure 10 The effect of cigarette smoke exposure in A549 epithelial cells on (a) glutathione (GSH), (b) gamma-glutamylcysteine synthetase (γGCS) mRNA by RTPCR, and (c) AP-1 nuclear binding by gel mobility shift assay. (From Ref. 193.)

doubt about their effectiveness in reducing airway inflammation in COPD (197). Interestingly, dexamethasone also causes a decrease in intracellular glutathione in airspace epithelial cells, but no rebound increase compared with the effects of TNF (196). Moreover, the rebound increase in gluta-thione produced by TNF in epithelial cells is prevented by co-treatment with dexamethasone (196). These effects may have relevance for the treatment of COPD patients with corticosteroids.

Gilks and coworkers (198) have shown increased expression of a number of antioxidant genes in the bronchial epithelial cells in rats exposed to whole cigarette smoke for up to 14 days. Whereas mRNA of manganese superoxide dismutase (MnSOD) and metallothionein (MT) was increased at

1–2 days and returned to normal by 7 days, mRNA for glutathione peroxidase did not increase until 7 days, suggesting the importance of the glutathione redox system as a mechanism for chronic protection against the effects of the cigarette smoke (198).

The *cfos* gene belongs to a family of growth and differentiation-related immediate early genes, the expression of which generally represents the first measurable response to a variety of chemical and physical stimuli (185). Studies in various cell lines have shown enhanced gene expression of the *cfos* in response to cigarette smoke condensate (199). These effects of cigarette smoke condensate can be mimicked by peroxynitrite and smoke-related aldehydes in concentrations that are present in cigarette smoke condensate (199). The effects of cigarette smoke condensate can be enhanced by pretreatment of the cells with buthionine sulfoximine to decrease intracellular glutathione and can be prevented by treatment with the thiol antioxidant *N*-acetylcysteine (199). These studies emphasize the importance of intracellular levels of the antioxidant glutathione in regulating gene expression.

Thus, oxidative stress, including that produced by cigarette smoke, causes increased gene expression of both pro-inflammatory genes by oxidant-mediated activation of transcription factors such as NF-κB, but also activation of protective genes such as γ-glutamylcysteine synthetase (γ-GCS) through other transcription factors, which in the case of γ-GCS is the transcription factor AP-1. A balance may therefore exist between pro- and anti-inflammatory gene expression in response to cigarette smoke, which may be critical for whether cell injury is induced by cigarette smoking. Knowledge of the molecular mechanisms that regulate these events may open new therapeutic avenues in the treatment of COPD.

XI. Oxidatives Stress and Susceptibility to COPD

Only 15–20% of cigarette smokers appear to be susceptible to the effects of cigarette smoke, showing a rapid decline in FEV_1 and developing COPD (200). There has been considerable interest in identifying those who are susceptible and the mechanisms of that susceptibility (200–202), since this would provide an important insight into the pathogenesis of COPD as did the recognition of the association between α_1-antitrypsin and COPD.

Polymorphisms of various genes have been shown to be more prevalent in smokers who develop COPD (201). A number of these polymorphisms may have functional significance, such as the association between the TNFα gene polymorphism (TNF2), which is associated with increased TNF levels in response to inflammation, and the development of chronic bronchitis (203). Relevant to the effects of cigarette smoke is a polymorphism in the gene for microsomal epoxide hydrolase, an enzyme involved in the metabolism of highly reactive epoxide intermediates which are present in cigarette smoke (204). The proportion of individuals with slow microsomal epoxide hydrolase activity was significantly higher in patients with COPD and a subgroup of patients shown pathologically to have emphysema (COPD 22%; emphysema 19%), compared with control subjects (6%) (204). It may be that a panel of "susceptibility" polymorphisms, of functional significance in enzymes involved in xenobiotic metabolism or antioxidant enzyme genes, may allow individuals to be identified as being susceptible to the effects of cigarette smoke.

XII. Therapeutic Options to Redress the Oxidant/Antioxidant Imbalance in COPD

There is now convincing evidence for an oxidant/antioxidant imbalance in smokers and a probable role for this imbalance in the pathogenesis of COPD. However, proof of concept of the role of oxidative stress in the pathogeneis of COPD will come with studies of effective antioxidant therapy. Various approaches have been tried to redress the oxidant/antioxidant imbalance. One approach is to target the inflammatory response by reducing the sequestration or migration of leukocytes from the pulmonary circulation into the airspaces. Possible therapeutic options for this are drugs that alter cell deformability, preventing neutrophil sequestration or the migration of neutrophils either by interfering with the adhesion molecules necessary for migration or preventing the release of inflammatory cytokines such as IL-8 or leukotrine B_4, which result in neutrophil migration. It should also be possible to use agents to prevent the release of oxygen radicals from activated leukocytes or to quench those oxidants once they are formed by enhancing the antioxidant screen in the lungs.

Recent preliminary studies of a phosphodiesterase 4 inhibitor (PDE4) have shown some therapeutic benefit in patients with COPD (205). The mechanism by which such drugs act is by increasing cAMP, which decreases neutrophil activation. In particular, the release of ROS by neutrophils may be decreased, since increasing cAMP blocks the assembly of NADPH oxidase (206).

There are various options to enhance the lung antioxidant screen. One approach would be to use specific spin traps such as α-phenyl-*N-tert*-butyl nitrone to react directly with ROS and RNS at the site of inflammation. However, considerable work is needed to demonstrate the efficacy of such drugs in vivo. Inhibitors that have a double action, such as the inhibition of lipid peroxidation and quenching radicals, could be developed (207). Another approach could be the molecular manipulation of antioxidant genes, such as glutathione peroxidase or genes involved in the synthesis of glutathione, such as γGCS, or by developing molecules with activity similar to these antioxidant enzymes.

Recent animal studies have shown that recombinent SOD treatment can prevent the neutrophil influx to the airspaces and IL-8 release induced by cigarette smoking through a mechanism involving downregulation of NF-κB (208) (Fig. 11). This holds great promise if compounds can be developed with antioxidant enzyme properties that may be able to act as novel anti-inflammatory drugs by regulating the molecular events in lung inflammation.

Another approach would be to simply administer antioxidant therapy. This has been attempted in cigarette smokers using various antioxidants such as vitamin C and vitamin E (75–77). The results have been rather disappointing, although, as described above, the antioxidant vitamin E has been shown to reduce oxidative stress in patients with COPD (178). Attempts to supplement lung glutathione have been made using glutathione

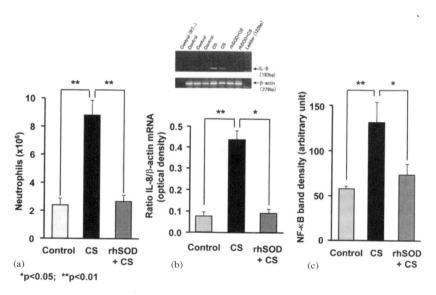

Figure 11 The effect of a recombinant SOD (rhSOD) on cigarette smoke–induced (a) neutrophil influx, (b) IL-8 mRNA by RPTCR, and (c) NF-κB nuclear binding in guinea pig lungs. $^*p < 0.05$; $^{**}p < 0.01$. (From Ref. 208.)

or its precursors (209). Glutathione itself is not efficiently transported into most animal cells, and an excess of glutathione may be a source of the thiyl radical under conditions of oxidative stress (210). Nebulized glutathione has also been used therapeutically, but this has been shown to induce bronchial hyperreactivity. The thiol cysteine is the rate-limiting amino acid in GSH synthesis (211). Cysteine administration is not possible since it is oxidized to cystine, which is neurotoxic (212). The cysteine donating compound *N*-acetylcysteine (NAC) acts as a cellular precursor of GSH and is deacetylated in the gut to cysteine following oral administration. It reduces disulfide bonds and has the potential to interact directly with oxidants. The use of *N*-acetylcysteine in an attempt to enhance GSH in patients with COPD has met with varying success (213–215). NAC given orally in low doses of 600 mg per day to normal subject results in very low levels of NAC in the plasma for up to 2 hours after administration (216).

Bridgeman and colleagues (217) showed after 5 days of NAC 600 mg 3 times daily that there was a significant increase in plasma GSH levels. However, there was no associated significant rise in BAL GSH or in lung tissue. These data seem to imply that producing a sustained increase in lung GSH is difficult using NAC in subjects who are not already depleted of glutathione. Continental European studies have shown that NAC reduces the number of exacerbation days in patients with COPD (213,214). This was not confirmed in a British Thoracic Society study of NAC (215). However, recent meta-analysis of all of the studies with NAC have suggested beneficial effects in reducing exacerbations in COPD patients (218). Recently a study of *N*-isobutyrylcysteine, a derivative of *N*-acetylcysteine, also failed to reduce exacerbation rates in patients with COPD (219).

Nacystelyn (NAL) is a lysine salt of *N*-acetylcysteine. It is also a mucolytic and oxidant thiol compound that, in contrast to NAC, which is acid, has a neutral pH. NAL can be aerosolized into the lung without causing significant side effects (220). Studies comparing the effects of NAL and NAC found that both drugs enhance intracellular glutathione in alveolar epithelial cells (218) and inhibit hydrogen peroxide and superoxide anion release from neutrophils harvested from peripheral blood from smokers and patients with COPD (221).

Molecular regulation of glutathione synthesis by targeting γGCS has great promise as a means of treating oxidant-medicated injury in the lungs. Recent work by Manna and coworkers (222) has shown that recombinant γGCS in rat hepatoma cells completely protected against the TNFα-induced activation of NF-κB, AP-1, and the apoptosis/inflammatory process. Cellular GSh may be increased by increasing γGCS activity, which may be possible by gene transfer techniques, although this would be an expensive treatment that may not be considered for a condition such as COPD.

However, knowledge of how γGCS is regulated may allow the development of other compounds that may act to enhance GSH.

In summary, there is now very good evidence for an oxidant/antioxidant imbalance in COPD and increasing evidence that this imbalance is important in the pathogenesis of this condition. Oxidative stress may also be critical to the inflammatory response to cigarette smoke, through the upregulation of redox-sensitive transcription factors and hence pro-inflammatory gene expression, but it is also involved in the protective mechanisms against the effects of cigarette smoke by the induction of antioxidant genes. Inflammation itself induces oxidative stress in the lungs, and polymorphisms in genes for inflammatory mediators or antioxidant genes may have a role in the susceptibility to the effects of cigarette smoke. Knowledge of the mechanisms of the effects of oxidative stress should in the future allow the development of potent antioxidant therapies that can be used to test the hypothesis that oxidative stress is involved in the pathogenesis of COPD, not only by direct injury to cells, but also as a fundamental factor in the inflammation in smoking-related lung disease.

References

1. Halliwell B. Antioxidants in human health and disease. Ann Rev Nutr 1996; 16:33–50.
2. Sies H. Oxidative stress. NewYork: Academic Press, 1985.
3. Halliwell B. Free radicals, antioxidants, and human disease: curiosity, cause, or consequence? Lancet 1994; 344:721–724.
4. British Thoracic Society Guidelines for the management of chronic obstructive pulmonary disease. Thorax 1997; 52 (suppl 5) S1–S28.
5. American Thoracic Society Standards for the diagnosis and care of patients with chronic obstructive pulmonary disease. Am J Respir Crit Care Med 1995; 152:S77–S120.
6. MacNee W, Donaldson K. Pathogenesis of chronic obstructive pulmonary disease. In: Wardlaw AJ, Hamid Q, eds. Textbook of Respiratory Cell and Molecular Biology. Martin Dunitz, London. 2002; pp. 99–132.
7. Peto R, Lopez AD, Boreham J, Thun M, Heatch C. Mortality from tobacco in developed countries: indirect estimation from national vital statistics. Lancet 1992; 339:1268–1278.
8. Church T, Pryor WA. Free-radical chemistry of cigarette smoke and its toxicology implications. Environ Health Perspect 1985; 64:111–126.
9. Rahman I, MacNee W. Role of oxidants/antioxidants in smoking-induced lung diseases. Free Rad Biol Med 1996; 21:669–681.
10. Repine JE, Bast A, Lankhorst I, and the Oxidative Stress Study Group. Oxidative stress in chronic obstructive pulmonary disease. Am J Respir Crit Care Med 1997; 156:341–357.

11. Pryor WA, Stone K. Oxidants in cigarette smoke: radicals hydrogen peroxides peroxynitrate and peroxynitrite. Ann NY Acad Sci 1993; 686:12–28.

12. Zang KY, Stone K, Pryor WA. Detection of free radicals in aqueous extracts of cigarette tar by electron spin resonance. Free Rad Biol Med 1995; 19:161–167.

13. Nakayama T, Church DF, Pryor WA. Quantitative analysis of the hydrogen peroxide formed in aqueous cigarette tar extracts. Free Rad Biol Med 1989; 7:9–15.

14. Cross CE, Van der Vliet A, Eiserich JP, Wong J. Oxidative stress and antioxidants in respiratory tract lining fluids. In: Clerch LB, Massaro DJ, eds. Oxygen, Gene Expression, and Cellular Function. New York: Marcel Dekker, Inc., 1997:367–398.

15. Beckman JS, Beckman TW, Chen J, Marshall PA, Freeman BA. Apparent hydroxyl radical production by peroxynitrite: implications for endothelial injury from nitric oxide and superoxide. Proc Natl Acad Sci USA 1990; 87:1620–1624.

16. Moreno JJ, Foroozesh M, Church DF, Pryor WA. Release of iron from ferritin by aqueous extracts of cigarette smoke. Chem Res Toxicol 1992; 5:116–123.

17. Eidelman D, Saetta MP, Nai-San Wang HG, Hoidal JR, King M, Cosio MG. Cellularity of the alveolar walls in smokers and its relation to alveolar destruction. Am Rev Respir Dis 1990; 141:1547–1552.

18. Jeffery PK. Structural and inflammatory changes in COPD; a comparison with asthma. Thorax 1998; 53:129–136.

19. Saetta M, Stefano A, Maestrelli P, Ferraresso A, Drigo R, Potena A, Cicaccia A, Fabbri LM. Activated T-lymphocytes and macrophages in bronchial mucosa of subjects with chronic bronchitis. Am Rev Respir Dis 1993; 147:301–306.

20. Hunninghake GW, Crystal RG. Cigarette smoking and lung destruction: accumulation of neutrophils in the lungs of cigarette smokers. Am Rev Respir Dis 1983; 128:833–838.

21. Bosken CH, Hards J, Gatter K, Hogg JC. Characterization of the inflammatory reaction in the peripheral airways of cigarette smokers using immunocytochemistry. Am Rev Respir Dis 1992; 145:911–917.

22. Rasp FL, Clawson CC, Hoidal JR, Repine JE. Reversible impairment of the adherence of alveolar macrophages from cigarette smokers. Am Rev Respir Dis 1978; 119:979–986.

23. Costabel U, Guyman J. Effect of smoking on bronchoalveolar lavage constituents. Eur Respir J 1992; 5:776–779.

24. Morrison D, Rahamn I, Lannan S, MacNee W. Epithelial permeability, inflammation and oxidant stress in the air spaces of smokers. Am J Respir Crit Care Med 1999; 159:473–479.

25. Hoidal JR, Fox RB, LeMarbe PA, Perri R, Repine JE. Altered oxidative metabolic responses *in vitro* of alveolar macrophages from asymtomatic cigarette smokers. Am Rev Respir Dis 1981; 123:85–89.

26. Nakashima H, Ando M, Sugimoto M, Suga M, Soda K, Araki S. Receptor-mediated O_2^- release by alveolar macrophages and peripheral blood monocytes from smokers and nonsmokers. Am Rev Respir Dis 1987; 136:310–315.

27. Schaberg T, Haller H, Rau M, Kaiser D, Fassbender M, Lode H. Superoxide anion release induced by platelet-activating factor is increased in human alveolar macrophages from smokers. Eur Respir J 1992; 5:387–393.

28. Drath DB, Larnovsky ML, Huber GL. The effects of experimental exposure to tobacco smoke on the oxidative metabolism of alveolar macrophages. J Reticul Soc 1970; 25:597–604.

29. Schaberg T, Klein U, Rau M, Eller J, Lode H. Subpopulation of alveolar macrophages in smokers and nonsmokers: relation to the expression of CD11/CD18 molecules and superoxide anion production. Am J Respir Crit Care Med 1995; 151:1551–1558.

30. Saetta M, Di Stefano A, Maestrelli P, Turato G, Ruggieri MP, Roggeri A, Calcagni P, Mapp CE, Ciaccia A, Fabbri LM. Airway eosinophilia in chronic bronchitis during exacerbations. Am J Respir Crit Care Med 1994; 150:1646–1652.

31. Lacoste JY, Bousquet J, Chanez P, Van Vgve T, Simony-Lafontaine J, Lequeu N, Vic P, Enander I, Godard P, Michel FB. Eosinophilic and neutrophilic inflammation in asthma, chronic bronchitis, and chronic obstructive pulmonary disease. J Allergy Clin Immunol 1993; 149:803–810.

32. Lebowitz MD, Postma DS. Adverse effects of eosinophilic and smoking on the natural history of newly diagnosed chronic beonchitis. Chest 1995; 108:55–61.

33. Sedgwick JB, Vrtis RF, Gourley MF, Busse WW. Stimulus-dependent differences in superoxide anion generation by normal human esinophils and neutrophils. J Allergy Clin Immunol 1988; 81:876–883.

34. Pinamonti S, Muzzuli M, Chicca C, Papi A, Ravenna F, Fabri LM, Ciaccia A. Xanthine oxidase activity in bronchoalveolar lavage fluid from patients with chronic obstructive lung disease. Free Radical Biol Med 1996; 21:147–155.

35. Toth KM, Burthon LL, Berger EM, Beehler CJ, Rodell TC, Cheronis JC, Halek MM, White CW, Repine JE. Cigarette smoke exposure increases erythrocyte (RBC) and lung antioxidant levels and lung xanthine oxidase (XO) activities (abstr). Clin Res 1987; 35:172A.

36. Halliwell B, Gutteridge JMC. Role of free radicals and catalytic metal ions in human disease: an overview. Methods Enzymol 1990; 186:1–85.

37. Gutteridge JMC. Lipid peroxidation and antioxidants as biomarkers of tissue damage. Clin Chem 1995; 41/12:1819–1828.

38. Mateos F, Brock JF, Perez-Arellano JL. Iron metabolism in the lower respiratory tract. Thorax 1998; 53:594–600.

39. Thompson AB, Bohling T, Heries A, Linder J, Rennard SI. Lower respiratory tract iron burden is increased in association with cigarette smoking. J Lab Clin Med 1991; 117:494–499.

40. Wesselius LJ, Nelson ME, Skikne BS. Increased release of ferritin and iron by iron loaded alveolar macrophages in cigarette smokers. Am J Respir Crit Care med 1994; 150:690–695.

41. Wallaert B, Gressier B, Marquette CH, Gosset P, Remy-Jardin M, Mizon J, Tonnel AB. Inactivation of alpha-1 proteinase inhibitor by alveolar inflammatory cells from smoking patients with or without emphysema. Am Rev Respir Dis 1993; 147:1537–1543.

42. Halliwell B, Gutteridge JMC, Cross CE. Free radicals, antioxidants, and human disease: Where are we now? J Lab Clin Med 1992; 119:598–620.

43. van der Vliet A, Eiserich JP, Shigenaga MK, Cross CE. Reactive nitrogen species and tyrosine nitration in the respiratory tract. Am J Respir Crit Care Med 1999; 160:1–9.

44. Beckman JS, Koppenol WH. Nitric oxide, superoxide, and peroxynitrite: the good, the bad, and the ugly. Am J Physiol 1996; 271:C1424–C1437.

45. Kaminsky DA, Janssen YMW. Evidence for peroxynitrite formation in severe human asthma (abstr). Am J Respir Crit Care Med 1998; 157:A876.

46. Saleh D, Ernst P, Lim S, Barnes PJ, Giaid A. Increased formation of the potent oxidant peroxynitrite in the airways of asthmatic patients is associated with induction of nitric oxide synthase: effects of inhaled glucocorticoid. FASEB J 1998; 12:929–937.

47. Rochelle LG, Fischer BM, Adler KB. Concurrent production of reactive oxygen and nitrogen species by airway epithelial cells in vitro. Free Rad Biol Med 1998; 24:863–868.

48. MacNee W. Chronic obstructive pulmonary disease from science to the clinic: role of glutathione in oxidant-antioxidant balance. Monaldi Arch Chest Dis 1997; 52:479–485.

49. Rahman I, MacNee W. Oxidant/antioxidant imbalance in smokers and in chronic obstructive pulmonary disease. Thorax 1996; 51:348–350.

50. Cross CE, van der Vliet A, O' Neil CA, Louie S, Halliwell B. Oxidants, antioxidants, and respiratory tract lining fluids. Environ Health Perspect 1994; 102:185–191.

51. Gutteridge JMC. Biological origin of free radicals, and mechanisms of antioxidant protection. Chemico-Biol Interact 1994; 91:133–140.

52. Hatch GE. Comparative biochemistry of the airway lining fluid. In: Parent RA, ed. Treatise on Pulmonary Toxicology, Vol 1, Comparative Biology of the Normal Lung. Boca Raton, FL: CRC Press, 1991:617–632.

53. Sies H, Stahl W, Sundquist AR. Antioxidant functions of vitamins (vitamins E and C, beta-carotene, and other carotenoids). In: Machlin LF, Sauberlich HE, eds. Beyonds Deficiency: New Views on the Function and Health Benefits of Vitamins. Ann NY Acad Sci 1992; 669:7–20.

54. Halliwell B, Gutteridge JMC. The antoxidants of human extracellular fluids. Arch Biochem Biophys 1990; 280:1–8.

55. Frei B, Stocker R, Smes BN. Small molecule antioxidant defenses in human extracellular fluids. In: Scandalois J, ed. The Molecular Biology of Free Radical Scanvenging Systems. Cold Spring Harbor, NY: Cold Spring Harbor Laboratory Press, 1992:23–45.

56. Cantin AM, Fells GA, Hubbard RC, Crystal RG. Antioxidant macromolecules in the epithelial lining fluid of the normal human lower respiratory tract. J. Clin Invest 1990; 86:962–971.

57. Gum JR. Mucin genes and the proteins they encode: structure, divesity and regualtion. Am J Respir Cell Mol Biol 1992; 7:557–564.

58. Cross CE. Halliwell B, Allen A. Antioxidant protection: a function of tracheobranchial and gastrointestinal mucus. Lancet 1984; 1:1328–1330.

59. Hu M-L, Louie S, Cross CE, Motchnik P, Halliwell B. Antioxidant protection against hypochlorous acid in human plasma. J Lab Clin Med 1993; 121:257–262.

60. Cooper B, Creeth JM, Donanld ASR. Studies of the limited degradation of mucus glycoproteins: the mechanism of the peroxide reaction. Biochem J 1985; 228:615–626.

61. Adler KB, Holden-Stauffer WJ, Repine JE. Oxygen metabolites stimulate release of high-molecular-weight glycoconjugates by cell and organ cultures of rodent respiratory epithelium via an arachidonic acid-dependent mechanism. J Clin Invest 1990; 85: 75-85.

62. Lucey EC, Stone PJ, Breuer R, Christensen TG, Calore JD, Catanese A, Franzblau C, Snider GL. Effect of combined human neutrophil cathepsin G and elastase on induction of secretory cell metaplasia and emphysema in hamsters with *in vitro* observations on elastolysis by these enzymes. Am Rev Respir Dis 1985; 132:362–366.

63. Sommerhoff CP, Nadel JA, Basbaum CB, Caughey GH. Neutrophil elastase and cathepsin G stimulate secretion from cultured bovine airway gland serous cells. J Clin Invest 1990; 85:682–689.

64. Morrison D, Lannan S, Langridge A, Rahman I, MacNee W. Effect of acute cigarette smoking on epithelial permeability, inflammation and oxidant status in the airspaces of chronic smokers (abstr). Thorax 1994; 49:1077.

65. Cantin AM, North SL, Hubbard RC, Crystal RG. Normal alveolar epithelial lung fluid contains high levels of glutathione. J Appl Physiol 1987; 63:152–157.

66. Linden M, Hakansson L, Ohlsson K, Sjodin K, Tegner H, Tunek A, Venge P. Glutathione in bronchoalveolar lavage fluid from smokers is related to humoral markers of inflammatory cell activity. Inflammation 1989; 13:651–658.

67. Li XY, Donaldson K, Rahman I, MacNee W. An investigation of the role of glutathione in the increased epithelial permeability induced by cigarette smoke in vivo and in vitro. Am J Respir Crit Care med 1994; 149:1518–1525.

68. Rahman I, Li XY, Donaldson K, MacNee W, Cigarette smoke, glutathione metabolism and epithelial permeability in rat lungs. Biochem Soc Trans 1995; 23:235S.

69. Rahman I, Li XY, Donaldson K, Harrison DJ, MacNee W. Glutathione homeostasis in alveolar epithelial cells in vitro and lung in vivo under oxidative stress. Am J Physiol Lung Cell Mol Biol 1995; 269 L285-L292.

70. Li XY, Rahman I, Donaldson K, MacNee W. Mechanisms of cigarette smoke induced increased airspace permeability. Thorax 1996; 51:465–471.
71. Pacht ER, Kaseki H, Mohammed JR, Cornwell DG, Davis WR. Deficiency of vitamin E in the alveolar fluid of cigarette smokers, influence on alveolar macrophage cytotoxicity. J Clin Invest 1988; 77:789–796.
72. Bui MH, Sauty A, Collet F, Leuenberger P. Dietary vitamin C intake and concentrations in the body fluids and cells of male smokers and nonsmokers. J Nutr 1992; 122:312–336.
73. McGowan SE, Parenti CM. Hoidal JR, Niewoehner DW. Differences in ascorbic acid content and accumulation by alveolar macrophages from cigarette smokers and nonsmokers. J Lab Clin Med 1984; 104:127–134.
74. McCusker K, Hoidal J. Selective increase of antioxidant enzyme activity in the alveolar macrophages from cigarette smokers and smoke-exposed hamsters. Am Rev Respir Dis 1990; 141:678–682.
75. Kondo T, Tagami S, Yoshioka A, Nishumura M, Kawakami Y. Current smoking of elderly men reduces antioxidants in alveolar macrophages. Am J Respir Crit Care Med 1994; 149:178–182.
76. York GK, Pierce TH, Schwartz LS, Cross CE. Stimulation by cigarette smoke of glutathione peroxidase system enzyme activities in rat lung. Arch Environ Health 1976; 31:286–290.
77. Toth KM, Berger EM, Buhler CJ, Repine JE. Erythrocytes from cigarette smokers contain more glutathione and catalase and protect endothelial cells from hydrogen peroxide better than do erythrocytes from non-smokers. Am Rev Respir Dis 1986; 134:281–284.
78. Drost EM, Skwarski KM, Soler N, Suleda J, Roca J, Agusti AG, MacNee W. Oxidative stress and airway inflammation in healthy smokers and COPD patients. Eur Respir J 2002; 20:95s.
79. Nowak D, Kasielski M, Pietras T, Bialasiewicz P, Antczak A. Cigarette smoking does not increase hydrogen peroxide levels in expired breath condensate of patients with stable COPD. Monaldi Arch Chest Dis 1998; 53:268–273.
80. Nowak D, Antczak A, Drol M, Pietras T, Shariati B, Bialasiewicz P, Jeockowski K, Kula P. Increased content of hydrogen peroxide in expired breath of cigarette smokers. Eur Respir J 1996; 9:652–657.
81. Dekhuijzen PNR, Aben KKH, Dekker I, Aarts LP, Wielders PL, van Herwaarden CL, Bast A. Increased exhalation of hydrogen peroxide in patients with stable and unstable chronic obstructive pulmonary disease. Am J Respir Crit Care Med 1996; 154:813–816.
82. Maziak W, Loukides S, Culpitt S, Sullivan P, Kharitonov SA, Barnes PJ. Exhaled nitric oxide in chronic obstructive pulmonary disease. Am J Respir Crit Care Med 1998; 157:998–1002.
83. Corradi M, Majori M, Cacciani GC, Consigli GF, de'Munari E, Pesci A. Increased exhaled nitric oxide in patients with stable chronic obstructive pulmonary disease. Thorax 1999; 54:576–680.
84. Rutgers SR, van der Mark TW, Coers W, Moshage H, Timens W, Kauffman HF, Koeter GH, Postama DS. Markers of nitric oxide metabolism

in sputum and exhaled air are not increased in chronic obstructive pulmonary disease. Thorax 1999; 54:576–680.

85. Robbins RA, Millatmal T, Lassi K, Rennard S, Daughton D. Smoking cessation is associated with an increase in exhaled nitric oxide. Chest 1997; 112:313–318.

86. Choi AM, Alam J. Heme oxygenase-1: function, regulation, and implication of a novel stress-inducible protein in oxidant-induced lung injury. Am J Respir Cell Mol Biol 1996; 15:9–19.

87. Maziak W, Loukides S, Culpitt S, Sullivan P, Kharitonov SA, Barnes PJ. Exhaled nitric oxide in chronic obstructive pulmonary disease. Am J Respir Crit Care Med 1998; 157:998–1002.

88. Morrow JD, Roberts LJ. This isoprostanes: Unique bioactive products of lipid peroxidation. Prog Lipid Res 1997; 36:1–21.

89. Zayasu K, Sekizawa K, Okinaga S, Yamaya M, Ohrui T, Sasaki H. Increased carbon monoxide in exhaled air of asthmatic patients. Am J Respir Crit Care Med 1997; 156:1140–1143.

90. Kharitonov SA, Chung FK, Evans D, O'Connor BJ, Barnes PJ. Increased exhaled nitric oxide in asthma is mainly derived from the lower respiratory tract. Am J Respir Crit Care Med 1996; 153:1773–1780.

91. Reilly M, Delanty N, Lawson JA, FitzGerald GA. Modulation of oxidant stress in vivo in chronic cigarette smokers. Circulation 1996; 94:19–25.

92. Pratico D, Basili S, Vieri M, Cordova C, Violi F, FitzGerald GA. Chronic obstructive pulmonary disease is associated with an increase in urinary levels of isoprostane $F_{2\alpha}$-III, an index of oxidant stress. Am J Respir Crit Care Med 1998; 158:1709–1714.

93. Montuschi P, Corradi M, Ciabattoni G, Nightingale J, Kharitonov SA, Barnes PJ. Increased 8-isoprostane, a marker of oxidative stress, in exhaled condensate of asthma patients. Am J Respir Crit Care Med 1999; 160:216–220.

94. Sonowaka D. Kasielski M, Antczak A, Pietras T, Bialasiewicz P. Increased content of thiobarbiturate reactive acid substances in hydrogen peroxide in the expired breath condensate of patients with stable chronic obstructive pulmonary disease: no significant effect of cigarette smoking. Respir Med 1999; 93:389–386.

95. Fahn HJ, Wang LS, Kao SH, Chang SC, Huang MH, Wei YH. Smoking-associated mitochondrial DNA mutations and lipid peroxidation in human lung tissues. Am J Respir Cell Mol Biol 1998; 19:901–909.

96. Knaapen ADM, Seiler F, Schilderman PA, Nehls P, Bruch J, Schins RPF, Borm AJA. Neutrophils cause oxidative DNA damage inalveolar epithelial cells. Free Rad Biol Med 1999; 27:234–240.

97. Rahman I, van Schadewijk AAM, Crowther AJL, Hiemstra PS, Stolk J, MacNee W, De Boer WI. 4-Hydroxy-2-nonenal, a specific lipid peroxidation product, is elevated in lungs of patients with chronic obstructive pulmonary disease. Am J Respir Crit Care Med 2002; 166:490–495.

98. Agusti AG, Noguera A, Sauleda J, Sala E, Pons J, Busquets X. Systemic effects of chronic obstructive pulmonary disease. Eur Respir J 2003; 21:347–360.

99. Schols AM, Slagen J, Volovics L, Wouters EF. Weight loss is a reversible factor in the prognosis of chronic obstructive pulmonary disease. Am J Respir Crit Care Med 1998; 157:1791–1797.

100. MacNee W, Wiggs B, Belzberg AS, Hogg JC. The effect of cigarette smoking on neutrophil kinetics in human lungs. N Engl J Med 1989; 321(14):924–928.

101. Selby C, Drost E, Lannan S, Wraith PK, MacNee W. Neutrophil retention in the lungs of patients with chronic obstructive pulmonary diseases. Am Rev Respir Dis 1991; 143:1359–1364.

102. Rahman I, Morrison D, Donaldson K, MacNee W. Systemic oxidative stress in asthma, COPD, and smokers. Am J Respir Crit Care Med 1996; 154:1055–1060.

103. Rahman I, Skwarska E, MacNee W. Attenuation of oxidant/antioxidant imbalance during treatment of exacerbations of chronic obstructive pulmonary disease. Thorax 1997; 52:565–568.

104. Noguera A, Busquets X, Sauleda J, Villaverde JM, MacNee W, Agusti AG. Expression of adhesion molecules and g-proteins in circulating neutrophils in COPD. Am J Respir Crit Care Med 1998; 158:1664–1668.

105. Brown DM, Drost E, Donaldson K, MacNee W. Deformability and CD11/CD18 expression of sequestered neutrophils in normal and inflamed lungs. Am J Respir Cell Mol Biol 1995; 13:531–539.

106. Duthie GG, Arthur JR, James WPT. Effects of smoking and vitamin E on blood antioxidant status. Am J Clin Nutr 1991; 53:1061S-1063S.

107. Morrow JD, Frei B, Longmire AW, Gaziano JM, Lynch SM, Shyr Y, Strauss WE, Oates JA, Roberts LJ II. Increase in circulating products of lipid peroxidation (F_2-isoprostanes) in smokers. N Engl J Med 1995; 332:1198–1203.

108. Lapenna D, Mezzetti A, Giola SD, Pierdomenico F, Daniele F, Cuccurullo F. Plasma copper and lipid peroxidation in cigarette smokers. Free Rad Biol Med 1995; 19:849–885.

109. Uchida K, Shiraishi M, Naito Y, Torii Y, Nakamura Y, Osawa T. Activation of stress signaling pathways by the end product of lipid peroxiation J Biol Chem 1999; 274:2234–2242.

110. Page S, Fischer C, Baumgartner B, Haas M, Kreusel U, Loidl G, Hayn M, Ziegler-Hetbrock HWL, Neumeier D, Brand K. 4-Hydrozynonenal prevents NF-κB activation and tumor necrosis factor expression by inhibiting IκB phosphorylation and subsequent proteolysis. J Biol Chem 1999; 274:11611–11618.

111. Cross CE, O'Neill CA, Reznick AZ, Hu ML, Marcocci L, Packer L, Frei B. Cigarette smoke oxidation of human plasma constituents. Ann N Y Acad Sci USA 1993; 656:72–90.

112. Eiserich JP, Vossen V, O'Neil CA, Halliwell B, Cross CE, Van der Viliet A. Molecular mechanisms of damage by excess nitrogen oxides: nitration of tyrosine by gas-phase cigarette smoke. FEBS Lett 1994; 353:53–56.

113. Petruzzelli S, Hietanen E, Bartsch H, Camus AM, Mussi A, Angeletti CA, Saracci R, Giuntini C. Pulmonary lipid peroxidation in cigarette smokers and lung patients. Chest 1990; 98:930–935.

114. Bridges AB, Scott NA, Parry GJ, Belch JJF. Age, sex, cigarette smoking and indices of free radical activity in healthy humans. Eur J Med 1993; 2:205–208.

115. Duthie GG, Arthur JR, James WPT. Effects of smoking and vitamin E on blood antioxidant status. Am J Clin Nutr 1991; 53:1061S-1063S.

116. Mezzetti A, Lapenna D, Pierdomenico SD, Calafiore AM, Costantini F, Riario-Sforza G, Imbastaro T, Neri M, Cuccurullo F. Vitamins E, C and lipid peroxidation in plasma and arterial tissue of smokers and non-smokers. Atherosclerosis. 1995; 112:91–99.

117. Antwerpen LV, Theron AJ, Myer MS, Richards GA, Wolmarans L, Booysen U. Cigarette smoke-mediated oxidant stress, phagocytes, vitamin C, vitamin E and tissue injury. Ann NY Acad Sci USA 1993; 686: 53–65.

118. Pelletier O. Vitamin C status of cigarette smokers and nonsmokers. Am J Clin Nutr 1970; 23:520–528.

119. Chow CK, Thacker R, Bridges RB, Rehm SR, Humble J, Turbek J. Lower levels of vitamin C and carotenes in plasma of cigarette smokers. J Am Coll Nutr 1986; 5:305–312.

120. Bridges RB, Chow CK, Rehm SR. Micronutrients and immune functions in smokers. Ann N Acad Sci USA. 1990; 587:218–231.

121. Theron AJ, Richards GA, Rensburg AJ, Van der Merwe CA, Anderson R. Investigation of the role of phagocytes and antioxidant nutrients in oxidant stress mediated by cigarette smoke. Int J Vitam Nutr Res 1990; 60:261–266.

122. Barton GM, Roath OS. Leukocytic ascorbic acid in abnormal leukocyte states. Int J Vitam Nutr Res 1976; 46:271–274.

123. Hemilla H, Roberts P, Wilstrom M. Activated polymorphonuclear leukocytes consume vitamin C FEBS Lett 1984; 178:25–30.

124. Van der Vliet A, Smith D, O'Neill CA. Kaur H, Darley-Usmar V, Cross CE, Helliwell B. Interactions of peroxynitrite and human plasma and its constituents: oxidative damage and antioxidant depletion. Biochem J 1994; 303:295–301.

125. Petruzzelli S, Puntoni R, Mimotti P, Pulera N, Baliva F, Fornai E, Giuntini C. Plasma 3-nitrotyrosine in cigarette smokers. Am J Respir Crit Care Med 1997; 156:1902–1907.

126. Dye JA, Adler KB. Effects of cigarette smoke on epithelial cells on the respiratory tract. Thorax 1994; 49:825–834.

127. Cantin A, Crystal RG. Oxidants, antioxidants and the pathogenesis of emphysema. Eur J Respir Dis 1985; 66 (suppl 139):7–17.

128. Laurent P, Janoff A, Kagan HM. Cigarette smoke blocks cross-linking of elastin in vitro. Am Rev Respir Dis 1983; 127: 189–192.

129. Jones JG, Lawler P, Crawley JCW, Minty BD, Hulands G, Veall N. Increased alveolar epithelial permeability in cigarette smokers. Lancet 1980; 1:66–68.

130. Lannan S, Donaldson K, Brown D, MacNee W. Effects of cigarette smoke and its condensates on alveolar cell injury in vitro. Am J Physiol 1994; 266:L92–L100.

131. Li XY, Donaldson K, Brown D, MacNee. W. The role of tumour necrosis factor in increased airspace epithelial permeability in acute lung inflammation. Am J Resp Cell Mol Biol 1995; 13:185–195.

132. MacNee W, Selby C. Neutrophil traffic in the lungs: role of haemodynamics, cell adhesion, and deformability. Thorax 1993; 48:79–88.

133. Selby C, Drost E, Wraith PK, MacNee W. In vivo neutrophil sequestration within the lungs of man is determined by in vitro 'filterability'. J Appl Physiol 1991; 71:1996–2003.

134. Selby C, MacNee W. Factors affecting neutrophil transit during acute pulmonary inflammation: minireview. Exp Lung Res 1993; 19:407–428.

135. Drost EM, Selby C, Lannan S, Lowe GDO, MacNee W. Changes in neutrophil deformability following in vitro smoke exposure: mechanism and protection. Am J Respir Cell Mol Biol 1992; 6:287–295.

136. Drost E, Selby C, Bridgeman MME, MacNee W. Decreased leukocyte deformability following acute cigarette smoking in smokers. Am Rev Respir Dis 1993; 148:1277–1283.

137. Terashima T, Klut ME, English D, Hards J, Hogg JC, van Eeden SF. Cigarette smoking causes sequestration of polymorphonuclear leukocytes released from the bone marrow in lung microvessels. Am J Respir Cell Mol Biol 1999; 20:171–177.

138. Lehr HA, Kress E, Menger MD, Friedl HP, Hubner C, Arfors KE, Messmer K. Cigarette smoke elicits leukocyte adhesion to endothelium in hamsters: inhibition by CuZnSOD. Free Rad Biol Med 1993; 14:573–581.

139. Klut DE, Doerschuk CM, Van Eeden JF, Burns AF, Hoff JC. Activation of neutrophils within the pulmonary microvasculature of rabbits exposed to cigarette smoke. Am J Respir Cell Mol Biol 1993; 39:82–90.

140. Nathan C, Srimal S, Farber C, Sanchez E, Kabbash L, Asch A, Gailit J, Wright S. Cytokine-induced respiratory burst of human neutrophils, dependence on extracellular matrix proteins and CD11/CD18 integrins. J Cell Biol 1989; 109:1341–1349.

141. Kokura S, Wolf RE, Yoshikawa T, Granger DN, Aw TY. Molecular mechanisms of neutrophil-endothelial cell adhesion induced by redox imbalance. Circ Res 1999; 84:516–524.

142. Selby C, Drost E, Brown D, Howie S, MacNee W. Inhibition of neutrophil adherence and movement by acute cigarette smoke exposure. Exp Lung Res 1992; 18:813–827.

143. Stockley RA. Biochemical and cellular mechanisms. In: Calverley P, Pride N, eds. Chronic Obstructive Pulmonary Diseases. London, Chapman & Hall, 1995:93–133.

144. Morrison D, Strieter RM, Donnelly SC, Burdick MD, Dunkel SL, MacNee W. Neutrophil chemokines in bronchoalveolar lavage fluid and leukocyte-conditioned medium from nonsmokers and smokers. Eur Respir J 1998; 12:1067–1072.

145. Bosken CH, Doerschuk CM, English D, Hogg JC. Neutrophil kinetics during active cigarette smoking in rabbits. J Appl Physiol 1991; 71:830–837.

146. Brumwell ML, MacNee W, Doerschuk CM, Wiggs B, Hogg JC. Neutrophil kinetics in normal and emphysematous regions of human lungs. Ann NY Acad Sci 1991; 624:30–39.

147. Gadek J, Fells GA, Crystal RG. Cigarette smoking induces functional antiprotease deficiency in the lower respiratory tract of humans. Science 1979; 206:1315–1316.

148. Carp H, Janoff A. Inactivation of bronchial mucous proteinase inhibitor by cigarette smoke and phagocyte-derived oxidants. Exp Lung Res 1980: 1:225–237.

149. Hubbard RC, Ogushi F, Fells GA, Cantin AM, Jallat S, Courtney M, Crystal RG. Oxidants spontaneously released by alveolar macrophages of cigarette smokers can inactivate the active site of α-1-antitrypsin rendering it ineffective as an inhibitor of neutrophil elastase. J Clin Invest 1987; 80,1289–1295.

150. Kramps JA, Rudolphus A, Stolk J, Willems LNA, Dijkman JH. Role of antileukoprotease in the lung. Ann NY Acad Sci USA. 1991; 624:97–108.

151. Kramps JA, van Twisk C, Dijkman DH. Oxidative inactivation of antileukoprotease is triggered by polymorphonuclear leucocytes. Clin Sci 1988; 75:53–62.

152. Johnson D, Travis J. The oxidative inactivation of human α1-proteinase inhibitor. Further evidence for methionine at the reactive center. J Biol Chem 1979; 254:4022–4026.

153. Carp H, Janoff A. Possible mechanisms of emphysema in smokers: in vitro suppression of serum elastase-inhibitory capacity by fresh cigarette smoke and its prevention by anti-oxidants. Am Rev Respir Dis 1978; 118:617–621.

154. Carp H, Miller F, Hoidal JR, Janoff A. Potential mechanisms of emphysema: α1-proteinase inhibitor recovered from lungs of cigarette smokers contains oxidised methionine and has decreased elastase inhibitory capacity. Proc Natl Acad Sci 1982; 79:2041–2045.

155. Stone P, Calore JD, McGowan SE, Bernardo J, Snider GL, Franzblau C. Functional alpha-1-protease inhibitor in the lower respiratory tract of smokers is not decreased. Science 1983:221:1187–1189.

156. Boudier C, Pelletier A, Pauli G, Beith JG. The functional activity of alpha1-proteinase inhibitor in bronchoalveolar lavage fluids from healthy human smokers and non smokers. Clin Chim Acta 1983; 131:309–315.

157. Abboud RT, Fera T, Richter A, Tabona MZ, Johal S. Acute effect of smoking on the functional activity of alpha-1-protease inhibitor in bronchoalveolar lavage fluid. Am Rev Respir Dis 1985; 131:1187–1189.

158. Gadek JE, Hunninghake GW, Fells GA, Zimmerman RL, Keogh BA, Crystal RG. Evaluation of the protease-antiprotease theory of human destructive lung disease. Bull Eur Physiopathol Respir 1980; 16(suppl):27–40.

159. Takeyama K, Jung B, Shim JJ, Burgel PR, Dao-Pick T, Ueki IF, Protin U, Kroschel P, Nadel JA. Activation of epidermal growth factor receptors is

responsible for mucin synthesis induced by cigarette smoke. Am J Physiol Lung Cell Mol Physiol 2001; 280:L165-L172.

160. Nadel JA, Burgel PR. The role epidermal growth factor in mucus production. Curr Opin Pharmacol 2001; 1:254–258.

161. Nakajima Y, Aoshiba K, Yasui S, Nagai A H_2O_2 induces apoptosis in bovine tracheal epithelial cells in vitro. Life Sci 1999; 64:2489–2496.

162. Aoshiba K, Yasui S, Nagai A. Apoptosis of alveolar macrophages by cigarette smoke. Proceedings of Aspen Lung Conference 1999. Chest. 2000; 117 (suppl 1):3205.

163. Hall AG. Review: The role of glutathione in the regulation of apoptosis. Eur J Clin Invest 1999; 29:238–245.

164. Tuder RM, Wood K, Tarasevicience L, Flores S, Voelkel NF. Cigarette smoke extract decreases the expression of vascular endothelial growth factor by cultured cells and triggers apoptosis of pulmonary endothelial cells. Chest 2000; 117:241S–242S.

165. Kasahara Y, Tuder RM, Cool CD, Lynch DA, Flores SC, Voelkel NF. Endothelial cell death and decreased expression of vascular endothelial growth factor and vascular endothelial growth factor receptor 2 in emphysema. Am J Respir Crit Care Med 2001;163:737–744.

166. Kasahara Y, Tuder RM, Taraseviciene-Stewart L, Le Cras TD, Abman S, Hirth PK, Waltenberger J, Voelkel NF. Inhibition of VEGF receptors causes lung cell apoptosis and emphysema. J Clin Invest 2000; 106:1311–1319.

167. Tuder RM, Zhen L, Cho CY, Taraseviciene-Stewart L, Kasahara Y, Salvemini D, Voelkel NF, Flores SC. Oxidative stress and apoptosis interact and cause emphysema due to vascular endothelial growth factor receptor blockade. Am J Respir Cell Mol Biol 2003;29:88–97.

168. Chan-Yeung M, Dybuncio A. Leucocyte count, smoking and lung function. Am J Med 1984; 76:31–37.

169. Chan-Yeung M, Abboud R, Dybuncio A, Vedal S. Peripheral leucocyte count and longitudinal decline in lung function. Thorax 1988; 43:426–468.

170. Richards GA, Theron AJ, van der Merwe CA, Anderson R. Spirometric abnormalities in young smokers correlate with increased chemiluminescence responses of activated blood phagocytes. Am Rev Respir Dis 1989; 139:181–187.

171. Anderson R, Theron AJ, Richards GA, Myer MS, van Rensburg AJ. Passive smoking by humans sensitizes circulating neutrophils. Am Rev Respir Dis 1991; 144:570–574.

172. Schunemann HJ, Muti P, Freudenheim JL, Armstrong D, Browne R, Klocke RA, Trevisan M. Oxidative stress and lung function. Am J Epiderm 1997; 146:939–948.

173. Britton JR, Pavord ID, Richards KA, Knox AJ, Wisniewski AF, Lewis SA, Tattersfield AE, Weiss ST. Dietary antioxidant vitamin intake and lung function in the general population. Am J Respir Crit Care Med 1995; 151:1383–1387.

174. Grievink L, Smit HA, Ocke MC, van't Veer P, Kromhout D. Dietary intake of antioxidant (pro)-vitamins, respiratory symptoms and pulmonary function: the MORGEN study. Thorax 1998; 53:166–171.

175. Shahar E, Folsom AR, Melnick SL, Tockman MS, Comstock GW, Gennaro V, Higgins MW, Sorlie PD, Ko WJ, Szklo M. Dietary n-3 polyunsaturated fatty acids and smoking-related chronic obstructive pulmonary disease. Atherosclerosis Risk in Communities Study Investigators. N Engl J Med 1994; 331:228–233.

176. Shahar E, Boland LL, Folsom AR, Tockman MA, McGovern PG, Eckfeldt JH. Docosahexaenoic acid and smoking related chronic obstructive pulmonary disease. Atherosclerosis Risk in Communities Study Investigators. Am J Respir Crit Care Med 1999;159:1780–1785.

177. Sridhar MK, Galloway A, Lean MEJ, Banham SW. An out-patient nutritional supplementation programme in COPD patients. Eur Respir J 1994; 7:720–724.

178. Steinberg FM, Chait A. Antioxidant vitamin supplementation and lipid peroxidation in smokers. Am J Clin Nutr 1998; 68:319–327.

179. Rabinovich RA, Ardite E, Trooster T, Carbo N, Alonso J, Gonzalex de Suso JM, Vilaro J, Barbera JA, Polo MF, Argiles JM, Fernandez-Checa JC, Roca J. Reduced muscle redox capacity after endurance training in patients with chronic obstructive pulmonary disease. Am J Respir Crit Care Med 2001; 164:1114–1118.

180. Sauleda J, Garcia-Palmer FJ, Gonzalez G, Palou A, Agusti AG. The activity of cytochrome oxidase is increased in circulating lymphocytes of patients with chronic obstructive pulmonary disease, asthma, and chronic arthritis. Am J Respir Crit Care Med 2000; 161:32–35.

181. Engelen MP, Schols AM, Does JD, Deutz NE, Wouters EF. Altered glutamate metabolism is associated with reduced muscle glutathione levels in patients with emphysema. Am J Respir Crit Care Med 2000; 161: 98–103.

182. Heunks LM, Dekhuijzen PN. Respiratory muscle function and free radicals: from cell to COPD. Thorax 2000; 55:704–716.

183. Keatings VM, Collins PD, Scott DM, Barnes PJ. Differences in interleukin 8 and tumour necrosis factor α in induced sputum from patients with chronic obstructive pulmonary disease or asthma. Am J Respir Crit Care Med 1996; 153:530–534.

184. Rahman I, MacNee W. Role of transcription factors in inflammatory lung diseases. Thorax 1998; 53:601–612.

185. Parmentier M, Hirani N, Rahman I, Drost EM, MacNee W, Antonicelli F. Regulation of LPS-mediated interleukin-1β release by N-acetylcysteine in THP-1 cells. Eur Respir J. 2000; 16:933–939.

186. Parmentier M, Drost ME, Hirani N, Rahman I, Donaldson K, MacNee W, Antonicelli F. Thiol antioxidants inhibit neutrophil chemotaxis by decreasing release of IL-8 from macrophases and pulmonary epithelial cells. Br J Pharmacol. In press.

187. Jimenez LA, Thomson J, Brown DA, Rahman I, Antonicelli F, Duffin R, Droot EM, Hay RT, Donaldson K, MacNee W. Activation of NF-κB by PM_{10} via an iron-mediated mechanism in the absence of 1κB degradation. Toxical App Pharmacol 2000; 166:101–110.

188. Galter D, Mihm S, Droge W. Distinct effect of glutathione disulphide on the nuclear transcription factor kappa B and the activator protein-1. Eur J Biochem 1994; 221:639–648.

189. Ginn-Pease ME, Whisler RL. Optimal NF kappa B mediated transcriptional responses in Jurkat T cells exposed to oxidative stress are dependent on intracellular glutathione and costimulatory signals. Biochem Biophys Res Commun 1996; 226:695–702.

190. Cho S, Urata Y, Iida T, Goto S, Yamaguchi M, Sumikawa K, Kondo T. Glutathione downregulates the phosphorylation of I kappa B: autoloop regulation of the NF-kappa B-mediated expression of NF-kappa B subunits by TNF-alpha in mouse vascular endothelial cells. Biochem Biophys Res Commun 1998; 253:104–108.

191. Janssen-Heininger YMW, Macara I, Mossman BT. Cooperativity between oxidants and tumour necrosis factor in the activation of neuclear factor (NF)-κB. Requirement of Ras/Mitogen-activated protein kinases in the activation of NF-κB by oxidants. Am J Respir Cell Mol Biol 1999; 20:942–952.

192. Rahman I, Li XY, Donaldson K, Harrison DJ, MacNee W. Glutathione homeostatis in alveolar epithelial cells *in vitro* and lung *in vivo* under oxidative stress. Am J Physiol Lung Cell Mol Biol 1995; 269 L285-L292.

193. Rahman I, Smith CAD, Lawson M, Harrison DJ, MacNee W. Induction of gamma-glutamylcysteine synthetase by cigarette smoke condensate is associated with AP-1 in human alveolar epithelial cells. FEBS Lett 1996; 396:21–25.

194. Rahman I, Bel A, Mulier B, Lawson MF, Harrison DJ, MacNee W, Smith CAD. Transcriptional regulation of γ-glutamylcysteine synthetase-heavy subunit by oxidants in human alveolar epithelial cells. Biochem Biophys Res Commun 1996; 229:832–837.

195. Rahman I, Smith CAD, Antonicelli F, MacNee W. Characterisation of γ-glutamylcysteine synthetase-heavy subunit promoter: a critical role for AP-1. FEBS Let 1998; 427:129–133.

196. Rahman I, Antonicelli F, MacNee W. Molecular mechanisms of the regulation of glutathione synthesis by tumour necrosis factor-α and dexamethasone in human alveolar epithelial cells. J Biol Chem 1999; 274:5088–5096.

197. Keatings VM, Jatakanon A, Worsdell YM, Barnes PJ. Effects of inhaled and oral glucocorticoids on inflammatory indices in asthma and COPD. Am J Respir Crit Care Med 1997; 155:542–548.

198. Gilks CB, Price K, Wright JL, Churg A. Antioxidant gene expression in rat lung after exposure to cigarette smoke. Am J Path 1998; 152:269–278.

199. Muller T, Gebel S. The cellular stress response induced by aqueous extracts of cigarette smoke is critically dependent on the intracellular glutathione concentration. Cardiogenesis 1998; 19:797–801.

200. Silverman EK, Speizer FE. Risk factors for the development of chronic obstructive pulmonary disease. Med Clin North Am 1996; 80:501–522.

201. Sandford AJ, Weir TD, Pare PD. Genetic risk factors for chronic obstructive pulmonary disease. Eur Respir J 1997; 10:1380–1391.

202. Barnes PJ. Genetics and pulmonary medicine. 9. Molecular genetics of chronic obstructive pulmonary disease. Thorax 1999; 54:245–252.

203. Huang S-L, Su C-H, Chang S-C. Tumour necrosis factor-α gene polymorphism in chronic bronchitis. Am J Respir Crit Care Med 1997; 156:1436–1439.

204. Smith CAD, Harrison DJ. Association between polymorphism in gene for microsomal epoxide hydrolase and susceptibility to emphysema. Lancet 1997; 350:630–633.

205. Compton CH, Gubb J, Cedar E, Nieman RB, Amit O, Brambila C, Ayres J. SB 207499, a second generation oral PDE4 inhibitor, first demonstration of efficacy in patients with COPD. Eur Respir J 1999; 14(suppl 30): 281s.

206. Torphy TJ. Phosphodiesterase isozymes. Am J Respir Crit Care Med 1998; 157:351–370.

207. Chabrier PE, Auguet M, Spinnewyn B, Auvin S, Cornet S, Demerle-Pallardy C, Guilmard Favre C, Marin J-G, Pignol B, Gillard-Roubert V, Roussillot-Charnet C, Schulz J, Voissat I, Bigg d, Monca S. BN 80933, a dual inhibitor of neuronal nitric oxide synthase and lipid peroxidation: a promising neuroprotective strategy. Proc Natl Acad Sci USA 1999; 96:10824–10829.

208. Nishikawa M, Kakemizu N, Ito T, Kudo M, Kaneko T, Suzuki M, Udaka N, Ikeda H, Okubo T. Superoxide mediates cigarette smoke-induced infiltration of neutrophils into the airways through nuclear factor-κB activation and IL-8 mRNA expression in guinea pigs in vivo. Am J Respir Cell Mol Biol 1999; 20:189–198.

209. MacNee W, Bridgeman MME, Marsden M, Drost E, Lannan S, Selby C, Donaldson K. The effects of N-acetylcysteine and glutathione on smoke-induced changes in lung phagocytes and epithelial cells. Am J Med 1991; 90:60s–66s.

210. Ross D, Norbeck K, Moldeus P. The generation and subsequent fate of glutathionyl radicals in biological systems. J Biol Chem 1985; 260:15028–15032.

211. Marrades RM, Roca J, Barbera JA, Jover L de, MacNee W, Rodriguez-Roisin, R. Nebulized glutathione induces bronchoconstriction in patients with mild asthma. Am J Respir Crit Care Med 1997; 156:425–430.

212. Meister A, Anderson ME. Glutathione. Ann Rev Biochem 1983; 52:711–760.

213. Bowman G, Backer U, Larsson S, Melander B, Wahlander L. Oral acetylcysteine reduces exaceration rate in chronic bronchitis: report of a trial organized by the Swedish Society for Pulmonary Diseases. Eur J Respir Dis 1983; 64:405–415.

214. Rasmusse JB, Glennow C. Reduction in days of illness after long-term treatment with N-acetylcysteine controlled-release tablets in patients with chronic bronchitis. Eur J Respir Dis 1988; 1:351–355.

215. British Thoracic Society Research Committee. Oral N-acetylcysteine and exacerbation rates in patients with chronic bronchitis and severe airways obstruction. Thorax 1985; 40:823–835.

216. Bridgeman MME, Marsden M, MacNee W, Flenley DC, Kyle AP. Cysteine and glutathione concentrations in plasma and bronchoalveolar lavage fluid after treatment with N-acetylcysteine. Thorax 1991; 46:39–42.

217. Bridgeman MME, Marsden M, Selby C. Effect of N-acetyl cysteine on the concentrations of thiols in plasma bronchoalveolar lavage fluid and lining tissue. Thorax 1994; 49:670–675.

218. Stey C, Steurer J, Bachmann S, Medici TC, Tramer MR. The effect of oral N-acetylcysteine in chronic bronchitis: a quantitative systemic review. Eur Respir J 2000; 16:253–262.

219. Ekberg-Jansson A, Larson M, MacNee W, Tunek A, Wahlgren L, Wouters EFM, Larsson S for the N-Isobutyrylcysteine Study Group. N-Isobutyrylcysteine, a donor of systemic thiols, does not reduce the exacerbation rate in chronic bronchitis. Eur Respir J 1999; 13:829–834.

220. Gillissen A, Jaworska M, Orth M, Coffiner M, Maes P, App EM, Cantin AM, Schultze-Werninghous G. Nacystelyn a novel lysine salt of N-acetylcysteine to augment cellular antioxidant defence in vitro. Respir Med 1997; 91:159–168.

221. Nagy AM, Vanderbist F, Parij N, Maes P, Fondu P, Neve J. Effect of the mucoactive drug Nacystelyn on the respiratory burst of human blood polymorphonuclear neutrophils. Pulm Pharmacol Ther 1997; 10:287–292.

222. Manna SK, Tien Kuo M, Aggarwal BB. Overexpression of γ-glutamylcysteine synthetase suppresses tumor necrosis factor-induced apoptosis and activation of nuclear transcription factor-kappa B and activator protein-1. Oncogene 1999; 18:4371–4382.

12

Pathogenesis of Infections in COPD Patients

MURIEL VAN SCHILFGAARDE and LOEK VAN ALPHEN

Netherlands Vaccine Institute
Bilthoven, The Netherlands

PETER VAN ULSEN

Utrecht University
Utrecht, The Netherlands

JACOB DANKERT

University of Amsterdam
Amsterdam, The Netherlands

I. Introduction

Bacterial infections of the lower airways in chronic obstructive pulmonary disease (COPD) patients have been investigated extensively for over 50 years now. Although the precise role of these infections in the pathogenesis of COPD is still not fully established, many data have become available on the bacteriology, immunology, pathogenesis of the disease, and the pathogenic repertoire of the infecting microorganisms.

In this chapter the bacterial infections in COPD patients, their role in disease, the pathogenic potential of the bacteria causing infection, their persistence, and their potential to escape immune defense of the host are described. We will focus on infections by *Haemophilus influenzae* since these have been characterized most extensively.

II. Role of Bacterial Infection in COPD

The presence of bacteria in the lower airways does not correlate very well with the appearance of clinical symptoms, although sputum cultures are often positive during exacerbations of the disease. Some COPD patients seem to be prone to bacterial infection (1).

The observation that during bacterial infection pulmonary function acutely worsens in chronic bronchitis indicates that bacteria are harmful for the lower airways. From long-term, carefully designed prospective studies, the progression of disease appeared associated with an increased number of episodes of infection only in patients having multiple exacerbations per year (2–5).

A second approach to assess the importance of infection for disease is by comparing the outcome of antibiotic therapy on disease symptoms in treated and not treated patients. Although most of these studies are hampered by the poor definition of the patients, a reduction in the frequency of exacerbations was observed among antibiotic-treated patients compared to placebo-treated patients in about half of the studies. Such an effect was only observed for patients with more than two exacerbations per year (6,7). Ant*h*onissen et al. (8) demonstrated prevention of deterioration of lung function by antibiotics. A meta-analysis of nine placebo-controlled antibiotic trials in COPD established a small but significant benefit from antibiotic therapy (9). These data indicate a pathogenic role for bacterial infections in COPD.

III. Bacterial Pathogens

Haemophilus influenzae, *Streptococcus pneumoniae*, and *Moraxella (Branhamella) catarrhalis* have long been recognized as the major pathogens from sputum specimens of COPD patients, especially from purulent sputum (10,11). *H. influenzae* isolates are nonencapsulated (nontypable), *S. pneumoniae* is encapsulated with a variety of capsule types, and *M. catarrhalis* is nonencapsulated. Using protected brush specimens for microbial sampling, Monso et al. (12) compared the presence of bacteria in the lower airways of outpatients with stable COPD and patients with exacerbations. Both groups had *H. influenzae*– and *S. pneumoniae*–positive cultures, but the prevalence of these bacteria and the bacterial concentrations were higher for patients with exacerbated COPD. Sethi et al. (13) reported that the isolation of a new strain of *H. influenzae*, *S. pneumoniae*, or *M. catarrhalis* was associated with a significantly increased risk of an exacerbation, supporting the causative role of these bacteria in exacerbations in COPD.

In addition to *H. influenzae*, *S. pneumoniae*, and *M. catarrhalis*, a variety of microorganisms is isolated from sputum cultures, which are most likely contaminants (12). In severe cases, like in patients with bronchiectasis,

Pseudomonas aeruginosa is an additional pathogen. In the last decade, some attention has been given to *Chlamydia pneumoniae* as a pathogen in COPD. Soler et al. (14) and Miyashita et al. (15) demonstrated that *C. pneumoniae* was more frequently present in sputum of COPD patients than in controls, independent of other pathogens. Based on the few studies until recently, Sethi and Murphy (16) estimate that 5–10% of exacerbations of COPD are associated with *C. pneumoniae*.

The bacteria isolated from COPD patients are normal inhabitants of the nasopharynx of healthy individuals. In COPD patients they are also successful in colonizing and infecting the lower respiratory tract by surviving and proliferating in the mucus layer and the bronchial epithelium without being expelled by mucociliary clearance mechanisms. The three major pathogens are able to adhere to epithelial cells, to survive humoral defense mechanisms in the absence of specific antibodies, and to degrade IgA by expressing IgA protease.

IV. *H. influenzae*, *S. pneumoniae*, and *M. catarrhalis* in Health: Nasopharyngeal Carriage

Colonization of the upper respiratory tract is generally considered the first step of infections by *H. influenzae*, *S. pneumoniae*, and *M. catarrhalis*. The carrier rate for *H. influenzae* is up to 80% (7,17) and a few percent for the other pathogens. After initial colonization, nontypable *H. influenzae* elicits specific antibodies directed against the infecting strain. The mucosal immune response is associated with reduction or elimination of *H. influenzae* strains from the respiratory tract (18–20). A high turnover of *H. influenzae* strains colonizing the nasopharynx contributes to the high incidence of carriership despite antibodies on the respiratory mucosa (18,21). The targets of antibodies present in human serum and on mucosal surfaces against nontypable *H. influenzae* strains are outer membrane proteins (OMPs), lipooligosaccharide (LOS), and IgA proteases (22–24).

V. Colonization of the Lower Respiratory Tract: Binding to Mucus

In healthy persons binding to mucus is of importance for clearance of bacteria from the lower respiratory tract, since mucus is rapidly removed by mucociliary clearance. In COPD patients conditions in the lower respiratory tract are altered due to chronic inflammation, which is characterized by infiltration of neutrophils and the upregulation of the production of cytokines and other inflammatory mediators leading to airway obstruction and impaired mucociliary clearance (25). In these patients association of *H. influenzae* with mucus may allow bacterial multiplication, resulting in persistent colonization (7,26).

H. influenzae associates with mucus strands produced by cultured human epithelial cells (27–29). Mucins are high molecular weight glycoproteins and major constituents of mucus. Adherence of *H. influenzae* to mucus sol phase or to purified preparations of mucins has been described (30–33). Fimbriae of *H. influenzae* may be involved in adherence to mucus (30). There was, however, no evidence that the fimbriae interacted with mucins on the cells. Using intact bacteria, only a subset of nontypable *H. influenzae* strains adhered to mucins in a specific manner (32).

Reddy et al. (33) found that sialic acid containing oligosaccharides in mucins bound to the P2 and P5 OMPs of outer membrane preparations from all *H. influenzae* strains tested. In addition, of two nontypable *H. influenzae* strains, other unidentified proteins bound mucin with a greater affinity than OMPs P2 and P5. Since in this study isolated OMPs were used, it remains to be shown whether these OMPs are available for adherence to mucus in vivo. OMP P5 seems available for mucus binding since OMP P5-mediated binding of intact *H. influenzae* was demonstrated to mucus in the chinchilla Eustachian tube and middle ear (34).

VI. Adherence to Epithelial Cells

Adherence of bacteria to human epithelial cells is important for establishment and outgrowth of the bacteria on the epithelial cells. Isolates of *H. influenzae*, *S. pneumoniae*, and *M. catarrhalis* adhere to these cells. Several adhesins with affinity for various receptors on the eukaryotic cell surface may determine tissue tropism (28,29).

Adherence of *H. influenzae* to epithelial cells may occur in a fimbriae-mediated as well as a fimbriae-independent way. Fimbriae are long filamentous organelles that extend from the bacterial surface. Fimbriae of the long thick hemaglutination-positive (LKP) family are involved in the adherence to oropharyngeal epithelial cells and the agglutination of human erythrocytes (35,36). The agglutination is mediated via the AnWj blood group antigen (37) and the receptor for the *H. influenzae* fimbriae on human epithelial cells is a sialic acid–containing lactosylceramide localized in the cell membrane. Fimbriae-mediated adherence to epithelial cells can be demonstrated in vitro in binding assays with nasopharyngeal epithelial cells and can be inhibited with purified ganglioside GM2 (38). Fimbriae-mediated adherence seems to be especially relevant for adherence of encapsulated *H. influenzae* strains to different cells during infection (39–42), since adherence through nonfimbrial adhesins is blocked by capsule, in contrast to fimbriae-mediated adherence (43,44).

Only a minority of nontypable *H. influenzae* strains from COPD patients contains a fimbriae gene cluster (45), suggesting a minor role for fimbriae in the colonization of nontypable *H. influenzae* in the respiratory tract. In addition, several nonfimbrial proteins have been described to mediate attachment of nontypable *H. influenzae* to different cell lines (46–48). Barenkamp and Leininger (49) identified two immunogenic high molecular weight adhesins designated HMW1 and HMW2, that are expressed by 70–80% of nontypable *H. influenzae* strains isolated from otitis media (43,50). These proteins show homology to filamentous hemagglutinin (FHA), an adhesin of *Bordetella pertussis*, that plays a critical role in colonization of the lower respiratory tract. The two HMW proteins mediate a high level of binding to distinct human epithelial cells indicating different receptor specificity (43,47,51–53). HMW1 recognizes a sialylated glycoprotein, and HMW1-mediated adherence can be inhibited by heparin or dextran sulfate (54–56). Nontypable *H. influenzae* isolates lacking the HMW proteins and still showing efficient in vitro adherence to Chang epithelial cells instead express an adhesin named Hia (48). Characterization of adherence of *H. influenzae* isolates from COPD patients showed that 37% of the isolates did not show this high-level adherence due to HMW or Hia proteins (53). Possibly, the ability of *H. influenzae* for high-level adherence is more relevant for the onset of acute upper respiratory tract infections than for lower respiratory tract infection in COPD patients.

Several other proteins of *H. influenzae* mediating lower levels of adherence to epithelial cells have been described. The Hap protein mediates low-level but intimate adherence to Chang epithelial cells, thereby leading to invasion of *H. influenzae* into epithelial cells (46). More recently OapA (57) and OMP P5 (in this context sometimes described as "P5-homologous fimbriae") have been identified as adhesins (58). OMP P5–mediated attachment of *H. influenzae* to the A549 lung epithelial cell line is enhanced after infection with the respiratory syncytial virus (59). Hill et al. (60) show that OMP P5 interacts with CEACAM1 molecules on the cell surface and suggest that A549 cells accommodate *H. influenzae* via these receptors.

Furthermore, adherence can be mediated by the expression of phosphorylcholine (ChoP) on *H. influenzae* LOS (61) as well as teichoic acid on the surface of *S. pneumoniae* (62). The ChoP decoration of the LOS on *H. influenzae* is phase-variable (63), and although it contributes to adherence it renders the bacteria susceptible to killing by C-reactive protein.

In organ culture studies, adherence of nontypable *H. influenzae* is enhanced on injured epithelial cells (27,29). Recently we described that adherence of nontypable *H. influenzae* to human airway epithelial cell is enhanced in the presence of neutrophil defensins (64). Neutrophil defensins are released upon neutrophil degranulation and are present in high concentrations in purulent airway secretions from patients with COPD (65). The interaction seems to involve the secondary fatty acids of lipid A of LOS (66). All nontypable *H. influenzae* strains tested showed this phenomenon irrespective of the presence of adhesins and the phenomenon was also shown for *M. catarrhalis* (67). Therefore, defensin-stimulated adherence may be an important factor in recurrent infections in the airways of COPD patients.

VII.   Bacterial Invasion into the Airway Epithelium (Table 1)

During incubation of *H. influenzae* with organ cultures of respiratory epithelium bacterial products, including the ciliotoxic LOS, disorganize the ciliairy beating and damage the respiratory epithelium (29,68,69), thereby inhibiting mucociliary clearance. Mucus production is stimulated by *H. influenzae*, presumably through the bacterial production of histamine (70). Pneumococci produce pneumolysin that damages cells, thereby allowing the bacteria to enter the subepithelial tissue (71,72). Translocation through epithelial cells was reported to occur by the interaction of CpbA with the polymeric immunoglobulin receptor (73). *M. catarrhalis* also enters into lung tissues and may cause damage of the epithelial lining (74), but the mechanism responsible is not known.

Several in vivo studies indicate that nontypable *H. influenzae* penetrates the respiratory epithelium during carriage and invasive disease. *H. influenzae* penetration of the upper respiratory tract after colonization was shown in vivo by in situ hybridization and bacterial viability assays of adenoid tissue from young children who were clinically infection-free (75). Subepithelial localization of *H. influenzae* was demonstrated in lungs of COPD patients analyzed postmortem (76), and in lung explants from COPD and cystic fibrosis (CF) patients obtained during lung transplantation (77). Nontypable *H. influenzae* bacteria resided diffusely in the epithelium and the submucosa and were localized mostly extracellularly. More recently, examination of bronchial biopsies by in situ hybridization and immuno-fluorescence microscopy showed *H. influenzae* within and between cells of acutely ill and stable chronic bronchitis patients (78).

Using an in vitro model of confluent human lung epithelial cell layers on permeable supports, we showed that *H. influenzae* passed mainly between the epithelial cells, since clusters of bacteria were localized in the large intercellular spaces of the cell layer (79). A picture of this process named paracytosis is shown in Fig. 1. In this model intracellular bacteria were seen

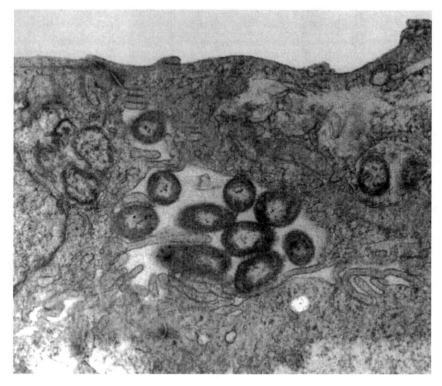

Figure 1 Electron micrograph showing the intercellular location of nontypable *H. influenzae* in lung epithelial cell layers of the NCI-H292 cell line.

only occasionally, and these seemed to be degraded. Highly adherent strains of *H. influenzae* showed greater paracytosis than nonadherent *H. influenzae*, revealing a larger number of bacterial clusters and eventually more cell damage.

Forsgren et al. (75) found viable *H. influenzae* in macrophage-like cells and Bandi et al. (80) showed intracellular location of *H. influenzae* in the submucosa. *H. influenzae* may enter epithelial cells by macropinocytosis (81) or through the interaction of phosphorylcholine with the human PAF receptor (61). For entry of *H. influenzae* in monocytic cells, the β-glucan receptor is invovled, indicating a phagocytosis-like process (82).

In organ cultures incubated with *H. influenzae*, progressive damage of the respiratory tissue allowed interaction of *H. influenzae* with the underlying basal cells and the epithelial basement membrane (27,40,83). In vitro, *H. influenzae* adheres to the extracellular matrix via specific interactions with laminin, fibronectin, and various collagens (84). The Hap adhesin was shown to bind with high affinity to these components (85). In addition, binding of plasmin to *H. influenzae* potentiated penetration of bacteria through a basement membrane preparation (84). These mechanisms are likely relevant for spread of *H. influenzae* into subepithelial tissue.

In vitro experiments with cultured epithelial cells showed that presence of *H. influenzae* leads to production of pro-inflammatory mediators such as IL-8, IL-6, and TNF-α by the epithelial cells, and subsequently to increased neutrophil chemotaxis (86,87). Upregulation of cytokine production may result from activation of NF-κB by OMP P6 of *H. influenzae* through Toll-like receptor 2 (TLR2) (88). *H. influenzae* also exploits the TGF-β signaling pathway, resulting in upregulation of mucin production (89). More epithelial cell-signaling events due to *H. influenzae* are reviewed by Li (90). *H. influenzae* strains persisting in patients elicited lower IL-8 and IL-6 responses than strains isolated on only one occasion (91). These results suggest that *H. influenzae* may affect epithelial cell function and influence inflammation of the airway mucosa via induction of pro-inflammatory mediators.

VIII. Persistence of *H. influenzae* in the Lower Airways of COPD Patients (Table 2)

Longitudinal bacteriological follow-up studies indicated that nontypable *H. influenzae* persists in the lower respiratory tract of COPD and CF patients. Genotyping of *H. influenzae* isolates by DNA restriction fragment length polymorphism (RFLP) or random amplified polymorphic DNA (RAPD) patterns, and phenotyping by OMP analysis were used to characterize the isolates. Persistence of particular *H. influenzae* strains in the lungs of these patients was shown for periods up to 2 years (92–95), despite antibiotic treatment of the patients and specific antibodies in the sputum and sera of these patients (96–98). Although usually one or two different strains are isolated from sputum samples, multiple strains can occur concomitantly in some patients (99). Similar results were found for CF patients (98).

Using DNA-based typing techniques, an average persistence of *M. catarrhalis* of 2.3 months was determined in bronchiectasis patients (100). Persistence of pneumococci was determined by capsular typing of sputum isolates. Also, this pathogen was isolated for many months from the same patient (101).

IX. Humoral and Cellular Immunity Against *H. influenzae*, *S. pneumoniae*, and *M. catarrhalis*

Many studies have been performed on the amounts and antigen specificity of antibodies elicited after natural infection and various immunization schedules. The reader is referred to reviews by Murphy and Sethi (11), Foxwell et al. (102), and Van Alphen et al. (103) for *H. influenzae*, AlonsoDeVelasco et al. (104) for *S. pneumoniae*, and Verduin et al. (105) and Murphy (106) for *M. catarrhalis*. In general, COPD patients respond strongly to a variety of antigens of the bacteria infecting the patient. The most prominent antibody responses are strain specific. T-cell immunity against these pathogens after infection is ill defined, but recent studies show that T-cell immunity plays an important role in the reduction of the number and density of *H. influenzae*–positive sputum cultures (107,108) (Fig. 2).

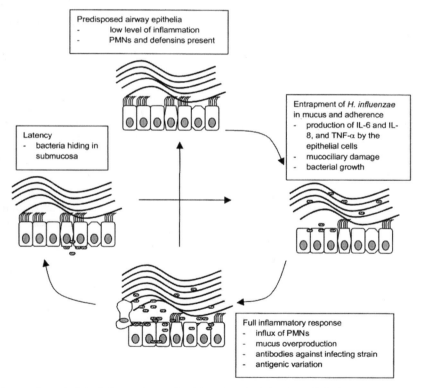

Figure 2 Model of the steps required for chronic infection of the lower respiratory tract of COPD patients by nontypable *Haemophilus influenzae*.

In support of this, King et al. (109) reported that subjects with severe chronic infection with *H. influenzae* had a predominant humoral response to *H. influenzae* compared to a cell-mediated response in healthy controls, indicating that only the cell-mediated immune response is protective against chronic *H. influenzae* infection.

X. Escape from Immune Defense Mechanisms of the Host During Persistent Infection

An effective mechanism for microorganisms to evade the immune defenses of the host is antigenic variation of surface proteins. Of nontypable *H. influenzae* strains with a defined genotype isolated at different time points from the lower respiratory tract of COPD and CF patients, the electrophoretic mobility of OMPs P2 and P5 showed variation (92,98,110). Preexisting antibodies were unable to kill the new variants in a bactericidal assay. Sequence analysis revealed that these changes are always associated with amino acid substitutions due to nonsynonymous point mutations in surface exposed loops. This antigenic drift is indicative for strong immunological pressure (98,111,112).

The effect of immunological pressure on antigenic drift was studied in a rabbit model using subcutaneous tissue cages. *H. influenzae* inoculated in these tissue cages persisted up to 3 years. Antigenic drift similar to that observed in COPD and CF patients was shown for these persisting strains (113). The OMP variants appeared spontaneously and vaccination with the infecting strain resulted in earlier appearance of OMP variants due to antibody-mediated strain-specific bactericidal activity. Therefore, antigenic drift is suggested to be a mechanism to escape the antibody-dependent immune response and as a consequence to promote persistence of *H. influenzae*.

Despite the immunological pressure, the parental strain coexisted with its variants in the subcutaneous tissue cages. Apparently, the clearance mechanisms in the tissue cages are ineffective for the complete removal of bacteria, and immune escape by antigenic drift is not a prerequisite for persistence of *H. influenzae*.

Exacerbations in COPD patients were associated with re-infection by either exogenous strains with a different genotype, or endogenous variants, with the same genotype but a different OMP pattern (93). The appearance of OMP variants in COPD patients soon after exacerbations suggests that immunological selective pressure is effective during exacerbations (Table 3). In support of this hypothesis, Yi et al. (114) showed that during an exacerbation, COPD patients made new antibodies to a number of antigenic determinants, including strain-specific epitopes of P2.

Antigenic variation of *H. influenzae* antigens was also observed for *H. influenzae* LOS, another major target for bactericidal antibodies against *H. influenzae* (97). The molecular basis for this variation is the switching on and off of genes encoding glycosyltransferases and thereby antigenic determinants (115,116). Diversity in LOS is also caused by phase-variable decoration of the molecule with either phosphorylcholine or a terminal galactose molecule. The phosphorylcholine contributes to adherence to epithelial cells, and the terminal galactose confers resistance to killing of the bacteria by C-reactive protein–mediated defense mechanisms (63,117).

The observation that a particular strain of *H. influenzae* persists in COPD patients indicates a general inefficiency in the immune defense mechanisms operating on *H. influenzae*. Opsonizing antibodies against *H. influenzae* are most likely not capable of stimulating effective eradication of the bacteria, since viable nontypable *H. influenzae* were reported to be poorly opsonophagocytozed in the presence of specific antibodies and complement (118). Since the presence of sialic acid on the surface of bacteria is known to inhibit humoral defense mechanisms, this may be relevant for *H. influenzae* survival in the host.

The mechanisms responsible for persistence of pneumococci are not known. Immune defense against pneumococci is dependent on the presence of antibodies specific for the capsular polysaccharides and complement. However, vaccination studies using the 23-valent pneumococcal polysaccharide vaccine showed efficacy in only two of the five studies. Vaccination in the elderly does not provide a major advantage. For an overview of these studies, the reader is referred to Sethi and Murphy (16).

Complement-mediated humoral defense mechanisms against *M. catarrhalis* may be impaired by binding of vitronectin from the tissue fluids to receptors on the bacterial surface (119). Clinical isolates from COPD patients expressed this vitronectin receptor in contrast to the majority of carrier strains (120).

XI. Host Factors Affecting Bacterial Persistence

From all the data discussed above it is clear that the major pathogens in COPD patients have virulence factors contributing to infection. However, host factors must also be important, since the same bacteria colonize the upper respiratory tract of healthy individuals without causing disease. One predisposing factor is tobacco smoking, but not all smokers develop chronic bronchitis and even fewer eventually develop COPD. As mentioned, recurrent infections with these pathogens may be the result of nonclearing adaptive immunity (109). While it is uncertain why bacteria are not eradicated from the lungs of COPD-prone patients, it is apparent that once bacterial pathogens have gained access to the lower respiratory tract, the bacteria persist by further stimulating the inflammation and impairing the mucociliairy clearance. In COPD patients the lower respiratory tract is often chronically colonized with pathogenic bacteria, leading to a continuous elevated level of inflammation.

One of the consequences of inflammation is excessive production of mucus in these patients, even further stimulated during infection. The bacteria from COPD patients are in close interaction with mucus, which contains a variety of compounds including nutrients for the bacteria. Mucus is a diffusion barrier for antibodies and complement and is impermeable for inflammatory cells. In addition, the low penetration of compounds through mucus may also contribute to inefficient killing of *H. influenzae* by antibiotic treatment although selection of isolates with increased antimicrobial resistance during persistance in the respiratory tract occurs at low frequency (121). However, mucus is most likely not the reservoir where *H. influenzae* persists in COPD patients, since persistence occurs despite long periods in which *H. influenzae* cannot be detected in sputum and throat swabs by culturing and immunochemical staining (32,93,98,103).

Bacteria may escape eradication by hiding in subepithelial tissues of the lungs of COPD patients. The localization of *H. influenzae* in the cell layer protects the bacterium from the bactericidal activity of several antibiotics and against antibody-mediated killing (122), indicating that bacteria in the intercellular space may form a reservoir for recurrent infection. *H. influenzae* bacteria that reside inside or bound to macrophages may also provide a reservoir, since bacteria were found localized intracellularly in macrophages in adenoid tissue of young children (75) and in close contact with tissue macrophages in the lungs of CF and COPD patients (77). *H. influenzae* bound to macrophages via HMW proteins in vitro remained largely extracellular and viable, indicating that efficient killing of bacteria by macrophages requires additional serum opsonization (56). In addition, survival of *H. influenzae* in a mouse macrophage cell line for over 72 hours has been reported (123).

XII. Summary

The lower respiratory tract of COPD patients is predisposed to bacterial infections, especially by *H. influenzae*, *S. pneumoniae*, and *M. catarrhalis*.

These bacteria have an extensive repertoire of virulence properties, allowing these to attach to and invade host tissues of the respiratory tract. Once present, these bacteria are not easily eradicated from the lungs of the patients, despite the host response elicited and antibiotics prescribed. Poor opsonophagocytosis, antigenic drift and variation, and "hiding" in submucosal tissue are likely important factors contributing to persistence. Furthermore, the inflammatory response may favor bacterial infection by more progressive damage to the mucosal cells and overproduction of mucus, thereby contributing to a vicious circle of infection.

Table 1   Invasive Strategies of Bacteria Causing Infections in COPD Patients

Haemophilus influenzae: passage between epithelial cells, mechanism unknown
Streptococcus pneumoniae: pneumolysin-mediated passage between epithelial cells; CpbA (PspC) + pIgR interaction promotes translocation across the mucosal barrier through epithelial cells
Moraxella catarrhalis: invasive into cells (?); colonization promotes microabsesses, cell destruction, and discontinuity of epithelial lining
Pseudomonas aeruginosa: elastase and alkaline protease are toxic for epithelial cells (124); defective epithelial cell internalization promotes survival in respiratory tract (125)
Chlamydia pneumoniae: obligate intracellular organism, circumvents the endocytic pathway and prevents apoptosis of host cell (80,126)

Table 2   Persistence of *H. influenzae* in COPD Patients

Each patient is infected by a distinct set of strains.
Distinct strains differ in outer membrane protein composition.
Strains persist up to 2 years.
Bacterial colonization promotes inflammation and further impairment of mucociliairy clearance.
Variants of distinct strains differ in outer membrane proteins (OMPs) P2 and P5 during persistence, especially in connection with exacerbations.
Strains hide from antibiotics and antibody-mediated defense by localization in submucosa.
Multiple variants and strains coexist.

Table 3   Model for the Appearance of Antigenic Variants of *Haemophilus influenzae*

During persistence of bacteria in the lung, the number of bacteria is high (10^8–10^{10}/ mL) for prolonged periods of time.

The number of bacteria allows for appearance of spontaneous mutants.

Antibody-mediated defense mechanisms select for mutants; only antibodies to loop 6 of OMP P2 cause killing of the original strain.

The defense mechanism is rather ineffective; therefore, selection takes a long time.

Vaccination with the infecting strain (and exacerbations of the disease) leads to antibody-mediated defense and promotes selection.

Mutations not under selective pressure are not detected (e.g., antibiotic resistance in the absence of antibiotics).

References

1. Taylor DC, Clancy RL, Cripps AW, Butt H, Bartlett L, Murree-Allen K. An alteration in the host-parasite relationship in subjects with chronic bronchitis prone to recurrent episodes of acute bronchitis. Immunol Cell Biol 1994; 72:143–151.

2. Howard P. A long term follow-up of respiratory symptoms and ventilatory function in a group of working man. Br J Industr Med 1970; 27:326–333.

3. Bates DV. The fate of the chronic bronchitic: a report of the ten-year follow-up in the Canadian Department of Veteran's Affairs coordinated study of chronic bronchitis. Am Rev Respir Dis 1973; 108:1043–1065.

4. Fletcher C, Petro R. The natural history of chronic bronchitis airflow obstruction. Br Med J 1977; 1:1645–1648.

5. Kanner RE, Renzetti ADj, Klauber MR, Smith CB, Golden CA. Variables associated with changes in spirometry in patients with obstructive lung diseases. Am J Med 1979; 67:44–50.

6. Davies AL, Grobow EJ, Tomsett R, McClement JH. Bacterial infection and some effect of chemoprophylaxis in chronic pulmonary emphysema. I. Chemoprophylaxis with intermittent tetracyclin. Am J Med 1961; 1:297–303.

7. Murphy TF, Sethi S. Bacterial infection in chronic obstructive pulmonary disease. Am Rev Respir Dis 1992; 146:1067–1083.

8. Anthonisen NR, Manfreda J, Warren CPW, Hersfield ES, Harding GKM, Nelson NA. Antibiotic therapy in exacerbations of chronic obstructive pulmonary disease. Ann Intern Med 1987; 106:196–204.

9. Saint S, Bent S, Vittinghoff E, Grady D. Antibiotics in chronic obstructive pulmonary disease exacerbations: a meta-analysis. JAMA 1995; 73:957–960.

10. Tager I, Speizer FE. Role of infection in chronic bronchitis. N Engl J Med 1975; 292:563–571.

11. Murphy TF, Apicella MA. Nontypable *Haemophilus influenzae*: a review of clinical aspects, surface antigens, and the human immune response to infection. Rev Infect Dis 1987; 9:1–15.

12. Monso E, Ruiz J, Rosell A, Manterola J, Fiz J, Morera J, Ausina V. Bacterial infection in chronic obstructive pulmonary disease. Am J Respir Crit Care Med 1995; 152:1316–1320.

13. Sethi S, Evans N, Grant BJ, Murphy TF. New strains of bacteria and exacerbations of chronic obstructive pulmonary disease. N Engl J Med 2002; 347:465–471.

14. Soler N, Torres A, Ewig S, Gonzalez J, Celis R, El-Ebiary M, Hernandez C, Rodriguez-Roisin R. Bronchial microbial patterns in severe exacerbations of chronic obstructive pulmonary disease (COPD) requiring mechanical ventilation. Am J Respir Crit Care Med 1998; 157:1498–1505.

15. Miyashita N, Niki Y, Nakajima M, Kawane H, Matsushima T. *Chlamydia pneumoniae* infection in patients with diffuse panbronchiolitis and COPD. Chest 1998; 114:969–971.

16. Sethi S, Murphy TF. Bacterial infection in chronic obstructive pulmonary disease in 2000: a state-of-the-art review. Clin Microbiol Rev 2001; 14:336–363.

17. Turk DC. The pathogenicity of *Haemophilus influenzae*. J Med Microbiol 1984; 18:1–16.

18. Faden H, Duffy L, Williams A, Krystofik DA, Wolf J. Epidemiology of nasopharyngeal colonization with nontypeable *Haemophilus influenzae* in the first 2 years of life. J Infect Dis 1995; 172:132–135.

19. Harabuchi Y, Faden H, Yamanaka N, Duffy L, Wolf J, Krystofik D. Nasopharyngeal colonization with nontypeable *Haemophilus influenzae* and recurrent otitis media. J Infect Dis 1994; 170:862–866.

20. Sakamoto N, Kurono Y, Suzuki M, Kerakawauchi H, Mogi G. Immune responses of adenoidal lymphocytes specific to *Haemophilus influenzae* in the nasopharynx. Laryngoscope 1998; 108:1036–1041.

21. Murphy TF, Bernstein JM, Dryja DM, Campagnari AA, Apicella MA. Outer membrane protein and lipooligosaccharide analysis of paired nasopharyngeal and middle ear isolates in otitis media due to nontypable *Haemophilus influenzae*: pathogenetic and epidemiological observations. J Infect Dis 1987; 156:723–731.

22. Campagnari AA, Gupta MR, Dudas KC, Murphy TF, Apicella MA. Antigenic diversity of lipooligosaccharides of nontypable *Haemophilus influenzae*. Infect Immun 1987; 55:882–887.

23. Troelstra A, Vogel L, van Alphen L, Eijk P, Jansen H, Dankert J. Opsonic antibodies to outer membrane protein P2 of nonencapsulated *Haemophilus influenzae* are strain specific. Infect Immun 1994; 62:779–784.

24. Lomholt H, van Alphen L, Kilian M. Antigenic variation of immunoglobulin A1 proteases among sequential isolates of *Haemophilus influenzae* from healthy children and patients with chronic obstructive pulmonary disease. Infect Immun 1993; 61:4575–4581.

25. Jansen HM, Sachs AP, van Alphen L. Predisposing conditions to bacterial infections in chronic obstructive pulmonary disease. Am J Respir Crit Care Med 1995; 151:2073–2080.

26. Moxon ER, Wilson R. The role of *Haemophilus influenzae* in the pathogenesis of pneumonia. Rev Infect Dis 1991; 13:S518–527.

27. Read RC, Wilson R, Rutman A, Lund V, Todd HC, Brain APR, Jeffery PK, Cole PJ. Interaction of nontypable *Haemophilus influenzae* with human respiratory mucosa in vitro. J Infect Dis 1991; 163:549–558.

28. Stephens DS, Farley M. Pathogenic events during infection of the human nasopharynx with *Neisseria meningitidis* and *Haemophilus influenzae*. Rev Infect Dis 1991; 13:22–33.

29. Wilson R, Read R, Cole P. Interaction of *Haemophilus influenzae* with mucus, cilia and respiratory epithelium. J Infect Dis 1992; 165:S100–S102.

30. Barsum W, Wilson R, Read RC, Rutman A, Todd HC, Houdret N, Roussel P, Cole PJ. Interaction of fimbriated and nonfimbriated strains of unencapsulated *Haemophilus influenzae* with human respiratory tract mucus in vitro. Eur Respir J 1995; 8:709–714.

31. Kubiet M, Ramphal R. Adhesion of nontypeable *Haemophilus influenzae* from blood and sputum to human tracheobronchial mucins and lactoferrin. Infect Immun 1995; 63:899–902.

32. Davies J, Carlstedt I, Nilsson AK, Hakansson A, Sabharwal H, van Alphen L, van Ham M, Svanborg C. Binding of *Haemophilus influenzae* to purified mucins from the human respiratory tract. Infect Immun 1995; 63:2485–2492.

33. Reddy MS, Bernstein JM, Murphy TF, Faden HS. Binding between outer membrane proteins of nontypeable *Haemophilus influenzae* and human nasopharyngeal mucin. Infect Immun 1996; 64:1477–1479.

34. Miyamoto N, Bakaletz LO. Selective adherence of non-typeable *Haemophilus influenzae* (NTHi) to mucus or epithelial cells in the chinchilla eustachian tube and middle ear. Microb Pathog 1996; 21:343–356.

35. Forney LJ, Gilsdorf JR, Wong DC. Effect of pili-specific antibodies on the adherence of *Haemophilus influenzae* type b to human buccal cells. J Infect Dis 1992; 165:464–470.

36. van Alphen L, van den Berghe N, Geelen-van den Broek L. interaction of *Haemophilus influenzae* with human erythrocytes and oropharyngeal epithelial cells is mediated by a common fimbrial epitope. Infect Immun 1988; 56:1800–1806.

37. van Alphen L, Poole J, Overbeeke M. The Anton blood group antigen is the erythrocyte receptor for *Haemophilus influenzae*. FEMS Microbiol Lett 1986; 37:69–71.

38. van Alphen L, Geelen-van dB, Blass L, van Ham M, Dankert J. Blocking of fimbria-mediated adherence of *Haemophilus influenzae* by sialyl gangliosides. Infect Immun 1991; 59:4473–4477.

39. Farley MM, Stephens DS, Kaplan SL, Mason Jr EO. Pilus and non-pilus-mediated interactions of *Haemophilus influenzae* type b with human

erythrocytes and human nasopharyngeal mucosa. J Infect Dis 1990; 161:274–280.

40. Loeb MR, Connor E, Penney D. A comparison of the adherence of fimbriated and nonfimbriated *Haemophilus influenzae* type b to human adenoids in organ culture. Infect Immun 1988; 56:484–489.

41. Sterk LM, van Alphen L, Geelen-van dB, Houthoff HJ, Dankert J. Differential binding of *Haemophilus influenzae* to human tissues by fimbriae. J Med Microbiol 1991; 35:129–138.

42. St. Geme JW3, Cutter D. Evidence that surface fibrils expressed by *Haemophilus influenzae* type b promote attachment to human epithelial cells. Mol Microbiol 1995; 15:77–85.

43. St. Geme JW3. Molecular determinants of the interaction between *Haemophilus influenzae* and human cells. Am J Respir Crit Care Med 1996; 154:S192–S196.

44. St. Geme JW3, Cutter D. Influence of pili, fibrils, and capsule on in vitro adherence by *Haemophilus influenzae* type b. Mol Microbiol 1996; 21:21–31.

45. Geluk F, Eijk PP, van Ham SM, Jansen HM, van Alphen L. The fimbria gene cluster of nonencapsulated *Haemophilus influenzae*. Infect Immun 1998; 66:406–417.

46. St. Geme JW3, de la Morena ML. Falkow S. A *Haemophilus influenzae* IgA protease-like protein promotes intimate interaction with human epithelial cells. Mol Microbiol 1994; 14:217–233.

47. St Geme JW3, Falkow S, Barenkamp SJ. High-molecular-weight proteins of nontypable *Haemophilus influenzae* mediate attachment to human epithelial cells. Proc Natl Acad Sci 1993; 90:2875–2879.

48. Barenkamp SJ, St Geme JW3. Identification of a second family of high-molecular-weight adhesion proteins expressed by non-typable *Haemophilus influenzae*. Mol Microbiol 1996; 19:1215–1223.

49. Barenkamp SJ, Leininger E. Cloning, expression, and DNA sequence analysis of genes encoding nontypeable *Haemophilus influenzae* high-molecular-weight surface-exposed proteins related to filamentous hemagglutinin of *Bordetella pertussis*. Infect Immun 1992; 60:1302–1313.

50. Barenkamp SJ, St. Geme JW3. Identification of surface-exposed B-cell epitopes on high molecular-weight adhesion proteins of nontypeable *Haemophilus influenzae*. Infect Immun 1996; 64:3032–3037.

51. St. Geme JW, Kumar VV, Cutter D, Barenkamp SJ. Prevalence and distribution of the hmw and hia genes and the HMW and Hia adhesins among genetically diverse strains of nontypeable *Haemophilus influenzae*. Infect Immun 1998; 66:364–368.

52. Hultgren SJ, Abraham S, Caparon M, Falk P, St. Geme JW3, Normark S. Pilus and nonpilus bacterial adhesins: assembly and function in cell recognition. Cell 1973; 73:887–901.

53. van Schilfgaarde M, van Ulsen P, Eijk P, Brand M, Stam M, Kouame J, van Alphen L, Dankert J. Characterization of adherence of nontypeable *Haemophilus influenzae* to human epithelial cells. Infect Immun 2000; 68:4658–4665.

54. St. Geme JW3. The HMW1 adhesin of nontypeable *Haemophilus influenzae* recognizes sialylated glycoprotein receptors on cultured human epithelial cells. Infect Immun 1994; 62:3881–3889.

55. Noel GJ, Love DC, Mosser DM. High-Molecular-Weight proteins of Nontypeable *Haemophilus influenzae* mediate bacterial adhesion to cellular proteoglycans. Infect Immun 1994; 62:4028–4033.

56. Noel GJ, barenkamp SJ, St Geme JW3, Haining WN, Mosser DM. High-molecular-weight surface-exposed proteins of *Haemophilus influenzae* mediate binding to macrophages. J Infect Dis 1994; 169:425–429.

57. Prasadarao NV, Lysenko E, Wass CA, Kim KS, Weiser JN. Opacity-associated protein A contributes to the binding of *Haemophilus influenzae* to Chang epithelial cells. Infect Immun 1999; 67:4153–4160.

58. Novotny LA, Jurcisek JA, Pichichero ME, Bakaletz LO. Epitope mapping of the outer membrane protein P5-homologous fimbrin adhesin of nontypeable *Haemophilus influenzae*. Infect Immun 2000; 68:2119–2128.

59. Jiang Z, Nagata N, Molina E, Bakaletz LO, Hawkins H, Patel JA. Fimbria-mediated enhanced attachment of nontypeable *Haemophilus influenzae* to respiratory syncytial virus-infected respiratory epithelial cells. Infect Immun 1999; 67:187–192.

60. Hill DJ, Toleman MA, Evans DJ, Villullas S, van Alphen L, Virji M. The variable P5 proteins of typeable and non-typeable *Haemophilus influenzae* target human CEACAM1. Mol Microbiol 2001; 39:850–862.

61. Swords WE, Buscher BA, Versteeg Lik S, I, Preston A, Nichols WA, Weiser JN, Gibson BW, Apicella MA. Non-typeable *Haemophilus influenzae* adhere to and invade human bronchial epithelial cells via an interaction of lipooligosaccharide with the PAF receptor. Mol Microbiol 2000; 37:13–27.

62. Zhang JR, Idanpaan-Heikkila I, Fischer W, Tuomanen EI. Pneumococcal licD2 gene is involved in phosphorylcholine metabolism. Mol Microbiol 1999; 31:1477–1488.

63. Weiser JN, Pan N, McGowan KL, Musher D, Martin A, Richards J. Phosphorylcholine on the lipopolysaccharide of *Haemophilus influenzae* contributes to persistence in the respiratory tract and sensitivity to serum killing mediated by C-reactive protein. J Exp Med 1998; 187:631–640.

64. Gorter A, Eijk PP, van Wetering S, Hiemstra PS, Dankert J, van Alphen L. Stimulation of adherence of *Haemophilus influenzae* to human lung epithelial cells by antimicrobial neutrophil defensins. J Infect Dis 1998; 178:1067–1074.

65. Panyutich AV, Hiemstra PS, van Wetering S, Ganz T. Human neutrophil defensin and serpins form complexes and inactivate each other. Am J Respir Cell Mol Biol 1995; 12:351–357.

66. Gorter AD, Oostrik J, van der LP, Hiemstra PS, Dankert J, van Alphen L. Involvement of lipooligosaccharides of *Haemophilus influenzae* and *Neisseria meningitidis* in defensin-enhanced bacterial adherence to epithelial cells. Microb Pathog 2003; 34:121–130.

67. Gorter AD, Hiemstra PS, de Bentzmann S, van Wetering S, Dankert J, van Alphen L. Stimulation of bacterial adherence by neutrophil defensins varies

among bacterial species but not among host cell types. FEMS Immunol Med Microbiol 2000; 28:105–111.

68. Johnson AP, Inzana TJ. Loss of ciliary activity in organ cultures of rat trachea treated with lipo-oligosaccharide from *Haemophilus influenzae*. J Med Microbiol 1986; 22:265–268.

69. Wilson R, Roberts D, Cole P. Effect of bacterial products on human ciliary function in vitro. Thorax 1985; 40:125–131.

70. Sheinman BD, Devalia JL, Davies RJ, Crook SJ, Tabaqchali S. Synthesis of histamine by *Haemophilus influenzae*. Br Med J Clin Res 1986; 292:857–858.

71. Rayner CF, Jackson AD, Rutman A, Dewar A, Mitchell TJ, Andrew PW, Cole PJ, Wilson R. Interaction of pneumolysin-sufficient and –deficient isogenic variants of *Streptococcus pneumoniae* with human respiratory mucosa. Infect Immun 1995; 63:442–447.

72. Paton JC. The contribution of penumolysin to the pathogenicity of *Streptococcus pneumoniae*. Trends Microbiol 1996; 4:103–106.

73. Zhang JR, Mostov KE, Lamm ME, Nanno M, Shimida S, Ohwaki M, Tuomanen E. The polymeric immunoglobulin receptor translocates pneumococci across human nasopharyngeal epithelial cells. Cell 2000; 102:827–837.

74. Jorgensen F, Hansson HA, Petruson B, Andersson B. Nasal mucosal changes in children treated with gammaglobulin. Aspects on middle ear pathology and nasopharyngeal bactgeriology. Acta Otolaryngol 1991; 111:785–796.

75. Forsgren J, Samuelson A, Ahlin A, Jonasson J, Rynnel-Dogöö B, Lindberg A. *Haemophilus influenzae* resides and multiplies intracellularly in human adenoid tissue as demonstrated by in situ hybridisation and bacterial viability assay. Infect Immun 1994; 62:673–679.

76. Hers JFP, Mulder J. The mucosal epithelium of the respiratory tract in mucopurulent bronchitis caused by *Haemophilus influenzae*. J Pathol Bacteriol 1953; 66:103–108.

77. Moller LV, Timens W, van der Bij W, Kooi K, de Wever B, Dankert J, van Alphen L. *Haemophilus influenzae* in lung explants of patients with end-stage pulmonary disease. Am J Respir Crit Care Med 1998; 157:950–956.

78. Bandi V, Apicella MA, Mason E, Murphy TF, Siddiqi A, Atmar RL, Greenberg SB. Nontypeable *Haemophilus influenzae* in the lower respiratory tract of patients with chronic bronchitis. Am J Respir Crit Care Med 2001; 164:2114–2119.

79. van Schilfgaarde M, van Alphen L, Eijk P, Everts V, Dankert J. Paracytosis of *Haemophilus influenzae* through cell layers of NCI- H292 lung epithelial cells. Infect Immun 1995; 63:4729–4737.

80. Al Younes HM, Rudel T, Meyer TF. Characterization and intracellular trafficking pattern of vacuoles containing *Chlamydia pneumoniae* in human epithelial cells. Cell Microbiol 1999; 1:237–247.

81. Ketterer MR, Shao JQ, Hornick DB, Buscher B, Bandi VK, Apicella MA. Infection of primary human bronchial epithelial cells by *Haemophilus influenzae*: macropinocytosis as a mechanism of airway epithelial cell entry. Infect Immun 1999; 67:4161–4170.

82. Ahren IL, Williams DL, Rice PJ, Forsgren A, Riesbeck K. The importance of a beta-glucan receptor in the nonopsonic entry of nontypeable *Haemophilus influenzae* into human monocytic and epithelial cells. J Infect Dis 2001; 184:150–158.

83. Cereijido M, Robbins ES, Dolan WJ, Rotunno CA, Sabatini DD. Polarized cell layers formed by epithelial cells on a permeable and translucent support. J Cell Biol 1978; 77:853–880.

84. Virkola R, Lahteenmaki K, Eberhard T, Kuusela P, van Alphen L, Ullberg M, Korhonen TK. Interaction of *Haemophilus influenzae* with the mammalian extracellular matrix. J Infect Dis 1996; 173:1137–1147.

85. Fink DL, Green BA, St GJ, III. The *Haemophilus influenzae* Hap autotransporter binds to fibronectin, laminin, and collagen IV. Infect Immun 2002; 70:4902–4907.

86. Khair OA, Devalia JL, Abdelaziz MM, Sapsford RJ, Tarraf H, Davies RJ. Effect of *Haemophilus influenzae* endotoxin on the synthesis of IL-6, IL-8, TNF-alpha and expression of ICAM-1 in cultured human bronchial epithelial cells. Eur Respir J 1994; 7:2109–2116.

87. Khair OA, Davies RJ, Devalia JL. Bacterial-induced release of inflammatory mediators by bronchial epithelial cells. Eur Respir J 1996; 9:1913–1922.

88. Shuto T, Imasato A, Jono H, Sakai A, Xu H, Watanabe T, Rixter DD, Kai H, Andalibi A, Linthicum F, Guan YL, Han J, Cato AC, Lim DJ, Akira S, Li JD. Glucocorticoids synergistically enhance nontypeable *Haemophilus influenzae*-induced Toll-like receptor 2 expression via a negative cross-talk with p38 MAP kianse. J Biol Chem 2002; 277:17263–17270.

89. Jono H, Shuto T, Xu H, Kai H, Lim DJ, Gum JR, Jr., Kim YS, Yamaoka S, Feng XH, Li JD. Transforming growth factor-beta-Smad signaling pathway cooperates with NF-kappa B to mediate nontypeable *Haemophilus influenzae*-induced MUC2 mucin transcription. J Biol Chem 2002; 277:45547–45557.

90. Li JD. Exploitation of host epithelial signaling networks by respiratory bacterial pathogens. J Pharmacol Sci 2003; 91:1–7.

91. Bresser P, van Alphen L, Habets FJ, Hart AA, Dankert J, Jansen HM, Lutter R. Persisting *Haemophilus influenzae* strains induce lower levels of interleukin-6 and interleukin-8 in H292 lung epithelial cells than nonpersisting strains. Eur Respir J 1997; 10:2319–2326.

92. Groeneveld K, van Alphen L, Eijk PP, Jansen HM, Zanen HC. Changes in outer membrane proteins of nontypable *Haemophilus influenzae* in patients with chronic obstructive pulmonary disease. J Infect Dis 1988; 158:360–365.

93. Groeneveld K, van Alphen L, Eijk PP, Visschers G, Jansen HM, Zanen HC. Endogenous and exogenous reinfections by *Haemophilus influenzae* in patients with chronic obstructive pulmonary disease: the effect of antibiotic treatment on persistence. J Infect Dis 1990; 161:512–517.

94. Moller LV, Ruijs GJ, Heijerman HG, Dankert J, van Alphen L. *Haemophilus influenzae* is frequently detected with monoclonal antibody 8BD9 in sputum samples from patients with cystic fibrosis. J Clin Microbiol 1992; 30:2495–2497.

95. Moller LV, van Alphen L, Grasselier H, Dankert J. N-Acetyl-D-glucosamine medium improves recovery of *Haemophilus influenzae* from sputa of patients with cystic fibrosis. J Clin Microbiol 1993; 31:1952–1954.

96. Brandtzaeg P. Humoral immune response patterns of human mucosae: induction and relation to bacterial respiratory tract infections. J Infect Dis 1992; 165:S167–176.

97. Groeneveld K, Eijk PP, van Alphen L, Jansen HM, Zanen HC. *Haemophilus influenzae* infections in patients with chronic obstructive pulmonary disease despite specific antibodies in serum and sputum. Am Rev Respir Dis 1990; 141:1316–1321.

98. Moller LV, Regelink AG, Grasselier H, Dankert-Roelse JE, Dankert J, van Alphen L. Multiple *Haemophilus influenzae* strains and strain variants coexist in the respiratory tract of patients with cystic fibrosis. J Infect Dis 1995; 172:1388–1392.

99. Murphy TF, Sethi S, Klingman KL, Brueggemann AB, Doern GV. Simultaneous respiratory tract colonization by multiple strains of nontypeable *Haemophilus influenzae* in chronic obstructive pulmonary disease: implications for antibiotic therapy. J Infect Dis 1999; 180:404–409.

100. Klingman KL, Pye A, Murphy TF, Hill S. Dynamics of respiratory tract colonization by *Moraxella (Branhamella) catarrhalis* in bronchiectasis. Am J Respir Crit Care Med 1995; 152:1072–1078.

101. Calder MA, Schonell ME. Pneumococcal typing and the problem of endogenous or exogenous reinfection in chronic bronchitis. Lancet 1971; I:1156–1159.

102. Foxwell AR, Kyd JM, Cripps AW. Nontypeable *Haemophilus influenzae*: pathogenesis and prevention. Microbiol Mol Biol Rev 1998; 62:294–308.

103. van Alphen L, Jansen HM, Dankert J. Virulence factors in the colonization and persistence of bacteria in the airways. Am J Respir Crit Care Med 1995; 151:2094–9.

104. AlonsoDeVelasco E, Verheul AMF, Verhoef J, Snippe H. *Streptococcus pneumoniae*: virulence factors, pathogenesis and vaccines. Micobiol Rev 1995; 59:591–603.

105. Verduin CM, Hol C, Fleer A, van Dijk H, van Belkum A. *Moraxella catarrhalis*: from emerging to established pathogen. Clin Microbiol Rev 2002; 15:125–144.

106. Murphy TF. Lung infections. 2. *Branhamella catarrhalis*: epidemiological and clinical aspects of a human respiratory tract pathogen. Thorax 1998; 53:124–128.

107. Foxwell AR, Kyd JM, Karupiah G, Cripps AW. CD8+T cells have an essential role in pulmonary clearance of nontypeable *Haemophilus influenzae* following mucosal immunization. Infect Immun 2001; 69:2636–2642.

108. Abe Y, Murphy TF, Sethi S, Faden HS, Dmochowski J, Harabuchi Y, Thanavala YM. Lymphocyte proliferative response to P6 of *Haemophilus influenzae* is associated with relative protection from exacerbations of

chronic obstructive pulmonary disease. Am J Respir Crit Care Med 2002; 165:967–971.

109. King PT, Hutchinson PE, Johnson PD, Holmes PW, Freezer NJ, Holdsworth SR. Adaptive immunity to nontypeable *Haemophilus influenzae*. Am J Respir Crit Care Med 2003; 167:587–592.

110. Groeneveld K, van Alphen L, Voorter C, Eijk PP, Jansen HM, Zanen HC. Antigenic drift of *Haemophilus influenzae* in patients with chronic obstructive pulmonary disease. Infect Immun 1989; 57:3038–3044.

111. Duim B, Bowler LD, Eijk PP, Jansen HM, Dankert J, van Alphen L. Molecular variation in the major outer membrane protein P5 gene of nonencapsulated *Haemophilus influenzae* during chronic infections. Infect Immun 1997; 65:1351–1356.

112. Duim B, van Alphen L, Eijk P, Jansen HM, Dankert J. Antigenic drift of nonencapsulated *Haemophilus influenzae* major outer membrane protein P2 in patients with chronic bronchitis is caused by point mutations. Mol Microbiol 1994; 11:1181–1189.

113. Vogel L, Duim B, Geluk F, Eijk P, Jansen H, Dankert J, van Alphen L. Immune selection for antigenic drift of major outer membrane protein P2 of *Haemophilus influenzae* during persistence in subcutaneous tissue cages in rabbits. Infect Immun 1996; 64:980–986.

114. Yi K, Sethi S, Murphy TF. Human immune response to nontypeable *Haemophilus influenzae* in chronic bronchitis. J Infect Dis 1997; 176:1247–1252.

115. Roche RJ, Moxon ER. Phenotypic variation in *Haemophilus influenzae*: the interrelationship of colony opacity, capsule and lipopolysaccharide. Microb Pathogen 1995; 18:129–140.

116. Weiser JN. Relationship between colony morphology and the life cycle of *Haemophilus influenzae*: the contribution of lipopolysaccharide phase variation to pathogenesis. J Infect Dis 1993; 168:672–680.

117. Weiser JN, Pan N. Adaptation of *Haemophilus influenzae* to acquired and innate humoral immunity based on phase variation of lipopolysaccharide. Mol Microbiol 1998; 30:767–775.

118. Vogel L, van Alphen L, Geluk F, Troelstra A, Martin E, Bredius R, Eijk P, Jansen H, Dankert J. Quantitative flow cytometric analysis of opsonophago-cytosis and killing of nonencapsulated *Haemophilus influenzae* by human polymorphonuclear leukocytes. Clin Diagn Lab Immunol 1994; 1:394–400.

119. Verduin CM, Jansze M, Hol C, Mollnes TE, Verhoef J, van Dijk H. Differences in complement activation between complement-resistant and complement-sensitive *Moraxella (Branhamella) catarrhalis* strains occur at the level of membrane attack complex formation. Infect Immun 1994; 62:589–595.

120. Hol C, Verduin CM, van Dijke E, Verhoef J, van Dijk H. Complement resistance in *Branhamella (Moraxella) catarrhalis*. Lancet 1993; 341:1281.

121. Moller LV, Regelink AG, Grasselier H, van Alphen L, Dankert J. Antimicrobial susceptibility of *Haemophilus influenzae* in the respiratory

tracts of patients with cystic fibrosis. Antimicrob Agents Chemother 1998; 42:319–324.

122. van Schilfgaarde M, Eijk P, Regelink A, van Ulsen P, Everts V, Dankert J, van Alphen L. *Haemophilus influenzae* localized in epithelial cell layers is shielded from antibiotics and antibody-mediated bactericidal acitivity. Microb Pathogen 1999; 26:249–262.

123. Craig JE, Cliffe A, Garnett K, High NJ. Survival of nontypeable *Haemophilus influenzae* in macrophages. FEMS Microbiol Lett 2001; 203:55–61.

124. Heck LW, Morihara K, Abrahamson DR. Degradation of soluble laminin and depletion of tissue-associated basement membrane laminin by *Pseudomonas aeruginosa* elastase and alkaline protease. Infect Immun 1986; 54:149–153.

125. Pier GB, Grout M, Zaidi TS, Goldberg JB. How mutant CFTR may contribute to *Pseudomonas aeruginosa* infection in cystic fibrosis. Am J Respir Crit Care Med 1996; 154:S175–S182.

126. Rajalingam K, Al Younes H, Muller A, Meyer TF, Szczepek AJ, Rudel T. Epithelial cells infected with *Chalamydophila pneumoniae (Chlamydia pneumoniae)* are resistant to apoptosis. Infect Immun 2001; 69:7880–7888.

13

Extrapulmonary Effects of COPD

NICHOLAS J. GROSS

Stritch-Loyola School of Medicine
Chicago, Illinois, U.S.A.

I. Introduction

Patients with chronic obstructive pulmonary disease (COPD) present to a physician in their 50s and 60s and may live for another 20–30 years. During this long period while the disease progresses inexorably, the clinician's focus is naturally on the patient's lungs. However, it has become clear in recent years that many systems other than the respiratory system may be involved by COPD. To this extent, COPD can be regarded as a systemic disorder.

In this chapter we review current information about three extra-pulmonary effects of COPD, namely skeletal muscle dysfunction, osteoporosis, and weight loss. We focus on these because they are common, because there is now substantial information about them, and because they may ultimately contribute as much to the patient's overall disability as their lung disease—a fact that the clinician may initially overlook. Moreover, there are grounds for optimism that each of them may be, at least in part, reversible, making it particularly important that they be recognized. One hopes also that early treatment of these extrapulmonary aspects of COPD will improve the quality of life during the long course of the patient's disease and may even prolong life.

II. Skeletal Muscle Dysfunction

Abnormalities in the function of the respiratory muscles in COPD have been recognized for many years (1) and will not be addressed here. Evidence is growing, however, that abnormalities of other skeletal muscles are equally common. Most such studies have focused on the function of limb muscles. [In reviewing this section we have relied extensively on an excellent recent joint statement by the American Thoracic Society and the European Respiratory Society, to which the reader is referred for fuller details (2).]

A. Muscle Mass

The mass of individual skeletal muscles, although difficult to measure accurately, is probably decreased in COPD as compared to matched control subjects (3). It is unclear whether the atrophy is due to specific loss of either type I (slow-twitch, aerobic) or type II (fast-twitch, anaerobic) muscle fibers, or a switch from the former toward the more fatigable latter fiber type (3a). The capillarity of skeletal muscles was lower in COPD patients than in age-matched controls, as was their myoglobin content (4), both of which features would tend to reduce oxygen supply to mitochondria in these muscles. Enzymes of oxidative metabolism are reduced, while enzymes of anaerobic glycolysis are normal in the muscles of COPD patients (5,6).

B. Muscle Strength

It is clear that the strength of some muscles (e.g., the quadriceps) is reduced by 20–30% in subjects with COPD (7–9), an effect that correlates with maximal oxygen uptake and the 6-minute walking distance. In contrast, upper limb muscle strength appears to be relatively well preserved (7,9,10), possibly because these, being accessory muscles of respiration, are exercised more in patients with COPD. But it is not clear whether the endurance of skeletal muscles is impaired; both normal (11) and impaired endurance (12) having been reported for the vastus lateralis muscles, for example. However, muscle training improves both strength and exercise tolerance (13).

C. Bioenergetics

Patients with COPD show overall reductions in both peak O_2 uptake and work rate at peak exercise, but the ratio of these is similar to that seen in healthy subjects, suggesting that the efficiency of oxygen utilization is preserved while muscle mass is reduced (14,15). Moreover, cardiac output also remains tightly coupled to oxygen uptake (at least at submaximal effort). What then explains the reduction in their exercise capacity? Which of these three factors is primarily responsible? Although the answer is uncertain, and possibly different among patients, the reduction in ventilatory capacity due to mechanical abnormalities in the chest wall is considered to be the likeliest explanation (2). Where cardiac failure due to cor pulmonale is present, low cardiac output is a likely alternative.

D. Muscle Biochemistry

The biochemistry of skeletal muscles during exercise in patients with COPD is altered in that oxygen extraction becomes limited at relatively low work rates and lactic acid production increases earlier during exercise (16). Increased lactic acid production would lead, by conversion of bicarbonate ions to CO_2, to acidosis and transient hypercapnia (16a). However, these changes can be explained at least in part by deconditioning and could be reversible by training (6,17). Further analysis of the possibility that exercise limitation in COPD is due to skeletal muscle dysfunction *per se* will require studies of regional oxygen transport, oxygen extraction, blood flow, and work capacity, which are at present lacking.

Studies of skeletal muscle energy metabolism using ^{31}P-magnetic resonance spectroscopy suggest that forearm skeletal muscle oxidative metabolism is impaired in patients with COPD (18–21), and that the time to recovery after exercise is prolonged (3,21). These data are consistent with the deficit in the level of oxidative (mitochondrial) enzymes mentioned above.

In patients with or without COPD, corticosteroids can have both acute and chronic effects on skeletal muscle function, the chronic effects being more common. Proximal muscles are preferentially affected, with selective atrophy of type II fibers. Recovery occurs upon withdrawal, albeit slowly and possibly not completely. In patients with airways obstruction, large studies have not been performed. However, in smaller studies, COPD patients with myopathy were likely to have received doses of methylprednisolone greater than 4 mg/day in the previous 6 months (22). Serum lactic dehydrogenase and 24-hour urinary creatinine excretion were significantly greater than in matched COPD patients without myopathy, and their survival was significantly worse (23).

Corticosteroids inhibit the synthesis of myofibrillar protein, primarily in type II fibers (24), and also may increase myofibrillar catabolism (25), possibly by downregulating insulin-like growth factor 1 (IGF-1). This effect seems to be more marked with fluorinated steroids, namely almost all the currently available inhaled steroids, than with nonfluorinated steroids.

They also have effects on carbohydrate metabolism and energy production in skeletal muscle (26–28) that may or may not be clinically detrimental. It is not clear whether the effects of corticoids on skeletal muscle are compounded by comorbidities such as poor nutritional status and low levels of physical activity, but this is possible.

E. Mechanisms of Skeletal Muscle Dysfunction

The above skeletal muscle abnormalities in COPD could, in large part, be plausibly explained by inactivity or physical deconditioning. Because of dyspnea on effort, these patients have usually altered their lifestyle to reduce their physical activity, and this might account for many of the biochemical and structural abnormalities that have been found. In support of this explanation is the fact that muscles of the lower limbs are more severely affected than either upper limbs (28a), or the diaphragm (28b), both of which latter muscle groups are involved in ventilatory efforts. In part these changes are reversible by physical retraining, although the improvements are lost if and when retraining and exercise are not continued indefinitely (29). However, this is probably an incomplete explanation of skeletal muscle dysfunction in COPD.

Patients with moderate to severe COPD tend to have elevated circulatory levels of inflammatory chemokines such as tumor necrosis factor-alpha (TNF-α), or its soluble receptors, and interleukin-6 (IL-6), each of which has catabolic effects on muscle proteins (29a,29b). The same patients also tend to have frequent exacerbations of their COPD, during which circulating inflammatory chemokines tend to be elevated (29c–29e) with similar possible effects. The same patients are also frequently malnourished and may also receive oral corticosteroids for acute exacerbations. It is also notable that relief of COPD-related airways obstruction by lung transplantation improves lung function but only partially improves effort capacity (30,31). Evidently, skeletal muscle weakness in COPD has many potential causes, of which deconditioning is only one. The roles of inflammatory mediators in its pathogenesis and pulmonary rehabilitation in its correction require further research.

F. Clinical Implications

A decade ago, limitation of physical activity in patients with COPD was usually attributed to dyspnea secondary to impaired lung function, a cause that is difficult to treat (32) and even more difficult to correct. Today, there is evidence that skeletal muscle dysfunction contributes substantially to the limitation of effort tolerance experienced by many patients with COPD. In fact, effort tolerance of COPD patients shows only a weak relation to lung function (33). Moreover, unlike impaired lung function, skeletal muscle dysfunction may be partially remediable by appropriate training (34,35). Pulmonary rehabilitation programs have been shown to enhance endurance and muscle strength in patients with COPD (29,36,37) and should be included in the total therapeutic program for patients with this disease, as advocated in recent guidelines (37b). It is probable, however, that attempts to correct the systemic inflammation will also be necessary in order to reverse the muscle weakness due to COPD.

III. Osteoporosis

It is easily appreciated clinically that overt osteoporosis is common in patients with severe COPD. Among those patients who have progressed to the stage of lung transplantation, radiological and biochemical evidence of osteoporosis is almost so common as to be the rule (38,39). However, by end stage, the COPD patient has accumulated a large number of well-known risk factors for osteoporosis. These include age, chronic disease, reduced mobility, and corticosteroid use, among others. Not surprisingly, therefore, osteoporosis is common in patients with COPD. But is osteoporosis more common in patients with COPD than in matched individuals who do not have COPD? Is COPD itself a risk factor for osteoporosis? Studies of appropriate size that control for the many possible variables have not been performed, to our knowledge. However, there are relevant data, albeit inconclusive.

Riancho et al. (40) compared a group of 44 male COPD patients with 27 "healthy" control subjects of similar age. None of the COPD patients were receiving long-term corticosteroid therapy, although 7 had received short courses for acute exacerbations up to 3 times per year. No differences were found with respect to radiological vertebral or metacarpal deformities or a variety of biochemical markers including serum osteocalcin (as a marker of bone formation) and urinary hydroxyproline (as a marker of bone resorption). The authors concluded that osteoporosis was not more common in COPD *per se*. In contrast, Praet and coworkers found decreases in both trabecular bone density and serum osteocalcin in patients with COPD as compared to matched subjects without COPD, even when the COPD patients had not received oral corticosteroids (41). Similarly, Meeran and colleagues found that osteocalcin levels of patients with asthma or COPD who had not taken long-term corticosteroids (by any route) were lower than in normal volunteers (42). None of these studies can be called definitive, and, being contradictory in outcome, they do not permit one to conclude whether or not COPD itself is a risk factor for osteoporosis.

However, in related studies, vertebral fractures were found to be significantly more common in males who smoked cigarettes (relative risk 2.3 : 1) (43) and among postmenopausal women who smoked cigarettes (44). In both studies the risk of osteoporosis increased with age and, interestingly, was greater in nonobese subjects. Neither study was controlled for the presence or absence of COPD. Thus, the verdict is open as to whether smoking itself or smoking-induced COPD is associated with osteoporosis.

A.   The Effect of Corticosteroids

Systemic Steroids

Corticosteroid use has long been known to be a potent risk factor for osteoporosis (45). Many patients with COPD receive short courses of systemic corticosteroids for acute exacerbations. In addition, many COPD patients receive long-term inhaled corticosteroids, whose benefit is reportedly modest (46,47), and patients with advanced COPD often receive long-term oral corticosteroids. Indeed, their use is discussed in current guidelines for the management of COPD (48). Although multifactorial, their predominant effect on bone mass appears to be the inhibition of bone formation, particularly in trabecular bones such as the vertebral bodies and ribs, resulting in progressive loss of bone from these structures, but also from cortical bone.

Inhaled Steroids

Many studies have shown that inhaled as well as orally administered corticosteroids have measurable effects on bone metabolism. Thus, in healthy volunteers (mean age 29 years), administration of either oral prednisolone 15 mg daily for 7 days or inhaled budesonide 500 μg twice daily for 7 days resulted in significant decreases in serum osteocalcin by 40% and 17%, respectively (42). In subjects with either asthma or COPD who were receiving long-term oral prednisolone (mean 10.1 mg daily), serum osteocalcin levels were 25% lower than in comparable patients who were not receiving steroids (42). Kerstjens and coworkers questioned the significance of reduced serum osteocalcin levels (49). Using two novel telopeptide markers of bone formation and resorption, they found no evidence of detrimental effects on bone metabolism other than a decrease in osteocalcin over the initial 4 weeks of inhaled steroid therapy. Nor, in a large, controlled 2.5-year study, did they find differences in the novel markers of bone metabolism between patients who received bronchodilators plus inhaled corticosteroids versus those who received only bronchodilators. [Perhaps relevantly, their patients were designated as having "asthma and COPD" and their mean age was 40 years. They cite several studies of the short- and long-term effects of corticosteroids in asthmatics (49).]

Effects of corticosteroids on bone mineral content and radiological density are perhaps more clinically important, but there are relatively few publications on patients with COPD. In a recent study of 312 men with COPD, McEvoy and colleagues found prevalences of radiological vertebral fractures of 49% in those patients who had never received corticosteroids, 57% in those who were receiving long-term inhaled steroids (mean of 11.8 puffs per day for 3.5 years), and 63% in those receiving oral steroids (mean of 17.1 mg prednisone per day for 3.1 years), with only the latter group being significantly different from never-users (50). Fractures were not only more frequent in those patients receiving oral steroids, but were more likely to be multiple and more severe. In a subgroup analysis, oral steroid users were further divided into intermittent and continuous steroid users on the basis of continuous use for 6 months. Intermittent users (mean life-time cumulative dose of 2.8 g prednisone over a mean of 16.6 weeks) had an adjusted odds ratio of 1.55 (95% CI 0.72–3.32) compared to never-users. Continuous users (mean cumulative dose of 31.2 g prednisone, or a mean of 16.5 mg per day over a mean of 5.2 years) had an adjusted odds ratio of 2.99 (95% CI 1.38–6.49) compared to never-users and thus accounted for most of the risk of being on oral steroids.

In a brief report on patients with sarcoidosis that had remitted, the withdrawal of oral corticosteroids was followed by apparently complete normalization of bone mass (51).

McEvoy and Niewoehner reviewed the literature on many adverse effects of corticosteroids in COPD (52). They concluded that continuous use of systemic corticosteroids probably results in significant loss of trabecular bone, but that it is unknown whether this effect contributes to overall morbidity. Prospective long-term studies that are controlled for confounding factors are needed.

While one can certainly agree with these conclusions regarding systemic steroid use, it is equally important to know whether long-term use of inhaled steroids carries similar risks. From the data cited above, one tentatively concludes that changes in bone metabolism can be detected in the first few weeks following initiation of inhaled steroids, following which bone metabolism probably stabilizes. One prospective study in patients with mild COPD showed that 3-year treatment with budesonide 800 μg/day via Turbuhaler had no clinically significant effects on bone mineral density or fracture rates (52a). However, it is so far not certain whether there is a threshold of inhaled steroid dose and duration of use below which the risks are clinically insignificant. Other risk factors that may have bearing on the development of osteoporosis in patients with COPD are greater age (53), a decline in mobility and physical activity (54), lower levels of anabolic steroids such as testosterone (55,56) and poor nutritional status (below).

B. Clinical Implications

Clearly there are many factors that put patients with COPD at high risk for osteoporosis. Subtle changes in bone mass, such as most of the metabolic and imaging derangements reviewed here, probably have little effect on the quality of life. However, they probably presage more serious problems, such as collapse of vertebral bodies, which can have a major effect on quality of life and the consumption of health care. Some of these risk factors are at least theoretically reversible (e.g., smoking, physical deconditioning, and poor nutritional status). Where this is impractical (e.g., steroid use) or impossible (e.g., age), a strong suspicion that osteoporosis is likely to occur or is already present should prompt the clinician to perform appropriate investigations [e.g., dual energy x-ray absorptometry (DEXA) scan] and to institute prophylactic therapy.

IV. Weight Loss

Weight loss has long been recognized as a feature of advanced COPD and has been taken as an indication of a poor prognosis (57). It was considered to be an unavoidable consequence of severe airways disease, perhaps resulting from increased energy utilization by respiratory muscles (58). The clinician's approach, therefore, was to attempt to improve airways function, rather than to seek other possibly remediable explanations for weight loss.

Indeed, a longitudinal study of 348 men with severe COPD suggested that a low body mass index (BMI) was associated with shorter survival (59); however, the effect of low BMI appeared to be independent of at least some other correlates of COPD such as abnormal pulmonary mechanics. In a similar but larger longitudinal study, the IPPB trial (60), body weight (expressed as a percent of ideal body weight) was an independent predictor of mortality, adjustments having been made for the strong association between body weight and FEV_1. Recent epidemiological studies support the latter notion (60a). These, among other studies, suggest that weight loss, far from being a consequence of airways obstruction *per se*, might independently contribute to a poor prognosis.

Nor is higher mortality the only outcome associated with low body weight in COPD. Low body weight has been shown, for example, to be an independent predictor of both peripheral and respiratory muscle weakness (61,62), exercise capacity (63), and quality of life (64), all of which are strong reasons to understand its mechanism and to try to correct it.

If low body weight is an independent factor that contributes to the morbidity and mortality of COPD, increasing body weight should ameliorate these outcomes. As discussed below, regimens that increase body weight, particularly fat-free mass, do appear to have a favorable effect on COPD outcomes, although they do not improve the underlying airways disease. This evidence, therefore, provides proof-of-concept, namely that weight loss itself contributes to worse outcomes in COPD.

A. Mechanisms of Weight Loss in COPD

These are quite poorly understood. Former notions were that it was due to a combination of chronic disease, poor nutritional intake possibly compounded by depression, and the increased energy expended by respiratory muscles in performing the increased work of breathing. There is probably some truth to these notions. Baarends and coworkers, for example, have shown that total daily energy expenditure of patients with moderate to severe COPD was almost 20% higher than in age- and weight-matched normal controls, the difference being attributable to an increase in the nonresting component (65). Jounieaux and Mayeux (66) compared the oxygen cost of breathing in ventilated patients with either predominant emphysema or predominant bronchitis, both groups having similarly severe airways obstruction. The emphysema patients as a group had significantly lower BMI and decreases in muscle mass, and their oxygen cost of breathing was more than twice as great as in the group with bronchitis. Similarly, Mannix and colleagues (67) found that COPD patients with a low BMI had a significantly higher oxygen cost of breathing than COPD patients with a normal BMI, and both were higher than that of a group of healthy control subjects (means of 16.4, 9.7, and 2.4 ml O_2/L of minute ventilation, respectively). Moreover, the oxygen cost of breathing was inversely related to BMI and inversely related to the severity of airways obstruction.

Several authors have recently drawn attention to another aspect of energy metabolism in COPD—the impact of pulmonary rehabilitation on energy balance in COPD (67a–67c). Patients who are borderline underweight before entering a rehabilitation program are quite likely to lose weight during it, presumably because of increased expenditure.

These findings can be constructed into a plausible scenario in which airways obstruction and mechanical disadvantage of the respiratory muscles requires the respiratory muscles to work harder and longer, thus increasing their utilization of oxygen and energy. The extra energy consumed by the respiratory muscles becomes so high that total energy expenditure, metabolic rate, and thus energy requirements increase, creating a hypermetabolic state. Unless caloric intake increases accordingly, weight loss occurs.

There are suggestions however, that this scenario may not be a full explanation (68) and that other mechanisms of weight loss may also be present (69–72). Evidence of increased circulating levels of several acute phase reactants and inflammatory mediators has been reported in COPD patients with increased resting energy expenditure and low fat-free body mass (69). Similarly, Di Fracia and colleagues found that elevated levels of TNF-α were an order of magnitude higher in the serum of COPD patients with weight loss than in COPD patients without weight loss (70). The two groups did not differ significantly in terms of severity of airflow limitation, blood gases, or other indices of lung function. Similar evidence for excess production of TNF-α production by monocytes of weight-losing as compared to weight-stable patients with COPD has also been published (71). Recently, too, Takabatake and colleagues (72) reported that serum leptin, an obesity gene product, was lower by more than 50% in patients with COPD and low BMI than in age-matched healthy controls. Their serum TNF-α and TNF-α receptor levels were also higher than those of the controls.

As far as we know, there is not yet a satisfactory explanation for the alternations in these and other circulating mediators in COPD, although they could potentially result in weight loss in this condition. The authors frequently mention airways inflammation as a potential source of catabolic mediators. However, airways inflammation is not nearly so prominent in COPD as in asthma, so one wonders why patients with asthma do not experience as much weight loss, if any at all, as do patients with COPD. Probably weight loss in COPD is multifactorial, and no doubt other mediator abnormalities will come to light in the future, and their role as sufficient and necessary correlates of weight loss in patients with COPD will be tested.

B. Therapeutic Approaches

Is it possible to reverse low body weight in COPD, and if so, does this have beneficial effects on the morbidity and mortality of COPD? Early controlled trials of refeeding in malnourished COPD patients, which were relatively aggressive and short-term, showed that it was possible by increasing caloric intake to reverse nitrogen imbalance and to increase body weight (73–75). Moreover, these effects were associated with improvements in some aspects of respiratory muscle function and exercise capacity. However, the interventions in these early studies were quite aggressive, requiring in-hospital treatment at least for their initiation, and were consequently expensive and impractical for the large numbers of patients that might require them in everyday practice.

Trials of nutritional supplementation in the outpatient setting have generally met with less success (76,77), for which there are several possible explanations. These have to do, in part, with the difficulty of administering sufficient nutritional support over the long-term. Success in terms of an increase in muscle strength is probably dependent on substantial weight gain, say more than 4–5 kg in 2–3 months. Yet the high daily caloric intake requirements for weight gain of this amount are hard for patients to accept (65,78). Even if a fairly aggressive approach is adopted, patients tend to stop eating their regular meals in favor of the supplements. However, the science of nutritional support in COPD has advanced. Recent reports, as reviewed by Schols and Brug (78a), suggest the importance of appropriate management of nutrition in the COPD patient.

Schols and colleagues studied the effect of adding an anabolic steroid or placebo to a program in which all subjects received modest nutritional supplementation (420 kcal/day) plus pulmonary rehabilitation (79). Although overall weight gain was similar in both groups (and only 2.6 kg over 8 weeks), only the group that received anabolic steroids experienced an increase in muscle mass and an improvement in inspiratory muscle strength. Moreover, in a 4-year follow-up study (80), those patients that gained more than 2 kg experienced improved survival (Fig. 1). But in a similar study, Ferreira and coworkers (81) found similar increases of body weight and muscle mass in underweight COPD patients who received an anabolic steroid for 6 months, but no significant improvement in inspiratory muscle strength or exercise capacity. Probably, nutritional supplementation and physical rehabilitation needs to be complemented by one or more biochemical factors which have yet to be identified.

D. Clinical Implications

Weight loss can be viewed as a surrogate for decreased muscle strength and a poor prognosis in patients with COPD. A low or falling body mass index should trigger efforts to increase caloric intake by regular administration of feeding supplements. But, as this measure alone is unlikely to achieve consistent improvement in weight and muscle strength, it should be combined with a pulmonary rehabilitation program. Even so, it may be difficult to achieve sustained weight gain. Possibly, other therapy such as anabolic hormones and/or growth factors, in addition to refeeding and rehabilitation, may offer greater benefits. Further studies are

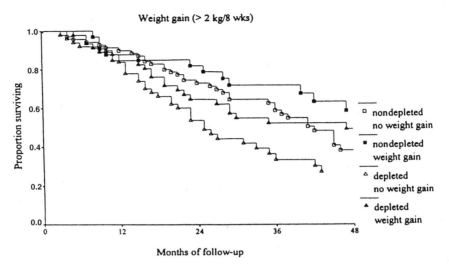

Figure 1   Weight gain after an intervention predicts improved survival in patients with COPD. Patients with COPD ($n = 203$; average $FEV_1 = 34\%$ predicted) undergoing an 8-week pulmonary rehabilitation program were randomized to receive nutritional supplementation, anabolic steroid administration, or neither intervention. In a post hoc survival analysis, patients were divided into four groups based on their initial nutritional status (depleted or nondepleted) and their response (weight gain or no weight gain). Both higher initial body weight and weight gain during the 8-week intervention predicted better survival. (From Ref. 80.)

required to identify the causes and potential remedies of weight loss in severe COPD.

References

1.   De Troyer A, Pride NB. The chest wall and respiratory muscles in chronic obstructive pulmonary disease. In: Roussos C, ed. The Thorax, Part C: Disease, 2nd ed. Marcel Dekker: New York. 1995:1975–2006.
2.   American Thoracic Society/European Thoracic Society. Skeletal muscle dysfunction in chronic obstructive disease. Am J Respir Crit Care Med 1999; 159(suppl): S1–S40.
3.   Wuyam B, Payen JF, Levy P, Bensaidane H, Reutenauer H, Le Bas F, Benabid AL. Metabolism and aerobic capacity of skeletal muscle in chronic respiratory failure related to chronic obstructive pulmonary disease. Eur Respir J 1992; 5:157–162.

3a. Jakobsson P, Jorfeldt L, Brundin A. Skeletal muscle metabolites and fibre types in patients with advanced chronic obstructive pulmonary disease, with and without chronic respiratory failure. Eur Respir J 1990; 3:192–196.

4. Simard C, Maltais F, Leblanc P, Simard PM, Jobin J. Mitochondrial and capillarity changes in vastus lateralis muscle of COPD patients, electron microscopic study. Med Sci Sports Exerc 1996; 28:S95.

5. Jakobsson P, Jordfeldt L, Henriksson J. Metabolic enzyme activity in the quadriceps femoris muscle in patients with severe chronic obstructive pulmonary disease. Am J Respir Crit Care Med 1995; 151:374–377.

6. Maltais F, Simard AA, Simard C, Jobin J, Desgagnes P, Leblanc P. Oxidative capacity of the skeletal muscle and lactic acid kinetics during exercise in normal subjects and in patients with COPD. Am J Respir Crit Care Med 1996; 153:288–293.

7. Gosselink R, Troosters, T, Decramer M. Peripheral muscle weakness contributes to exercise limitation in COPD. Am J Respir Crit Care Med 1996; 153:976–980.

8. Hamilton AL, Killian KJ, Summers E, Jones NL. Muscle strength, symptom intensity and exercise capacity in patients with cardiorespiratory disorders. Am J Respir Crit Care Med 1995; 152:2021–2031.

9. Bernard S, Leblanc P, Whittom F, Carrier G, Jobin J, Belleau R, Maltais F. Peripheral muscle weakness in patients with chronic obstructive pulmonary disease. Am J Respir Crit Care Med 1998; 158:629–634.

10. Newell SZ, McKenzie DK, Gandevia SC. Inspiratory and skeletal muscle strength and endurance and diaphragmatic activation in patients with chronic airflow limitation. Thorax 1989; 44:903–912.

11. Zattara-Hartmann MC, Badier M, Guillot C, Tomei C, Jammes Y. Maximal force and endurance to fatigue of respiratory and skeletal muscles in chronic hypoxemic patients, the effects of oxygen breathing. Muscle Nerve 1995; 18:495–502.

12. Serres I, Gautier V, Varray AL, Prefaut CG. Impaired skeletal muscle endurance related to physical inactivity and altered lung function in COPD patients. Chest 1998; 113:900–905.

13. Simpson K, Killian KJ, McCartney N, Stubbing DG, Jones NL. Randomised controlled trial of weightlifting exercise in patients with chronic airflow limitation. Thorax 1992; 47:70–75.

14. Agusti AGN, Cotes J, Wagner PD. Responses to exercise in lung disease. In: Whipp BJ, Roca J, eds. Clinical Exercise Testing. Eur Respir Monograph 1997; 6:32–50.

15. Wehr KL, Johnson RL. Maximal oxygen consumption in patients with lung disease. 1976; 56:880–890.

16. Sala E, Roca J, Marrades RM, Alonso J, Gonzales de Suso JM, Moreno A, Barbera JA, Nadal J, de Jover L, Rodriguez-Roisin R, Wagner PD. Effects of endurance training on skeletal muscle bioenergetics in chronic obstructive pulmonary disease. Am J Respir Crit Care Med 1999; 159: 1726–1734.

16a. Polkey MI, Hawkins P, Kyroussis D et al. Inspiratory pressure support prolongs exercise induced lactataemia in severe COPD. Thorax 2000; 55:547–549.

17. Maltais F, Leblanc P, Simard C, Jobin J, Berube C, Bruneau J, Carrier L, Belleau R. Skeletal muscle adaptation to endurance training in patients with chronic obstructive pulmonary disease. Am J Respir Crit Care Med 1996; 154:442–447.

18. Kutsuzawa T, Shioya S, Kurita D, Haida M, Ohta Y, Yamabayashi H. Muscle energy metabolism and nutritional status in patients with chronic obstructive pulmonary disease, a ^{31}P magnetic resonance study. Am J Respir Crit Care Med 1995; 152:647–652.

19. Tada H, Kato H, Misawa T, Sasaki F, Hayashi S, Takahashi H, Kutsumi Y, Ishizaki T, Nakai T, Miyabo S. ^{31}P-nuclear magnetic resonance evidence of abnormal skeletal muscle metabolism in patients with chronic lung disease and congestive heart failure. Eur Respir J 1992; 5:163–169.

20. Thompson C, Davies R, Kemp G, Taylor D, Radda G, Rajagopalan B. Skeletal muscle metabolism during exercise and recovery in patients with respiratory failure. Thorax 1993; 48:486–490.

21. Payen JF, Wuyam B, Levy P, Reutenauer H, Steiglitz P, Paramelle B, Le Bais JF. Muscular metabolism during oxygen supplementation in patients with chronic hypoxemia. Am J Respir Crit Care Med 1993; 147:592–598.

22. Decramer M, Lacquet LM, Fagard R, Rogiers P. Corticosteroids contribute to muscle weakness in chronic airflow obstruction. Am J Respir Crit Care Med 1994; 150:11–16.

23. Decramer M, de Bock V, Dom R. Functional and histologic picture of steroid-induced myopathy in chronic obstructive pulmonary disease. Am J Respir Crit Care Med 1996; 153:1958–1964.

24. Lieu F, Powers SK, Herb RA, Criswell D, Martin D, Wood C, Stainsby W, Chen CL. Exercise and glucocorticoid-induced diaphragmatic myopathy. J Appl Physiol 1993; 75:763–771.

25. Mayer M, Rosen F. Interaction of glucocorticoids and androgens with skeletal muscle. Metabolism 1977; 26:937–962.

26. Shoji S, Takagi A, Sugita H, Toyokura Y. Muscle glycogen metabolism in steroid-induced myopathy of rabbits. Exp Neurol 1974; 45:1–7.

27. Ferguson GT, Irvin CG, Cherniack RM. Effects of corticosteroids on diaphragm function and biochemistry in the rabbit. Am J Respir Crit Care Med 1990; 141:156–163.

28. Fernandez-Sola J, Cusso R, Picado C, Vernet M, Grau JM, Urbanomarquez A. Patients with chronic glucocorticoid treatment develop changes in muscle glycogen metabolism. J Neurol Sci 1993; 117:103–106.

28a. Man WDC, Soliman MGG, Nikoletou D, et al. Non-volitional assessment of skeletal muscle strength in patients with chronic obstructive pulmonary disease. Thorax 2003; 58:665–669.

28b. Polkey MI, Kyroussis D, Hamnegard C-H, et al. Diaphragm strength in chronic obstructive pulmonary disease. Am J Respir Crit Care Med 1996; 154:1310–1317.

29. Reis A, Kaplan R, Limberg T, Prewit L. Effects of pulmonary rehabilitation on physiologic and psychosocial outcomes in patients with chronic obstructive pulmonary disease. Ann Int Med 1995; 122:823–832.

29a. Creutzberg EC, Schols AM, Weling-Scheepers CA, et al. Characterization of non-response to high caloric oral nutritional therapy in depleted patients with chronic obstructive pulmonary disease. Am J Respir Crit Care Med 2000; 161:745–752.

29b. Eid AA, Ionescu AA, Nixon LS, et al. Inflammatory response and body composition in chronic obstructive pulmonary disease. Am J Respir Crit Care Med 2001; 164:1414–1418.

29c. Spruitt MA, Gooselink R, Troosters, T, et al. Muscle force during an acute exacerbation in hospitalized COPD patients and its relationship with CXCL8 and IGF-1. Thorax 2003; 58:752–756.

29d. Wedzicha JA, Seemungal TA, MacCallum PK, et al. Acute exacerbations of chronic obstructive pulmonary disease are accompanied by elevations of plasma fibrinogen and serum IL-6 levels. Thromb Haemost 2000; 84:210–215.

29e. Dentener MA, Creutzberg EC, Schols AM, et al. Systemic anti-inflammatory mediatory in COPD, increase in soluble interleukin 1 receptor II during treatment of exacerbations. Thorax 2001; 56:721–726.

30. Casaburi R. Deconditioning. In: Fishman AP, ed. Pulmonary Rehabilitation. Marcel Dekker, New York. 1996:213–230.

31. Low DE, Trulock EP, Kaiser LR, Pasque MK, Dresler C, Ettinger N, Cooper DJ. Morbidity, mortality, and early results of single versus bilateral lung transplantation for emphysema. J Thorac Cardiovasc Surg 1992; 103:1119–1126.

32. Grove A, Lipworth BJ, Reid P, Smith RP, Ingram RJ, Jenkins RJ, Winter JH, Dhillon DP. Effects of regular salmeterol on lung function and exercise capacity in patients with chronic obstructive pulmonary disease. Thorax 1996; 51:689–693.

33. Wasserman K, Sue DY, Casaburi R, Moricca RB. Selection criteria for exercise training in pulmonary rehabilitation. Eur Respir J 1989; 7(suppl): 604s–610s.

34. Casaburi R. Exercise training in chronic obstructive lung disease. In: Casaburi R, Petty TL, eds. Principles and Practice of Pulmonary Rehabilitation. Saunders, Philadelphia. 1993:204–224.

35. Reis AL, Carlin BW, Carrieri-Kohlman V, Casaburi R, Celli BR, Emery CF, Hodgkin JE, Mahler DA, Make B, Skolnick J. Pulmonary rehabilitation, evidence based guidelines. Chest 1997; 112:1363–1396.

36. Casaburi R, Patessio A, Ioli F, Zanaboni S, Donner CF, Wasserman K. Reductions in exercise lactic acidosis and ventilation as a result of exercise training in patients with obstructive lung disease. Am Rev Respir Dis 1991; 143:9–18.

37. Casaburi R. Mechanisms of the reduced ventilatory requirement as a result of exercise training. Eur Respir Rev 1995; 5:42–46.

37b. Executive Summary. Global Initiative for Chronic Obstructive Lung Disease. 2003. www.goldcopd.com

38. Shane, E, Silverberg SG, Donovan D, Papodopoulos A, Staron RB, Addesso V, Jogesen B, McGregor C, Schulman L. Osteoporosis in lung transplantation candidates with end-stage pulmonary disease. Am J Med 1996; 101:262–269.

39. Aris RM, Neuringer IP, Weiner MA, Egan TM, Ontjes D. Severe osteoporosis before and after lung transplantation. Chest 1996; 109:1176–1183.

40. Riancho JA, Gonzalez Macias J, Del Arco C, Amado JA, Freijanes J, Anton MA. Thorax 1987; 42:962–966.

41. Praet JP, Peretz A, Rozenberg S, Famaey JP, Bourdoux P. Risk of osteoporosis in men with chronic bronchitis. Osteoporosis Int 1992; 2:257–261.

42. Meeran K, Hattersley A, Burrin J, Shiner R, Ibbertson K. Oral and inhaled corticosteroids reduce bone formation as shown by serum osteocalcin levels. Am J Respir Crit Care Med 1995; 151:333–336.

43. Seeman E, Melton LJ, O'Fallon WM, Riggs BL. Risk factors for spinal osteoporosis in men. Am J Med 1983; 75:977–983.

44. Daniell HW. Osteoporosis of the slender smoker, vertebral compression fractures and loss of metacarpal cortex in relation to postmenopausal cigarette smoking and lack of obesity. Arch Int Med 1976; 136:298–304.

45. Reid IR. Pathogenesis and treatment of steroid osteoporosis. Clin Endocrinol 1989; 30:83–103.

46. Pauwels RA, Lofdahl CG, Laitinen LA, Schouten JP, Postma DS, Pride NB, Ohlsson SV. Long-term treatment with inhaled budesonide in persons with mild chronic obstructive pulmonary disease who continue smoking, European Respiratory Society Study on Chronic Obstructive Pulmonary Disease. N Engl J Med 1999; 340:1948–1953.

47. Renkema TEJ, Schouten JP, Koeter GH, Postma DS. Effects of long-term treatment with corticosteroids in COPD. Chest 1996; 109:1156–1162.

48. American Thoracic Society. ATS Statement: standards for the diagnosis and care of patients with chronic obstructive pulmonary disease. Am J Respir Crit Care Med 1995; 152:S77–S121.

49. Kerstjens HAM, Postma DS, van Doormaal J, van Zanten AK, Brand PLP, Dekhuijzen PNR, Koeter GH. Effects of short term and long term treatment with inhaled corticosteroids on bone metabolism in patients with airways obstruction. Thorax 1994; 49:652–656.

50. McEvoy CE, Ensrud KE, Bender E, Genant HK, Yu W, Griffith JM, Niewoehner DE. Association between corticosteroid use and vertebral fractures in older men with chronic obstructive pulmonary disease. Am J Respir Crit Care Med 1998; 157:704–709.

51. Rizzato G, Montemurro L. Reversibility of exogenous corticosteroid-induced bone loss. Eur Respir J 1993; 6:116–119.

52. McEvoy CE, Niewohner DE. Adverse effects of corticosteroid therapy for COPD. Chest 1997; 111:732–743.

52a. Johnell O, Pauwels R, Lofdahl CG, Laitinen LA, Postma DS, Pride NB, Ohlsson SV. Bone mineral density in patients with chronic obstructive pulmonary disease treated with budesonide Turbuhaler. Eur Respir J 2002; 19(6):1058–1063.

53. Kiel DP, Hannan MT, Genant HK, Felson DT. Prevalence and incidence of vertebral fractures in the elderly: initial results from the Framingham study. J Bone Miner Res 1995; 9:S129–S132.

54. Sinaki M. Osteoporosis, Etiology, Diagnosis. Raven Press, New York 1988:457–465.

55. Gow SM, Seth J, Beckett GJ, Douglas G. Thyroid function and endocrine abnormalities in elderly patients with severe chronic obstructive lung disease. Thorax 1987; 42:520–525.

56. Kamische A, Kemper DE, Castel MA, Luthke M, Rolf C, Behre HM, Magnussen H, Nieschlag E. Testosterone levels in men with chronic obstructive pulmonary disease with or without glucocorticoid therapy. Eur Respir J 1998; 11:41–45.

57. Nandenbergh E, Van de Woestijne KP, Gyselen A. Weight changes in the terminal stages of chronic obstructive pulmonary disease. Am Rev Respir Dis 1992; 146:1511–1517.

58. Braun SR, Kiem NL, Dixon RM, Clagnaz P, Anderegg A, Shrago ES. Chest 1984; 86:558–563.

59. Gray-Donald K, Gibbons L, Shapiro SH, Macklem PT, Martin JG. Nutritional status and mortality in chronic obstructive pulmonary disease. Am J Respir Crit Care Med 1996; 153:961–966.

60. Wilson DO, Rogers RM, Wright EC, Anthonisen NR. Body weight in chronic obstructive pulmonary disease, the National Institute of Health Intermittent Positive-Pressure Breathing Trial. Am Rev Respir Dis 1989; 139:1435–1438.

60a. Prescott E, Almdal T, Mikkelsen KL, et al. Prognostic value of weight change in chronic obstructive pulmonary disease, results from the Copenhagen City Heart Study. Eur Respir J 2002; 20:539–544.

61. Engelen MAM, Schols AMWJ, Baken WC, Wesseling GJ, Wouters EFM. Nutritional depletion in relation to respiratory and peripheral skeletal muscle function in an outpatient population with COPD. Eur Respir J 1994; 7:1793–1797.

62. Arora NS, Rochester DF. Respiratory muscle strength and maximal voluntary ventilation in undernourished patients. Am Rev Respir Dis 1982; 126:5–8.

63. Baarends EM, Schols AMWJ, Mostert R, Wouters EFM. Peak exercise in relation to tissue depletion in patients with chronic obstructive pulmonary disease. Eur Respir J 1997; 10:2807–2813.

64. Shoup R, Dalsky G, Warner G, Davies H, Connors M, Khan M, Khan F, Zuwallack R. Eur Respir J 1997; 10:1576–1580.

65. Baarends EM, Schols AMWJ, Pannemans DLE, Westerterp KR, Wouters EFM. Total free-energy expenditure in severe chronic obstructive pulmonary disease. Am J Respir Crit Care Med 1997; 155; 549–554.

66. Jounieaux V, Mayeux I. Oxygen cost of breathing in patients with emphysema or chronic bronchitis in acute respiratory failure. Am J Respir Crit Care Med 1995; 152:2181–2184.

67. Mannix ET, Manfredi F, Farber MO. Elevated O_2 cost of ventilation contributes to tissue wasting in COPD. Chest 1999; 115:708–713.

67a. Wouters EFM. Eat well to get well. Thorax 2003; 58:739–740.

67b. Steiner MC, Barton RL, Singh SJ, et al. Nutritional enhancement of exercise performance in chronic obstructive pulmonary disease, a randomized controlled trial. Thorax 2003; 58:745–751.

67c. Goris AHC, Vermeeren MAP, Wouters EFM, et al. Energy balance in depleted ambulatory patients with chronic obstructive pulmonary disease, the effect of physical activity and oral nutritional supplementation. Br J Nutr 2003; 89:725–729.

68. Sridhar MK, Carter R, Lean ME, Banham SW. Resting energy expenditure and nutritional state of patients with increased oxygen cost of breathing due to emphysema, scoliosis, and thoracoplasty. Thorax 1994; 49:781–785.

69. Schols AM, Buurman WA, Staal van den Brekel AJ, Dentener MA, Wouters EF. Evidence for a relation between metabolic derangements and increased levels of inflammatory mediators in a subgroup of patients with chronic obstructive pulmonary disease. Thorax 1996; 51:819–824.

70. Di Francia M, Barbier D, Mege JL, Orehek J. Tumor necrosis factor-alpha levels and weight loss in chronic obstructive pulmonary disease. Am J Respir Crit Care Med 1994; 150:1453–1455.

71. De Godoy I, Donahoe M, Calhoun WJ, Mancino J, Rogers RM. Elevated TNF-alpha production by peripheral blood monocytes of weight-losing COPD patients. Am J Respir Crit Care Med 1996; 153:633–637.

72. Takabatake N, Nakamura H, Abe S, Hino T, Saito H, Yuki H, Kato S, Tomoike H. Circulating leptin in patients with chronic obstructive pulmonary disease. Am J Respir Crit Care Med 1999; 159:1215–1219.

73. Goldstein SA, Thomashow BM, Kvetan V, Askanazi JM, Kinney JM, Elwyn DH. Nitrogen and energy relationships in malnourished patients with emphysema. Am Rev Respir Dis 1988; 138:636–644.

74. Whittaker JS, Ryan CF, Buckley PA, Road JD. The effects of refeeding on peripheral and respiratory muscle function in malnourished chronic obstructive pulmonary disease patients. Am Rev Respir Dis 1990; 142:283–288.

75. Rogers RM, Donahoe M, Costantino J. Physiologic effects of oral supplemental feeding in malnourished patients with chronic obstructive pulmonary disease, a randomized control study. Am Rev Respir Dis 1992; 146:1511–1517.

76. Efthimiou J, Fleming J, Gomes C, Spiro SG. The effect of supplementary oral nutrition in poorly nourished patients with chronic obstructive pulmonary disease. Am Rev Respir Dis 1988; 137:1075–1082.

77. Sridhar MK, Gallaway A, Lean ME, Banham SW. An outpatient nutritional supplementation programme in COPD patients. Eur Respir J 1994; 7:720–724.
78. Rochester DF. Nutritional repletion. Semin Respir Med 1992; 13:44–52.
78a. Schols AMWJ, Brug J. Efficacy of nutritional intervention in chronic obstructive pulmonary disease. Eur Respir Monogr 2003; 8(monograph 24): 142–152.
79. Schols AM, Soeters PB, Mostert R, Pluymers RJ, Wouters EF. Physiologic effects of nutritional support and anabolic steroids in patients with chronic obstructive pulmonary disease, a placebo controlled randomized trial. Am J Respir Crit Care Med 1995; 152:1268–1274.
80. Schols AM, Slangen J, Volovics A, Wouters EFM. Weight loss is a reversible factor in the prognosis of COPD. Am J Respir Crit Care Med 1998; 157:1791–1797.
81. Ferreira IM, Verreschi IT, Nery LE, Goldstein RS, Zamel N, Brooks D, Jardim JR. The influence of 6 months of oral anabolic steroids on body mass and respiratory muscles in undernourished COPD patients. Chest 1998; 114:19–28.

14

Smoking Cessation

PHILIP TØNNESEN

Gentofte University Hospital
Hellerup, Copenhagen, Denmark

I. Introduction

The first part of this chapter reviews the literature about smoking cessation with nicotine-replacement therapy (NRT) and bupropion in healthy smokers. Readers familiar with the smoking cessation literature can skip the first part. The last part focuses on identification of smokers with chronic obstructive pulmonary disease (COPD) and smoking cessation trials in this group of patients, ending with a recommendation about smoking cessation for COPD patients.

It should be remembered that cigarette smoking is an addiction, and for that reason smoking cessation cannot be compared with treatment of other medical conditions. NRT will produce low success rates when used without adjunctive behavioral support. However, as most smokers quit by their own and buy NRT over the counter (OTC), even this low success rate will have an important influence on public health. The degree of supportive adjunctive behavioral therapy parallels the factual success rate, while the relative success rate (i.e., the odds ratio between NRT and placebo) remains more or less unchanged around a factor of 2 (1).

Smoking cessation is one of the only interventions that affects the decline in FEV_1 in patients with COPD and thus its prognosis. Fletcher et al.'s prospective epidemiological long-term study (2,3) showed in a large cohort that cessation of smoking changed the annual decline in FEV_1 to normal and that most smokers did not develop airway obstruction. Also, smoking cessation is one of the most cost-effective treatments compared to more than 300 other medical therapies (4).

Many physicians have neglected the issue of smoking cessation, and advice to quit has not been delivered systematically to all smoking patients. Many physicians are much more likely to prescribe bronchodilators and inhaled steroids to COPD patients than recommend they stop smoking. The EUROSCOP and ISOLDE studies have focused on less important factors for prognosis, i.e., use of inhaled steroids for smoking COPD patients, instead of on getting patients to stop smoking.

From smoking cessation studies, solid scientific documentation exists that NRT and bupropion are effective tools, along with multicomponent programs, with a doubling of the 1-year sustained quit rate in healthy smokers. However, the efficacy of NRT and bupropion has been far less often investigated in COPD patients.

II. Motivation to Quit

The motivation to quit is important to the individual outcome of a smoking cessation attempt. Hospitalization provides an opportunity for the patient to try to stop smoking.

Some smokers are contented smokers. The cigarette may be the only "friend" left for a lonesome COPD patient with a low quality of life and without the ability to leave the house due to physical disability. Although many smokers would like to quit, some need a push from others. Motivation to quit can be regarded as a cyclic process of change, as described by Prochaska and Goldstein (5). They proposed five stages of motivation to quit: precontemplation, contemplation, preparation, action, and maintenance. Using three questions it is possible to classify the individual smoker's motivation to quit (Table 1).

The action stage can be divided into two parts: the first 3 months after quitting, or the relapse stage, and the period 3–6 months after quitting, or the consolidation stage. During the first 3 months more than 75% of initial quitters will start smoking again. Thus, it is during this initial period that we must intensify our interventions if we want to increase the long-term success rate in smoking cessation.

Table 1 Prochaska's Modified Stages of Motivation to Quit Smoking

1. Do you plan to quit smoking in the next 6 months?
Answer No: Precontemplation stage

2. Do you plan to quit smoking in the next month?
Answer No and Yes to 1: Contemplation stage

3. Have you tried to quit in the last year?
Answer Yes and Yes to 2: Preparation stage

4. Subjects who have already quit:
Did you quit less than 6 months ago?
Answer Yes: Action stage (1–3 months, relapse stage; 4–6 months,
    consolidation stage)
Did you quit more than 6 months ago?
Answer Yes: Maintenance stage

Source: Modified from Ref. 5.

Some smokers may move through all five stages, and some may skip one or more stages. The approach to the smoker depends on the stage: in the preparation stage, support and advice about NRT and the golden rules of smoking cessation are relevant, while relapse prevention strategies and support are adequate in the action stage. Use of the above questions is an easy and quick way to classify the motivational stage of the individual smoker and then apply the right treatment.

It might also be relevant to ask if the smoker has decided to quit completely or to simply cut down. In the latter case the stage can be considered as precontemplation. However, whenever a COPD patient is hospitalized, regardless of the motivational stage, a quit attempt should be initiated. It is important never to miss an opportunity to intervene with a smoker. The Prochaska stages are only a poorly documented theory.

III. Basic Principles

A. Complete Abstinence from Cigarettes Predicts Success

Some basic principles related to successful smoking cessation should always be considered. Smokers must stop smoking completely at quit day (even 1–2 cigarettes per day during the first 1–2 weeks of cessation are usually followed by relapse); use of NRT lessens withdrawal symptoms and improves cessation outcomes; follow-up should be arranged to prevent relapse during the first 3–6 weeks, when relapse is highest. The most important point is to get the smoker to understand that stopping smoking means "no cigarettes or failure." This is supported by findings from several smoking cessation trials.

In the CEASE study comprising 3575 subjects, initial cessation was a very strong predictor of long-term success. Of the first-week abstainers, 25% attained 12-month success versus only 3% of the subjects still smoking in the first week (6).

In a multicenter study comprising 1686 smokers using nicotine patches, early abstinence from smoking was the strongest predictor of sustained abstinence (7). Of first-week abstainers, 25% of 277 in the active group and 28% of 182 in the placebo group achieved long-term success as opposed to first-week smokers—4% of 565 in the active group and 2% of 662 in the placebo group. In a similar study comprising 1200 subjects, all but one of the 96 subjects achieving long-term abstinence quit during the first week of cessation (8). Observations in the three above studies emphasize that the first weeks after quit day are the most important for long-term outcome. Use of the patch for a few weeks, or longer if abstinence is achieved, may be an effective policy and might be a more cost-effective way to administer the nicotine patch.

B. Nicotine Replacement Therapy

Nicotine appears to be responsible for the hemodynamic effects and coronary vasoconstriction caused by smoking cigarettes. It has sympathomimetic effects that lead to increased heart rate (HR) and increased blood pressure and cause coronary vasoconstriction (9). Nicotine is liberated from the acid cigarette smoke as a gas, inhaled into the lungs, and transferred via the alveoli to the blood. It is measurable in the central nervous system less than 8 seconds after inhalation. All nicotine products used in the area of smoking cessation are alkaline and therefore absorbed through the skin or mucous membranes. This route is much slower than that by inhalation and does not give the quick plasma concentration that cigarette smoking does. Six hours after a transdermal patch of 21 mg is applied, the blood level is approximately 10–17 ng/mL, in contrast to approximately 15–25 ng/mL within minutes after a cigarette (10).

It is likely that nicotine from cigarettes is more toxic than nicotine delivered from NRT products like patches. The rapid absorption from cigarette smoke results in a transient high blood concentration with a greater biological effect compared with the equivalent dose of nicotine delivered from gums or patches (11). Compared with cigarette smoking, NRT produces lower plasma nicotine levels, i.e., one-third to one-half the levels attained over several hours, and without high peak levels. The slower absorption of nicotine from these products does not produce the same cardiovascular stimulation as does cigarette smoke (12).

The rationale for nicotine substitution is as follows: the administration of nicotine decreases withdrawal symptoms in the first months, allowing the subject to cope with the behavioral and psychological aspects of smoking. Withdrawal symptoms (craving for cigarettes, irritability, anxiety, depression, drowsiness, difficulty concentrating, restlessness, headache, hunger, sleep disturbances) are usually assessed on a 4-point scale (0 = not at all; 1 = mild; 2 = moderate; 3 = severe) (13,14). Withdrawal symptoms often appear 4–8 hours after quitting, peak during the first week (days 3–5), and then gradually decline over the next 2–4 weeks. Nicotine dependence is measured by the Fagerström Test of Nicotine Dependence (FTND) with a possible scoring of 0–10 (most dependent) (Table 2) (15). NRT products are weaned gradually (usually over 2–6 weeks) concomitant with the decrease in withdrawal symptoms. The average 12-month success rate reported in most studies is about 15–25% (16).

Nicotine is the drug of choice to assist smoking cessation. Results reported in a recent meta-analysis of 108 trials indicated that NRT doubled long-term (6–12 months) quit rates (1). The odds ratio for success of nicotine-replacement therapy compared with controls was 1.73 (95% CI 1.62–1.85). The odd ratios for the different nicotine replacement products were 1.66 for gum, 1.76 for patch, 2.27 for nasal spray, 2.08 for inhaler, and 1.73 for sublingual tablet (NS). The nicotine-replacement products described above are self-dosing systems to be used ad libitum, in contrast to the patch, which infuses about 1 mg of nicotine per hour at a constant rate.

The classical relapse curve shows that approximately 50% of smokers having failed within the first 6 weeks after quit day on active drug compared to almost 75% on placebo. This underscores that health care providers should focus on an increase of NRT dose during the first weeks after quit day.

Nicotine Transdermal Patch

The nicotine patch is a fixed nicotine-delivery system, which releases about 1 mg of nicotine per hour for 16 hours (daytime patch) or for 24 hours (24-hour patch). Nicotine substitution is about 50% of the smoking level (21 mg patch/24 h and 15 mg patch/16 h). It is much easier to administer and use the patch than the gum, but it is not possible to self-titrate (17). The recommended treatment duration is 18–12 weeks. In a U.S. multicenter smoking cessation trial examination the effect of 0, 7, 14, and 21 mg nicotine

Table 2 Fagerström Test for Nicotine Dependence

Item	Answers	Score
1. How soon after you wake up do you smoke your first cigarette?	Within 5 min	3
	6–30 min	2
	31–60 min	1
	61–	0
2. Do you find it difficult to refrain from smoking in places where it is forbidden, e.g., in church, at the library, in the cinema, etc.?	Yes	1
	No	0
3. Which cigarette would you hate most to give up?	The first one in the morning	1
	All others	0
4. How many cigarettes per day do you smoke?	1–10	0
	11–20	1
	31 or more	3
5. Do you smoke more frequently during the first hours after waking than during the rest of the day?	Yes	1
	No	0
6. Do you smoke if you are so ill that you are in bed most of the day (or absent from work)?	Yes	1
	No	0
Total score		0–10

Source: Ref. 15.

patches, a dose-response effect of increasing nicotine dosages was reported (18).

Two large placebo-controlled trials comprising 1200 and 1686 smokers have recently been published. These studies were conducted in general practice with minimal behavioral support (19,20). A 1-year success rate of 9.3% in the active patch group versus 5.0% in the placebo patch group was reported in the first study (19), and a 3-month success rate of 14.4% versus 8.6% was reported in the other study (20). Among eight studies examining long-term smoking cessation success, five showed a significant outcome in favor of the nicotine patch (17). The main side effect is mild local skin irritation, occurring in 10–20% of subjects. In 2% of subjects, the patch was terminated due to more persistent and severe skin irritation at the location of the nicotine patch (17).

In the CEASE trial it was found that 8 weeks of full-dose treatment followed by 4 weeks of dose tapering was as effective as 22 weeks, and this is also supported in meta-analyses comparing studies with different treatment durations. The only study comparing different treatment durations in the same group is CEASE (1,6). Wearing the patch during waking hours (approximately 16 hours/day) has been found to be as effective as wearing it for 24 hours/day. Also, there is no evidence that tapered therapy is better than abrupt withdrawal (1). Due to its ease of use, the patch may be the first choice of nicotine-delivery systems today.

While the patch is a fixed-delivery system, the delivered dose from the gum, inhaler, nasal spray, and lozenge is dependent on the frequency of dosing. A basic advantage of these four products is the ability to self-titrate the dose as opposed to the patch, which delivers a fixed dose. Thus, it is possible to administer a dose whenever wanted or needed during the day, while the principal disadvantage is potential underdosing. Also, these products may replace some of the habit patterns associated with smoking (e.g., handling reinforcement) along with providing nicotine replacement.

Nicotine Chewing Gum

Using nicotine gum throughout the day, blood levels of one third (for 2 mg gum) and two thirds (for 4 mg gum) of the nicotine obtained through smoking are achieved (21–23). In most studies gum has been used for at least 6–12 weeks and up to one year. Individualization of treatment duration is recommended. Ten percent of successful quitters will still use the gum after 12 months.

Gum users should chew a piece of gum 5–10 times until they can taste the nicotine, then let the gum rest in the cheek for a few minutes, and then chew again to expose a new surface of the gum. Free nicotine can then be absorbed and reduce side effects due to swallowed nicotine. The gum can be chewed for about 20–30 minutes. About 0.8–1.0 mg of nicotine is absorbed from a piece of 2 mg nicotine gum and 1.2–1.4 mg of nicotine from a 4 mg piece. The approximate dose equivalent for most nicotine patches is approximately 20 pieces of 2 mg gum, whereas the mean number of pieces of gum used daily is only around 5–6 in most studies. Thus, underdosing is a plausible explanation for the lack of efficacy in several studies (24,25).

From these observations it would be logical to attempt to raise the consumed dose either by increasing the number of pieces of gum chewed or by using the higher-dose gum (4 mg). In four comparison studies, the 4 mg gum was superior to the 2 mg gum for short-term outcome. Another way to increase the amount of consumed gum might be to administer the gum in fixed dosage schedules, as shown by Killen et al. (26). The odds ratio for success in trials that directly compared 2 and 4 mg gums in highly dependent smokers found a significantly higher abstinence rate with the 4 mg gum (odds ratio 2.67; 95% CI 1.69–4.22) (1).

Side effects of the gum consist mainly of mild, transient local symptoms in the mouth, throat, and stomach due to swallowed nicotine (e.g., nausea, vomiting, indigestion, and hiccups). After adequate instruction most smokers can learn to use the gum properly. However, without instructions many will discontinue use or underdose themselves. In the Lung Health Study, among 3094 smokers followed for 5 years, use of the 2 mg gum appeared safe and did not produce cardiovascular problems or other adverse events even in subjects who continued to smoke and still use nicotine gum (27).

It is suggested that smokers be instructed to stop smoking completely, use the nicotine gum on a fixed schedule (i.e., every hour, from early morning, for at least 8–10 hours) and use extra pieces of gum whenever needed. The optimal duration of treatment is not known; in most studies the gum has been used for at least 6–12 weeks and up to one year. Individualization of treatment duration is recommended.

Nicotine Inhaler

An inhaler consists of a mouthpiece and a plastic tube with a porous plug impregnated with nicotine, which release nicotine vapor when air is drawn through the plug. Most of the nicotine is absorbed through the mouth and throat. Each inhaler contains 10 mg of nicotine and can release approximately 4–5 mg of nicotine. In clinical use each inhaler releases approximately 2.0–3.0 mg of nicotine, and the number of inhalers used daily averages 5–6. Thus, nicotine levels comparable to those found with use of the 2 mg nicotine gum are attainable (i.e., relatively low concentrations). The mean nicotine substitution based on determinations after 1–2 weeks of therapy was 38–43% of smoking levels (28).

Four controlled trials have been conducted with the nicotine inhaler. The efficacy and safety of the nicotine inhaler were examined in several double-blind, clinical smoking cessation studies (28–30).

The first published study was a 1-year randomized, double-blind, placebo-controlled trial, which enrolled 286 smokers. The success rate for smoking cessation was 15% and 5% at 12 months ($p < 0.001$) for active and placebo, respectively. The mean nicotine substitution based on determinations after 1–2 weeks of therapy was 38–43% of smoking levels. The treatment was well accepted, and no serious adverse events were reported. Three other studies have confirmed the above findings, with odd ratios in favor of active treatment of 1.6, 2.2, and 1.6 (31). The inhaler may replace some of the habit patterns associated with smoking (e.g., oral and handling reinforcement) along with providing nicotine replacement. At least 4 inhalers should be used per day; the optimal number is 4–10 per day, and the duration of use is 3 months, with another 3 months of downtitration if needed. With rapid and frequent puffing it is possible to increase the delivered dose of nicotine. The number of puffs on the inhaler should be around 10 times the usual puffing on a cigarette to get a similar amount of nicotine.

Nicotine Nasal Spray

Nicotine nasal spray (NNS) consists of a multidose, hand-driven pump spray containing a nicotine solution. Each puff contains 0.5 mg of nicotine; thus, a 1 mg dose is delivered if both nostrils are sprayed as recommended. NNS is a strong and rapid means of delivering nicotine into the human body with a pharmacokinetic profile closely approximating cigarettes. After a single dose of 1 mg nicotine, the peak level is reached within 5–10 minutes with average plasma trough levels of 16 ng/mL (32–34). Three published studies with nicotine nasal spray reported 1-year success rates for active NNS versus placebo of 26% versus 10%, 27% versus 15%, and 27% versus 17%, respectively (32–34).

This strong spray induces localized side effects, such as sneezing, nasal secretion and irritation, congestion, watery eyes, and coughing. Up to 5% of subjects rate these side effects as unacceptable; however, most symptoms decrease within a few days after the spray is initiated. Highly nicotine-dependent smokers might be the target group for this delivery mode.

Careful instruction in the use of the NNS should be given and a test dose administered under supervision during the consultation to correct spray use. The NNS should be used for 3 months (it was used up to 1 year in some studies). The dose is 10–40 puffs in each nostril per day.

Nicotine Lozenge (Sublingual Tablet)

This is the latest marketed nicotine administration system. One to two sublingual tablets placed under the tongue will disintegrate within 20–30 minutes, and then the free nicotine will be absorbed through the oral mucous membrane. With regard to delivered dose, the tablet is comparable with the 2 mg nicotine chewing gum. One tablet per hour is the recommended dosage up to 20 per day (i.e., up to 2 tablets per hour). In highly dependent subjects a maximum dose of up to 40 tablets per day can be used. Two trials have been conducted with 247 and 241 smokers, respectively. The 6-month success rates were significantly higher with active treatment than placebo in both trials (33 vs. 18% and 20 vs. 11%; $p < 0.05$), while the 1-year success rate did not reach a statistical significant difference (23 vs. 15% and 17 vs. 10%; NS). Hiccups (13 vs. 0.4%), nausea (17 vs. 5%), and dyspepsia (13 vs. 7%) were observed more often among active than placebo treatments. Local adverse events were gingival bleeding (3.3 vs. 1.6%) and gastritis (5 vs. 2.9%). All adverse events were mild and transient during the first week as with most other nicotine replacement products (35,36).

The tablet should be used up to 3 months. The dose is 8–20 (40) tablets per day or 1–2 tablets per hour depending on withdrawal symptoms and craving.

Combination of NRT Products and Dose-Response Effects

Table 3 contains a summary of the principal differences between the five different NRT products and some suggestions for their use. Side effects are generally mild and related to the local irritative effect of nicotine. Side effects are generally transient, and most reported side effects are acceptable to the user.

A logical question would be whether it is possible to combine several NRT products. Laboratory studies have shown that the combination of nicotine gum and patch might relieve withdrawal symptoms to the same degree as when smoking and more effective than a single NRT (37). Three studies have been published about combining two NRT products. A short-term increase in success has been observed in some, but no statistically significant 12-month increase has been found (38). Thus, although the combination of nicotine patch and gum seems to be safe, there is no strong evidence for an increase in the long-term success rate.

A dose-response effect has been observed with both nicotine gum and the patch. Both 22 and 44 mg patches have been tested with promising results after 4 weeks of treatment (success rates of 45 and 68%, respectively). In two studies the degree of nicotine substitution was compared to outcome, and in both studies higher success rates were found with increasing degree of substitution. In the CEASE study comprising 3575 subjects, a higher success rate was achieved with 25 mg 16-hour patches compared with 15 mg nicotine patches (6).

C. Bupropion

Bupropion (Zyban) is an older antidepressant drug—an amino-ketone agent—with an inhibitory effect on noradrenaline and dopamine reuptake.

Table 3 Recommendations for Use of 5 Different Nicotine-Replacement Products

	Patch	Gum	Inhaler	Nasal spray	Lozenge
Absorption	Skin	Mouth	Mouth, throat	Nasal	Mouth
Principle	Fixed	Ad lib	Ad lib	Ad lib	Ad lib
Daily dose	1 patch, 15–25 mg	1 piece/hr 10–15 mg	6–10, 10–15 mg	2 puff/×40, 10–40 mg	8–20 tablets, 16–40 mg
Dose per piece	15 mg/16 hr 21 mg/24 hr	2 mg/4 mg	10 mg	0.5 mg per puff	2 mg/dose
Duration	3 M*	3 M(12 M)	3 M(6 M)	3 M(12 M)	3 M(6 M)
Side effects	Skin irritation	Hiccups Irritation in mouth Dyspepsia	Irritation in throat	Sneezing Secretion	Irritation in mouth Hiccups Dyspepsia
Precautions	Eczema	Dentures	Pharyngitis	Rhinitis Nose bleeding	Oral disease
Low dependent	+++	+++	+++	−	++
High dependent	+	+++	++	+++	++

*M = months

Some years ago its potential effect as a smoking cessation agent was reported (39). Several placebo-controlled studies with bupropion have been published (40–42).

In the first published study with bupropion, a total of 615 smokers (>14 cigarettes/day) were assigned to receive placebo, 100, 150, and 300 mg of slow-release (SR) bupropion for 7 weeks. Moderately intensive counseling was provided at baseline, weekly for 8 weeks, and at months 2, 6, 12. Eight telephone calls were used monthly from the third month after quit day. Thus, the adjunctive support was considerable. The point prevalence success rate after 1 year was significantly higher for 300 mg bupropion compared with placebo, i.e., 23.1% versus 12.4% ($p = 0.01$). The success rate for 100 mg and 150 mg bupropion was 19.6% and 22.6%, respectively (Table 4). From this study 300 mg bupropion was chosen as the optimal dose for further trials. It is known that with dosage higher than 300 mg the risk for seizures increases. Weight gain was inversely associated with the dose of bupropion. After 1 year the average weight gain was 2.9 kg in the placebos, 2.3 kg in the 100 and 150 mg, and 1.5 kg in the 300 mg dose group ($p = 0.02$). In contrast to other smoking cessation studies this well-respected paper did not report the sustained quit rate in spite of being published in a journal. It is important to remember that "point prevalence" is not comparable with "sustained success rate." From presentations in conference talks the sustained quit rate was approximately 14% for 300 mg bupropion versus 10% for placebo (NS).

In another study, bupropion SR 300 mg was compared with nicotine patch 21 mg for 24 hours, placebo, and the combination of bupropion and

Table 4 Sustained 1-Year Success Rate from 2 Published Placebo-Controlled Trials with Bupropion and Nicotine Patch

| | Subject no. | Success (%) | | | |
		Placebo	Nicotine patch, 21 mg/24 hr	Bupropion 300 mg	Bupropion + nicotine patch
Point prev.	309	12.4	$p < 0.01$	23.1	
Sustained	309	10[a]		14[a]	
Point prev.	894	15.6	NS 16.4, $p < 0.001$	30.3 NS	35.5
Sustained	894	5.6, $p < 0.001$	9.8, $p < 0.001$	18.4 NS	22.5

[a]Estimated success rate from conference discussion.
Source: Refs. 40,41.

nicotine patch. Bupropion was used for 9 weeks and nicotine patches for 8 weeks. A total of 893 smokers (>14 cigarettes/day) from four centers were enrolled. Weekly sessions were scheduled with up to 15 minutes of counseling for 9 weeks followed by visits after 10, 12, 26, and 52 weeks and 8 telephone calls from month 3 on. The sustained quit rate after 1 year was 5.6% (placebo), 9.8% (nicotine patch), 18.4% (bupropion), and 22.5% (bupropion + nicotine patch), respectively (Table 4). The two bupropion groups achieved a higher success rate compared with placebo and nicotine patch.

A meta-analysis of 16 controlled trials reported an odds ratio of 1.97 (95% CI 1.67–2.34) for bupropion versus placebo for 1-year success (43). A sustained success rate of 18–23% is in accordance with the success rates found in many studies with NRT with support in the same range as in the above studies. Further comparative studies are needed before the relative potency of NRT and bupropion can be determined.

In one recent published RCT, bupropion SR was used as relapse prevention in 461 of 784 participants who were abstainers after 7 weeks of bupropion open-label treament (44). Subjects were randomized to bupropion SR or placebo for 45 weeks and followed up to the 2-year timepoint. Weekly point prevalence abstinence and continuous abstinence were consistently greater in the bupropion SR treatment group compared to placebo from randomization through follow-up. However, the differences in continuous abstinence rates between the bupropion SR group and the placebo group, did not reach statistical significance from week 36 through to month 24. Thus, 7 weeks of treatment with bupropion seems an adequate treatment duration for smoking cessation, although longer treatment prolongs time to relapse.

Recycling (i.e., repeated treatment with bupropion in smokers treated previously with bupropion) should be tried, as this increased success rates in a recently published randomized controlled trial (RCT) with 450 smokers, with a 6-month continuous success rate of 12% for the bupropion group and 2% for the placebo group (45). Several large randomized, controlled studies with bupropion are ongoing, and preliminary reports in the form of conference abstracts confirm the above efficacy in smoking cessation.

The most common adverse events from bupropion are insomnia (42%) and dry mouth (11%) (Table 5). Aggravation of hypertension is also reported as well as allergic rash. In approximately 10–12%, the treatment was stopped due to adverse events. The most serious adverse event is seizures, which have been reported in 0.1% of depressed patients treated with bupropion, but not yet reported during treatment for smoking

Table 5 Contraindications for Bupropion

Epilepsy
Excessive use of alcohol
Addiction to opiates, cocaine, stimulants
Abrupt withdrawal from alcohol or other sedatives
Family history of seizure disorder
History of infantile febrile seizures
Severe history of head trauma or prior seizure
Seizure disorders such as epilepsy
Predisposition to seizures (history of brain tumor or stroke)
EEG abnormalities
History or current diagnosis of anorexia nervosa or bulimia
Treatment with theophylline, systemic steroids, other antidepressants,
    antipsychotics, MAO inhibitors (at least 14 days between discontinuation of
    MAO inhibitors and initiation of burpropion), cimetidine, carbamazepine,
    phenobarbital, phenytoin, orphenadine, cyclophosphamide
Pregnancy, nursing mothers
Allergy to bupropion

Source: Modified from Ref. 49.

cessation. Postmarketing reports have been published with several cases of seizures even in subjects with no known disposition to seizures as well as intentional overdose (46–48).

In a prospective 105-site study with 3100 patients with depression treated with bupropion SR 150 mg b.i.d., the cumulative observed seizure rate was 0.08% for the first 8 weeks and 0.15% for both phases combined, which is well within the range observed with other marketed antidepressants (49). If the contraindications for use of bupropion are followed, one of every 1000 treated subjects can expect to experience seizures (Table 6). For that reason, it is important to (a) exclude subjects with an increased risk of seizures, (b) not to increase the dose above 300 mg, and (c) to administer the daily dose divided by an interval of at least 8 hours. The last dose should not be taken later than 6 p.m. to reduce insomnia. Weight gain was significantly lower during the drug treatment period for the bupropion group, but after week 7 there was no significant difference in weight change between groups.

In summary, bupropion SR is as least as efficacious as NRT and generally well tolerated in smoking cessation. It is regarded as first-line medication in some guidelines (16). As bupropion has a more severe side effect profile, more contraindications, and is only available by prescription, the author regards NRT as first-line medication and

Table 6 Side Effects from Bupropion Used in Smoking Cessation

Side effect	Percentage	
	Bupropion ($n = 399$)	Placebo ($n = 312$)
Insomnia	39	20
Dry mouth	12	5
Worsening hypertension	1	<1
Discontinuation of drug	12	8
Urticaria	2	0
Seizure	0.1[a]	0

[a]Not observed in any of the smoking-cessation studies.
Source: Refs. 40,41, and drug-prescribing information from Zyban®.

bupropion as a second-line drug. This is a matter of personal judgment, and some physicians will use bupropion as a first-line medication. Because another antidepressant, nortriptyline, has been shown effective in smoking cessation, it is not clear if the effect on smoking cessation of these two agents is drug specific or a class effect. On the other hand, several other antidepressants have not been found to be effective in smoking cessation (e.g., doxepin, fluoxetine, sertraline, moclobemide, and venlafaxine) (43).

D. Weight Gain

Weight gain can be regarded as a withdrawal symptom due to increased hunger and increased caloric intake. But the low and flat nicotine levels produced by NRT are only able to partially prevent a decrease in metabolic rate after cessation of cigarette use. A weight gain of 4–5 kg for abstainers after 1 year is found in most studies. About half of the participants are afraid of gaining weight, and it may be a more prominent problem for females. Both NRT, especially nicotine gum, and bupropion SR can reduce postcessation weight gain to 2–3 kg. However, when NRT or bupropion is stopped, the ex-smoker ends up with a weight gain similar to that of quitters who had not used medication (16).

In the Lung Health Study, sustained quitters gained 5.2 kg (women) and 4.9 kg (men) in year 1 and another 3.4 kg (women) and 2.6 kg (men) in years 1–5. Over 5 years, 33% of the abstainers gained 10 kg (50). Weight gain prevention using caffeine plus ephedrine or a serotonergic anorexic drug, diphenfluramine, did not increase the success rate (51).

Diet intervention and daily exercise might be an effective way to control excessive weight gain in the long term.

E. Harm Reduction

This new concept needs close investigation. It could be applied to smokers not able to quit or not motivated to quit completely (i.e., recalcitrant smokers). The concept is that a reduction in the number of daily cigarettes maintained by sustained use of NRT or bupropion SR will reduce the health risks from smoking (52). The following questions arise from this approach: Is it possible to maintain, say, a 50% reduction in number of daily smoked cigarettes for more than 2–3 months? How much compensation will occur over time (i.e., higher inhalation of toxic substances per cigarette smoked)? Could the motivation to quit be increased by this approach? Would the concept interfere with ordinary smoking cessation and confuse the important message about complete cessation in the first week to attain long-term success? Is this a cost-effective approach, i.e., would the cost per saved life be higher than with ordinary smoking cessation?

Only one RCT is published enrolling smokers not motivated to quit smoking but to reduce. This study comprised 400 smokers who used nicotine or placebo inhalers for 1 year. They reported a low but significant sustained reduction (defined as smoking fewer than 50% of the cigarettes smoked at baseline) after 2 years (active 9.5% vs. placebo 3%) (53). There was no statistically significant difference in point prevalence abstinence between active and placebo group beyond month 4. Nevertheless, almost 10% of subjects were smoke-free after 2 years. In another study with nicotine gum, we found a smoking cessation rate of approximately 10% after 2 years and a low reduction rate of 6% (54). There is no consistent evidence that smoking reduction per se will be followed by harm reduction. In a prospective population study, self-reported smoking reduction was not associated with lower risk of hospital admission for COPD, while quitting smoking was associated with a relative hazard of 0.57 for hospitalization (55). In the same population with a 16-year follow-up, it was observed that smoking cessation reduces mortality and morbidity risk while smoking reduction did not (56).

COPD smokers not motivated to quit should be prescribed NRT—nicotine gum or inhaler—for 1 year and recommended to reduce the number of cigarettes by at least 50% during the first 1–2 weeks and then try to reduce further, although this concept has only been tested in healthy smokers.

Several ongoing studies will clarify the utility of smoking reduction. Without long-term NRT or bupropion it is most unlikely that a permanent reduction can be maintained. From two published studies, it seems that by applying this concept to smokers with low motivation to quit, around 10% will eventually quit smoking. This is a surprising but promising aspect.

F. Verifying Abstinence with Carbon Monoxide

Smokers have elevated levels of carbon monoxide (CO) in the blood and expiratory air, while subjects using smokeless tobacco and/or NRT have levels indicative of nonsmoking. The plasma half-life of CO is about 4–6 hours. The CO level in expired air is 1–4 ppm in most nonsmokers compared to 10–20 ppm in regular smokers with an increase in CO levels concomitant with increasing cigarette consumption. By exposure to environmental tobacco smoke (ETS), nonsmokers can attain expiratory CO levels of 6–9 ppm (57). The cut-off between nonsmokers and smokers in most smoking cessation studies is 9–10 ppm.

The correlation between arterial blood CO levels and expiratory air CO levels are high, but in more severe COPD patients with decreased diffusion capacity, expiratory air CO might underestimate the blood levels. In light smokers smoking 3–6 cigarettes daily, CO levels might be 10 ppm (420 mmol/L). Thus, the discriminative power of CO is less in light smokers, who might present with CO levels of 6–9 ppm. Plasma or saliva nicotine or cotinine levels might then be used for categorization in smokers and nonsmokers, but only in subjects not using NRT.

The CO analyzer is a relatively simple, inexpensive, and quick method to assess the CO level in expiratory air. It is important to hold the breath for 15–20 seconds to attain an equilibrium between capillary CO and alveolar CO levels. The result is displayed immediately. False-positive values might be observed in subjects with lactose malabsorption. Although an ethanol filter is present, high concentrations in the breath might interfere with measurements. Drifting of the zero-point might be observed if many smokers are tested consecutively. Calibration of the CO analyzer is indicated every 4–6 months with a 50 ppm CO test gas. Without CO monitoring up to 10% of failures might state that they do not smoke.

A portable CO analyzer (Bedfont Monitor, Bedfont Technical Instruments, Sittingbourne, United Kingdom) should be available at every hospital unit. Because quitting smoking is one of the only factors to influence the decline of lung function in a positive way in COPD, it would be common sense to include assessment of CO for all COPD patients at admittance to the hospital. Whenever an arterial blood sample is obtained in COPD patients in LTOT (Long Term Oxygen Treatment), the CO level should also be examined to identify smokers and encourage them to stop smoking.

The baseline expiratory air CO level in the CEASE study was 27 ppm (mean) (SD 10 ppm) in 3575 smokers from 37 centers in Europe with a mean consumption of 27 cigarettes/day (SD 10), all smokers using >14 cigarettes/day (6). In 550 consecutive patients with COPD and 100 patients on LTOT in Italy, arterial carboxyhemoglobin was >2% (= 10 ppm) in 25.8% of the 550 COPD patients and in 21% of the patients on LTOT indicative of smoking (58).

IV. Smoking Cessation in Patients with Special Attention to COPD

The short-term quit rate for patients hospitalized for acute myocardial infarction is very high, but the one-year outcome is often below 50% (59). In a prospective study in 63 smokers hospitalized with myocardial infarction or angina pectoris, we found a 6- and 12-month quit rate of 20.7% and 15.5%, respectively (60). The high initial quit rate is not surprising, as myocardial infarction is often a dramatic event accompanied by fear. In comparison, the acute hospitalization of patients with COPD might also be quite dramatic and thus an opportunity for smoking cessation. With nurse-conducted follow-up by phone it is possible to maintain the high quit rate for 12 months (61% success rate), while a substantial relapse was observed in a control group (32% success rate) without follow-up in a well-conducted study with 173 patients with acute myocardial infarction (61). This very effective intervention consisted of nurse-managed relapse prevention initiated in the hospital followed by telephone contacts weekly for 3 weeks and then monthly for the next 4 months. The patients received a booklet and audiotapes. When indicated, nicotine gum was prescribed. A total of 3.5 hours were spent on the intervention per patient. Patients who expressed low motivation to quit and subjects who resumed smoking in the first 3 weeks after the acute event had a low probability to have stopped smoking after 1 year.

In ambulatory patients with cardiovascular disease, a much lower success rate has been found, and the efficacy of nicotine patches has been evaluated in two randomized trials. In a large multicenter trial enrolling 584 male patients with different cardiovascular diseases, the 14-week success rate was 21% for nicotine patch versus 9% for placebo, but after 6 months the difference was not statistically different. In the other trial 156 patients with coronary artery disease received nicotine patch or placebo for 5 weeks, and the 5-week abstinence rate was 36% versus 22% ($p < 0.05$). In conclusion, these two trials showed that the use of the nicotine patch in this group of males with cardiovascular disease appeared safe, with an increase in short-term outcome but not in long-term success. The success rate was also much lower than that reported after acute myocardial infarction (62–64).

The goal is that all smokers admitted to hospital be identified, advised to stop smoking, and offered a smoking cessation program. Why is contact with a hospital such an excellent opportunity for smoking cessation? First, 51–79% of hospitalized smokers remain abstinent throughout their hospital stay, even without hospital policies restricting smoking (65). Second, in one survey, 79% of hospitalized smokers for medical illness expressed a desire to stop smoking (63). Third, brief intervention for inpatient smokers has produced high and clinically important long-term quit rates of 25–70% (67). The efficacy of inpatient smoking cessation programs versus none from five studies was reported in the AHCPR (the Agency for Health Care Policy and Research, U.S. Department of Health and Human Services) guideline paper with an estimated odds ratio of 1.4 (1.1–1.7) or an estimated cessation rate of 23% (19–29) versus 18% (10–28). Thus, admittance to the hospital is a window of opportunity for smoking cessation as many smokers are motivated to quit tobacco and because cessation programs are cost-effective.

A. Systematic Identification of Smokers

The AHCPR Guidelines suggest that every medical setting should implement a smoker-identification system. Meta-analysis of nine studies showed that estimated intervention rate by clinicians with their patients who smoke increased from 39 to 66% (95% CI) with a screening system in place to identify smoking status. The impact of an identification system versus none ($n = 3$ studies) reported an estimated cessation rate of 6.4% (1.3–11.6) vs. 3.1% (NS), based on a small number of studies (13). The identification system should be included in the vital signs in the patient records (preprinted, a vital signs stamp, preprinted progress notepaper) or be included in the computerized records (Table 7). Actual smoking status should be recorded: i.e., smoker, ex-smoker, never-smoker, age when started to smoke, average number of cigarettes smoked daily, estimated pack-years (number of cigarettes per day × years smoked/20 = pack-years), and quit date. The quit date is important, as many patients might have stopped smoking shortly before referral (hours to days) and thus should be offered relapse prevention. The inclusion of smoking status as vital signs might get the clinician more interested and involved in smoking cessation. This is important, as a physician's strong advice to a patient who smokes to quit has been shown to increase cessation rate from 7.9 to 10.2% (8.5–12.0) with an estimated odds ratio of 1.3 (1.1–1.6) in a meta-analysis of seven studies, while insufficient data exist to assess the efficacy of advice to quit by

Table 7 Intervention for Hospitalized Smoking COPD Patients

Identification of smokers:	*Ask*: Do you smoke?
	Examine patient for smell of tobacco/yellow nails/fingers
	Assess: Carbon monoxide in expired air; if >10 ppm = a smoker
	Document smoking status in patient records
Intervention:	Physician: *Advise* all smokers to quit (clear, strong, and personalized)
	Referral to a smoking-cessation program: use stickers in patient chart to increase percentage of referrals or computer reminders
	Provide *assistance* with NRT whenever indicated
	Implement smoke-free units/smoke-free hospitals
Follow-up:	List smoking as a discharge diagnosis and note "advise to quit"
	Arrange phone calls to patients within first month after quitting
	Request patient's G.P. to *arrange* follow-up and support for smoking cessation/relapse prevention
	Provide smoking-cessation intervention when patient attends outpatient clinic (measure CO)
Quality control:	Perform audits: At regular intervals (at least yearly) calculate percentage of smokers identified/smokers referred to treatment/ "smoking" as a discharge diagnosis/patients with CO assessed/percentage smoking cessation counselors on staff

Source: Modified from Ref. 16.

nonphysician clinicians. Thus, all clinicians should advise patients to stop smoking, as it is reasonable to believe that such advice is effective.

Effective alternatives are to place tobacco-use reminders on all patient charts. In a 27-bed inpatient unit receiving acute cardiopulmonary patients, posted memos reminded the nurses to refer smokers for a 4-week period followed by stickers in all patient charts for 4 weeks and then posted memos for 4 weeks. The referral rate to a smoking-cessation program was 1 of 29 (3.4%), 18 of 52 (34.6%), and 1 of 47 (2.1%) smokers, respectively, in the three periods above. This system seems to be a simple, low-cost strategy to identify and refer smokers to a cessation program, but it is in fact alarming how few patients are offered treatment even with this method (68). In the next few years, more and more records will be computerized, and smoking status should be incorporated as well as reminder systems. It will then be much easier to perform quality-assurance control and continuously monitor the degree of implementation.

A meta-analysis of 55 studies showed multiple sessions to increase cessation rates compared with one session (AHCPR), i.e., estimated cessation rates of 10% for one session versus 19% for two to three sessions. Thus, at least one follow-up should be arranged after discharge as either a telephone call or a clinic visit. Many patients are seen at the outpatient clinic 1–2 months after discharge, and this is an excellent opportunity for follow-up on smoking (16).

To increase the rate of implementation of smoking cessation in patients with COPD, including this in the quality control of COPD care might be helpful. When assessing the degree of smoking intervention in the different hospital units, this might motivate the staff to intervene more in this area.

B. Older Smoking Cessation Studies in Patients with Pulmonary Diseases

Ten studies of smoking cessation among patients with pulmonary diseases were published between 1969 and 1983 enrolling a total of 1021 patients, varying from 35 to 308 subjects with a success rate of 12.5–51% (mean 30%) after 3 months up to 5 years (69). However, these studies did not fulfill the criteria for randomized controlled studies today, as most of these older studies had no control group or no biochemical verification of abstinence. In most studies "physician advice" to stop smoking was the main intervention. In a chest clinic ($n = 204$), Williams in 1969 reported a 6-month quit rate of 23% (70), and in another study among 308 newly diagnosed pulmonary patients, a 6-month quit rate of 13% was found (71).

C. Hospitalized Smokers

Surprisingly few randomized controlled studies about smoking cessation for COPD patients have been published. Campell et al. (72) enrolled 219 hospital patients with smoking-related disease—50% with lung disease—in a placebo-controlled trial with nicotine chewing gum up to 3 months with follow-up sessions after 2, 3, and 5 weeks and 3 and 6 months. Success was defined as CO-verified nonsmoking at 6 and 12 months. No difference was found between active and placebo gum in success, i.e., 20% and 20%, respectively. The quit rate was lower for patients with lung disease (13%) compared with subjects with heart disease (32%) (Table 8). The 13% quit rate in patients with respiratory disease is the same as the quit rate of 13% for outpatients with COPD in the British Thoracic Society (BTS) second study.

Table 8   One-Year Success in Hospital Patients with Nicotine Gum[a]

	Success 6 + 12 months (%)	
	Placebo gum	Nicotine gum
Lung disease ($n = 111$)	11	15
Heart disease ($n = 85$)	34	29

[a]$n = 219$.
Source: Data from Ref. 72.

In a study among 185 hospital inpatients motivated to quit with a wide range of diagnoses, three conditions were compared: physician advice only (2–3 min), counseling plus nicotine patch, and counseling plus placebo patch for 6 weeks and phone follow-up at weeks 1, 3, 6, and 24. The 6-month abstinence rates (point prevalence) were 4.9, 6.5 and 9.7% (NS), respectively. The use of nicotine patches appeared to be safe, but the dose was reduced from 22 to 11 mg per 24 hours after 3 weeks, which might have been too low a dose. There was a trend toward higher success rate in the nicotine patch group, although not statistically significant, which might be due to lack of power due to the small sample size (73). Patients with respiratory disease were more likely to quit than patients with other diagnoses. However, only 13 patients with respiratory disease were enrolled, and this small sample lacked statistical power.

In a small study, 74 inpatients with COPD received advice to quit versus advice, a self-help manual, and 3–8 counseling sessions. The success rate after 6 months was 21.4% for advice only versus 33.3% for intervention (NS). This sample was too small to give any valid information about efficacy.

Because of the above disappointing findings, we need a large placebo, controlled trial among inpatients with COPD to evaluate if NRT has any relevant efficacy in this patient group.

In a large randomized trial, admitted patients from four hospitals were allocated to (a) usual care (i.e., physician advice to quit smoking plus a booklet), (b) minimal intervention, consisting of physician advice, a 30-minute nurse-mediated bedside smoking intervention, a 16-minute video, a contract, NRT when indicated, and a single 10-minute phone call 2 days after discharge, and (c) intensive intervention, with an extra four phone calls after 2, 7, 21, and 90 days. NRT was used when indicated.

The 12-month point prevalence was 27, 22, and 20% for the intensive, minimal, and usual care groups, respectively ($p < 0.01$ for intensive vs. usual care) (Table 9) (67). Subjects who used NRT (35%) had a lower success rate than nonusers, perhaps due to self-selection bias, as they seemed

Table 9 One-Year Point Prevalence Quit Rates Among Different Diagnoses for Hospitalized Patients

Diagnosis group	No. of patients	Intensive	Minimal	Usual care
All diagnoses (sum)	1942	27[*a]	22	20[*]
Pulmonary disorders	226	25	37	35
Cardiovascular disease	630	34[*b]	28	24[*]
Other internal medicine	536	27[*c]	19	15[*]

[*]Odds ratio and 95% CI for intensive vs. usual care: 1.4 (1.1–1.8),[a] 1.6 (1.1–2.5),[b] and 2.0 (1.2–3.4).[c]
Source: Data from Ref. 67.

to be more nicotine addicted (i.e., higher FTQ scores and smoked more cigarettes). Also, NRT prescription did not follow a randomized design. The cessation rate was high for the 226 patients with pulmonary diseases, with no significant effect of intervention, in contrast to patients with other medical diagnoses, such patients with cardiovascular diseases (Table 9). Overall, this model consisting of strong physician advice at bedside plus nurse-mediated bedside counseling and telephone follow-up proved very effective. However, no effect of the intervention was found for patients with pulmonary disorders.

In a study comprising 185 in-hospital smoking patients, three conditions were used: physician advice, counseling both bedside and via telephone plus nicotine patch for 6 weeks, and counseling plus placebo patch (74). The success rate after 6 months was not statistically significant among the three groups (4.9% vs. 6.5% vs. 9.7%, respectively). However, patients with respiratory attained a higher quit rate than patients with other diagnoses (75). In another well-conducted randomized, placebo-controlled study, 234 hospitalized and ambulatory patients (75% with COPD) were allocated to nicotine patch for 12 weeks or placebo plus 4 visits of 15–30 minutes duration during the first 12 weeks after quit day. The 1-year success rate was 21% versus 14% (NS), an increase of 50% in relative terms. Although this finding was not statistically significant, this study would call for the conductance of a larger study with greater power to examine if this result was due to chance.

In another study, all hospitalized smokers were enrolled in a smoking-cessation study regardless of motivation to quit. In total, 1119 patients were allocated to either usual-care blinded for the staff or intervention consisting of counseling for 20 minutes by smoking counselors, a 12-minute videotape, two phone calls 1 and 2–3 weeks after the quit day, and 6 letters every second week and nicotine gum (76). The sustained quit rate after 12 months was 9.2% versus 13.5% ($p = 0.023$), not biochemically verified. The study population contained 95 (8%) patients with pulmonary disease, but the quit rate was not calculated across diagnoses. Although there was an effect of intervention in this study, the results from this trial cannot be generalized to the population of acute hospitalized COPD patients.

A meta-analysis of 17 trials of smoking-cessation interventions for hospitalized patients showed that "intensive intervention," i.e., inpatient contact plus follow-up for at least a month, was associated with higher quit rates than in controls (odds ratio 1.82; 95% CI 1.49–2.22; six trials). Results of NRT treatment in this group of patients were compatible with data from other trials, suggesting that NRT increases quit rates (77).

D. Ambulatory Patients

The first BTS study comprised 1618 outpatients with respiratory disease attending a chest clinic. Four methods were evaluated: physician advice, plus a booklet, plus placebo gum, and plus 2 mg nicotine chewing gum. For all treatment groups, follow-ups were scheduled after 1, 3, 6, and 12 months. The overall 1-year success rate was 9.7% (95% CI 8.3–11.3%) with no significant difference between the four treatment groups, i.e., no effect of nicotine chewing gum.

Of the patients claiming to be nonsmokers at 6 and 12 months, 27 and 25%, respectively, had CO and thiocyanate levels suggestive of smoking (Table 10) (78).

The British Thoracic Society's second smoking cessation study consisted of two multicenter trials with patients attending hospital or chest clinics (79). A total of 87% of the enrolled patients suffered from respiratory disease, mainly chronic bronchitis and emphysema.

In Study A, the effect of the physician's advice to stop smoking was compared with the same advice plus a signed agreement to stop smoking by a target quit day plus two visits by a health visitor plus several letters. These two interventions were found to be equally effective (Table 11). In Study B,

Table 10 One-Year Outcome of Physician Advice: BTS Study I[a]

	Physician advice	Physician advice + booklet	Physician advice + placebo gum	Physician advice + nicotine gum
Success 6 + 12 months	8.9%	8.5%	11.4%	9.8%

[a]$n = 1550$.
Source: Ref. 78.

Table 11 One-year Outcome of Physician Advice and Letters: BTS Study II

Study A ($n = 1462$)			
	Physician advice	Physician advice +signed agreement, letters week 1, month 2,3,5,9 2 health visitor contacts	
Success 12 months:	7.0%	9.0%	($p = 0.17$)
Study B ($n = 1392$)			
	Physician advice + signed agreement	Physician advice +signed agreement +6 letters	
Success 12 months:	5.1%	8.7%	($p = 0.011$)

Secondary stratification[a] Study A + B ($n = 2854$)			
	Physician advice	Intervention	Outpatient visits
Success 12 months:	5%	9%	None
	9%	13%	One or more

[a]Estimates of effects of intervention and outpatient visits on cessation rate.
Source: Data from Ref. 79.

four groups were compared: physician advice vs. advice plus a signed agreement vs. advice plus letters vs. advice plus letters plus a signed agreement. Signed agreement did not effect outcome, while letters increased outcome from 5.1 to 8.7%. A secondary stratification and analysis of the two studies combined found that 5% would stop by advice alone and that postal encouragement would increase the success rate by more than half as much again. Also, outpatient visits seemed to increase the success rate (Table 11). In conclusion, physician advice supported by encouraging letters was found to be more effective than advice alone in a group of outpatients with respiratory disease, although the overall success rate of 13% might seem low. This group of smokers might be a group of committed smokers, because less heavily committed smokers would probably have stopped smoking at an earlier stage of their disease. This is supported by a retrospective study in 107 COPD patients referred for pulmonary rehabilitation (80). Most (67%) were ex-smokers at the time of hospital admission, which is in accordance with another study reporting a rate of 76% (81). A prediction that all COPD patients would stop smoking would be accurate in two out of three cases, while psychosocial factors and pack-years were of no benefit in identifying smokers who quit following hospitalization.

E. Newer Studies in COPD

The Lung Health Study was a multicenter randomized study of smoking intervention versus usual care also testing an inhaled anticholinergic bronochodilator enrolling a total of 5887 subjects. The subjects suffered from mild to moderate airway obstruction. They had a mean age of 48 years, with a smoking history of 40 pack-years. Five years of follow-up was scheduled (82). Initially, an intensive 12-session smoking-cessation program was planned with the use of nicotine chewing gum plus adjunct behavioral modification with a relapse-prevention program every 4 months during the 5 years. At entry, strong physician advice to quit was given, and a target quit day was set. Nicotine gum was used aggressively. The mean FEV_1 was 2.7 L (SD 0.6 L), i.e., 75% of predicted normal.

The sustained quit rate was high in the intervention group and declined as usual over the study period, from 35% after 1 year to 22% after 5 years compared with 10% after 1 year and 5% after 5 years in the usual-care group (Table 12). The cross-sectional quit rate increased slightly during the 5 years to 39% in the intervention group and 22% in the usual-care group. The other important finding was that smoking cessation significantly reduced the age-related decline in FEV_1.

Overall, this large well-conducted study showed that aggressive and intensive smoking-cessation programs can produce high long-term quit rates in smokers with mild airway obstruction. Also, the effect on the decline of FEV_1 supports that smoking cessation is the first and most important intervention in smokers with mild "subclincal COPD." Because nicotine gum was not administered in a randomized way, it is not possible to judge its efficacy separately in this study.

Table 12 Smoking Cessation Rates in Lung Health Study ($n = 5887$)

	Cessation rate (%)				
	1 year	2 year	3 year	4 year	5 year
Sustained abstinence rates					
SI	35	28	25	23	22
UC	9	7	7	6	5
Cross-sectional success rates					
SI	35	34	36	37	38
UC	9	12	15	18	22

SI: smoking intervention; UC: usual care.
Source: Data modified from Ref. 82.

In a hospital chest unit, 74 smoking inpatients with COPD were randomized to usual care, i.e., physician advice to quit, versus intervention, i.e., 3–8 counseling sessions of 15–20 minutes every second day when hospitalized. The 6-month point prevalence quit rate was 33 vs. 21% (NS), perhaps due to lack of statistical power (83). In 49 severe COPD patients, daily home visits for 85 days were combined with different motivational methods. The quit rate after 6 months was only 14% (84). The motivational aspect might be of major importance in smoking COPD patients, and further studies in this field should be encouraged.

Overall, there is no evidence from these trials that NRT increase success rate in patients with moderate or severe COPD (Table 13). In the Lung Health Study an effect of nicotine gum was observed, although nicotine gum was administered in a nonrandomized design. Given the

Table 13 Success Rates from Smoking Cessation Studies in COPD Patients

Number of pts.	Sustained success (%)		p-Value	Ref.
	Intervention	Control/usual care		
	Hospitalized patients			
111	15 (+NRT/placebo)	11	NS	72
234	21 (+NRT/placebo)	14	NS	75
1402[a]	14 (+NRT)	13	NS	67
1482[b]	19 (+NRT)	13	<0.01	67
74[cd]	33	21	NS	83
185[d]	6.5 (+Placebo)	4.9	NS	73
185[d]	9.7 (+NRT)	4.9	NS	73
	Ambulatory patients			
1550	9.8 (+NRT/placebo)	8.9	NS	78
1462	9.0	7.0	NS	79
1392	8.7	5.1	<0.01	79
5817	28 (+NRT)	7	<0.001	82
49[d]	14 (+NRT)	14	NS	84
1119 (95 pulm. dis.)	13.5	9.2	<0.05	76
507	3.1	1.2	NS	85
446	5.6 (+NRT/placebo[e])	1.8	<0.01	86
404	10%	8%	NS	87

[a]Low intervention.
[b]High intervention.
[c]Point prevalence
[d]6-month success rate.
[e]5 mg nicotine patch used as placebo.

importance of smoking cessation in this patient population, we should perform larger well-designed studies with NRT in COPD. Until scientific evidence for the efficacy of NRT in COPD patients is available, NRT should be used whenever it is indicated. This is based on the massive documentation of efficacy of NRT in healthy smokers.

Is it possible to perform smoking cessation in chest clinics by recruitment of healthy smokers? A multicenter, multinational study with 37 centers in 17 European countries enrolled 3575 healthy smokers (>14 cigarettes/day). Two doses of nicotine patch were used as well as two treatment durations: 25 mg/16 hours and 15 mg/16 hours and 8 and 22 weeks of treatment, respectively. The subjects were seen at clinic visits 9 times, at weeks 0, 1, 2, 4, 8, 12, 22, 26, and 52, respectively. The time used at each visit per subject was approximately 15–20 minutes. The 1-year sustained success rate was 16% for the 25 mg group, 13% for the 15 mg group, and 10% for the placebo group, respectively ($p < 0.05$). There was no difference in success rate between short and long treatment duration (Table 14) (6).

We have tried to implement smoking cessation as routine in our lung clinic based on the following study. We enrolled light smokers (<10 cigarettes/day) and smokers (>10 cigarettes/day) not interested in participating in a formal smoking cessation program. The lung clinic nurses applied minimal intervention consisting of nurse advice to quit of 5 minutes duration, CO assessment, an informational booklet, and an encouraging letter after 4–6 weeks. The control group was asked a few questions about smoking and had a CO assessment. The 1-year point prevalence of abstinence was 8.7% versus 3.6% ($p = 0.025$), while the sustained success rate was 3.1% versus 1.2% (NS) (85).

In another part of this study, smokers (>10 cigarettes/day) were enrolled in a RCT with NRT. We compared four different nicotine regimens

Table 14 Sustained Success Rate % for 3575 Smokers in CEASE Trial for 3 Treatment Groups

	Success rate (%)		
	25 mg nicotine patch ($n = 1430$)	15 mg nicotine patch ($n = 1431$)	Placebo ($n = 714$)
2 weeks	74	68	50
3 months	32	25	21
1 year	16	13	10

Source: Data from Ref. 6.

in this open randomized trial in daily routine in a lung clinic. The 446 subjects were referred to a lung clinic by their physicians for routine chest x-ray, lung function testing, or evaluation of COPD. Smokers were allocated to a nurse-conducted smoking cessation program with follow-up visits after 2 and 6 weeks and 3, 6, 9, and 12 months. The 12-month sustained success rate was 1.8% for the 5 mg nicotine patch group (placebo), 8.7% for 15 mg nicotine patch group, 5.1% for the nicotine inhaler group, and 3.5% for the nicotine inhaler plus 15 mg nicotine patch group, and for the sum of the three active treatments 5.6% ($p < 0.01$) (Table 13) (86).

An 11-center RCT with bupropion SR in 464 COPD patients has recently been published (87). Mild to moderate COPD patients with a mean consumption of 28 cigarettes per day were allocated to either bupropion SR 300 mg or placebo for 12 weeks with weekly visits. The sustained success rate was 16% for bupropion and 9% for placebo after 6 months ($p < 0.05$). Bupropion SR doubled absolute smoking abstinence rates, although the absolute success rate were somewhat lower in this COPD population. Bupropion was relatively well tolerated; 5 had to stop medication due to anxiety and 4 due to insomnia. After 1 year the significance was lost, with a success rate of 10% versus 8%, which is much lower compared to similar studies with bupropion in healthy subjects (88).

Table 15 Pulmonary Unit Requirements

Item	Comment
CO analyzer	Test every patient
	Calibrations with CO test gas 50 ppm
FTND	Should be completed by every smoker
Booklets	To different target groups
NRT	Knowledge about patch, gum, inhaler, tablet, nasal spray
Bupropion	Knowledge about dose, duration, and contraindications
Smoking-cessation counselor	Continue to educate counselors as staff change
Multicomponent program	Physician advice, counseling, NRT, follow-up (i.e., phone, letter, clinic visits, etc.)
Teaching	Regular teaching of all staff members about smoking cessation
Audit	Regularly in patient records, questionnaires to patients

One staff member should be appointed as responsible for smoking-cessation program including practical aspects.

In a Cochrane meta-analysis, five studies in COPD patients were included, two of which were of high quality (82,87). It was concluded that a combination of psychosocial and pharmacological intervention was superior to no treatment or psychosocial therapy alone (89).

V. Implementation of Smoking Cessation

How can we implement this important knowledge in our clinical work? First, we must change our institutions (i.e., hospital in- and outpatient clinics and units) to offer smoking cessation programs. We should take the leading role as pulmonary physicians because so many of our patients suffer from smoking-related disease. Certain requirements should be fulfilled in each clinic unit (Table 15). Second, we must train our health care workers and clinicians about smoking cessation and convince them of the importance of this topic. A smoking cessation program is shown in Table 16, with

Table 16 COPD and Smoking Cessation

1. A smoking cessation program should be included in all rehabilitation programs.
2. Identify all smokers: use carbon monoxide measurement for monitoring.
3. Consider nicotine substitution or bupropion (both first-line drugs in COPD):

≥ 10 *cigarettes daily*	<10 *cigarettes daily*
NRT: Nicotine patches	NRT: Nicotine patches
Dose: 15 mg/16 hr or 21 mg/24 hr	10 mg/16 hr or 14 mg/24 hr
Patients who have not smoked for the last days: 10 mg/16 hr or 14 mg/24 hr for 2 days, then dose as mentioned above	
Duration: 8(–12) weeks	
Nicotine chewing gum	Nicotine gum
Dose: 2 mg, 5–15 pieces daily	2 mg, 5–10 pieces daily
Duration: 12–24 weeks	
Nicotine inhaler	Nicotine inhaler
Dose: 10 mg, 4–10 containers/day	10 mg, 1–5 daily
Duration: 12–24 weeks	
Nicotine lozenges: 12–24 weeks	
Dose: 10–20 tablets, 2 mg/day	
Bupropion SR: no contraindication	(Bupropion SR: second-line)
150 mg daily in 7 days, then 150 mg b.i.d. for 12 weeks	

4. Alternatively, consider smokeless tobacco in the recalcitrant smoker.
5. Arrange follow-up (telephone, mail, and clinic visit).

suggestions for the use of NRT in the individual smoking COPD patient. Bupropion has been tested and found efficacious in COPD patients. Thirdly, stopping smoking is the single most important way of affecting outcome in patients at all stages of COPD. The program used in the Lung Health Study with an intensive initial smoking-cessation program with NRT, followed by boosters during subsequent visits, seems to be a design with a high sustained quit rate.

Clinical guidelines for smoking cessation with a special focus on COPD and patients with other pulmonary diseases should be worked out. Such guidelines might be a necessary step to incorporate the above knowledge about smoking cessation into daily clinical practice. Today, we have effective treatment tools, including specific pharmacotherapy, to interfere with smoking. These treatments are very cost-effective, and with regard to COPD, smoking cessation is the only intervention to improve survival and decrease the decline in lung function.

References

1. Silagy C, Mant D, Fowler G, Lancaster T. Nicotine replacement therapy for smoking cessation (Cochrane review). In: The Cochrane Library, 3, 2001. Oxford: Update Software.
2. Fletcher C, Peto R. The natural history of chronic airflow obstruction. Br Med J 1977; 1:1645–1648.
3. Fletcher C, Peto R, Tinker C, Speizer FE. The natural history of chronic bronchitis and emphysema. Oxford, Oxford University Press, 1976.
4. Raw M, McNeil A, West R. Smoking cessation guidelines for health professionals. A guide to effective smoking cessation intervention for the health care system. Thorax 1998; 53(suppl 5):S1–S38.
5. Prochaska JO, Goldstein MG: Process of smoking cessation. Implications for clinicans. Clin Chest Med 1991; 12:727–735.
6. Tønnesen P, Paoletti P, Gustavsson G, Russell MA, Sarracci R, Gulsvik A, Rijcken B, Säwe U, members of the steering committee of CEASE on behalf of the European Respiratory Society. Higher dosage nicotine patches increase one-year smoking cessation rates: results from the European CEASE trial. Eur Respir J 1999; 13:238–246.
7. Yudkin PL, Jones L, Lancaster T, Fowler GH. Which smokers are helped to give up smoking using transdermal nicotine patches? Results from a randomized, double-blind, placebo-controlled trial. Br J Gen Pract 1996; 46:145–148.
8. Stapleton JA, Russell MAH, Feyerabend C, Wiseman SM, Gustavsson G, Säwe U, Wiseman D. Dose effects and predictors of outcome in a randomized trial of nicotine patches in general practice. Addiction 1995; 90(1):31–42.
9. Kajser L, Berglund B. Effects of nicotine on coronary blood-flow in man. Clin. Physiol. 1985; 5:541–552.

10. Palme KJ, Brickley MM, Faulds D. Transdermal nicotine. A review of its pharmacodynamic and pharmacokinetic properties and therapeutic efficacy as an aid to smoking cessation. Drugs 1992; 44(3):498–529.

11. Porchet HC, Benowitz NL, Scheiner LB, Copeland JR. Apparent tolerance to the acute effect of nicotine results in part from distribution kinetics. J Clin Invest 1987; 80:1466–1467.

12. Benowitz MD. Smoking-induced coronary vasoconstriction: implications for therapeutic use of nicotine. J Am Coll Cardiol 22 (3):648–649.

13. APA. Diagnostic and Statistical Manual of Mental or Mental Disorders—IV. Washington D.C.: American Phychiatric Association, 1994.

14. Hughes JR, Gust SW, Skoog K, Keenan RM, Fenwick JW. Symptoms of tobacco withdrawal. A replication and extension. Arch Gen Phychiatry 1991; 48:52–59.

15. Fagerström KO, Heatherton TF, Kozlowski LT. Nicotine addiction and its assessment. Ear Nose Throat 1991; 69:763–768.

16. Fiore MC, Bailey SJ, Cohen SJ, Dorfman SF, Goldstein MG, Gritz ER, Heyman RB, Jaen CR, Kottke TE, Lando HA, Mecklenburg R, Mullen PD, Nett LM, Robinson L, Stitzer ML, Tommasello AC, Villejo L, Wewers ME. Treating Tobaccouse and Dependence. Clinical Practice Guideline. Rockville, MD: No.U.S. Department of Health and Human Services. Public Health Services, June 2000.

17. Fagerström KO, Säwe U, Tønnesen P. Therapeutic use of nicotine patches: efficacy and safety. J Smoking-Related Dis 1992; 3:247–261.

18. Transdermal Nicotine Study Group. Transdermal nicotine for smoking cessation. IAMA 1991; 22:3133–3138.

19. Russell MAH, Stableton JA, Feyerabend C, Wiserman SM, Gustavasson G, Säwe U, Connor P. Targeting heavy smokers in general practice: randomised controlled trial of transdermal nicotine patches. Br Med J 1993; 306:1308–1312.

20. Imperial Cancer Research Fund General Practice Research Group. Effectiveness of a nicotine patch in helping people to stop smoking: results of a randomized trial in general practice. Br Med J 1993; 306:1304–1308.

21. McNabb ME, Ebert RV, McCusker K. Plasma nicotine levels produced by chewing nicotine gum. JAMA 1982; 248:865–868.

22. McNabb ME. Chewing nicotine gum for 3 months: What happens to plasma nicotine levels? Can Med Assoc J 1984; 131:589–592.

23. Tønnesen P, Fryd V, Hansen M, Helsted J, Gunnersen AB, Forchammer H, Stockner M. Two and four mg nicotine chewing gum and group counseling in smoking cessation: an open, randomized, controlled trial with a 22 month follow-up. Addict Behav 1988; 13:17–27.

24. Tønnesen P, Fryd V, Hansen M, Helsted J, Gunnersen AB, Forchammer H, Stockner M. Effect of nicotine chewing gum in combination with group counseling on the cessation of smoking. N Engl J Med 1988; 318:15–18.

25. Puska P, Bjorkqvist S, Koskela K. Nicotine containing chewing gum in smoking cessation: a double-blind trial with half year follw-up. Addict Behav 1979; 4:141–146.

26. Killen JD, Fortmann SP, Newman B, Varady A. Evaluation of a treatment approach combining nicotine gum with self-guided behavioral treatments for smoking relapse prevention. Consult Clin Phychol 1990; 58:85–92.

27. Murray RP, Bailey WC, Daniels K, Bjrnson WM, Kurnow K, Connett JE, Nides MA, Kiley JP. Safety of nicotine polacrilex gum used by 3,094 participants in the Lung Health Study. Chest 1996; 109:438–445.

28. Tønnesen P, Nørregaard J, Mikkelsen K, Jørgensen S, Nilsson F. A double-blind trial of a nicotine inhaler for smoking cessation. JAMA 1993; 269:1268–1271.

29. Hjalmarsson A, Nilsson F, Sjöstrom L, Wiklund O. The nicotine inhaler in smoking cessation. Arch Intern Med 1997; 157:1721–1728.

30. Leischow JJ, Nisson F, Franzon M, Hill A, Otte P, Merikle ED. Efficacy of the nicotine inhaler as an adjunct to smoking cessation. Am J Health Behav 1996; 20:264–271.

31. Schneider NG, Olmstead R, Nilsson F, Vaghaiwalla Mody F, Franzon M, Doan K. Efficacy of a nicotine inhaler in smoking cessation: a double-blind, placebo-controlled trial. Addiction 1996; 91(9):1293–1306.

32. Sutherland G, Stapleton JA, Russell MAH, Jarvis MJ, Hajek P, Belcher M, Feyerabend C. Randomized controlled trial of a nasal nicotine spray in smoking cessation. Lancet 1992; 340:324–329.

33. Blöndal T, Franzon M, Westin A, Olafsdottir I, Gudmundosdottir S, Gunnarsdottir R. A double-blind randomized trial of nicotine nasal spray as an aid in smoking cessation. Eur Respir J 1997; 10:1585–1596.

34. Schneider HG, Olmstead R, Vaghaiwall MF, Doan K, Franzon M, Jarvik ME, Steinberg C. Efficacy of a nasal nicotine spray in smoking cessation placebo controlled double-blind trial. Addiction 1995; 90:1671–1682.

35. Wallström M, Nilsson F, Hirch JM. A randomized, double-blind, placebo-controlled clinical evaluation of a nicotine sublingual tablet in smoking cessation. Addiction 2000; 95:1161–1171.

36. Glover ED, Glover PN, Franzon M, Sullivan CR, Cerullo CC, Howell RM, Keyes GG, Nilsson F, Hobbs GR. A comparison of a nicotine sublingual tablet and placebo for smoking cessation. Nicotine Tob Res 2002; 4:441–450.

37. Fagerström KO, Schneider NG, Lunnel E. Effectiveness of nicotine patch and nicotine gum as individual versus combined treatment for tobacco withdrawal symptoms. Psychopharmacology 1993; 110:251–257.

38. Puska P, Bjorkqvist S, Koskela K. Nicotine containing chewing gum in smoking cessation: a double-blind trial with half year follow-up. Addict Behav 1979; 4:141–146.

39. Gawin F, Comptom M, Byck R. Buspirone reduces smoking. Arch Gen Psychiatry 1989; 46:288.

40. Hurt RD, Sachs DPL, Glover ED, Offord KP, Johnston JA, Dale LC, Khayrallah MA, Schroeder DR, Glover PN, Sullivan CR, Croghan IT, Sullivan P. A comparison of sustained release bupropion and placebo for smoking cessation. N Engl J Med 1997; 337:1195–1120.

41.   Jorenby DE, Leischow SJ, Nides MA, Rennard SI, Johnston JA, Hughes AR, Smith SS, Muramoto ML, Daughton DM, Doan K, Fiore MC, Baker TB. A controlled trial of sustained-release bupropion, a nicotine patch, or both for smoking cessation. N Engl J Med 1999; 340:685–691.
42.   Holm KJ, Spencer CM. Bupropion. A review of its use in the management of smoking cessation. Drugs 2000; 59:1007–1024.
43.   Hughes JR, Stead LF, Lancaster T. Antidepressants for smoking cessation (Cochrane review). In: The Cochrane Library, 2, 2003. Oxford: Update Software.
44.   Hays JT, Hurt RD, Rigotti NA, Nidura R, Gonzales D, Durcan MJ, Sachs DP, Wolter TD, Buist AS, Johnston JA, White JD. Sustained-release bupropion for pharmacologic relapse prevention after smoking cessation. A randomized, controlled trial. Ann Intern Med 2001; 18:423–433.
45.   Gonzales DH, Nides MA, Ferry LH, Kustra RP, Jamerson BD, Segal N, Herrero LA, Krishen A, Sweeney A, Buaron K, Metz A. Bupropion SR as an aid to smoking cessation in smokers treated previously with bupropion: a randomized placebo-controlled study. Clin pharmacol Ther 2001; 69:438–444.
46.   Kwan AL, Meiners AP, van Groorheest AC, Lekkerkerker JF. Risk of convulsions due to use of burpropion as an aid for smoking cessation. Ned Tijdschr Geneeskd 2001;145: 277–278.
47.   Humma LM, Swims MP. Bupropion mimics a transient ischemic attack. Ann Pharmacother 1999; 33:305–307.
48.   Bhattacharjee C, Smith M, Todd F, Gillespie M. Bupropion overdose: a potential problem with the new "miracle" anti-smoking drug. Int J Clin Pract 2001; 55:221–222.
49.   Dunner DL, Zisook S, Billow AA, Batey SR, Johnston JA, Ascher JA. A prospective safety surveillance study for bupropion sustained-release in the treatment of depression. J Clin Psychiatry 1998; 59:366–373.
50.   O'Hara P, Connett JE, Lee WW, Nides M, Murray R, Wise R. Early and late weight gain following smoking cessation in the lung health study. Am J Epidemiol 1998; 148:821–830.
51.   Nørregaard J, Jørgensen S, Mikkelsen KL, Tønnesen P, Iversen E, Sørensen T, Søeberg B, Jakobsen HB. The effect of ephedrine plus caffeine on smoking cessation and postcessation weight gain. Clin Pharmacol Ther 1996; 60:679–686.
52.   Fagerström KO, Tejding R, Westin Å, Lunell E. Aiding reduction of smoking with nicotine replacement medications: hope for the recalcitrant smoker? Tobacco Control 1997; 6:311–316.
53.   Bolliger CT, Zellwegar JP, Danielsson T, van Biljon X, Robidou A, Westin Å, Perruchoud AP, Säwe U. Smoking reduction with oral nicotine inhalers: double blind, randomised clinical trial of efficacy and safety. BMJ 2000; 321:329–333.
54.   Wennike P, Danielsson T, Landfeldt B, Westin Å, Tønnesen P. Smoking reduction promotes smoking cessation: a double blind, randomized, placebo-controlled trial of nicotine gum with 2-year follow-up. Addiction 2003; 98:1395–1402.

55. Godfredsen NS, Vestbo J, Osler M, Prescott E. Risk of hospital admission for COPD following smoking cessation and reduction: a Danish population study. Thorax 2002; 57:967–972.

56. Godfredsen NS, Holst C, Prescott E, Vestbo J, Osler M. Smoking reduction, smoking cessation and mortality: a 16-year follow-up of 19,732 men and women from the Copenhagen Centre for Prospective Population Studies. Am J Epidemiol 2002; 156:994–1001.

57. Jarvis MJ, Russell MA, Saloojee Y. Expired air carbon monoxide: a simple breath test of tobacco smoke intake. Br Med J 1980; 281:484–485.

58. Rizzi M, Andreoli A, Greco M, Bamberga M, Petrigni G, Sergi M. Smoking habits in severe respiratory insufficiency (abstr). Eur Respir J 1995; 8(suppl), 214s.

59. Burling TA, Singleton EG, Bigelow GE. Smoking following myocardial infarction critical review of the literature. Health Pyschol 1989; 3:83–96.

60. Kollerup G, Tønnesen P, Åbom B, Søndergård. Cessation of smoking and smoking habits in patients with ischaemic heart disease. J Smoking-Related Dis 1992; 3:5–10.

61. Barr Taylor C, Huston-Miller N, Killen JD, DeBusk RF. Smoking cessation after acute myocardial infarction: effects of nurse-managed intervention. Ann of Intern Med 1990; 113:118–123.

62. Pissinger C, Wennike P, Tønnesen P. Nicotine replacement therapy in patients with coronary heart disease. Recommendations for effective use. CNS Drugs 1999; 12:99–110.

63. Joseph AM, Norman SM, Ferry LH, Prochazka AV, Westman EC, Steele BG, Sherman SE, Cleveland M, Antonnucio DO. The safety of transdermal nicotine as an aid to smoking cessation in patients with cardiac disease. N Engl J Med 1996; 335:1792–1798.

64. Working Group for the Study of Transdermal Nicotine in Patients with Coronary Artery Disease. Nicotine replacement therapy for patients with coronary artery disease. Arch Intern Med 1994; 154: 989–995.

65. Glasgow RE, Stevens VJ, Vogt TM, Mullooly JP, Lichtenstein E. Changes in smoking associated with hospitalization: quit rates, predictive variables, and intervention implications. Am J Health Promotion 1991; 6:24–29.

66. Emmons KM, Goldstein MG. Smokers who are hospitalized: a window of opportunity for smoking cessation. Prev Med 1992; 21:262–269.

67. Miller H, Smith PM, DeBusk RF, Sobel DS, Taylor CB. Smoking cessation in hospitalized patients: results of a randomized trial. Arch Intern Med 1997; 157:409–415.

68. McDaniel AM, Kristeller JL, Hudson DM. Chart reminder increase referrals for inpatients smoking cessation intervention. Nicotine Tobacco Res 1999; 1:175–180.

69. US Department of Health and Human Services. The Health Consequences of Smoking: Chronic Obstructive Lung Disease. A Report of the Surgeon General. U.S. Department of Health and Human Services. Public Health Service. Office on Smoking and Health. Rockville, Maryland, 1984.

70. Williams HO. Routine advice against smoking. A chest clinic pilot study. Practitioner 1969; 202:672–676.
71. Pederson LL, Baskerville JC, Wanklin JM. Multivariate statistical models for predicting change in smoking behavior following physician advice to quit smoking. Prevent Med 1982; 11:536–549.
72. Campell IA, Prescott RJ, Tjeder-Burton SM. Smoking cessation in hospital patients given repeated advice plus nicotine or placebo chewing gum. Respir Med 1991; 85:155–157.
73. Lewis SF, Piasecki TM, Anderson JE, Baker TB. Transdermal nicotine replacement for hospitalized patients randomized clinical trial. Prev Med 1998; 27:296–303.
74. Lewis SF, Piasecksi TM, Fiore MC, Anderson JE, Baker TB. Transdermal nicotine replacement for hospitalized patients: a randomized clinical trial. Prev Med 1998; 27:296–303.
75. Cambell IA, Prescott RJ, Theder-Burton SM. Transdermal nicotine plus support in patients attending hospital with smoking-related diseases placebo-controlled study. Respir Med 1996: 90:47–51.
76. Stevens VJ, Glasgow RS, Hollis JF, Lichtenstein E, Vogt TM. A smoking-cessation intervention for hospital patients. Med Care 1993; 31:65–72.
77. Rigotti NA, Munafo MR, Murphy MFG, Stead LF. Interventions for smoking cessation in hospitalized patients (Cochrane review). In: The Cochrane Library 2003, Issue 2. Oxford: Update Software.
78. British Thoracic Society. Comparison of four methods of smoking withdrawal in patients with smoking related diseases. Br Med J 1983; 286:595–597.
79. Research Committee of the British Thoracic Society. Smoking cessation in patients: two further studies by the British Thoracic Society. Thorax 1990; 45:835–840.
80. Daughton DM, Fix AJ, Kass I, and Patil KD. Smoking cessation among patients with chronic obstructive pulmonary disease (COPD). Addict Behav 1980; 5:125–128.
81. Dudley DL, Aickin M, Martin CV. Cigarette smoking in a chest clinic population—psychophysiologic variable. J Psychosom Res 1977; 21:367–375.
82. Anthonisen NR, Connett JE, Kiley JP, Aldose MD, Bailey WC, Buist AS, Conway WA, Enoright PL, Kammer RE, O'Hary P, Owens GR, Scanlon PD, Tashkin DP, Wise RA, for The Lung Health Study Research Group. Effects of smoking intervention and the use of an inhaled anticholinergic bronchodilator on the rate of decline of FEV1. The Lung Health Study. JAMA 1994; 272:1497–1505.
83. Pederson LL, Wanklin JM, Lefcoe NM. The effects of counseling on smoking cessation among patients hospitalized with chronic obstructive pulmonary disease randomized clinical trial. Int J Addict 1991; 26:107–119.
84. Crowley TJ, Macdonald MJ, Walter MI. Behavioral anti-smoking trial in chronic obstructive pulmonary disease. Psychopharmacology(Berl) 1995; 119:193–204.

85. Tønnesen P, Mikkelsen KL. Routine smoking cessation with 4 nicotine regimens in a lung clinic. Eur Respir J 2000; 16:714–722.
86. Tønnesen P, Mikkelsen KL, Markholst C, Ibsen A, Bendixen M, Pedersen L, Fuursted R, Hansen LH, Stensgaard H, Schiøtz R, Petersen T, Breman L, Clementsen P, Evald T. Nurse-conducted smoking cessation with minimal intervention in a lung clinic randomized controlled study. Eur Respir J 1996; 9:2351–2355.
87. Taskin D, Kanner R, Bailey W, Buist S, Anderson P, Nides MA, Gonzales D, Dozier G, Patel MK, Jamerson BD. Smoking cessation in patients with chronic obstructive pulmonary disease: a double-blind, placebo-controlled, randomised trial. Lancet 2001; 357:1571–1575.
88. Jarvis MJ, Powell Sr, Marsh HS. A meta-analysis of clinical studies confirms the effectiveness of bupropion SR in smoking cessation. Poster. 8th Annual Meeting Society for Research on Nicotine and Tobacco, Savannah (GA), 20–23.02.2002.
89. van der Meer RM, Wagena EJ, Ostelo RWJG, Jacobs JE, van Schayck CP. Smoking cessation for chronic obstructive pulmonary disease (Cochrane review). In: The Cochrane Library, Issue 2, 2003.Oxford: Update Software.

15

Anticholinergics

MICHAEL BRUNSON and WILLIAM C. BAILEY

University of Alabama at Birmingham
Birmingham, Alabama, U.S.A.

I. Introduction

Modern quaternary anticholinergic bronchodilators are descendants of the early botanical preparations of the nightshade family (Solanaceae). The stems, roots, and seeds of these plants contain alkaloids, which have been used for millennia in religious ceremonies, assassinations, recreational hallucinations, and medical remedies. Inhalation therapy for obstructive pulmonary disease with various compounds containing the belladonna alkaloids has been used for centuries. The effectiveness of these preparations can be attributed to their containing atropine, a tertiary ammonium structure. The use of these "medications" fell out of favor within the medical community in the early twentieth century with the development of long-acting methyxanthines and β_2-agonists for obstructive disease. However, in the 1970s, the pharmaceutical industry developed synthetic congeners of atropine, which exhibited fewer systemic side effects. These newer quaternary ammonium compounds have reestablished the place of anticholinergic agents in the treatment of obstructive airways disease.

II. History

Datura is a genus of the Solanaceae family of plants. Various species of *Datura* grow worldwide. *Datura stramonium* is the most commonly mentioned botanical source for treatment of obstructive disease, and is the most common species found in North America. It is also called Jimson weed, thornapple, and stinkweed. *D. meteloides* is found in Africa and Asia and was likely the species used in medicinal and religious preparations by the ancient Greeks. *D. inoxia, D. candida, D. sanguinea,* and *D. aurea* may be found in South America and were used by the Aztecs and Incas for religious and medicinal purposes (1).

D. stramonium is a tall, coarse, annual weed with rank-smelling foliage and large white trumpet-shaped flowers succeeded by globose prickly fruits. Because of its worldwide distribution, this belladonna alkaloid has found its way into many medicinal, religious, and nefarious uses. The *Datura* species contains not only atropine, but hyoscyamine and scopolamine as well.

The earliest reference to the effects of *Datura* is felt to be documented during Odysseus's encounter with Circe. When Odysseus arrived at the island of Aeaea, Circe offered his crew food mixed with drugs so that they would forget their homeland. She then magically turned the men into pigs. It is felt that the major ingredient of her poison was derived from *D. meteloides.* The drugs could have caused the men to become forgetful and could have caused a delusional state in which they thought they were pigs (2). Setting out to save his crew, Odysseus met the god Hermes, who offered Odysseus an antidote to the poison, a plant known as moly. Plaitakis and Duvoisin have argued that moly was in fact snowdrop (*Galanthus nivalis*), which contains galanthamine, a centrally acting anticholinesterase, which could have reversed some of the symptoms caused by Circe's poison (3).

Another, more substantiated account of the use of the effects of *Datura* species was recorded during the Roman era. During one of the campaigns of Mark Antony's legions (37–38 B.C.), *Datura* was added to the campfires of his army by his enemies. This was likely *D. meteloides,* the uses of which had been passed down from the Greeks. Those soldiers exposed to the smoke of the campfires were disabled by euphoria and hallucinations (4,5).

Peruvian healers and shamans employed the *Datura* species for a wide range of medicinal and religious purposes. The plants themselves were considered sacred, to be used only by the priest. The narcotic and anesthetic properties were well described during rituals or medicinal operations such as skull trepanation. The Conquistadors reported use of *Datura* species by the Aztecs in both initiation rituals and as a narcotic for the victims of ritual sacrifices (6).

In North America, the name Jimson weed is derived from the earlier name Jamestown weed (i.e., Jamestown, Virginia). British soldiers were present in 1679 to stop an uprising in the colony. *Datura* was added to their food, causing the soldiers to show classic signs of anticholinergic hallucinations. A report of the event described bizarre behavior, including one soldier sitting naked in a corner grinning like a monkey and making bows to the crowd (7).

The writings of Carlos Castenada and the teaching of his mentor Don Jaun describe in detail the preparation and uses of *Datura* species, including communication with the spirits of their forefathers (8). Many native Americans ate, drank, or smoked *D. stramonium* to enter the spirit world and communicate with the spirits of nature or of their ancestors.

The recreational use of Datura species has persisted throughout civilization. The effects of accidental overdose, including excitation, euphoria, hallucination, tachycardia, coma, and death, have been described in medical journals since the time of the Romans.

The drug culture of the 1960s in the United States saw a particular resurgence of *Datura* use. This phenomenon led to an increase in the number of persons seeking medical attention for accidental overdose. *Datura* species are easily identified throughout North and South America, and this ease of access probably accounts for many adolescents and young adults experimenting with the effects of this genus of plant.

III. Medical History

The physiological effects caused by the *Datura* species make it a natural choice for use as a medicinal agent. As with most of the concoctions from the botanical world, trial and error over the centuries led to its trial as a remedy for many common diseases, including depression and tuberculosis. The first recorded use of *Datura* for pulmonary disease has been attributed to the Egyptians. A second millennium B.C. papyrus describes a breathing disorder that may have been asthma. The various treatments included plants from the *Datura* species (9). The first definitive record of *Datura* for use in obstructive disease comes from the ayurvedic medicine of India. The symptoms of asthma, cough, wheezing, and dyspnea are well described in the seventeenth century *Yogaratnakara*. The preparation of the remedy is also quite specific: "One should powder together dry ginger, long pepper, black pepper, root of *Datura* plant (*Dhuttoramoola*) and red arsenic, prepare a paste out of it, turn it into a roll, dry it, and smoke it for three days" (10). The inhalation of smoke from the *Datura* species was recognized as an effective route of medication administration. This likely represented the early precursor to the asthma cigarettes sold to the public well into the twentieth century.

The use of *Datura* by the British has been traced to Indian origins. Dr. Anderson, a physician-general, stationed in Madras, learned of the Indian practice of smoking *Datura ferox* for the relief of asthma and adopted it in his own practice. His patients, a General Gent, brought the practice to England. Although *D. ferox* is not found in Britain, General Gent found *D. stramonium* to be an adequate substitute (10).

The London surgeon William English, 1811, recorded using *D. stramonium* in treating his own asthma. English's history of his disease reveals childhood asthma of some severity, with partial remission in early adulthood. He also recorded worsening of symptoms in later life leading to chronic cough and wheezing. English's record of his first use of *Datura* resulted in the famous quote: "[*Datura*] was wonderful even to me almost incredible—the irritation and constant cough ceased and I expectorated from the bronchia pieces of clear congealed phlegm, from half-an-inch to about an inch in length, and the thickness of a crow's quill, which enabled me to fill the chest with air" (11). Despite this glowing review, the use of *D. stramonium* in asthma was not overwhelmingly accepted by the medical community. Caution was recommended because General Gent was said to have become a victim of overuse of *Datura*. The side effects of the atropine were well documented, as well as the potentially addictive qualities of overuse.

In 1840 C. J. B. Williams demonstrated the contractility of the bronchial tree. He further demonstrated the antispasmodic effect of *D. stramonium* (12). Labelia, belladonna, and hyoscyamine were commonly used in the 1850s for asthma; however, *D. stramonium* was regarded as the most specific, antispasmodic for asthma (10). There were many preparations of *D. stramonium* for sale, most in the form of asthma cigarettes. Many of these remedies had as much potential for harm as good and included a large number of other substances, including nitrites, arsenic, tobacco, and cannabis. How each of these preparations was smoked was also known to be important. Salter recommended deep inhalation in order to enhance delivery to the lungs (13). The efficacy of each of these preparations was never tested using rigorous scientific method until the middle of the twentieth century, but their continued use by the medical community indicates that at least some patients benefited from their use.

In the 1950s, Ervenius and colleagues demonstrated that asthma cigarettes deposited 0.5 mg of atropine in the distal airway when patients inspired deeply and held their breath. Inadequate delivery was caused by poor inspiratory effort or inability to breath-hold (14). These findings are reminiscent of the use of metered-dose inhalers today. The use of anticholinergics in asthma waned in the middle of the twentieth century because of the advent of methyxanthines and β₂-agonists. The side effects of atropine limited the use of *D. stramonium* and other atropine-containing medications for use in asthma, and as the efficacy of methyxanthines and adrenergic agonists became more established, the role of anticholinergics in obstructive disease lessened (10).

The current use of anticholinergic medications stems from the development of quaternary anticholinergic agents. These drugs are absorbed poorly across mucous membranes and are free from most of the side effects of the atropine-containing compounds. These medications were first tested for use in asthma, but as our understanding of asthma has changed from a bronchoconstrictive disorder to a complex inflammatory disease, the use of anticholinergics has become an adjunctive therapy and not a first-line treatment. The role of anticholinergics as a first-line treatment in patients with chronic obstructive pulmonary disease (COPD) is now being recognized.

IV. Physiological Control of the Airways

Control of the airways involves a complicated interaction between the autonomic motor nerves and sensory receptors. Cholinergic nerve fibers originate from the nucleus ambiguous and the dorsal motor nucleus of the brainstem and travel down to the peripheral ganglia located in the walls of the airways (15). Short postaganglionic fibers travel to airway smooth muscles and submucosal glands. The vagus nerve is parasympathetic and acts as a bronchoconstrictor by its effect on smooth muscles and as a secretagogue by its effect on submucosal glands (16,17). The effects of cholinergic antagonists on bronchial smooth muscles and submucosal glands has established their role in the treatment of obstructive pulmonary disorders. The electrical stimulation of the vagus nerve causes the release of acetylcholine from the cholinergic nerve terminals, which in turn activate muscarinic receptors of both smooth muscles and submucosal glands (15). Animal studies have revealed that the concentration of muscarinic receptors is greater in the larger airways compared to the smaller peripheral airways (17,18). In humans, however, muscarinic receptors are also found in smaller airways. Studies have shown that cholinergic bronchoconstriction affects larger airways more than smaller airways. Studies have also revealed that adrenergic agonists cause bronchodilatation in both large and small airways (19). The clinical use of cholinergic antagonists may be limited in patients with bronchoconstriction of the smaller airways. The airways maintain some smooth muscle tone through cholinergic innervation. This has been demonstrated by showing that atropine will cause bronchodilatation in healthy subjects. Likewise, bronchoconstriction can be enhanced by a cholinergic agonist such as edrophonium (20). The control of airway tone is not solely determined by vagal innervation; local mediators also play a role.

A. Muscarinic Receptors

The cholinergic control of the airways is established through muscarinic receptors (Fig. 1). Five subtypes of muscarinic receptors have been established, three of which play a role in control of airway tone (21).

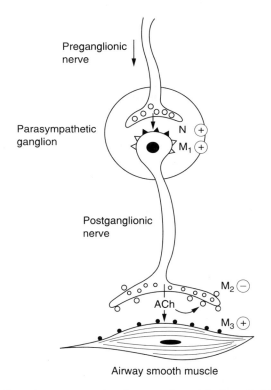

Figure 1 Cholinergic receptors in airways. Acetylcholine (Ach) released from preganglionic nerves acts on nicotinic receptors (N) on postganglionic neurons. Muscarinic M1 receptors may facilitate this neurotransmission in ganglia. In postganglionic nerves, M2 receptors may inhibit release of acetylcholine, and therefore reduce its effect on M3 receptors on airway smooth muscle. (From Ref. 21.)

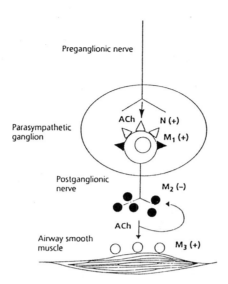

Figure 2 Muscarinic receptor subtypes in airways. Ganglionic transmission is mediated via nicotonic receptors (N), but M1 receptors may have a facilitatory role. M2 receptors at the postganglionic terminal may inhibit the release of acetylcholine (Ach), which acts on M3 receptors on airway smooth muscle.

Each of the receptor subtypes has been cloned (22,23). Three subtypes of receptors are now recognized phramacologically. M1 receptors are pirenzepine sensitive and are associated with ganglionic structures. M2 receptors are gallamine and AF-DX 116 sensitive and are found on the presynaptic terminals of the postganglionic parasympathetic fibers in the airways. M3 receptors are 4-DAMP (4-diphenylacetoxy-*N*-methyl-piperidine methiodide) and HHSiF (hexahydro-siladifenidol) sensitive and are located on smooth muscles, submucosal glands, and blood vessels (24). M4 and M5 receptors have not been found in the human lung (Fig. 2).

M1 Receptors

Acetylcholine is released from the preganglionic nerve in the airway, and its effects on the postganglionic nerve are mediated by nicotinic receptors. M1 receptors on the postganglionic nerve, when activated, enhance conduction at the parasympathetic ganglion. Hexamethonium, a nonspecific muscarinic inhibitor, will block this transmission. Pirenzepine and telenzepine are selective M1-receptor antagonists and inhibit the preganglionic stimulation of airway smooth muscle (25). The discovery of pirenzepine helped distinguish between two types of muscarinic receptors: those with a high affinity, designated M1 receptors, and low affinity, or M2 receptors. M1 receptors are found in the autonomic ganglion and cerebral cortex (26).

Pirenzepine given intravenously acts as a bronchodilator (27). The effect appears to be at the ganglionic site and was elucidated through several studies. Ipratropium bromide is a nonselective muscarinic antagonist and acts on all muscarinic receptors. In comparison with the effects of ipratropium bromide, pirenzepine did not block the bronchoconstrictive effects of methacholine as ipratropium did. However, both ipratropium bromide and pirenzepine were equally effective in inhibiting the bronchoconstrictor effect induced by the irritant sulfur dioxide (28). These studies suggest that pirenzepine acts on the parasympathetic ganglion on the airways and not directly on the airway smooth muscle receptors.

The role of M1 receptors in the airways is not clear, but it may involve the maintenance of vagal tone. Specific M1-receptor antagonists may play a role in treating obstructive pulmonary disease by reducing the cholinergic tone of the airways.

M2 Receptors

M2 muscarinic receptors have been described in the intestinal tract, heart, and airways. M2 muscarinic receptors have been described by their low affinity for pirenzepine. M2 receptors are located on the presynaptic terminal of the postganglionic nerve fibers. When stimulated, these receptors inhibit the release of acetylcholine and limit the contraction of smooth muscle. Pilocarpine is a selective M2-receptor agonist, and gallamine, AF-DX 116, and methoctramine are antagonists (21). Pilocarpine has been shown to inhibit both smooth muscle constriction in response to vagal stimulation and cholinergic reflex bronchoconstriction due to inhaled sulfur dioxide in normal subjects. However, bronchoconstriction due to inhaled histamine is not affected (29,30).

In patients with asthma, pilocarpine does not inhibit cholinergic reflex bronchoconstriction due to inhaled sulfur dioxide. This suggests that there may be some dysfunction in M2 receptors in this particular patient population (29). This may explain why some nonselective anticholinergic antagonists have an exaggerated bronchoconstrictive effect. This untoward bronchoconstriction has been reported in several patients taking ipratropium bromide. It may also explain why asthmatics may have such a pronounced bronchoconstrictive effect when given β-blockers.

The influenza virus may downregulate or inactivate the M2 receptor, and this may also explain the increased airway responsiveness in patients who have contracted the virus (31). It has been shown in guinea pigs that infection with the influenza virus increases bronchoconstriction, and this may occur in humans as well.

M3 Receptors

M3 receptors have been described by their response to 4-DAMP and HHSiF. These receptors have been demonstrated on smooth muscles, submucosal glands, and blood vessels by autoradiography and M3-selective cDNA probes (20,32). M3 receptors are activated by methacholine. Anticholinergic agents such as atropine and ipratropium bromide acting on the M3 receptors can prevent the effects of methacholine. The anticholinergic agents now in use are nonspecific, and a selective M3-receptor antagonist could play a large role in treating obstructive disease.

B. Relevance of Muscarinic Receptors

The anticholinergic drugs in use in the obstructive lung diseases act nonselectively on muscarinic receptors. The airway tone partially established by the vagus nerve is determined by the stimulation of the MI, M2, and M3 receptors. Effective and selective antagonists of the M3 receptor have not been approved for use in the United States. The paradoxical bronchoconstriction sometimes observed with nonselective anticholinergic agonist could theoretically be avoided with specific M3-receptor antagonists.

V. Pharmacology of Anticholinergic Medications

A. Atropine

Atropine (Fig. 3) is a naturally occurring tertiary amine muscarinic. It is the prototype of muscarinics. Atropine may be synthesized but is usually obtained by extraction from several plants of the Solananceae family: *Atropos belladonna*, *Datura stramonium*, or *Duboisia myoporoides*. Medications containing atropine served as the major treatment for obstructive pulmonary disease until the discovery of quaternary compounds by the pharmaceutical industry. The relative sensitivity of physiological function in descending order is secretions of the salivary, bronchial, and sweat glands; pupillary dilation, ocular accommodation, and heart rate; contraction of the detrusor muscle of the bladder and smooth muscle of the GI tract; and

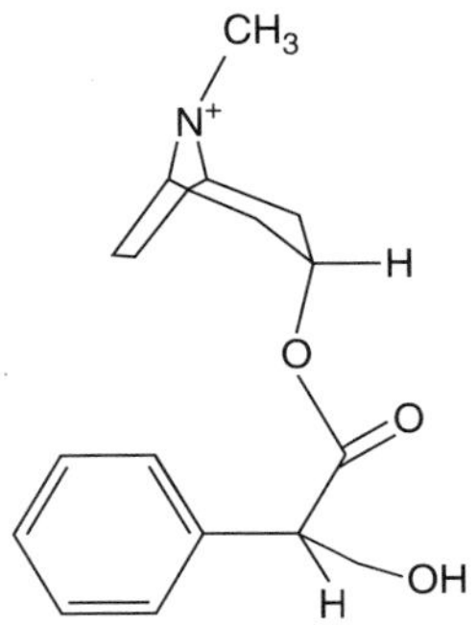

Figure 3 Structural formula of atropine.

gastric secretion and motility. The physiological effects of atropine are described below.

Respiratory

Atropine sulfate reduces the amount of secretions in the nose, mouth, pharynx, and bronchi. It also causes relaxation of the smooth muscles of the airway with a resultant decrease in airway resistance. Atropine is a potent bronchodilator, particularly of the large airways, and it was especially useful in preventing the bronchoconstriction caused by parasympathetic stimulation. Atropine reduces the incidence of laryngospasm caused by some general anesthetics.

Cardiovascular

Atropine sulfate has a dose-dependent effect on the cardiovascular system. Small doses act centrally and produce a slight decrease in heart rate attributable to central vagal stimulation. With larger doses, increased blocking of vagal stimulation of the sinoatrial node causes progressive tachycardia. Atropine has a positive chronotropic effect. Antropine is effective in reversing sinus bradycardia brought about by extracardiac causes but is not effective in treating bradycardia caused by intrinsic sinus node dysfunction.

Gastrointestinal

Atropine sulfate reduces salivation and causes xerostomia. It also causes a reduction in the volume of gastric secretions and a prolongation of gastrointestinal transit time. The doses required to produce a decrease in gastric acid production are not without significant side effects.

Central Nervous System

At small doses, atropine causes a centrally mediated reduction in heart rate. At larger doses, central stimulation of nicotinic receptors occurs and can cause restlessness, irritability, disorientation, hallucinations, and delirium. At toxic doses, depression, coma, medullary paralysis, and death may occur.

Genitourinary

Atropine decreases the tone and amplitude of smooth muscle contraction of the ureters and bladder. This results in a decreased urge to void and urinary retention.

The Eye

Atropine blocks the response of the sphincter muscle of the iris and the ciliary muscle of the lens to cholinergic stimulation, causing mydriasis and cycloplegia. Some medical uses of atropine include:

1. Preoperative administration to reduce salivation and excessive secretions in the respiratory tract
2. Adjunctive therapy in the treatment of peptic ulcer disease and irritable bowel syndrome
3. Assistance in the diagnosis of sinus node dysfunction and Wolff-Parkinson-White syndrome and the management of acute myocardial infarction and symptomatic bradycardia
4. Reducing the amplitude and frequency of uninhibited contractions of the bladder in patients with neurogenic bladder
5. Treatment of bronchospasm

The use of atropine is associated with anticholinergic side effects. This has limited the use of atropine for many therapeutic indications. The newer quaternary ammonium compounds offer fewer side effects because they are minimally absorbed from the gastrointestinal tract and do not cross the blood-brain barrier.

B. Ipratropium Bromide

Ipratropium bromide (Fig. 4) is a potent bronchodilator, particularly of the large airways. The degree of bronchodilatation is related to the cholinergic parasympathetic bronchomotor tone and the neural reflexes causing bronchomotor constriction. Ipratropium bromide (*N*-isopropylnoratropine

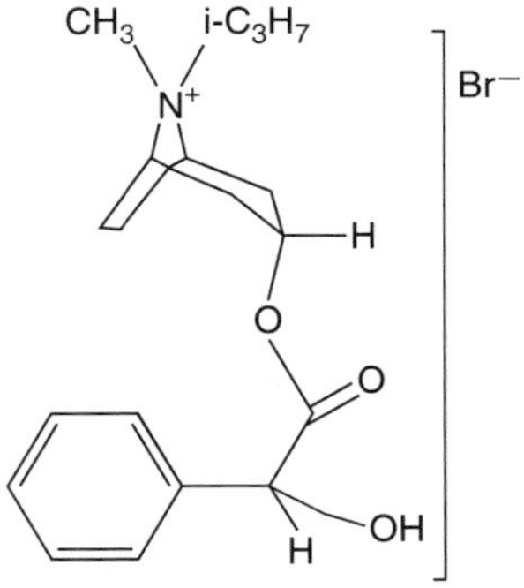

Figure 4 Structural formula of ipratropium bromide. Indication: chronic obstructive airways disease; asthma. Administration: inhalation. Itrop—indication: bradyarrhythmia. Administration: intravenous or oral.

methobromide) is the most widely studied quaternary compound used as a bronchodilator. It is a nonselective antagonist at muscarinic receptors present in airways and other organs. Ipratropium generally exhibits greater antimuscarinic activity on bronchial smooth muscle than on secretory glands. It is not significantly absorbed across mucous membranes, and most of the anticholinergic side effects associated with atropine use, such as tachycardia and dry mouth, are not seen (33).

Ipratropium bromide (Atrovent) is delivered by a metered-dose inhaler. The effective dose range is 0.6–8.0 mg/kg. The usual maintenance dose in COPD is 36 μg (two actuations of the metered dose inhaler) 4 times per day. If necessary, additional inhalations may be used up to 12 inhalations per 24 hours. Some clinicians feel that higher doses, 6 inhalations 4 times per day may be efficacious without side effects. After inhalation, blood levels are less than 1% of the inhaled dose. The half-life is 3 hours. The onset of bronchodilatation, as measured by an increase in the FEV_1 of 15%, occurs in 3–5 minutes; however, maximum effect is not reached for 1½–2 hours. Bronchodilatation generally last 4–5 hours but may last up to 7–8 hours. Combination therapy with β-adrenergic agonists in patients with COPD results in bronchodilatation for 5–7 hours, compared with 3–4 hours in patients given β-agonists alone (34). Combination therapy of ipratropium and β-agonists resulted in greater bronchodilatation than either drug alone.

Ipratropium bromide is generally well tolerated in the inhaled form. Plasma levels are approximately 1000 times higher following oral administration than inhalation. Side effects include dryness of the mouth, throat, or tongue in 5% of patients and nausea in 2% of patients. Blurred vision was reported in 1% of patients. Palpitations and chest pains were recorded in 3% of patients. Bronchitis or upper respiratory tract infection was reported in 13% of patients but was not necessarily related to the drug. Cough was noted in 6% of patients. None of these side effects was significantly different than placebo. The most common reported side effect was a bitter taste in 20–30% of patients. Only 7% of patients discontinued the drug due to side effects. Intravenous administration of ipratropium bromide results in similar physiological response to atropine. There has been no tolerance reported with the long-term use of ipratropium. The Lung Health Study evaluated the effectiveness for 5 years and reported continued bronchodilatation throughout the duration of the study. This is in contrast to studies with adrenergic agents, which have demonstrated significant tolerance in as little as one month of use.

C. Oxitropium Bromide

Oxitropium bromide (*N*-ethylnorscopolamine methobromide) (Fig. 5) is pharmacologically similar to ipratropium bromide. Oxitropium bromide (Oxivent) is delivered by metered-dose inhaler. The usual dosage is 200 μg (two actuations of the metered-dose inhaler). The optimal dose in chronic bronchitis is 400–600 μg (35). In comparison with ipratropium bromide, oxitropium has been shown to be equivalent in studies assessing the maximum response in regard to changes in FEV_1 and FVC. Oxitropium has been shown to have a longer duration of action than ipratropium bromide (36). Oxitropium is currently used as first-line therapy for COPD in Japan (37).

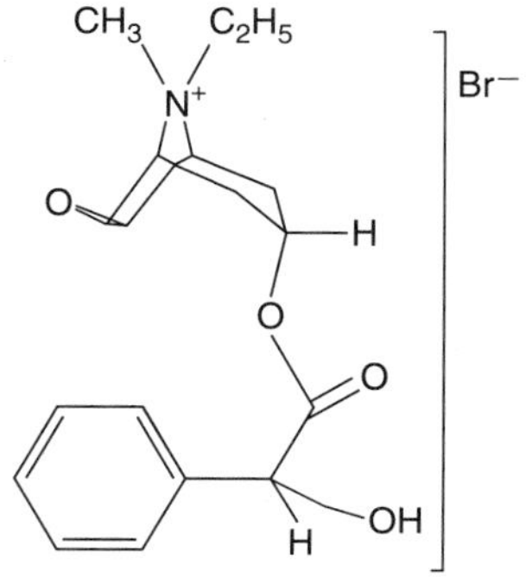

Figure 5   Structural formula of oxitropium bromide (Oxivent, Tersigat, Tersigan). Indication: chronic obstructive airways disease; asthma. Administration: inhalation.

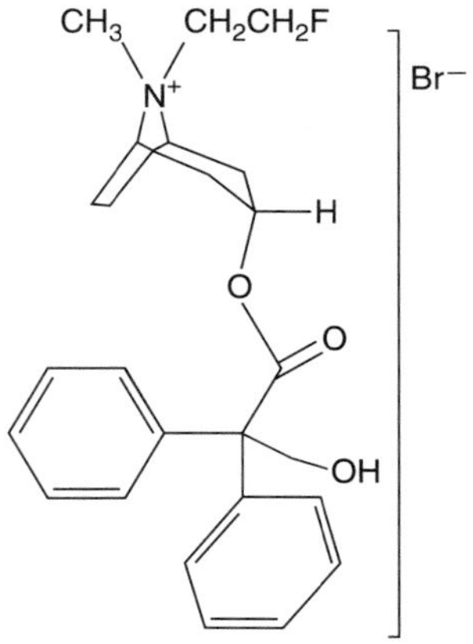

Figure 6 Structural formula of flutropium bromide (Flubron). Indication: antitussive expectorant for the relief of symptoms of asthma and chronic bronchitis, allergic rhinitis. Administration: inhalation.

D. Flutropium Bromide

Flutropium bromide (benzylic acid N-β-flouroethylnortropine ester methobromide (Fig. 6) is also pharmacologically similar to ipratropium bromide. The usual dose is 60 μg (two actuations of the metered-dose inhaler). Flutropium bromide has been shown to be equivalent to both ipratropium bromide and oxitropium bromide in studies assessing the maximum response to changes in both FEV_1 and FVC (38). Flutropium has been shown to have antihistamine effects in rats and has been reported to have improved symptoms in one case of lymphangioliomyomatosis (39).

E. Tiotropium Bromide

Tiotropium bromide, Ba 679 Br, is the latest quaternary ammonium compound developed by Boehringer Ingelheim labs. A 40 μg dose was effective against methacholine-induced bronchoconstriction for 48 hours. Doses up to 200 μg revealed no adverse effects in healthy individuals. Although the onset of action is slower than that of ipratropium bromide, the half-life of tiotropium is 540 minutes compared with 81 minutes for ipratropium. The peak effect has been shown to be 2 hours after inhalation in asthmatic volunteers. Tiotropium bromide affects M1, M2, and M3 receptors, but kinetic selectivity for M1 and M3 receptors over M2 receptors has been demonstrated (40). The clinical advantage of this selectivity has not yet been demonstrated. Tiotropium is 10-fold more potent than ipratropium bromide. Clinical studies reveal that it is a potent and long-lasting bronchodilator and is suitable for daily dosing (40a) at 18 μg (40b, 40c). The prolonged protection may be useful in nocturnal asthma symptoms.

In patients with COPD, tiotropium produced significant improvements in FEV_1, FVC, peak expiratory flow rate, peak mid-expiratory flows, improved dyspnea (40d), and long-term improvement in health outcomes (40e). In all these studies, tiotropium did not differ from placebo as to side effects (40f).

F. M3-Receptor-Specific Agents

Several M3-receptor-specific drugs are being studied at this time. Nonspecific action of anticholinergic medications such as atropine and ipratropium block both prejunctional (M2) and postjunctional (M3) receptors. The nonselective prejunctional increase in acetylcholine release on nerve stimulation may cause an increase in vagally mediated bronchoconstriction. This has been demonstrated with low-dose ipratropium bromide. M3-specific anticholinergic agents would avoid this prejunctional stimulation and may be more efficient bronchodilators.

Revatropate has been shown to have 50-fold increased M1 and M3 selectivity in guinea pig trachea and rabbit vas deferens over M2 subtype receptors (41). In studies, revatropate, in contrast to ipratropium bromide, did not potentiate bronchoconstrictor response induced by vagal nerve stimulation. This indicates that the inhibitory autoreceptors are still functional. Early studies in patients with chronic obstructive airways disease reveal that the medication is well tolerated.

Darifenacin is another agent being studied for its M3 selectivity. It has been shown to have a 100-fold selectivity for M3 receptors over M2 receptors in atria and a 30-fold increased selectivity over M1 receptors in rabbit vas deferens. M3 specific anticholinergic agents should not carry the risk of precipitating paradoxical bronchoconstriction.

VI. Anticholinergics and Bronchospastic Agents

A. Anticholinergic Agents

The usefulness of anticholinergic medications has been demonstrated to be effective against multiple stimuli. The airways have been demonstrated to have a vagally induced bronchomotor tone. The administration of anticholinergics in normal subjects causes bronchodilatation.

The anticholinergic medications provide protection against bronchoconstriction caused by cholinergic agents. This has been demonstrated with the use of several cholinergic agents, including methacholine and acetylcholine (42). The effectiveness of the anticholinergic medication given prior to the administration of a cholinergic agent has been demonstrated using atropine, ipratropium, tiotropium, or any other agent used. The effectiveness of anticholinergic agents in reversing bronchoconstriction when a subject has been given a prior cholinergic spamogen is reduced (43–45). This may be due to the release of other bronchospastic mediators into the airways after the administration of methacholine or acetylcholine that are not affected by anticholinergic medications.

B. Histamine

Histamine activates H1, H2, and H3 receptors and can, in varying dosages, cause tachycardia, bronchospasm, salivation, lacrimation, and increased gastric secretions. The anticholinergic agents have had mixed results in studies evaluating their effectiveness in preventing bronchoconstriction caused by histamine. Patient response to the administration of histamine is variable. Most of the studies evaluating the effectiveness of anticholinergic medication in preventing histamine-induced bronchospasm included both asthmatics and patients with COPD. Holtzman et al. demonstrated a protective effect of anticholinergic agents in patients with a history of (46). Rosenthal et al. demonstrated a protective effect of atropine in patients with hay fever but not in patients with asthma (47). The effectiveness of anticholinergic agents to prevent bronchoconstriction in patients exposed to histamine may depend on the population studied (48,49). Adrenergic agents have been shown to provide more protection than anticholinergic medications against histamine-induced bronchoconstriction (43,44). The bronchoconstriction caused by histamine is likely due to multiple factors and is not solely attributable to its vagal effect (44). Anticholinergics are at best partially effective at preventing the bronchoconstriction caused by histamine and are less effective than adrenergic agents.

C. β-Blockers

β-Blocking agents cause bronchoconstriction through the inhibition of β_2 receptors in the lung. β-Blockers, even in small doses such as eyedrops, have been shown to cause worsening bronchospasm in some patients. Patients with asthma are more affected than patients with chronic bronchitis or emphysema. Both atropine and ipratropium bromide have been shown to be effective in preventing the bronchoconstriction caused by β-adrenergic antagonist (42,50). They have also been shown to be effective in reversing the bronchoconstriction caused by inadvertent β-blocker usage. Anticholinergic agents presumably reverse the bronchoconstriction vagally induced by the β-adrenergic antagonist.

D. Irritants

The protective effect of anticholinergics against multiple airway irritants has been tested. Ipratropium bromide has been shown to be effective in preventing the bronchoconstrictive effects of cigarette smoke in asthmatic patients. Similar protective effect has been found in exposure to sulfur dioxide, ozone, carbon dust, and citric acid aerosol (51,54–58). Anticholinergic agents have demonstrated mixed results in protecting normal subjects or patients with obstructive airways disease when exposed to bradykinin (52,53). Likewise, anticholinergics offered little protection in young asthmatics exposed to serotonin (42,59). In patients exposed to PGF2-α, anticholinergics were shown to be only partially effective in preventing bronchoconstriction (59). In patients with gastroesophageal reflux disease, bronchospasm has been shown to be due to vagal reflex and not necessarily through direct irritation of the airway by stomach acid. Several studies have demonstrated that oral anticholinergic agents reduce esophageal reflux by limiting the frequency of lower esophageal sphincter relaxation through a central mechanism (60,61). No studies have yet demonstrated a reduction in bronchoconstriction in patients with gastroesophageal reflux treated with anticholinergic agents.

E. Exercise

The bronchoconstriction that occurs after exercise is felt to be due to a complex mechanism, of which airway cooling is a major factor (62). Studies of patients with both asthma and chronic bronchitis elicit a heterogeneous response in terms of the degree of bronchoconstriction when exercising. Several studies have demonstrated a reduction in bronchoconstriction in patients pretreated with anticholinergic medications, but not complete prevention (62–65). The protective effect of anticholinergic medications has been shown to be dose dependent and has required doses up to 10 times the amount needed for bronchodilatation alone in some studies. In other studies, no dose-dependent effect has been shown. When compared with adrenergic agents and cromolyn sodium, anticholinergics have been shown to be less effective in preventing exercise-induced bronchospasm (66,67).

When the use of anticholinergic medications is combined with other medications, the results have shown improvement with the combined regimen over either drug alone, as demonstrated by Tashkin et al. (67). Tsukino et al. also showed that theophylline and ipratropium were equally effective in increasing FEV_1 V_{O_2}, MMV, and several dyspnea ratios in patients with stable COPD during exercise (68). A combination of medications was demonstrated to be better than either drug alone. The varied response of patients to medications to prevent exercise-induced bronchospasm is indicative of the complex interactions of several mediators involved in the airways bronchoconstriction. Parasympathetic tone, the β- and α-adrenergic systems, and local mediators may all play a role in determining the airways response to exercise.

VII. Anticholinergics in Stable COPD

The efficacy of anticholinergic medications in stable COPD has been studied from many perspectives. Typical effects from a single dose of atropine include a rise in FEV_1 of 15–20%, a drop in the specific airways resistance of approximately 50%, a doubling of the airways conductance, and a reduction in the functional residual capacity (69–71). Patients with more severe airways obstruction obtain a relatively greater bronchodilatation than those with lesser airways disease (51,71). Anticholinergic medications may play several roles in improving airway diameter, including broncho- dilatation and reduction in airway secretions (73–76). The effects of ipratropium bromide and atropine, the two best studied anticholinergic agents, are similar (38,51,69).

The anticholinergic agents are generally used over a long period of time. Several studies have shown no decrease in the bronchodilatory effect of ipratropium (77,78). The Lung Health Study evaluated patients for 5 years and demonstrated no tolerance in the patient population (79). This is in contrast to the decline in responsiveness of patients to adrenergic therapy in as short a time as one month (80).

Most studies of patients with obstructive airways disease have included patients with both asthma and COPD. There is a subset of patients with COPD who will demonstrate a reversible component to their airways disease (81). In many early studies, the populations studied included patients with asthma, chronic bronchitis, and emphysema, grouping these patients as having obstructive airways disease. In these studies the groups of patients were often not separated, and the efficacy of drugs to provide bronchodilatation included the effects on patients with asthma and what is now considered COPD.

Several studies evaluated patients with obstructive airways disease to compare the efficacy of anticholinergic medications only and in combination with adrenergic agonists (72,80,82–85). In these studies, the combination of medications gave greater increases in FEV_1 than either drug alone. In two studies, salbuterol was given to patients until no further bronchodilatation could be elicited. With the addtion of 76 µg of ipratropium or atropine methonitrate, further increases in FEV_1 were demonstrated (86,87). When compared head to head, ipratropium bromide has been found to produce greater and more prolonged bronchodilatation than isoproterenol (88). Ipratropium bromide 36 µg has been found to be as effective a bronchodilator as salbutamol 200 µg in patients with pulmonary emphysema (89). Ipratropium bromide has also been shown to be as effective as 400 µg of fenoterol (82). Deptropine 200 µg and thiaziamium 300 mg were not as effective at bronchodilatation as ipratropium 36 µg (70,90). The combination of α-adrenergic agonist and anticholinergic agent generally reveals greater bronchodilatation effect than either agent alone, but in several studies it is difficult to determine whether the patients had asthma or COPD. The combination of ipratropium 36 µg and salbutamol 200 µg or fenoterol 400 µg produced a greater increase in FEV_1 than either drug alone (82,91).

When patients are separated into those with reversible airways disease and those without, as in a study by Braun and Levy, a comparison of the efficacy between albuterol and ipratropium can be made (84). In patients with COPD, ipratropium 36 µg produced a 25% greater increase in FEV_1 at 6 hours than 18 µg of albuterol and a 50% greater increase in FVC. However, in the study by Easton et al. the effects of 800 µg salbuterol and 80 µg of ipratropium were found to be equivalent (92).

The bronchodilating effects of ipratropium have been shown to be greater than that of oral theophylline, with a greater increase in FEV_1 and a longer duration of action (93). Ipratropium was also shown to be more effective than fenoterol 5 µg plus theophylline 250 µg (94).

Corticosteroids are often used as adjunctive treatment in COPD. The addition of anticholinergic agents to the medical regimen of patients with chronic bronchitis has been reported to produce a steroid-sparing effect, but has not been shown to produce an increase in bronchodilatation (95,96).

VIII. Anticholinergic Drugs in Asthma

First-line treatment of asthma is inhaled corticosteroids to decrease airways inflammation. β_2-Agonists are used for bronchodilatation on an as-needed basis but are often employed on a scheduled regimen or during a period of acute exacerbation. The benefit of anticholinergic medications as adjunctive therapy in both chronic asthma and during acute exacerbations has been extensively studied and reviewed elsewhere (51,97,98). There is a considerable amount of overlap of patients with asthma and COPD. In asthmatic patients with moderate to severe symptoms, anticholinergics represent a safe addition to their medical regimen. Likewise, in COPD patients with evidence of reversible airways disease there is a role for adrenergic agonists.

IX. Anticholinergics in Prevention of Obstructive Disease

The Lung Health Study Research Group performed a randomized clinical trial to determine if a program utilizing smoking cessation intervention and an inhaled bronchodilator could slow the rate of decline in FEV_1 in smokers aged 35–60 years with mild obstructive pulmonary disease (79). This landmark study was performed in 10 clinical centers and enrolled 5887 patients (99). The smoking cessation intervention included a 12-session smoking cessation program combining behavior modification and the use of nicotine gum with a 5-year maintenance program. A bronchodilator was provided by the use of ipratropium bromide, two puffs three times per day. The main outcome measured was the rate of change and the cumulative change of FEV_1 over the 5 years of the study. Participants in the study were divided into three arms: 1) usual care, 2) smoking cessation and bronchodilator therapy, and 3) smoking cessation and placebo (Fig. 7).

The results of the study indicate that smoking cessation is the intervention with the greatest effect on decline of FEV_1. As Fig. 7 demonstrates, the effect of bronchodilator intervention was evaluated by comparing the smoking cessation group who received bronchodilator therapy and the smoking cessation group who received placebo. There was a significant rise in FEV_1 in the group receiving bronchodilator therapy during the first year. This difference was maintained throughout the remaining 4 years of the study. The conclusion was thus drawn that bronchodilator therapy significantly improved FEV_1 during the first year and that this improvement is maintained. The rate of decline of FEV_1 in both groups who received smoking cessation is essentially the same, indicating that bronchodilator therapy with ipratropium bromide did not prevent progression of disease in asymptomatic individuals.

The study also included a washout period at the end of the study. The advantage of ipratropium bromide noted during the first year was reversed

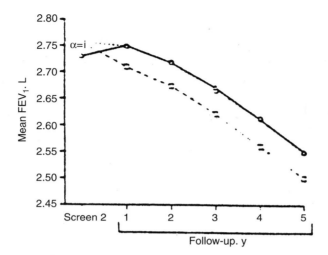

Figure 7 Mean postbronchodilator forced expiratory volume at 1 second (FEV_1) over the course of the study in all participants in whom the measurement was made. Circles/dotted lines represent the smoking-intervention and placebo group. Triangles/solid lines represent the smoking-intervention and ipratropium bromide group, and squares/dashed lines represent the usual-care group.

when patients stopped taking the medication for 40 hours or more at the end of the study. The first-year increase in FEV_1 (average 30 mL per patient) was followed by a comparable decrease when the medication was discontinued. Ipratropium bromide did not change the natural history of COPD but did act as a bronchodilator without the development of tolerance.

X.   Cost-Effectiveness

The cost of COPD has been estimated to be approximately $6.5 billion per year, both directly and indirectly. Clinical studies have revealed that long-term use of anticholinergics provides bronchodilator effects with little tolerance or side effects. With the skyrocketing cost of medical care, treating patients with chronic disease demands long-term cost-effective strategies. Ipratropium bromide was shown to reduce expenditures for physician care, hospital care, and total health services when compared with patients given a combination of theophylline, corticosteroids, and albuterol (100). These effects were measured during the first 6 months of therapy in patients with a new diagnosis of COPD.

Ipratropium has also been shown to be less costly than theophylline per patient therapy month in patients with COPD (101). In the same study ipratropium produced a greater number of complication-free therapy months as measured by the number of exacerbations and hospital and office visits.

Anticholinergic agents and adrenergic agonists are often used in combination. A pharmacoeconomic evaluation of ipratropium alone, albuterol alone, and ipratropium and albuterol combination revealed, as expected, a greater increase in FEV_1 for the combined regimen than for either drug alone (102). However, the ipratropium-only regimen resulted in the lowest cost per patient for the 85 days of the study. The combination therapy produced a decrease in the number of exacerbations, patient hospital hours, antibiotic use, and corticosteroid use.

XI. Anticholinergics in Acute Exacerbations of COPD

A large number of studies have evaluated the long-term use of anti-cholinergics in COPD in terms of bronchodilating effects, side effects, and cost. However, relatively few studies have evaluated the effectiveness of anticholinergic therapy in acute exacerbation of COPD. In contrast, there have been multiple studies evaluating the effectiveness of anticholinergics alone or in conjunction with adrenergic agents in the acute treatment of asthma.

Because of the number of emergency department visits per year for COPD exacerbation, it is important to evaluate the effectiveness of anticholinergics in terms of not only airway bronchodilatation, but also cost, hospital admission rate, and relapse rate (return visits to the emergency department). No study to date has evaluated all of these parameters.

Rebuck et al. evaluated 51 patients with COPD exacerbation given one of three regimens: 0.5 mg ipratropium, 1.25 mg fenoterol, or a combination of both medications (103). All patients had equal improvement in FEV_1. O'Driscoll et al. evaluated 47 patients in the emergency department given salbutamol 10 mg or a combination of salbutamol 10 mg and ipratropium 0.5 mg and found each regimen to be equally effective in improving FEV_1 (104). Karpel et al. studied 32 patients with COPD treated in the emergency department (105). Patients were enrolled in a crossover study utilizing ipratropium 54 µg or metaproterenol 1.94 mg initially. After 90 minutes patients were crossed over to receive the other medication. Both arms of the study were equivalent in terms of bronchodilatory effect, but the patients receiving initial therapy with ipratropium had a significant but unsustained increase in Pa_{O_2}.

Multiple studies in patients with asthma have demonstrated an additive effect with the combined use of adrenergic agonists and an anticholinergic agent. The study by Shrestha et al. is the only one in patients with COPD to show an improvement in patients receiving both medications (106). In this study 55 patients were evaluated in the emergency department and randomized to receive 0.5 mL isoetherine or 0.5 mL isoetherine plus ipratropium. The patients receiving both medications spent an average of 91 minutes less in the emergency department, significantly reducing the time patients spend there. One can surmise that decreased time would reduce costs, but this was not evaluated.

As these studies demonstrate, there were no additive effects when anticholinergic medications were given in combination with β_2-agonists. β_2-Agonists did exhibit a more rapid onset of action but were associated with more side effects. Anticholinergics alone are equally effective at bronchodilatation as combination therapy and may be more cost-effective with fewer side effects. Further investigation is needed in this area.

XII. Conclusions

Anticholinergic agents have a long history of use in the treatment of obstructive lung diseases. The continued development of quaternary ammonium compounds continues to improve treatment. As newer more specifically acting agents are developed for clinical use, physicians will have more options for treating their patients with COPD.

The role of anticholinergic medications in stable COPD is primarily one of symptomatic relief. The Lung Health Study has shown that ipratropium bromide is not effective in preventing the progression of disease in asymptomatic individuals. The role of anticholinergic therapy in acute exacerbation of COPD has not been as well studied as their role in acute exacerbation of asthma. Evidence suggests that anticholinergic agents are equally effective as β_2-agonists and have fewer side effects in treating COPD exacerbation.

The role of anticholinergic medications in the treatment of symptoms of specific aspects of COPD is continually evolving. Their effect in treating symptoms during exercise and sleep is being studied, as well as their role in preventing bronchospasm caused by gastroesophageal reflux. Nevertheless, the availability of tiotropium in a once-per-day dosing form has greatly increased therapeutic options. At this point, the one study comparing tiotropium once a day to salmeterol twice a day seems to indicate that tiotropium is superior in bronchodilatation and improvement of dyspnea (107).

References

1. Chapman KR. History of anticholinergic treatment in airways disease. In: Anticholinergic Therapy in Obstructive Airways Disease. Franklin Scientific Publications. 1993:9–17.
2. Graves R. The Greek Myths. Harmondsworth, UK: Penguin, 1960.
3. Plaitakis A. Duvoisin R.C. Homer's moly identified as *Galanthus nivalis* physiologic antidote to stramonium poisoning. Clin Neuropharmacol 1983; 6:1–5.
4. Thorwald J. Science and Secrets of Early Medicine. London: Thames and Hudson, 1962.
5. Hightower CE. Plants that kill and cure. Vet Human Toxicol 1979; 21:360–362.
6. Datura stramonium B and T. World seeds database output. The vaults of Erowid. WWW.Erowid.org.
7. Johnson C.E. Mystical force of the nightshade. Int J Neuropsychiatry 1967; 3:268–275.
8. Castenada C. The Teachings of Don Juan: A Yaqui Way of Knowledge. Los Angeles: University of California Press, 1968.
9. Brewis RAL. Classic Papers in Asthma. Vol. 1. London: Science Press, 1990.
10. Gandevia B. Historical review of the use of parasympathetic agents in the treatment of respiratory disorders. Postgrad Med J 1975; 51(suppl 7):13–20.
11. English W. Case of asthma cured by smoking the *Datura stramonium*. Edinb Med J 1811; 7:153.
12. (a) Williams CJB. The Pathology and Diagnosis of Diseases of the Chest 4th ed. London 1840:328; (b) Memories of Life and Work. London: Smith Elder, 1840:152.
13. Salter H.H. On Asthma: Its Pathology and Treatment. 2nd ed. London: Churchill 1860.
14. Ervenius O, Holmstedt B, Wallen O. Atropin und Stramoniumzigaretten. Nouyn-Schmiedeberg Arch Pharmakol Exp Pathol 1958; 234:343.
15. Barnes PJ. Neural control of human airways in health and disease. Am Rev Respir Dis 1986; 134:1289–1314.
16. Nadel JA, Barnes PJ, Holtzman MJ. Autonomic factors in the hyperreactivity of airway smooth muscle. In: Handbook of Physiology: The Respiratory System III. Washington, DC: American Physiological Society, 1986:693–702.
17. Barnes PJ. Cholinergic control of airway smooth muscle. Am Rev Respir Dis 1987; 136:s42–s45.
18. Richardson JB. Nerve supply to the lung. Am Rev Respir Dis 1979; 119:785–802.
19. Ingram RH, Wellman JJ, McFadden ER, Mead J. Relative contribution of large and small airways to flow limitation in normal subjects before and after atropine and isoproterenol. Clin Invest 1977; 59:693–703.

20. Barnes PJ. Neural control of airway function; new perspectives. Mol Aspects Med 1990; 11: 351–423.
21. Barnes PJ. Modulation of neurotransmission in airways. Physiol Rev 1992; 72:699–729.
22. Barnes PJ. Muscarinic receptors in the lung. Postgrad Med 1987; 63(suppl):13–19.
23. Barnes PJ. Muscarinic receptors in airways: recent developments. J Appl Physiol 1990; 68:1777–1785.
24. Widdicombe J. Neurohumoral mechanisms in obstructive airways disease. In: Anticholinergic Therapy in Obstructive Airways Disease. Franklin Scientific Publication 1993:33–47.
25. Bloom JW, Baumgartener-Folkerts C, Palmer JD, Yamamura HI, Halonen M. A muscarinic receptor subtype modulates vagally stimulated bronchial contraction. J Appl Physiol 1988; 65:2144–2150.
26. Hammer R, Berrie CP, Birdsall NJM, Burgen AS, Hulme EC. Pirenzepine distinguishes between different subclasses of muscarinic receptors. Nature 1980; 283:90–92.
27. Sertl K, Meryn S, Graninger W, Schlick W, Ramers H. Acute effects of pirenzepine on bronchospasm. Int J Clin Pharmacol Ther Toxicol 1986; 24:655–657.
28. Lammers JWJ, Minette P, McCusken K, Barnes PJ. The role of pirenzepine sensitive (M1) muscarinic receptors in vagally mediated bronchoconstriction in humans. A Rev Respir Dis 1989; 139:446–449.
29. Minette PA, Lammers J, Dixon CMS. A muscarinic agonist inhibits reflex bronchoconstriction in normal but not asthmatic subjects. J Appl Physiol 1989; 67:2461–2465.
30. Minette PA, Barnes PJ. Prejunctional inhibitory muscarinic receptors on cholinergic nerves in human and guinea pig airways. J Appl Physiol 1988; 64:2532–2537.
31. Fryer AD, Jacoby DB. Parainfluenza virus infection damages inhibitory M2 muscarinic receptors on pulmonary parasympathetic nerves in the guinea pig. Br Pharmacol 1991; 012:267–271.
32. Mak JCW, Baraniuk JN, Barnes PJ. Localization of muscarinic receptor subtype messenger RNA in human lung. Am Respir Cell Mol Biol 1992; 7:344–348.
33. Bauer R, Banholzer R, Grieben C. Ipratropium bromide. In: Goldberg ME, ed. Pharmacological and Biochemical Properties of Drug Substances. Washington, DC: American Pharmaceutical Association 1979; 485–515.
34. Barnes PJ. Rationale for use of antimuscarinics in obstructive airways disease. Rev Contemp Pharmacother 1992; 3:173–182.
35. Peel ET, Anderson G. A dose response study of oxitropium bromide in chronic bronchitis. Thorax 1984; 39(6):435–436.
36. Minette A, Marcq M. Oxitropium bromide (Ba 253) an advance in the field of anticholinergic bronchodilating treatments. Preliminary results. Rev Inst Hyg Mines 1979; 34(3):115–123.

37. Teramoto S, Ouchi Y. Inhaled oxitropium bromide is currently used as the first line therapy of patients with chronic pulmonary disease in Japan. Euro Respir J 13(2): 473–475, 1999.

38. Ikeda A, Nishimura K, Koyama H, Izumi T. Comparative dose response study of three anticholinergic agents and fenoterol using a metered dose inhaler in patients with chronic obstructive pulmonary disease. Thorax 1995; 50(1):62–66.

39. Mikami M, Nakamura S, Takizawa J, Kawakami M. Flutropium bromide was effective in relieving symptoms of lymphangioleiomyomatosis—a case report. Jpn J Thorac Dis 1997; 35(11):1223–1227.

40. Barnes PJ, Belvisi MG, Mak JCW, Haddad EB, O'Connor B. Tiotropium bromide (Ba 679 Br) A novel long-acting muscarinic antagonist for the treatment of obstructive airways disease. Life Sci 1995; 56(11/12):853–859.

40a. Disse B, Speck GA, Rominger KL, Witek Jr TJ, Hammer R. Tiotropium (Spiriva^{TM}) mechanical considerations and clinical profile in obstructive lung disease. Life Sci 1999; 64(6/7):457–464.

40b. Littner MR, Ilowite JS, Tashkin DP, Friedman M, Servy CW, Menjoge SS, Witek Jr TJ. Long-acting bronchodilation with one-daily dosing of tiotropium (Spiriva) in stable chonic obstructive pulmonary disease. Am J Respir Crit Care Med 2000; 161:1136–1142.

40c. vanNoord JA, Bantje ThA, Eland ME, Korducki L, Cornelissen PJG, on behalf of the Dutch Tiotropium Study Group. Thorax 2000; 55:289–294.

40d. Casaburi R, Mahler DA, Jones PW, Wanner A, San Pedro G, ZuWallack RL, Menjoge SS, Serby CW, Witek Jr T. A long-term evaluation of once-daily inhaled tiotropium in chronic obstructive pulmonary disease. Eur Respir J 2002; 19:217–224.

40e. Vincken W, van Noord JA, Greefhorst APM, Bantje ThA, Kesten S, Korducki L, Cornelissen PJG, on behalf of the Dutch Tiotropium Study Group. Eur Respir J 2002; 19:209–216.

40f. Casaburi R, Briggs Jr DD, Donohue JF, Serby CW, Menjoge SS, Witek Jr TJ, for the US Tiotropium Study Group. Chest 2000; 118:1294–1302.

41. Alabaster VA. Discovery and development of selective M3 antagonist for clinical use. Life Sci 1997; 60(13–14):1053–1060.

42. Devries K. The protective effect of inhaled SCH 1000 MDI on bronchoconstriction induced by seratonin, histamine, acetylcholine and propanolol (abstr) Post Grad Med J 1975; 51(suppl 7):106.

43. Frith PA, Ruffin RE, Cockcroft DW. A comparison of the protective effect of SCH 1000 and fenoterol against bronchoconstriction induced by histamine and methacholine (abstr). J Allergy Clin Immunol 1978; 61:175.

44. Bandouvakis J, Cartier A, Roberts R, Ryan G, Hargreave FE. The effect of ipratropium and fenoterol on methacholine and histamine induced bronchoconstriction. Br J Dis Chest 1981; 75:295–305.

45. O'Connor BJ, Towse LJ, Barnes PJ. Single dose of tiotropium provides protection from methacholine induced bronchoconstriction for 24–48 hrs. Am J Respir Crit Care Med 1996; 154(4 pt 1):876–880.

46. Holtzman MJ, Sheller JR, Dimeo M. Effect of ganglionic blockade on bronchial reactivity in atropine subjects. Am Rev Respir Dis 1980; 122:17–25.
47. Rosenthal RR, Bleeker ER, Laube B, Norman PS. Permutt Cholinergic response to histamine challenge (abstr). J Allergy Clin Immunol 1978; 61:139.
48. Itkin IH, Anand SC. The role of atropine as a mediator blocker of induced bronchial obstruction. J Allergy Clin Immunol 1970; 45:178–186.
49. Caterline CL, Evans R III, Ward GW. The effect of atropine and albuterol on the human response to histamine. J Allergy Clin Immunol 1976; 58:607–613.
50. Germouty J. The possible antagonism between SCH 1000 MDI and beta blocking agents (abstr). Postgrad Med J 1975;51(suppl):103.
51. Gross NJ, Skorodin MS. State of the art: anticholinergic antimuscarinic bronchodilators. Am Rev Respir Dis 1984; 129:856–879.
52. Simonsson BG, Skoogh BE, Bergh NP, Andersson R, Svedmyr N. In vivo and in vitro effects of bradykinin on bronchial motor tone in normal subjects and patients with airways obstruction. Respiration 1973; 30:378–388.
53. Fuller RW, Dixon CM, Cuss FM, Barnes PJ. Bradykinin-induced bronchoconstriction in humans. Mode of action. Am Rev Respir Dis 1987; 135(1):176–180.
54. Nadel JA, Salem H, Tamplin B, Tokiwa Y. Mechanisms of bronchoconstriction during inhalation of sulfur dioxide. J Appl Physiol 1965; 20:164–167.
55. Snashall PD, Baldwin C. Mechanism of sulfur dioxide induced bronchoconstriction in normal and asthmatic men. Thorax 1982; 37:118–123.
56. Tan WC, Cripps E, Douglas N, Sudlow MF. Protective effect of drugs on bronchoconstriction induced sulfur dioxide. Thorax 1982; 37:671–676.
57. Holtzman MJ, Cunnigham JH, Sheller JR, Irsigler GB, Nadel JA, Boushey HA. Effect of ozone on bronchial reactivity in atopic and nonatopic subjects. Am Rev Respir Dis 1979; 120:1059–1067.
58. Simonsson BG, Jacobs FM, Nadel J. Role of autonomic nervous system and the cough reflex in the increased responsiveness of airways in patients with obstructive airways disease. J Clin Invest 1967; 46:1812–1818.
59. Nolte D. The action of ACH 1000 MDI on experimental bronchoconstriction induced by various types of non specific and pharmacodynamic irritants in young asthmatics. Post Grad Med J 1975; 51(suppl):103.
60. Tang JC, Sarosiek I, Yamamoto Y. Cholinergic blockade inhibits gastroesophageal reflux and transient lower esophageal sphincter relaxation through a central mechanism. Gut 1999; 44(5):603–607.
61. Koerselman J, Pursani KG, Peghini P, Mohiuddin MA, Katzka D. Different effects of oral anticholinergic drug on gastroesophageal reflux in upright and supine position in normal, ambulatory subjects, a pilot study. Am J Gastroenterol 1999; 94(4):925–930.
62. McFadden ER, Jr. An analysis of exercise as a stimulus for the production of airway obstruction. Lung 1981; 159:3–11.
63. Deal EC Jr, McFadden ER Jr, Ingram RH, Jaeger JJ. Effects of atropine on protection of exercise-induced bronchospasm by cold air. J Appl Physiol 1978; 45:238–243.

64. Hartley JPR, Davis BH. Cholinergic blockade in the prevention of exercise-induced asthma. Thorax 1980; 35:680–685.

65. Chen WY, Brenner AM, Weiser PC, Chai R. Atropine and exercise-induced bronchoconstriction. Chest 1981; 79:651–656.

66. Thomson NC, Patel KR, Kerr JW. Sodium Chromoglycate and ipratropium bromide in exercise induced asthma. Thorax 1978; 33:694–699.

67. Tashkin DP, Katz RM, Kerschnar H, Rachelefsky GS, Siegel SC. Comparison of aerosolized atropine, isoproterenol, atropine plus isoproterenol, disodium chromoglycate and placebo on the prevention of exercise-induced asthma. Ann Allergy 1977; 39:311–318.

68. Tsukino M, Nishimura K, Ikeda A, Hajiro T, Koyama H, Izumi R. Effects of theophylline and ipratropium bromide on exercise performance in patients with stable chronic obstructive pulmonary disease. Thorax 1998; 53(4):269–273,.

69. Klock LE, Miller TD, Morris AH, Watanabe S, Dickman M. A comparative study of atropine sulfate and isoproterenol hydrochloride in chronic bronchitis. Am Rev Respir Dis 1975; 112:371–376.

70. Barber PV, Chatterjee SS, Scott R. A comparison of ipratropium bromide, deptropine citrate and placebo in asthma and chronic bronchitis. Br J Dis Chest 1977; 71:101–104.

71. Astin TW. Reversibility of airways obstruction in chronic bronchitis. Clin Sci 1972; 42:725–753.

72. Poppius H, Salorinne Y. Comparative trial of a new anticholinergic bronchodilator, SCH 1000 and salbutamol in chronic bronchitis. Br Med J 1973; 4:134–136.

73. Wanner A. Clinical aspects of mucociliary transport. Am Rev Respir Dis 1977; 116:73–125.

74. Foster WM, Bergofsky EH, Bohning DE, Lippman M, Albert RE. Effect of adrenergic agents and their mode of action in mucociliary clearance in man. J Appl Physiol 1976; 41:146–152.

75. Pavia D, Bateman JRM, Sheahan NF, Clark SW. Effect of ipratropium bromide on mucociliary clearance and pulmonary function in reversible airways obstruction. Thorax 1979; 34:501–507.

76. Clark SW, Pavia, D, Agnew JE, Newman SP. Lung mucociliary clearance and the deposition of therapeutic aerosols. Chest 1981; (suppl):921–924.

77. Cockcroft DW, Cotton DJ, Berscheid BA. Long term efficacy and safety of inhaled SCH 1000 on anticholinergic bronchodilator. Curr Ther Res 1982; 31:138–147.

78. Minette A. The effects of long term treatment with SCH 1000 MDI. Postgrad Med J 1975; 51(suppl):153–154.

79. Anthonisen NR, Connett JE, Kiley JP, Altose MD, Bailey WC, Buist AS, Conway WA, Enright PL, Kanner RE, O'Hara P, Owens GR, Scanlon PD, Tashkin DP, Wise RA. The Lung Health Study. Effects of smoking intervention and the use of an inhaled anticholinergic bronchodilator on the rate of decline of FEV$_1$. JAMA 1994; 272(19):1497–1505.

80. Braun SR, McKenzie WN, Copeland C, Knight L, Ellersiek M. A comparison of the effect of ipratropium and albuterol in the treatment of chronic obstructive airways disease. Arch Intern Med 1989; 149:544–547.

81. Sluiter HJ, Koeter GH, de Monchy JGR, Psotma DS, deVries K, Orie NGM. The Dutch hypothesis (chronic nonspecific lung disease) revisited. Eur Respir J 1991; 4:479–489.

82. Hughes JA, Tobin MJ, Bellamy D, Hutchinson DCS. Effects of ipratropium bromide and fenoterol aerosols in pulmonary emphysema. Thorax 1982; 37:667–670.

83. Dorinsky PM, Reisner C, Ferguson GT, Menjoge SS, Serby CW, Witek TJ Jr. The combination of ipratropium and albuterol optimizes pulmonary function reversibility testing in patients with COPD. Chest 1999; 115(4):966–971.

84. Braun SR, Levy SF. Comparison of ipratropium bromide and albuterol in COPD. A three center study. Am J Med 1991; 91(4a):285–325.

85. Campbell S. For COPD a combination of ipratropium bromide and albuterol sulfate is more effective than albuterol alone. Arch Intern Med 1999; 159(2):156–160.

86. Gross NJ, Skorodin MS. Role of the parasympathetic system in airway obstruction due to emphysema. N Engl J Med 1984; 311:421–425.

87. Douglas NJ, Davidson I, Sudlow MF, Flenley DC. Bronchodilation and the site of airway resistance in severe chronic bronchitis. Thorax 1979; 34:51–56.

88. Baigelman W, Chodosh S. Bronochodilator action of the anticholinergic drug, ipratropium bromide (SCH1000) as an aerosol in chronic bronchitis and asthma. Chest 1977; 71:324–328.

89. Petrie GR, Palmer KNV. Comparison of aerosol ipratropium bromide and salbutamol in chronic bronchitis and asthma. Br Med J 1975; 1:430–432.

90. Otto AJ. Comparison of ipratropium bromide and an oral anticholinergic drug in chronic bronchitis. Scand J Respir Dis 1979; 103(suppl):151–152.

91. Lightbody IM, Ingram CG, Legge JS, Johnston RN. Ipratropium bromide, salbutanol and prednisolone in bronchial asthma and chronic bronchitis. Br J Dis Chest 1978; 72:181–186.

92. Easton PA, Jadue C, Dhingra S, Anthonisen NR. A comparison of the bronchodilating effects of a beta 2 adrenergic agent (albuterol) and an anticholinergic agent (ipratropium bromide), given by aerosol alone or in sequence. N Engl J Med 1986; 315:735–739.

93. Blecker ER, Britt EJ. Acute bronchodilating effect of ipratropium bromide and theophylline in chronic obstructive pulmonary disease. Am J Med 1991; 91(4a): 245–275.

94. Lefcoe NM, Toogood JH, Blennerhassett G, Baskerville J, Patterson NAM. The addition of an aerosol anticholinergic to an oral beta agonist plus theophylline in asthma and bronchitis: a double blind single dose study. Chest 1982; 82:300–305.

95. Ajewski Z, Popiak B. The relation between permanent administration of Atrovent and the dose of steroids in chronic bronchitis (abstr). Scand J Respir Dis 1979; 103(supp):205.

96. Jilg J. Long term treatment with SCH 1000 MDI in outpatients with chronic bronchitis (abstr). Postgrad Med J 1975; 51(suppl):13.

97. Ward MJ. The role of anticholinergic drugs in acute asthma. In: Anticholinergic Therapy in Obstructive Airways Disease. Franklin Scientific Publications 1994.

98. Wolstenholme The role of anticholinergic drugs in chronic asthma. In: Antocholinergic Therapy in Obstructive Airways Disease. Franklin Scientific Publications 1994.

99. Connett JE, Kusek JW, Bailey WC, O'Hara P, Wu M. Lung Health Study Research Group. Design of the Lung Health Study. A Randomized Clinical Trial of Early Intervention for Chronic Obstructive Pulmonary Disease. Controlled Clinical Trials 14:3 S195, 1993. Elsevier Science Publishing 1993.

100. Sclar DA, Legge RF, Shaer T. Ipratropium bromide in management of chronic obstructive pulmonary disease: effects on health service expenditure. Clin Ther 16(3):595–601.

101. Jubram A, Gross N, Ramsdell J. Comparitive cost effectiveness analysis of theophylline and ipratropium bromide in chronic obstructive pulmonary disease. A Three Center Study. Chest 1993; 103(3):678–684.

102. Friedman M, Serby CW, Menjoge SS. The pharmacoeconomic evaluation of a combination of ipratropium plus albuterol with ipratropium alone and albuterol alone in COPD. Chest 1999; 115(3):635–641.

103. Rebuck AS, Chapman, KR, Abboud R, Pare PD, Kreisman H, Wolkove N. Nebulized anticholinergic and sympathomimetic treatment of asthma and chronic obstructive airways disease in the emergency room. Am J Med 1987; 82:59–64.

104. O'Driscoll BR, taylor RJ, Horsley MG, Chambers DK, Berstein A. Nebulised salbutamol with and without ipratropium bromide in acute airflow obstruction. Lancet 1989; 1:1418–1420.

105. Karpel JP, Appel D, Breidbart D, Fusco MJ. A comparison of atropine sulfate and metaproterenol sulfate in the emergency treatment of asthma. Am Rev Respir Dis 1986; 133:727–729.

106. Shrestha M, O'brien T, Haddox R, Goulay HS, Reed G. Decreased duration of emergency department treatment of chronic obstructive pulmonary disease exacerbations with the addition of ipratropium bromide to beta agonist therapy. Ann Emerg Med 1991; 20:1206–1209.

107. Donohue JF, van Noord JA, Bateman ED, Langley SJ, Lee A, Witek Jr TJ Kesten S, Towse L. A 6-month, placebo-controlled study comparing lung function and health status changes in COPD patients treated with tiotropium or salmeterol. Chest 2002; 121:1–9.

16

Long-Acting Beta-Adrenoreceptor Agonists for the Treatment of COPD

DIRKJE S. POSTMA

University Hospital Groningen
Groningen, The Netherlands

KLAUS F. RABE

Leiden University Medical Center
Leiden, The Netherlands

I. Introduction

Current national and international guidelines advocate the use of bronchodilators for the treatment of all degrees of severity of chronic obstructive pulmonary disease (COPD). While anticholinergics are preferred as initial therapy in some countries, the combination of beta-adrenoceptor agonists and anticholinergic drugs with a short or long duration of action are preferred and also more effective for moderate disease, sometimes supplemented with the use of theophylline.

Bronchodilators are generally prescribed to symptomatic patients with COPD either for relief of their persistent or worsening symptoms on a p.r.n. basis or regularly to prevent or reduce the development of symptoms, especially dyspnea during exercise. Further improvements by long-acting bronchodilators may include the reduction of mild exacerbations and the possible need for hospitalization and improvement of health status. Long-acting beta-adrenoreceptor agonists were initially introduced for the treatment of bronchial asthma. They have been shown to provide symptomatic benefit, to improve quality of life, and reduce the number of exacerbations and are advocated for use in combination with inhaled corticosteroids in case of asthma. The use of long-acting beta-agonists and long-acting anticholinergic drugs for the treatment of COPD has only been investigated over the past ten years. Since the precise role of inhaled corticosteroids for this disorder is still a matter of debate, it is necessary to assess the role of long-acting bronchodilators for this group of patients.

The response of FEV_1 following inhalation of a bronchodilator has been initially applied to assess its effect for clinical practice. Airflow limitation is a core characteristic of COPD patients and is generally used to define the severity of the disease. Moreover, FEV_1 is considered the best currently available predictor for long-term prognosis in COPD. However, for an individual patient it is important to perceive the acute effects of the drug used. Since a change in FEV_1 is not always associated with a change in symptoms, FEV_1 should not be the only parameter to assess drug effects in COPD. Thus, symptoms such as the severity of breathlessness, limitation of exercise capacity, and health status are important clinical endpoints in assessing drug efficacy, especially since they are not always related to airflow limitation. Additionally, the role of airway smooth muscle contraction as a contributing factor to airflow limitation may be highly variable between patients. O'Donnell et al. (1) evaluated the bronchodilator response in 84 patients with stable COPD who were considered irreversible, as defined by 10% change in FEV_1 after inhalation of 200 µg of salbutamol. They showed that 83% of this population had significant improvements in one or more lung volumes, especially those reflecting lung hyperinflation, even in the absence of changes in FEV_1 after bronchodilator treatment. These changes may simply reflect the frequently found improvements in dyspnea in COPD patients without significant spirometric changes. A study of Taube et al. (2) showed that measurement of forced inspiratory volume following a short-acting beta-agonist reflected symptomatic improvement better than measurements of forced expiratory volumes (Fig. 1). This may well also be the case for long-acting beta-agonists. Therefore, studies evaluating the clinical benefits of long-acting bronchodilators for COPD have to take several endpoints into consideration in addition to FEV_1, such as effort of independent lung function parameters, exercise capacity, parameters of quality of life, and frequency of exacerbations.

The preferred route of application for bronchodilators is inhalation, although in elderly patients with COPD coordinated drug application may pose a problem. Oral bambuterol is available for the treatment of COPD, but its clinical efficacy is poorly documented. In fact, the only published study was a double-blind, double-dummy, crossover, placebo-controlled and randomized trial study comparing the efficacy and safety of 20 mg oral bambuterol and 50 µg inhaled salmeterol in patients with "partially

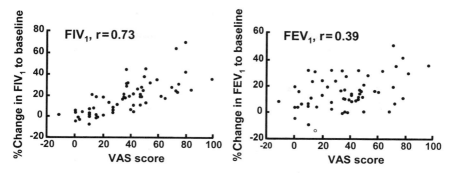

Figure 1 Perception of dyspnea as measured with VAS score in relation to inspiratory (left) and expiratory (right) volume in 1 second. (From Ref. 2.)

reversible" COPD (3). The onset and duration of action of bambuterol and salmeterol were compared in 16 patients. Lung function (FEV_1, FVC) and systemic effects such as tremor, heart rate, and blood pressure were monitored prior to the administration of the drug and for 12 hours after drug application. In this study, inhalation of salmeterol and bambuterol both induced a significant increase in lung function when compared with placebo. There was no significant difference between the overall effects of salmeterol and bambuterol. Notably, bambuterol, but not salmeterol, caused tremor in four patients and induced a greater increase in heart rate when compared with salmeterol; these differences were statistically significant after 9 and 12 hours. The authors concluded that both oral bambuterol and inhaled salmeterol resulted in a long-lasting bronchodilation in patients with stable COPD. However, bambuterol seemed to be associated with more systemic side effects.

Due to considerations of the preferred route of drug administration and the paucity of other data, this chapter aims to review the current literature on inhaled long-acting beta-adrenoceptor agonists, specifically formoterol and salmeterol, for patients with COPD.

II. Mechanism of Action

Beta-adrenoceptor agonists relax airways primarily through direct interaction with $beta_2$-adrenoceptors on smooth muscle. This interaction results ultimately in the elevation of intracellular cyclic adenosine monophosphate levels leading to relaxation and protection against subsequent bronchoconstrictor stimulation. The onset and duration of action of this class of drugs depends on the kinetics and time of agonist–receptor interaction and is partly related to the lipophilicity of a given drug and its chemical struture. Formoterol and salmeterol have both been shown—first in bronchial asthma and then in COPD—to have a duration of action of at least 12 hours, and although the underlying mechanism of the prolonged duration of these compounds may differ, a detailed discussion falls outside the scope of this chapter.

III. Studies with Formoterol

A. Lung Function

One of the first studies investigating formoterol in patients with COPD was performed by Schultze-Werninghaus (4) in 1990. In this open multicenter trial, performed in 242 subjects with chronic obstructive airways disease, 12 µg formoterol was given by metered-dose inhaler twice daily. Investigations were performed at days 0, 14, and subsequently at monthly intervals for one year. Airway resistance decreased by 43.5% at 1 year while the FEV_1 increased from 1.90 ± 0.80 to 2.54 ± 0.97 L or 33.7%. The global assessment of therapeutic efficacy was classified in arbitrary scales such as "very good" in 51% of patients and 47% of doctors, respectively, and as "good" in 38.7% and 42.0%, respectively. Tolerability was described as "very good" in 82.3% of patients and doctors, and "good" in 12.7% of patients and 13.7% of doctors. The treatment did not influence blood pressure or heart rate.

In single-dose experiments, Cazzola et al. (5) found a dose-dependent increase in spirometric parameters with (12, 24, and 36 µg), and in contrast to the study of Celik et al. (6) (see also below), the mean peak in bronchodilatation was more rapid than that observed with salmeterol. Maesen et al. (7) published the effects of formoterol on effort-dependent and effort-independent lung function parameters in patients with apparently poorly reversible COPD. This randomized, double-blind, placebo-controlled, crossover study investigated the effects of formoterol in 12 current or ex-smokers having COPD, with a mean FEV_1 of 47% of predicted and a poor reversibility after terbutaline sulfate inhalation. After inhaling a single dose of 6 or 24 µg formoterol or placebo via Turbuhaler, FEV_1, work of breathing (WoB), and airway resistance (Raw) were recorded over 12 hours on 3 test days. Compared to placebo, both doses of formoterol induced a clinically and statistically relevant improvement in WoB (>25%) and Raw (>20%). This occurred within 10 minutes and lasted over a period of 12 hours (Fig. 2). This signifies that inhaled formoterol causes long-lasting lung function improvements in patients with apparently poorly reversible COPD

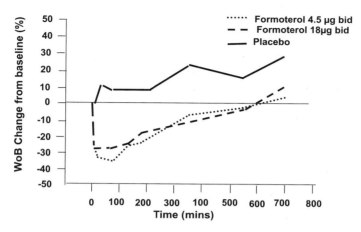

Figure 2 Formoterol reduces work of breathing. (From Ref. 7.)

and that additional lung function measurements during quiet breathing after forced expiration tests may be useful in COPD patients to assess beneficial effects of bronchodilators. DiMarco et al. (8) corroborated and extended these findings, describing a far greater improvement in inspiratory capacity than in FEV_1. The improvement in dyspnea correlated best with improvement in inspiratory capacity. Furthermore, formoterol elicited the greatest improvements in inspiratory capacity compared with salbutamol, salmeterol, and oxitropium, a finding that requires more studies.

Rossi et al. (9) investigated treatment during one year of follow-up. It appeared that FEV_1 improved similarly to a single dose of formoterol of 12 and 24 µg per dry powder inhalation via breath-activated inhaler. There was no tolerance development since this bronchodilator effect was still present after 3 and 12 months of treatment, and reversibility was similar throughout the study, and significantly better than with placebo (with on-demand salbutamol).

B. Combination of Formoterol with Other Bronchodilators

Since bronchodilator therapy for COPD is invariably not relying on a single agent, combination trials with anticholingeric drugs are warranted and some clinical data are already available in the literature. The study of Sichletidis and coworkers (10) investigated bronchodilator responses to formoterol, ipratropium, and their combination in 27 patients with stable COPD in a randomized, placebo-controlled trial. Each patient was assigned on 6 separate days to receive either 40 or 80 µg ipratropium bromide, 12 or 24 µg formoterol fumarate, or 12 µg formoterol plus 40 µg ipratoropium. Mean peak FEV_1 was maximal with the administration of the combination of ipratropium and formoterol, and it differed significantly from the observed peak changes following single administration of the two tested doses of ipratropium. Due to the different signal transduction mechanisms of beta-adrenoceptor agonists and anticholinergic drugs, these findings are not really surprising but underline the assertions that combination therapy with different (long-acting) bronchodilators yield the best functional results.

A further investigation of Cazzola et al. (11) investigated the effect of higher than conventional doses of oxitropium bromide on formoterol-induced bronchodilatation in COPD. Twenty outpatients inhaled 12 or 24 µg formoterol, and 2 hours later a dose-response curve to 100 µg inhaled oxitropium bromide or placebo was constructed up to a total cumulative dose of 600 µg oxitropium bromide. Doses were given at 20-minute intervals and measurements made 15 minutes after each dose. This study also demonstrated a small incremental benefit of high doses of oxitropium when added to formoterol in patients with stable COPD and a certain degree of reversibility. Almost the same conclusion was obtained through a further study from the same group of investigators (12) when conventional doses of oxitropium bromide (200 µg) were added to either 12 or 24 µg formoterol. In this group of 16 patients with COPD a dose difference between the two formoterol applications was observed.

C. Symptoms

Dahl et al. (13) reported that doses of 12 or 24 µg formoterol dry powder capsules via Foradil Aerolizer b.i.d. provided significant improvements in symptoms during a 12-week period in COPD patients with a mean FEV_1 of 45% predicted. This was accompanied by a concurrent reduction in rescue use of salbutamol. This was confirmed in a study by Aalbers et al. (14) investigating COPD patients with an FEV_1 of 54% predicted and variable reversibility (6.4% FEV_1 predicted in the mean) of airway obstruction following a beta-agonist. The average symptom score was 5.64 (range 1.0–14.2) at run-in, and a significant reduction of 13% was obtained with 18 µg formoterol inhaled via Turbuhaler, but not with 9 and 4.5 µg when compared to placebo over a 3-month treatment period. The number of days that patients were free of symptoms was 6.6% with placebo, and 21, 71, and 86% with treatment of 4.5, 9, and 18 µg of formoterol, respectively. The difference with placebo was significant for the two highest doses of formoterol, concurrent with a significant difference in reduction of the need for relief medication.

D. Exercise Performance

There are only a few recent studies on the effects of formoterol on exercise capacity. One study from Liesker et al. (15) investigated 47 COPD patients (mean FEV_1 55.6% predicted). They showed that both 1-week treatment with (4, 5, 9, or 18 μg formoterol via Turbuhaler) or ipratropium (80 μg via pMDI with spacer) resulted in prolonged time to exhaustion during a cycle ergometer exercise test compared to placebo. Interestingly there was a negative dose-response relationship for the three doses of formoterol (Fig. 3), the lowest dose corresponding with the longest exercise time, though the Borg scores reached were similar with the four different treatment strategies (approximately 7.6 out of a maximum of 10). This was not due to a better lung function with the lower dose of formoterol, since this showed in fact the dose-response effect. The authors suggest that increasing ventilation-perfusion mismatch at higher doses, due to vasodilatation, accounts for this effect but that this clearly needs further study.

Wadbo et al. (16) investigated 183 COPD patients with a mean FEV_1 of 40% predicted and a baseline incremental shuttle-walking test (SWT) of 325 m. A clinically significant improvement of 30 m in the SWT was

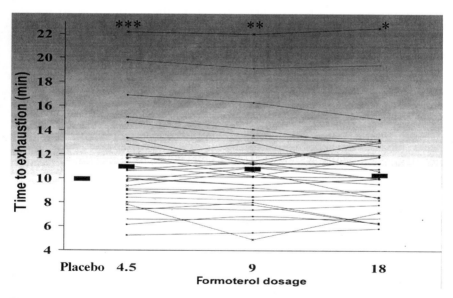

Figure 3 Formoterol prolongs the time to exhaustion compared with placebo: a significant dose-response effect (see text). (From Ref. 14.)

reached by similar percentages of patients during treatment with 18 μg of formoterol b.i.d., 80 μg ipratropium t.i.d., and placebo during 12 weeks. FEV_1 values, in contrast, improved similarly with formoterol and ipratropium and significantly better than with placebo.

The final available study was also published in 2002, with exercise being analyzed by SWT in 645 COPD patients (9). Formoterol improved lung function with treatment of 4.5, 9, and 18 μg after 3 months, yet this was not accompanied by SWT improvements, which appeared to be fairly small and variable both with treatment and placebo. The authors suggest that the lack of improvement was due to the large variability within the study population (60–102 m) and the fact that maximal performance had most likely not been reached, given the low Borg dyspnea scores reached (approximately 4 out of a maximum of 10).

E. Exacerbations

Dahl et al. suggested that that there were no significant differences between and placebo (12) in the number of days requiring additional therapy for exacerbations of COPD. Rossi et al. (16) found that the number of "bad days" (days with at least two individual symptom scores over 2 and/or reduction in Peak Expiratory Flour (PEF) more than 20% from run in) was significantly reduced by formoterol treatment during one year of follow-up. Also, the percentage of individuals receiving additional treatment for an exacerbation was reduced. Thus, 34% of COPD patients treated with placebo, 22% treated with formoterol 12 μg, and 34% treated with formoterol 24 μg experienced an exacerbation, a significant difference being reached for 24 μg and placebo treatment only. Finally, Szafranski et al. (17) showed that formoterol 6 μg b.i.d. significantly reduced the number of mild exacerbations significantly by 55% ($p < 0.001$), yet not the severe exacerbations (requiring oral steroid) compared with placebo treatment (Fig. 4).

F. Quality of life

Dahl et al. (12) showed that quality of life (QoL) improved with treatment of 12 and 24 μg during 12 weeks, in contrast to similar treatment duration with ipratropium 40 μg q.i.d. The dose of 12 μg provided a significant difference with ipratropium and placebo, whereas neither 24 μg nor ipratropium were significantly different from placebo or from each other. In contrast, Rossi et al. (16) showed a significant improvement in QoL with formoterol treatment (12 or 24 μg per dry powder via breath-activated inhaler).

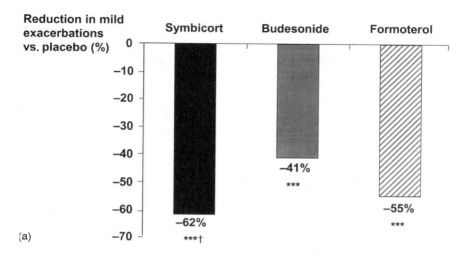

(a)

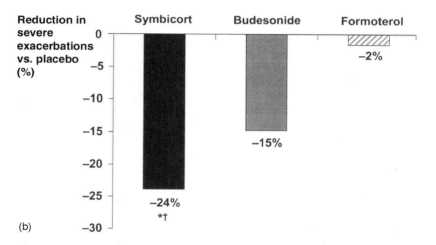

(b)

Figure 4 Long-term treatment with formoterol reduced the number of mild exacerbations (a) but not severe exacerbations (b). (a:***$p < 0.0001$ vs. placebo; †$p < 0.05$ Symbicort vs. budesonide. b:*$p < 0.05$ vs. placebo; †$p < 0.05$ Symbicort vs. formoterol.) (From Ref. 17.)

IV. Studies with Salmeterol

One of the first studies conducted with salmeterol for the treatment of COPD was published by Ulrik in 1995 (18,19). The efficacy of salmeterol

50 µg b.i.d. in smokers with moderate to severe COPD was investigated in a double-blind, randomized, crossover comparison in 63 patients with stable COPD with an FEV_1 of <60% of predicted and an improvement in FEV_1 of <15% following 400 µg inhaled salbutamol. Efficacy was measured as change in morning and evening peak expiratory flow rates, respiratory symptoms, and use of rescue salbutamol. Morning PEF values were higher during the salmeterol compared to the placebo period, although the mean treatment difference was small—12 L/min. No difference in mean evening PEF values was found, and the mean spirometric values obtained at the end of the two treatment periods were also similar. Compared with placebo, however, treatment with salmeterol was associated with fewer symptoms and less use of rescue salbutamol during both the day and the night. Many studies have supported these findings, and Rennard et al. (20) have recently shown that the effect of salmeterol treatment on FEV_1 and FVC cannot simply be predicted by the level of reversibility on a bronchodilator test with salbutamol.

A. Symptoms

Boyd et al. (21) investigated 647 COPD patients (baseline $FEV_1 \approx 1.30$ L) and concluded that symptoms improved both with 50 and 100 µg salmeterol b.i.d., but that the dose of 50 µg was better tolerated. Another study that addressed perception of dyspnea in COPD patients was performed in a small a group of 16 patients and published by Ramirez-Venegas et al. (22). The authors demonstrated improvements in lung function (FEV_1 and FVC at all time periods) and lower values for functional residual capacity and residual volume. Significantly lower dyspnea scores during resistive breathing accompanied these changes with salmeterol compared with placebo. Using a multidimensional instrument to measure dyspnea based on activities of living—the Transition Dyspnea Index (TDI)—Mahler et al. (23) showed that salmeterol reduced dyspnea after 2, 4, 8, and 10 weeks of treatment. However, in a similarly designed study, Rennard et al. (20) did not find significant differences. ZuWallack et al. (24) showed an improvement of 1.3 TDI units with salmeterol after 12 weeks of treatment compared with 1.1 and 1.9 TDI units improvement with treatment of theophylline or the combination of theophylline and salmeterol, respectively.

B. Exercise Capacity

Exercise capacity as an endpoint for interventions with long-acting bronchodilators in COPD was first measured in the study by Grove et al. (25). Twenty-nine patients with an FEV_1 of 42% of predicted and 5–15% reversibility to salbutamol 200 µg were randomized to receive salmeterol

50 µg twice daily for 4 weeks. In this study salmeterol produced a small improvement in spirometric values compared with placebo consistent with the degree of reversibility to salbutamol 200 µg originally shown by the subjects. This was not associated with improvements in adaptaion capacity measured with a cycle-ergometer test or in exercise capacity assessed by 6-minute walking distance, but there was some symptomatic benefit since patients were able to walk the same distance in 6 minutes with less perceived exertion. Boyd et al. (21) investigated the effects of salmeterol 50 and 100 µg b.i.d. for 16 weeks on symptoms, lung function, and exercise with a 6-minute walking test. They also found no improvement in exercise capacity with either of the doses used, but confirmed that treatment with 50 µg salmeterol b.i.d. resulted in less dyspnea with the same level of walking distance at 8 and 16 weeks of follow-up, possibly reflecting better tolerance than the use of 100 µg b.i.d. (see Sec. IV.A). Finally, Mahler et al. (23) and Rennard et al. (20) compared 50 µg salmeterol b.i.d. with placebo for 12 weeks, again without a significant difference in 6-minute walking distance.

C. Exacerbations

Rennard et al. (20) showed that the percentage of patients experiencing one or more COPD exacerbations over the 12-week treatment period were 30.4, 28.8, and 26.8% with placebo, salmeterol (50 µg b.i.d.), and ipratropium bromide (40 µg q.i.d.), respectively. Mahler et al. (23), in contrast, found a significant difference between salmeterol and placebo with regard to time to onset of first exacerbation (Fig. 5). One study investigated the effects of salmeterol over 12 months of follow-up, a period in which exacerbations can accurately be assessed. In this study (28), salmeterol improved the number of exacerbation significantly when compared with placebo, i.e., the number of exacerbation per patient per year was 1.04 with salmeterol and 1.30 with placebo. Interestingly Dowling et al. (26,27) reported that salmeterol reduced respiratory epithelial damage induced by *Haemophilus influenzae* and by *Pseudomonas aeruginosa*. They attributed this to the fact that salmeterol may maintain the intracellular concentrations of cyclic adenosine monophosphate. This clearly requires further investigation.

D. Quality of Life

Jones and Bosh (29) investigated the effects of 50 and 100 µg salmeterol on changes in health-related quality of life (HRQoL) using the Disease-Specific St. George's Respiratory Questionnaire (SGRQ) and the Medical Outcomes Study Short Form 36 (SF-36) in COPD patients. In a total of 283 patients, salmeterol 50 µg twice daily was associated with significant improvement in SGRQ scores. This exceeded the threshold for a clinically significant

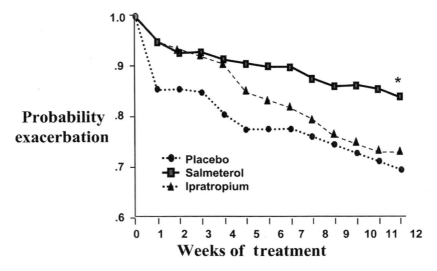

Figure 5   Significantly longer time to exacerbation with salmeterol treatment than with ipratropium bromide treatment. (*Significant vs. ip, $p = 0.0411$, and placebo, $p = 0.0052$.) (From Ref. 23.)

improvement in SGRQ (more than 4 units), but this effect was not seen with salmeterol 100 µg probably due to the side effects of the higher dose (Fig. 6). Changes in SGRQ and SF-36 scores correlated and also showed a weak but significant relationship with FEV_1.

Rennard et al. (20) found a beneficial effect of salmeterol on health status as well using a different measure of quality of life, the Chronic Respiratory Disease Questionnaire (CRDQ), but without a significant difference from placebo over 4 months of follow-up. They attributed this to the longer duration of measurements in the study by Jones (4 months) or the type of questionnaire used. Yet this is unlikely, since Mahler et al. (23) found an improvement in quality of life with the same CRDQ with 50 µg of salmeterol during 12-weeks treatment. The studies are difficult to compare since Rennard showed FEV_1 percent predicted values at baseline, whereas Mahler used absolute FEV_1 values, and baseline levels of CRDQ were not given in the study of Rennard et al. (20). It may thus well be that differences in outcome are determined by the severity of COPD and/or by the level of health status at baseline.

Finally, one study compared placebo, salmeterol (50 µg b.i.d.) with fluticasone and the combination of fluticasone and salmeterol over 12 months of follow-up in COPD patients with an FEV_1 of approximately

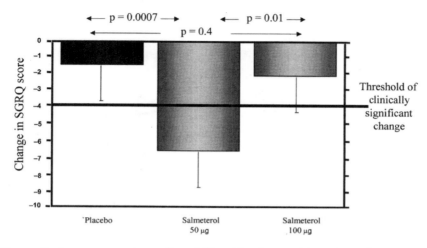

Figure 6 Improvement in quality of life with salmeterol in a dose of 50 µg twice daily yet not with 100 µg twice daily. (From Ref. 29.)

45% predicted (28). Salmeterol improved lung function, symptoms and health status and reduced the use of rescue medication and frequency of exacerbations (Fig. 7).

E. Comparison with Other Bronchodilators

A direct comparison between salmeterol and ipratropium bromide on breathlessness and gas exchange during exercise in 15 patients with COPD was performed by Patakas et al. (30). Compared to placebo, inhalation of both drugs resulted equally in small but significant improvement in airflow limitation and increase in walking distance. Notably, dyspnea decreased after salmeterol and after ipratorpium bromide to a similar extent, while another comparison by Mahler et al. (23) favored the use of salmeterol as first-line bronchodilator therapy for the long-term treatment of airway obstruction in patients with COPD (Fig. 7).

A direct comparison between salmeterol (50 µg b.i.d.) and the long-acting anticholinergic drug tiotropium bromide (8 µg once daily) in 623 patients with an FEV_1 of approximately 1.10 L (31) showed that FEV_1 increased significantly more in the tiotropium group (0.14 L) when compared to placebo than in the salmeterol arm (0.09 L). Tiotropium improved the TDI score by 1.02 units, whereas there was no significant difference between placebo and salmeterol. Both drugs reduced the need for additional bronchodilator use. Finally, tiotropium provided a significantly

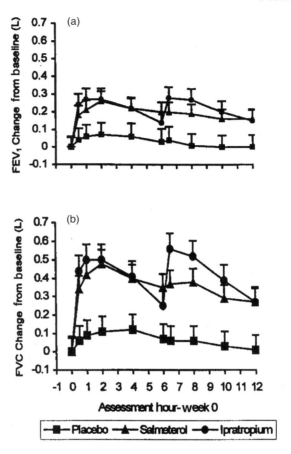

Figure 7 Salmeterol gives similar maximal bronchodilation as ipratropium bromide, but maintained with 12-hour duration: bronchodilation assessed with (a) FEV_1; (b) FVC. (From Ref. 20.)

better improvement in the HRQoL questionnaire than placebo—5.14 and 2.43 units, respectively (4 units being regarded as a clinically significant difference). Salmeterol improved HRQoL by 3.54 units, not significantly different from placebo (2.43 units).

A combined study in 1207 COPD patients comparing 6 months of treatment with tiotropium 18 µg (via Handihaler) once daily with salmeterol 50 µg twice daily via a metered-dose inhaler showed that both groups had significantly fewer days in hospital than patients taking placebo (32).

Tiotropium provided significantly fewer exacerbations per patient-year than placebo, without a significant difference between salmeterol and placebo. Whether this discrepancy with other studies is due to the patients enrolled or the inhaler used remains a matter of debate. Furthermore, a high proportion of the placebo-treated patients (39%) had a clinically meaningful improvement in health status, somewhat higher than in previous studies. A direct comparison of efficacy, tolerability, and effects on QoL of inhaled salmeterol 50 µg bio and titrated oral theophylline in patients with mild-to-moderate COPD was performed by Di Lorenzo et al. (33). One of the objectives of this study in 178 subjects was to assess changes in QoL using the SF-36 Health Survey. Both drugs improved QoL as measured by the SF-36 questionnaire, but salmeterol therapy was effective in more aspects, and the improvements seen in each were numerically greater than those seen with theophylline therapy. Statistically different changes between the two treatment groups were reported for physical functioning, changes in health perception, and social functioning.

In the meantime, a series of controlled clinical trials has been published underlining the usefulness of long-acting bronchodilator therapy in general (34), studying especially the effectiveness of salmeterol (35) and also comparing the effect of the drug to other accepted drug regimens for the treatment of COPD (36).

V. Trials Comparing Formoterol and Salmeterol

Several direct comparison trials of formoterol and salmeterol in patients with COPD have been published with single-dose bronchodilators (5,6,37). Two studies by Cazzola et al. (37,38) investigated the time course of inhaled salmeterol and formoterol on bronchodilation in comparison with that of inhaled salbutamol and placebo in 16 patients with moderate to severe COPD. The study was performed using a single-blind crossover randomized study. The bronchodilator effect of 200 µg salbutamol, 50 µg salmeterol, 24 µg formoterol, and placebo, all inhaled from a metered-dose inhaler, was investigated. Interestingly, and like the study of Celik et al. (6), similar times of onset to 15% improvement in FEV_1 were observed for salmeterol and formoterol, while salbutamol was faster in onset than any of the long-acting drugs. The duration of action showed clear differences between the two long-acting drugs and salbutamol. The results were interpreted as indicative that long-acting $beta_2$-agonists are effective in improving airway caliber in patients suffering from COPD. Although the onset of bronchodilation after inhaling salmeterol and formoterol was slightly delayed compared with salbutamol, the authors regarded this to be of little clinical relevance as they argued that these patients would receive these drugs for maintenance treatment and not immediate symptomatic relief, a statement that can be questioned.

The second study investigated the dose-response relation of salmeterol and formoterol in so-called partially reversible severe COPD and compared the time course of 25, 50, and 75 μg inhaled salmeterol and 12, 24, and 36 μg formoterol in a group of 12 patients with partially reversible, but severe COPD with an FEV_1 of 12–32% of predicted. All doses of salmeterol and formoterol induced a significant spirometric improvement over the 12-hour monitoring period when compared to the spirometric improvement after placebo. Interestingly, formoterol but not salmeterol induced a dose-dependent increase in FVC, FEV_1, and FEF40. Mean peak bronchodilation, expressed as increase in FEV_1 over baseline values, occurred 2 hours after inhalation of the three doses of salmeterol and 1 hour after inhalation of the three doses of formoterol. A comparison of 50 μg salmeterol with 12 or 24 μg formoterol showed that improvement of FEV_1 after salmeterol was statistically higher than that after the two doses of formoterol, although the mean peak bronchodilations were similar owing to the fact that in this study salmeterol had a longer duration of action than formoterol.

The long duration of action of long-acting beta-adrenoceptor agonists has also been shown in patients with COPD. Celik et al. (6) directly compared the onset and duration of action of a single inhalation of formoterol and salmeterol in COPD patients having "partially reversible" airway obstruction. In this double-blind, randomized, crossover and placebo-controlled study design, the respiratory functions of 22 patients with mild to severe COPD and a mean baseline reversibility of FEV_1 of $19.3 \pm 3.1\%$ were evaluated after inhalation of 12 and 50 μg salmeterol. Again, the onset of action of formoterol was not significantly quicker than that of salmeterol. At 20 minutes both formoterol (0.25 L) and salmeterol (0.20 L) produced a significant increase in FEV_1 compared to baseline and placebo. The duration of action, the 12-hour values of both formoterol (0.25 L) and salmeterol (0.22 L), was significantly higher than that of placebo (– 0.12 L). The area under the curve values of FEV_1 of formoterol and salmeterol over 12 hours were comparable and higher than placebo values. This study demonstrates that a single dose of 12 μg formoterol and 50 μg salmeterol provides comparable bronchodilation over 12 hours in patients with mild to severe COPD. It has to be said, however, that this study, as well as others described above, describe effects on airway caliber in COPD patients that have a marked bronchodilator response—a finding not shared by all patients, especially those with more severe disease.

VI. Side Effects

If long-acting bronchodilators such as formoterol and salmeterol were to be given to patients on a symptom-oriented basis, then side effects of higher doses of these drugs would be of particular concern. Additionally, due to the known cardiovascular comorbidity of COPD patients, unwanted effects on the cardiovascular system and serum potassium levels need to be closely investigated.

Maesen et al. (39) investigated the effect of maximal doses of formoterol and salbutamol from a metered-dose inhaler on pulse rate, ECG, and serum potassium concentrations in 13 patients with stable and reversible asthma. The maximal individual dose of formoterol administered was 84 µg in six patients, 132 µg in three patients, 180 µg in three patients, and 228 µg in one patient. For salbutamol, the maximal individual dose was 400 µg in three patients, 2200 µg in eight patients, 3000 µg in one patient, and 3800 µg in one patient. The mean maximal increase in FEV_1 was 36.0% after formoterol and 35.1% after salbutamol. Pulse rate increased from 73 to 83 beats/min after formoterol and from 75 to 84 beats/min with salbutamol. At these high doses, no changes in mean potassium levels were observed, and the lowest individual postassium level recorded was $3.1 \, \text{mmol} \times L^{-1}$. No clinically important changes in ECG were observed, and the authors concluded that even very high doses of formoterol and salbutamol administered from a metered-dose inhaler are safe for patients, a conclusion supported by another study in asthmatic patients by Tøtterman et al. (40).

The short-term cardiovascular effects of salmeterol were investigated by Tranfa et al. (41). Eight healthy subjects and eight patients with reversible airway obstruction and without cardiovascular alterations were treated with 50 µg of salmeterol twice a day for 3 days and then with 100 µg of salmeterol twice a day for a further 3-day period. The 24-hour ECG (Holter) monitoring and measurement of arterial BP, performed on the admission day and on the third and the sixth days of pharmacological treatment, showed that salmeterol did not produce any significant change in mean heart rate, number of supraventricular premature complexes, or BP. Furthermore, no ECG abnormality related to myocardial ischemia was recorded during 24-hour Holter monitoring. These data suggest that salmeterol, administered in regular and high doses for a short period, does not cause significant cardiovascular effects in either normal subjects or patients with reversible airway obstruction.

This may be different in patients suffering from COPD who have preexisting cardiac arrhythmias and hypoxemia. Another study by Cazzola et al. (42) was conducted with a randomized, crossover, and placebo-controlled design to assess the cardiac effects of two single doses of formoterol (12 and 24 µg) and one single dose of salmeterol (50 µg) in 12 patients suffering from COPD with preexisting cardiac arrhythmias and hypoxemia (Pa_{O_2} < 60 mmHg). Each patient was evaluated at screening visit including spirometery, blood gas analysis, serum potassium measurement, and 12-lead ECG. All patients underwent 24-hour Holter monitoring during each of the four treatments. Serum potassium level was measured before drug inhalation, at 2-hour intervals for 6 hours, and at 9, 12, and 24 hours following drug administration. Holter monitoring showed an increase in heart rate at 24 µg formoterol that differed from 12 µg formoterol and salmeterol 50 µg. Furthermore, supraventricular or ventricular premature beats occurred more often after formoterol 24 µg. Formoterol 24 µg also significantly reduced the serum potassium level at 9 hours when compared to placebo, while formoterol 12 µg was only different after 2 hours. Salmeterol 50 µg affected serum potassium from 4 to 6 hours. These results suggest that preexisting cardiac arrhythmias and hypoxemia need to be taken into consideration in patients with COPD, since long-acting beta-agonists may have adverse cardiac effect in susceptible individuals.

One recent study by Khoukaz and Gross (43) investigated one particular aspect of possible side effects of long-acting bronchodilators, namely their negative effect on blood oxygen levels, which has been attributed to the effect of these drugs on the pulmonary vasculature. The authors compared the acute effects on gas exchange of salmeterol with those of albuterol and the anticholinergic agent ipratropium in 20 patients with stable COPD. A small but statistically significant decline in Pa_{O_2}, the primary outcome variable, was found after administration of both salmeterol and albuterol. The decline in Pa_{O_2} after salmeterol was of lesser magnitude but was more prolonged than that after albuterol, the greatest mean change being -2.74 ± 0.89 mmHg at 30 minutes after salmeterol, and -3.45 ± 0.92 mmHg at 20 minutes. These declines, which were almost entirely attributable to an increase in the alveolar-arterial difference in oxygen tension tended to be more marked in subjects with higher baseline Pa_{O_2} values, and no subject experienced a decline in Pa_{O_2} to levels below 59 mmHg. There were no significant differences among the three drugs studied. The authors concluded that despite small decreases in Pa_{O_2} after each of the three drugs, the declines were small and of doubtful clinical significance.

Finally, the regular use of long-acting bronchodilators might interfere with the efficacy of short-acting bronchodilators such as salbutamol. The effects of formoterol, salmeterol, and oxitropium bromide on airway responses to salbutamol were evaluated in COPD (44). Sixteen outpatients with partially reversible, stable COPD received either 24 µg formoterol, 50 µg salmeterol, 200 µg oxitropium bromide, or placebo on

4 nonconsecutive days. A dose-response curve to inhaled salbutamol was then constructed using doses of 100, 100, 200, and 400 μg. The study demonstrated that pretreatment with a conventional dose of formoterol, salmeterol, or oxitropium bromide does not preclude the possibility of inducing a further bronchodilation with salbutamol in patients suffering from partially reversible COPD.

A similar study design investigating the acute effect of pretreatment with a single conventional dose of salmeterol on the dose-response curve to oxitropium bromide in COPD (45) also concluded that acute pretreatment with 50 μg salmeterol does not block the possibility of inducing further bronchodilation with an anticholinergic agent when a higher-than-normal dosage of the muscarinic antagonist (600 μg) is used.

VII. Economic Evaluation

One study evaluated the economic impact of formoterol dry powder (12 μg b.i.d.) versus ipratropium bromide pressurized metered-dose inhaler (40 μg q.i.d.) in the treatment of COPD (46). The cost analysis with respect to FEV_1 revealed an economic efficiency frontier formed by placebo, ipratropium, and formoterol, with cost-effectiveness ratios per FEV_1 change of $30.18, $53.50, and $142.04, respectively. Formoterol, however, provided better quality of life outcomes than ipratropium, with an additional cost of $554.28 per year. This represents the incremental cost to purchase 0.086 L additional FEV_1 change and 5.5 additional SGRQ points with formoterol 12 μg over ipratropium bromide. Outcomes were based on a 12-week study. This study was limited to drug and additional drug costs; it did not investigate hospital costs and other health care resources—the benefit might have been larger taking this into account. Thus, future studies must assess whether these short-term benefits would lead to long-term favorable health and economic outcomes.

Jones et al. (47) assessed the cost-effectiveness of salmeterol (50 μg b.i.d.) in patients with COPD (FEV_1 about 1.30 L, 45% predicted) in a 16-week study. Addition of salmeterol to COPD patients' current therapy improved lung function and health status at the expense of a modest increase in costs compared with usual therapy. The total health care costs were increased in the salmeterol group, but hospital and physician visit costs and concurrent COPD medication costs were lower. The reduction in hospital costs was sufficient to offset the substantial portion of acquisition costs of salmeterol. Since this study was performed over 16 weeks of follow-up, it was not possible to incorporate quality-adjusted life-years, a measure that would allow comparison between studies. Further studies are needed to assess whether the outcome is substantiated with longer follow-up periods.

VIII. Conclusion and Perspectives

Long-acting bronchodilators such as formoterol and salmeterol clearly have added to the therapeutic options in treating COPD. These drugs are effective in increasing airway caliber over a prolonged period of time and improve exercise capacity and parameters of quality of life. They furthermore reduce the number of (mild) exacerbations and add in certain aspects to the cost-effectiveness of COPD management. On-demand use appears to be possible since the safety data available so far are reassuring. Interestingly, the clear difference in the onset of action between formoterol and salmeterol is less obvious in patients with COPD. Data on the development of tolerance to the bronchodilator effects of formoterol and salmeterol in patients with COPD are, however, missing, and the potential protective role of steroids has not yet been addressed in this context.

Finally, while acute symptomatic relief and bronchodilatation are well documented for this class of drugs, their long-term effects, either alone or in combination with long-acting anticholinergic drugs, on airway caliber including the rate of lung function decline have not been extensively investigated. This clearly warrants further study, especially since the potential effects of these drugs might expand beyond bronchodilator efficacy.

References

1. O'Donnell DE, Forkert L, Webb KA. Evaluation of bronchodilator responses in patients with "irreversible" emphysema. Eur Respir J 2001; 18:913–920.
2. Taube C, Lehnigk B, Paasch K, Kirsten DK, Jones RA, Magnussen H. Factor analysis of changes in dyspnea and lung function parameters after bronchodilation in chronic obstructive pulmonary disease. Am J Respir Crit Care Med. 2000; 162(1):216–220.
3. Cazzola M, Calderaro F, Califano C, Dim Pema F, Vinciguerra A, Donner CF, Maters MG. Oral bambuterol compared to inhaled salmeterol in patients with partially reversible chronic obstructive pulmonary disease. Eur J Clin Pharmacol 1999; 54(11):829–833.
4. Schultze-Werninghaus G. Multicenter 1-year trial on formoterol, a new long-acting beta2-agonist, in chronic obstructive airway disease. Lung 1990; 168:83–89.
5. Cazzola M, Matera MG, Santangelo G, Vinciguerra A, Rossi F, D'Amato G. Salmeterol and formoterol in partially reversible severe chronic

obstructive pulmonary disease: a dose-response study. Respir Med 1995; 89(5):357–362.

6. Celik G, Kayacan O, Beder S, Durmaz G. Formoterol and salmeterol in partially reversible chronic obstructive pulmonary disease: a crossover, placebo-controlled comparison on onset and duration of action. Respiration 1999; 66(5):434–439.

7. Maesen BL, Wesermann CJ, Duurkens VA, van den Bosch JM. Effects of formoterol in apparently poorly reversible chronic obstructive pulmonary disease. Eur Respir J 1999; 13(5):1103–1108.

8. DiMarco, F. Millic-Emilli J, Boveri B, Carlucci P, Santus P, Casanova F, Cazzola M, Centanni S. Effect of inhaled bronchodilators in inspiratory capacity and dypnoea at rest in COPD. Eur Respir J 2003; 21:86–94.

9. Rossi A, Kristufek P, Levine BE, Thomson MH, Till D, Kottakis J, Della Cioppa G; for the Formoterol in Chronic Obstructive Pulmonary Disease (FICOPD) II Study Group. Comparison of the efficacy, tolerability, and safety of formoterol dry powder and oral, slow-release theophylline in the treatment of COPD. Chest 2002; 121:1058–1069.

10. Sichletidis L. Kottakis J, Marcou S, Constantinidis TC, Antoniades A. Bronchodilatory responses to formoterol, inpratropium, and their combination in patients with stable COPD. Int J Clin Pract 1999; 53(3):185–188.

11. Cazzola M, Matera MG, Di Perna E, Califano C, D'Amato M, Mazzarella G. Influence of higher than conventional doses of oxitropuim bromide on formoterol-induced bronchodilation in COPD. Respir Med 1999; 93(12):909–911.

12. Cazzola M, Di Perna F, Califano C, Vinciguerra A, D'Amato M, Incremental benefit of adding oxitropium bromide to formoterol in patients with stable COPD. Pulm Pharmacol Ther 1999; 12(4):267–271.

13. Dahl R, Greefhorst LAPM, Nowak D, Nonikov V, Byrne AM, Thomson ML, Till D, Della Cioppa G. Inhaled dry powder formoterol versus ipratropium bromide in chronic obstructive pulmonary disease. Am J Respir Crit Care Med 2001; 164:778–784.

14. Aalbers R, Ayres J, Backer V, Decramer M, Lier PA, Magyar P, Malolepszy J, Ruffin R, Sybrecht GW. Formoterol in patients with chronic obstructive pulmonary disease: a randomized, controlled, 3-month trial. Eur Respir J 2002; 19:936–943.

15. Liesker JJW, Van de Velde V, Meysman M, Vincken W, Wollmer P, Hansson L, Kerotjem HAM, Qvint U, Pauwels RA. Effect of formoterol (Oxis Turbuhaler) and ipratropium on exercise capacity in patients with COPD. Respir Med 2002; 96:559–566.

16. Wadbo M, Lofdahl C-G, Larsson K, Skoogh BE, Tornling F, Arwestrom E, Begtsson T, Strom L. Effects of formoterol and ipratropium bromide in COPD: a 3-month placebo-controlled study. Eur Respir J 2002; 20:1138–1146.

17. Szafranski W, Cukler A, Ramirez A, Menga G, Sansores R, Nahabedian, S, Peterson S, Olsson H. Efficacy and safety of budesonide/formoterol in the management of chronic obstructive pulmonary disease. Eur Respir J 2003; 21:74–81.

18. Ulrik CS. Efficacy of inhaled salmeterol in the management of smokers with chronic obstructive pulmonary disease: a single centre randomised, double blind, placebo controlled, crossover study [see comments]. Thorax 1995; 50(7):750–754.

19. Ulrik CS. [The effect of salmeterol in the treatment of smokers with chronic obstructive lung disease]. Ugeskr Laeger 1996; 158(25):3604–3607.

20. Rennard SI, Anderson W, ZuWallack R, Boughton J, Bailey W, Friedman M, Wisniewski M, Rickard K. Use of long-acting inhaled beta2-adrenergic agonist, salmeterol xinafoate, in patients with chronic obstructive pulmonary disease. Am J Respir Crit Care Med 2001; 163:1087–1092.

21. Boyd G, Morice AH, Pounsford JC, Siebert M, Peslis N, Crawford C. An evaluation of salmeterol in the treatment of chronic obstructive pulmonary disease (COPD) [published erratum appears in Eur Respir J 1997; 10(7):1696]. Eur Respir J 1997; 10(4):815–821.

22. Ramirez-Venegas A, Ward J, Lentine T, Mahler DA. Salmeterol reduces dyspnea and improves lung function in patients with COPD. Chest 1997; 112(2):336–340.

23. Mahler DA, Donohue JF, Barbee RA, Goldman MD, Gross NJ, Wisniewski ME, Yancee SW, Zaker BA, Richard KA, Anderson WH. Efficacy of salmeterol xinafoate in the treatment of COPD. Chest 1999; 115(4):957–965.

24. Van Noord JA, De Munck DR, Bantje TA, Hopa WCJ, Akveld MLM, Bommer AM. Long-term treatment of chronic obstructive pulmonary disease with salmeterol and the additive effect of ipratropium. Eur Respir J 2000; 15:878–885.

25. Grove A, Lipworth BJ, Reid P, Smith RP, Ramage L, Ingram CG, Jenkins RJ, Winter JH, Dhillon DP. Effects of regular salmeterol on lung function and exercise capacity in patients with chronic obstructive airways disease. Thorax 1996; 51(7):689–693.

26. Dowling RB, Rayner CFJ, Rutman A, Jackson AD, Kanrhakumar K, Dewar A, Taylor GW, Cole PJ, Johnson M, Wilson R. Effect of salmeterol in *Pseudomonas aeruginosa* infection of respiratory mucosa. Am J Respir Crit Care Med 1997; 114:327–336.

27. Dowling RB, Johnson M, Cole RJ, Wilson R. Effect of salmeterol on *Haemophilus influenzae* infection of respiratory mucosa in vitro. Eur Respir J 1998; 11:86–90.

28. Calverley P, Pauwels R, Vestbo J, Jones P, Pride N, Gulsvik A, Anderson J, Maden C. TRial of Inhaled STeroids ANd long-acting beta2 agonists study group. Combined salmeterol and fluticasone in the treatment of chronic obstructive pulmonary disease: a randomised controlled trial. Lancet 2003; 361:449–56.

29. Jones PW, Bosh YK in association with an international study group. Quality of life changes in COPD patients treated with salmeterol. Am J Respir Crit Care Med 1997; 155:1283–1289.

30. Patakas D, Andreadis D, Mavrofridis E, Argyropoulou P. Comparison of the effects of salmeterol and ipratropium bromide on exercise performance and

breathlessness in paients with stable chronic obstructive pulmonary disease [see comments]. Respir Med 1998; 92(9):1116–1121.

31. Donohue JF, Vn aNoord JA, Baeman ED, Langley SJ, Lee A, Witek TJ, Lesten S, Towse L. A 6-month, placebo-controlled study comparing long function and health status changes in COPD patients treated with tiotropium or salmeterol. Chest 2002; 122:47–55.

32. Brusaso V, Hodder R, Miravitlles M, Korducki L, Towse L, Kesten S. Health outcomes following treatment for six months with once daily tiotropium compared with twice daily salmeterol in patients with COPD. Thorax 2003; 58:399–404.

33. Di Lorenzo G, Morici G, Drago A, Pellitteri ME, Mansueto P, Melluso M, Norrits F, Squassante L, Fasolo A. Efficacy, tolerability, and effects on quality of life of inhaled salmeterol and oral theophylline in patients with mild-to-moderate chronic obstructive pulmonary disease. SLMT02 Italian Study Group. Clin Ther 1998; 20(6):1130–1148.

34. Cazzola M, Vinciguerra A, Di Perna F, Matera MG. Early reversibility to salbutamol does not always predict bronchodilation after salmeterol in stable chronic obstructive pulmonary disease. Respir Med 1998; 92(8):1012–1016.

35. Kaushik ML, Kashyap S, Bansal SK, Sharma A. Effectiveness of salmeterol in stable COPD. Indian J Chest Dis Allied Sci 1999; 41(4):207–212.

36. Matera MG, Cazzola M, Vinciguerra A, Di Perna F, Calderaro F, Caputi M, Roasi F. A comparison of the bronchodilating effects of salmeterol, salbutamol and ipratropium bromide in patients with chronic obstructive pulmonary disease. Pulm Pharmacol 1995; 8(6):267–271.

37. Cazzola M, Matera MG, Di Perna F, Calderaro F, Califano C, Vinciguerra A. A comparison of bronchodilating effects of salmeterol and oxitropium bromide in stable chronic obstructive pulmonary disease. Respir Med 1998; 92(2):354–357.

38. Cazzola M, Santagelo G, Piccolo A, Salzillo A, Matera MG, D'Amato G, Roasi F. Effect of salmeterol and formoterol in patients with chronic obstructive pulmonary disease. Pulm Pharmacol 1994; 7(2):103–107.

39. Maesen FP, Costongs R, Smeets JJ, Brombacher PK, Zweers PG. The effect of maximal doses of formoterol and salbutamol from a metered dose inhaler on pulse rates, ECG, and serum potassium concentrations. Chest 1991; 99(6):1367–1373.

40. Totterman KJ, Huhti L, Sutinen E, Backman R, Pietinalho A, Falck M, Larason P, Schood O. Tolerability to high doses of formoterol and terbutaline via Turbuhaler for 3 days in stable asthmatic patients. Eur Respir J 1998; 12(3):573–579.

41. Tranfa CM, Pelaia G, Grembiale RD, Naty S, Durate S, Borrello G. Short-term cardiovascular effects of salmeterol. Chest 1998; 113(5):1272–1276.

42. Cazzola M, Imperatore F, Salzillo A, Di Perna F, Calderaro F, Imperatore A, Matera MG. Cardiac effects of formoterol and salmeterol in patients suffering from COPD with preexisting cardiac arrhythmias and hypoxemia [see comments]. Chest 1998; 114(2):411–415.

43. Khoukaz G, Gross NJ. Effects of salmeterol on arterial blood gases in patients with stable chronic obstructive pulmonary disease. Comparison with albuterol and ipratropium. Am J Respir Crit Care Med 1999; 160(3):1028–1030.

44. Cazzola M, Di Perna F, Noschese P, Vinciguerra A, Calderaro F, Girbino G, Matera MG. Effects of formoterol, salmeterol or oxitropium bromide on airway responses to salbutamol in COPD [see comments]. Eur Respir J 1998; 11(6):1337–1341.

45. Cazzola M, Di Perna F, Centanni S, Califano C, Donner CF, D'Amato M, D'Amato G. Acute effect of pretreatment with single conventional dose of salmeterol on dose-response curve to oxitropium bromide in chronic obstructive pulmonary disease. Thorax 1999; 54(12):1083–1086.

46. Hogan TJ, Geddes R, Gonzalez ER. An economic assessment of inhaled formoterol dry powder versus ipratropium bromide pressurized metered dose inhaler in the treatment of chronic obstructive pulmonary disease. Clin Ther. 2003; 25(1):285–297.

47. Jones PW, Wilson K, Sondhi S. Cost-effectiveness of salmeterol in patients with chronic obstructive pulmonary disease: an economic evaluation. Respir Med 2003; 97:20–26.

17

The Role of Glucocorticosteroids in the Management of COPD

ROMAIN PAUWELS

Ghent University Hospital
Ghent, Belgium

I. Introduction

Glucocorticosteriods are undoubtedly the most effective controller medication for the treatment of asthma (1,2). They are also very effective in the treatment of acute severe asthma exacerbations. Chronic obstructive pulmonary disease (COPD) has many similarities with asthma, including common symptoms and airflow limitation. It is therefore not at all surprising that glucocorticosteroids have been and are being used extensively in the management of COPD, both in the long-term treatment and in the management of acute exacerbations (3). However, evidence supporting or refuting the use of glucocorticosteroids in COPD has so far been rather scarce. Controlled studies in a sufficient number of subjects have only recently become available, and evidence is still missing for a number of important clinical issues. The widespread use of glucocorticosteroids in COPD might reflect the confusion between asthma and COPD, the clinically perceived beneficial effect, or the need to do something for patients with COPD (3). Similar to other treatment for COPD, the assessment of the efficacy of glucocorticosteroids is hampered by the limited availability of clinically relevant, appropriately standardized, and reproducible outcome measures.

II. The Effect of Glucocorticosteroids on Airway Inflammation in COPD

The chronic airflow limitation in COPD is caused by a mixture of small airways abnormalities and parenchymal destruction (emphysema) (4,5). A chronic inflammation of the small airways and the lung parenchyma is thought to be the major pathogenic mechanism in COPD. The disease is characterized by the presence of an augmented number of activated neutrophils, macrophages, CD4+ and CD8+ T lymphocytes, B lymphocytes, and eosinophils in the airspaces and lung tissue (6). This inflammatory pathology in COPD is clearly different from that observed in asthma. The role of the different cell types and mediators involved in the pathogenesis of COPD is currently not well understood. Both the inflammatory changes in the small airways and the imbalance between destruction and repair in the lung parenchyma contribute to the no longer fully reversible airflow limitation in COPD.

Many studies have investigated the effect of glucocorticosteroids on inflammation in COPD. The conclusions of these studies are not unanimous. Thompson et al. (7) studied the effect of a 6-week treatment with 1000 μg beclomethasone per day on parameters of airway inflammation in subjects with mild COPD (mean FEV_1: 72% predicted). Beclomethasone treatment significantly decreased the visual evidence of inflammation as assessed via the fiberoptic bronchoscope. The active treatment also decreased the number of inflammatory cells in the bronchial lavage fluid and the concentration of albumin, lactoferrin, and lysosyme in the epithelial lining fluid. The significant decrease in parameters of airway inflammation was associated with an improvement in spirometry.

Llewellyn-Jones et al. (8) investigated the effects of 1.5 mg inhaled fluticasone propionate (FP) per day on sputum chemotactic activity, elastase inhibitory potential, albumin concentrations, and peripheral neutrophil function in a small group of patients with clinically stable, smoking-related chronic bronchitis and emphysema. Seventeen patients (50–75 years) were entered into a double-blind, placebo-controlled, parallel group study for 8 weeks. Following treatment with FP, the chemotactic activitity of the sputum sol phase was lower than the corresponding values for the placebo group. The neutrophil elastase inhibitory capacity of the sputum sol phase increased with treatment. Treatment with FP did not result in a change in the neutrophil functions studied or sputum albumin and myeloperoxidase (MPO) concentrations.

In the study performed by Keatings et al. (9), a 2-week course of inhaled budesonide (800 mg twice daily) in 13 patients with severe COPD did not modify significantly inflammatory indices in induced sputum. Total and differential cell counts, concentrations of tumor necrosis factor (TNF)-α, eosinophil activation markers eosinophil cationic protein (ECP) and eosinophil peroxidase (EPO), and neutrophil activation markers MPO and human neutrophil lipocalin (HNL) were not changed significantly. A 2-week course of oral prednisolone (30 mg/d) in the same patients did not modify the induced sputum markers.

A two-month course with inhaled beclomethasone 500 μg t.i.d. in 17 patients with clinically stable, smoking-related COPD reduced significantly neutrophil cell counts in induced sputum (10). The differences between the actively treated and placebo-control groups were significant for neutrophils, macrophages, and total cells. Culpitt et al. (11) examined the effect of fluticasone propionate (500 μg b.i.d.) on markers of inflammatory activity and protease/antiprotease inbalance in induced sputum. Thirteen patients with COPD were treated for 4 weeks in a double-blind crossover study. Induced sputum inflammatory cells, percentage neutrophils, and interleukin (IL)-8 levels were unchanged. Sputum supernatant elastase activity, matrix metalloproteinase (MMP)-1, MMP-9, and the antiproteases secretory leukoprotease inhibitor (SLPI) and tissue inhibitor of metalloproteinase (TIMP)-1 were similarly unaffected by treatment. In an open study, Balbi et al. (12) observed a decrease in the total number of cells, the percentage neutrophils, and the concentration of IL-8 and MPO in bronchoalveolar lavage fluid following 6 weeks of treatment with 1500 μg beclomethasone per day. Withdrawal during 6 weeks of beclomethasone in patients with moderate to severe COPD resulted in a deterioration of the ventilatory function and an increase in the exercise-induced dyspnea, but no change in the sputum total and differential cell counts (13).

Hattotuwa et al. performed a double-blind, placebo-controlled, randomized study to compare fluticasone propionate 500 μg twice daily via a dry powder inhaler and placebo (P) over a 3-month period in subjects with COPD (14). Using fiberbronchoscopic biopsies, the investigators found no significant reductions in the primary endpoints: CD8+, CD68+ cells, or neutrophils. However, there was a reduction in the CD8 : CD4 ratio in the epithelium and of the numbers of subepithelial mast cells in the fluticasone propionate group. CD4+ cells were significantly raised in the placebo group in both subepithelium and epithelium. Symptoms significantly improved, and there were significantly fewer exacerbations in subjects on fluticasone propionate.

The reasons for the differences in results between these studies are not fully understood. The selection of the patients, the number of patients included, the dose and the potency of the inhaled corticosteroid and the duration of the treatment period might explain some of the discrepancies. The reason why Hattotuwa et al. (14) were successful in finding a clinical correlate for the changes in pathology was probably that they selected a study population and a treatment regimen that was similar to the population of the ISOLDE trial (15), where clear-cut benefits for inhaled glucocorticosteroids had been demonstrated.

We should be careful in the interpretation of the findings by Hattotuwa et al. (14). The association of a change in pathology with clinical efficacy does not necessarily mean that the two are causally related. The major site of the chronic airflow limitation in COPD is the small airways. Bronchial biopsies are unlikely to reflect the change in pathology at this peripheral location. Very few studies have investigated the pathology of acute exacerbations in COPD, and the data are again confined to larger airways (16,17). These studies suggest an increase in airway eosinophilia during a COPD exacerbation. A possible explanation for the effect of inhaled glucocorticosteroids on the exacerbation rate could thus be their well-known effects on eosinophilic inflammation. How inhaled glucocorticosteroids would prevent the increase in eosinophilic inflammation in COPD and how to link this hypothesis with the findings of the Hattotuwa et al. (14) study needs further mechanistic investigations. The role of mast cells in COPD is equally unclear. Their number is increased in the bronchiolar epithelium (18), and bronchial challenges with indirect mast cell activating agents cause airway narrowing in patients with COPD (19,20). There might thus be a link between the effect of inhaled glucocorticosteroids on mast cells and the symptomatic benefit in COPD.

It is, however, apparent that the effects of inhaled glucocorticosteroids on markers of airway inflammation in COPD are clearly less marked than in asthma. There might be a link between the effect on airflow limitation and the changes in eosinophilic airway inflammation as suggested by the study of Chanez et al. (21). Twenty-five unselected patients clinically diagnosed as having COPD received a daily oral dose of 1.5 mg/kg body weight of prednisolone for 15 days. A response to treatment was defined as an increase in FEV_1 of at least 12% from baseline values and an absolute value of at least 200 mL. Twelve of 25 patients responded to the treatment. By comparison with nonresponders, responders had a significantly larger number of eosinophils and higher levels of eosinophil cationic protein (ECP) in their bronchoalveolar lavage fluid (BALF). The responders had a thicker reticular basement membrane than the nonresponders.

The findings of Chanez et al. (21) were confirmed by Pizzichini et al. (22) and Fujimoto et al. (23). They found a significant relationship between sputum eosinophilia and therapeutic response to glucocorticosteroids in patients with COPD.

III. Oral Glucocorticosteroids in the Long-Term Management of COPD

A. Short-Term Response to Oral Glucocorticosteroids as Predictor for Long-Term Effects

Almost all studies on the use of oral glucocorticosteroids have focused on the short-term effects of these drugs on the FEV_1 (24). Some COPD guidelines still recommend the use of a short course (2 weeks) of oral glucocorticosteroids to identify the patients with COPD who might benefit form long-term treatment with oral or inhaled glucocorticosteroids. There is no good evidence for this recommendation, nor is it known what the risks are for such a course in a population of generally older people with a high prevalence of comorbidity.

A meta-analysis of the clinical studies on the response of the FEV_1 to oral glucocorticosteroids in patients with COPD shows a high variability from study to study (24). The percentage of patients who have an increase of 20% above baseline following a short course of oral glucocorticosteroids varies from 0 to 44% and a similar response is noted in 0–30% of the patients treated with placebo. The weighted mean effect size (responders in active minus responders in placebo) is 11%. The weakness of this meta-analysis is the concept of 20% reversibility. This concept is derived from the belief that the therapeutic effect of glucocorticosteroids in asthma is translated into increase in FEV_1. It has now become evident that other outcome measures besides FEV_1 reflect more appropriately the true beneficial effects of glucocorticosteroids in asthma. These include decrease in symptoms, decrease in exacerbations, improvement in quality of life, and possibly prevention of irreversible airflow obstruction.

Two studies have now shown that the spirometric response to a short course of oral corticosteroids is a poor predictor of the long-term response to inhaled corticosteroids in patients with COPD (25,26). The results of these two controlled studies contrast with the conclusions of an open study, where a predictive value for an oral steroid trial was suggested (27). Senderovitz et al. (26) demonstrated that the spirometric response to a short course of oral glucocorticosteroids is a poor predictor of the long-term spirometric response to inhaled glucocorticosteroids in COPD. In their study, 40 patients with stable COPD and an airflow limitation that was poorly reversible to a β_2-agonist received prednisolone (37.5 mg o.d. for 2 weeks). The patients were subsequently divided into steroid-reversible and irreversible, and both groups were randomized to budesonide 400 µg b.i.d. or placebo. Very few patients responded to prednisolone, and there was no difference in the response to budesonide between the prednisolone responders and nonresponders.

In the ISOLDE trial, oral prednisolone 0.6 mg/kg was given for 14 days to 524 patients with COPD before before randomized treatment for 3 years with fluticasone propionate or placebo (25). There was no relationship between the change in FEV_1 after prednisolone and the subsequent change in FEV_1 over the following 3 years on either placebo or fluticasone propionate. The significant effect of treatment on decline in health status was not predicted by the prednisolone response.

Davies et al. (27) reported in an observational study that a large response to an inhaled β_2-agonist or a short course of oral prednisolone was a good predictor of the one-year change in prebronchodilator FEV_1 following treatment with inhaled glucocorticosteroids.

B. Long-Term Treatment with Oral Glucocorticosteroids

Two retrospective studies (28,29) have analyzed the effects of treatment with oral glucocorticosteroids on the long-term changes of the FEV_1. These studies looked at the change in FEV_1 over many years in a clinic population with moderate to severe COPD. Four patterns of change in FEV_1 were identified: no change, a progressive decline, an initial increase followed by a decline, and an initial decrease followed by an increase. The increase and the stable pattern were associated with the use of oral and/or inhaled glucocorticosteroids. These observations therefore suggested that oral and/or inhaled glucocorticosteroids might beneficially affect the long-term decline of the FEV_1 in COPD. The retrospective nature of these studies, the lack of a true control group and the imprecise definition of COPD were of course reason for a cautious interpretation of the data and conclusions. In view of the well-known toxicity of long-term treatment with oral glucocorticosteroids, it is not at all surprising that no prospective studies have been performed on the long-term effects of these oral drugs in COPD.

An important side effect of long-term treatment with systemic glucocorticosteroids in patients with COPD is steroid myopathy (30,31). This myopathy does contribute to muscle weakness and decreased functionality in subjects with advanced COPD (32,33). The myopathy could potentially contribute to respiratory muscle dysfunction and further enhance respiratory insufficiency (34).

The lack of evidence of the long-term beneficial effect of chronic oral glucocorticosteroid therapy in COPD and the large body of evidence on the long-term side effects of this treatment, including the contribution of steroid myopathy to the respiratory insufficiency of COPD, must lead to the conclusion that oral glucocorticosteroid therapy is not justified in COPD. The use of oral systemic glucocorticosteroids in COPD should be restricted to the treatment of acute exacerbations.

IV. Systemic Glucocorticosteroids in the Treatment of Acute Exacerbations of COPD

Several controlled studies have now shown that treatment with oral or systemic glucocorticosteroids is beneficial in the management of acute exacerbations of COPD. Thompson et al. (35) evaluated in a randomized placebo-controlled study the effect of oral prednisone, in tapering doses of 60 to 20 mg over 9 days, in 27 outpatients presenting with an acute exacerbation. Patients also continued their previous medications and increased their use of β-agonists. Treatment with prednisone resulted in a more rapid improvement in arterial Pa_{O_2}, alveolar-arterial oxygen gradient, FEV_1, and peak expiratory flow compared to placebo. Prednisolone also resulted in fewer treatment failures and in a trend toward more rapid improvement in dyspnea scale scores. Niewoehner et al. (36) conducted a double-blind, randomized trial of systemic glucocorticosteroids (given for 2 or 8 weeks) or placebo in 271 patients hospitalized for an exacerbation of COPD. Eighty patients received an 8-week course of glucocorticosteroid therapy, 80 a 2-week course, and 111 placebo. Rates of treatment failure were significantly higher in the placebo-treated patients than in the groups treated with glucocorticosteroids. Systemic glucocorticosteroid therapy was associated with a shorter initial hospital stay and with an FEV_1 that was about 0.1 L higher than that in the placebo group after the first day of treatment. Significant benefits were no longer evident after 6 months. The 8-week regimen was not superior in efficacy to the 2-week treatment regimen but resulted in more patients having hyperglycemia requiring therapy.

Davies et al. (37) reported a double-blind, placebo-controlled trial on the effect of oral glucocorticosteroids in patients with a nonacidotic exacerbation of COPD requiring hospitalization. Patients were randomly assigned to oral prednisolone 30 mg or placebo for 14 days, in addition to standard treatment with nebulized bronchodilators, antibiotics, and oxygen. The postbronchodilator FEV_1 increased more rapidly and to a greater extent in the glucocorticosteroid-treated group, and their hospital stay was shorter. The treatment groups did not differ at the 6-week follow-up.

Aaron et al. (38) recently confirmed the beneficial effect of a short course of oral glucocorticosteroids in the treatment of an acute exacerbation in patients seen at an emergency department. One hundred and forty-seven patients who were being discharged from the emergency department after an exacerbation of COPD were randomly assigned to 10 days of treatment with 40 mg of oral prednisone once daily or identical-appearing placebo. All patients received oral antibiotics for 10 days, plus inhaled bronchodilators. The primary endpoint was relapse, defined as an unscheduled visit to a physician's office or a return to the emergency department because of worsening dyspnea, within 30 days after randomization. The overall rate of relapse at 30 days was lower in the prednisone group than in the placebo group, and the time to relapse was prolonged in those taking prednisone. After 10 days of therapy, patients in the prednisone group had greater improvements in FEV_1 and in dyspnea but not in health-related quality of life.

Oral or systemic glucocorticosteroid therapy thus significantly accelerates the recovery of dyspnea, lung function, and gas exchange following a COPD exacerbation. It also reduces the number of treatment failures or relapses. This treatment can thus be recommended as addition to bronchodilator therapy (plus eventually antibiotics and oxygen therapy) in the management of acute exacerbations of COPD. The exact dose that should be given is not known, but high doses are associated with a significant risk of side effects and no gain in efficacy. A daily oral dose of 30–40 mg of prednisolone or equivalent for 10–14 days is probably a reasonable compromise between efficacy and safety.

V. Inhaled Steroids in the Long-Term Management of COPD

A. Short-Term Effects on Lung Function

Many small studies have looked at the short-term effect of inhaled corticosteroids on pulmonary function parameters in COPD (7,39–43). Some studies did indeed show a significant improvement, whereas others did not. The reasons for the differences in outcome might be related to the selection of the subjects and the dose and type of inhaled glucocorticosteroid. The major problem with most studies is the small number of subjects and the short duration of the treatment. Paggiaro et al. studied the effect of inhaled fluticasone in a large group of patients with COPD (44). In a randomized, double-blind, placebo-controlled design 281 outpatients were randomly assigned to fluticasone 500 µg or placebo twice daily for 6 months. Significantly more patients had moderate or severe exacerbations in the placebo group than in the fluticasone propionate group (86% vs. 60%). Diary-card and clinic morning peak expiratory flows improved significantly in the fluticasone propionate group, as did clinic FEV, forced vital capacity, and mid-expiratory flow. Symptom scores for median daily cough and sputum volume were significantly lower with fluticasone propionate treatment than with placebo. At the end of treatment, patients on fluticasone propionate had increased their 6-minute walking distance significantly more than those on placebo.

Overall the short-term effect of inhaled glucocorticosteroids on lung function seems to be limited, but there is an improvement of FEV_1 in the majority of studies. The improvement is seen after 1–2 weeks of treatment, and the difference with placebo treatment is maintained over time (15,45–47). The bronchodilating activity of the inhaled glucocorticosteroid is additive to that of a long-acting β_2-agonist (45,46).

B. Effect on Long-Term Decline in Lung Function

A number of studies have now investigated the effect of inhaled gluco-corticosteroid treatment on the long-term change FEV_1 in COPD. The initial studies had rather small numbers of patients. Dompeling et al. (48,49) observed that daily treatment with 800 µg of beclomethasone caused an increase in prebronchodilator FEV_1 during the first 6 months of treatment followed by a decline during the remaining 18 months of the treatment period. In a 2-year controlled study in a small group of patients with COPD, Renkema et al. (50) did not find a significant influence of treatment with budesonide 800 µg twice daily alone or in combination with 5 mg prednisolone daily on the FEV_1 decline. The glucocorticosteroid treatment significantly decreased the symptoms.

A meta-analysis of three studies on the effect of inhaled corticosteroids on the FEV_1 showed that a significant beneficial effect on the change over time of both the pre-and postbronchodilator FEV_1 (51).

Four large studies have now been published looking at the long-term effects of inhaled corticosteroids in COPD (Copenhagen City Lung Study, EUROSCOP, and ISOLDE, Lung Health Study II). The Copenhagen City Lung Study investigated the effect of 3 years of treatment with budesonide on the decline in FEV_1 in subjects with very mild COPD recruited from the general population (52). All subjects with a reversible airflow limitation either by bronchodilator or by oral corticosteroids were excluded. No effect of budesonide was seen on FEV_1 decline or symptoms.

The EUROSCOP study evaluated the effect of the inhaled glucocorticosteroid budesonide on the decline in lung function in individuals with mild COPD who continued smoking (47). After a run-in period, 1277 subjects were randomized to twice-daily treatment with 400 μg of budesonide or placebo for 3 years. Budesonide improved the FEV_1 during the first 6 months of treatment, and this gain was maintained throughout the study. From 9 to 36 months of treatment, the FEV_1 in the budesonide group decreased at a rate comparable to the placebo group: −57 and −67 mL/yr, respectively. The median FEV_1 decline over 3 years was 180 mL or 5.3% predicted for the placebo group compared to 140 mL or 4.3% for the budesonide group. Budesonide treatment was not associated with systemic glucocorticosteroid-related side effects except for an increased incidence of skin bruising. Bone density measurements did not show any difference in change over time between the budesonide and the placebo-treated group (53).

The ISOLDE study evaluated in patients with moderate to severe COPD the effect of 3 years of treatment with fluticasone 500 μg b.i.d. (15). Most subjects received an initial 2-week course of oral prednisolone. Fluticasone significantly improved the postbronchodilator FEV_1 but did not modify the long-term decline of this lung function parameter. The effects on the postbronchodilator FEV_1 were very similar to the results of the EUROSCOP study (47), with an initial small gain in the corticosteroid-treated group that was maintained over 3 years. The annual rate of decline of the FEV_1 was 59 mL/yr in the placebo group and 50 mL/yr in the fluticasone group. More importantly, fluticasone treatment significantly reduced the number of exacerbations by 25% and inhibited the loss of health status in these patients. Health status deteriorated by 3.2 units per year on placebo and by 2 units per year on fluticasone (St. George's Respiratory Questionnaire). Withdrawals due to respiratory disease were also higher in the placebo group.

The Lung Health Study II enrolled 1116 persons with COPD with an FEV_1 between 30 and 90% predicted in a randomized trial comparing inhaled triamcinolone acetonide at a dose of 600 μg twice daily with placebo (54). The mean duration of follow-up was 40 months. The rate of decline in the FEV_1 after bronchodilator use was similar in the triamcinolone group and the placebo group (44.2 vs. 47.0 mL/yr). Members of the triamcinolone group had fewer respiratory symptoms during the course of the study and had fewer visits to a physician because of a respiratory. Those taking triamcinolone also had lower airway reactivity in response to methacholine challenge at 9 and 33 months. After 3 years, the bone density of the lumbar spine and the femur was significantly lower in the triamcinolone group.

C. Effect on Exacerbations of COPD

A major finding in both the study by Paggiaro et al. (14) and in the ISOLDE study (15) was that treatment with inhaled glucocorticosteroids decreased the frequency of exacerbations in patients with COPD. This finding is especially significant in the patients with more advanced disease, i.e., a baseline FEV_1 of less than 50% predicted. The exacerbation rate in both studies was not a primary outcome, but the effect of inhaled corticosteroids has now been confirmed in two large studies in which the exacerbation rate was a primary variable (45,46). Both studies included patients with a history of exacerbations. Calverley et al. (46) reported that treatment with fluticasone 500 µg b.i.d. reduced significantly the rate of exacerbations by 19%. The protective effect was more evident for more severe exacerbations requiring a course of oral glucocorticosteroids (34% reduction) and in patients with more advanced COPD ($FEV_1 < 50\%$ predicted). In the study reported by Szafranski et al. (45) on patients with severe to very severe COPD ($FEV_1 < 50\%$ predicted), treatment with budesonide 400 µg b.i.d. reduced the exacerbation rate by 15% (NS) and the rate of exacerbations requiring a course of oral glucocorticosteroids by 29% ($p = 0.045$).

VI. Conclusions

The role of inhaled glucocorticosteroids in the management of chronic obstructive pulmonary disease is debated, but evidence is accumulating to support therapeutic recommendations (55). The evidence is coming from well-controlled clinical trails and is supported by mechanistic studies.

Large-scale clinical studies have shown that inhaled glucocorticosteroids have no influence on the long-term decline in lung function in COPD, but a similar statement can be made for all pharmacological therapies that are currently used in this disease. The major benefits from inhaled glucocorticosteroids in COPD are a decrease in the number exacerbations, an inhibition of the progressive decline in health status, and an additive effect with long-acting inhaled β_2-agonists on lung function and symptoms. There is also indirect evidence that inhaled glucocorticosteroids might decrease mortality in COPD (56). A large prospective controlled study on this issue, the TORCH study, is currently ongoing, but we can only expect to have the results available 5 years from now. What should we do for now? There is currently very little evidence to support the generalized use of inhaled glucocorticosteroids in mild to moderate COPD. However, accumulating evidence supports their use in patients with more advanced COPD ($FEV_1 < 50\%$ predicted) with a history of repeated exacerbations.

References

1. Van Essen-Zandvliet EE, Hughes MD, Waalkens HJ, Duiverman EJ, Pocock SJ, Kerrebijn EF. Effects of 22 months of treatment with inhaled corticosteroids and/or beta2-agonists on lung function, airway responsiveness and symptoms in children with asthma. Am Rev Respir Dis 1992; 146:547–554.
2. Haahtela T, Jarvinen M, Kava T, Kiviranta K, Koskinen S, Lehtonen K, Nikander K, Persson T, Reinikainen K, Selroos O, Sovijarvi A, Stenius-Aarniala B, Svahn T, Tammivaara R, Laitinen L. Comparison of beta2-agonist, terbutaline, with an inhaled corticosteroid, budesonide, in newly detected asthma. N Engl J Med 1991; 325:388–392.
3. Jackevicius C, Joyce DP, Kesten S, Chapman KR. Prehospitalization inhaled corticosteroid use in patients with COPD or asthma. Chest 1997; 111:296–302.
4. Kuwano K, Bosken CH, Paré P, Bai TR, Wiggs BR, Hogg JC. Small airway dimensions in asthma and in chronic obstructive pulmonary disease. Am Rev Respir Dis 1993; 148:1220–1225.
5. Saetta M, Finkelstein R, Cosio MG. Morphological and cellular basis for airflow limitation in smokers. Eur Respir J 1994; 7:1505–1515.
6. Retamales I, Elliott WM, Meshi B, Coxson HO, Pare PD, Sciurba FC, Rogers RM, Hayashi S, Hogg JC. Amplification of inflammation in emphysema and its association with latent adenoviral infection. Am J Respir Crit Care Med 2001; 164:469–473.
7. Thompson AB, Mueller MB, Heires AJ, Bohling TL, Daughton D, Yancey SW, Sykes RS, Rennard SI. Aerosolized beclomethasone in chronic bronchitis. Improved pulmonary function and diminished airway inflammation. Am Rev Respir Dis 1992; 146:389–395.
8. Llewellyn Jones CG, Harris TA, Stockley RA. Effect of fluticasone propionate on sputum of patients with chronic bronchitis and emphysema. Am J Respir Crit Care Med 1996; 153:616–621.
9. Keatings VM, Jatakanon A, Worsdell YM, Barnes PJ. Effects of inhaled and oral glucocorticoids on inflammatory indices in asthma and COPD. Am J Respir Crit Care Med 1997; 155:542–548.
10. Confalonieri M, Mainardi E, DellaPorta R, Bernorio S, Gandola L, Beghe B, Spanevello A. Inhaled corticosteroids reduce neutrophilic bronchial inflammation in patients with chronic obstructive pulmonary disease. Thorax 1998; 53:583–585.
11. Culpitt SV, Maziak W, Loukidis S, Nightingale JA, Matthews JL, Barnes PJ. Effect of high dose inhaled steroid in cells, cytokines, and proteases in induced sputum in chronic obstructive pulmonary disease. Am J Respir Crit Care Med 1999; 160:1635–1639.
12. Balbi B, Majori M, Bertacco S, Convertino G, Cuomo A, Donner CF, Pesci A. Inhaled corticosteroids in stable COPD patients: do they have effects on cells and molecular mediators of airway inflammation? Chest 2000; 117:1633–1637.
13. O'Brien A, Russo-Magno P, Karki A, Hiranniramol S, Hardin M, Kaszuba M, Sherman C, Rounds S. Effects of withdrawal of inhaled steroids in men with

severe irreversible airflow obstruction. Am J Respir Crit Care Med 2001; 164:365–371.

14. Hattotuwa KL, Gizycki MJ, Ansari TW, Jeffery PK, Barnes NC. The effects of inhaled fluticasone on airway inflammation in COPD: a double blind, placebo-controlled biopsy study. Am J Respir Crit Care Med 2002; 195:1592–1596.

15. Burge PS, Calverley PMA, Jones PW, Spencer S, Anderson JA, Maslen TK. Randomised, double blind, placebo controlled study of fluticasone propionate in patients with moderate to severe chronic obstructive pulmonary disease: the ISOLDE trial. Br Med J 2000; 320:1297–1303.

16. Zhu J, Qiu YS, Majumdar S, Gamble E, Matin D, Turato G, Fabbri LM, Barnes N, Saetta M, Jeffery PK. Exacerbations of bronchitis: bronchial eosinophilia and gene expression for interleukin-4, interleukin-5, and eosinophil chemoattractants. Am J Respir Crit Care Med 2001; 164:109–116.

17. Saetta M, Di Stefano A, Maestrelli P, Turato G, Ruggieri MP, Roggeri A, Calcagni P, Mapp CE, Ciaccia A, Fabbri LM. Airway eosinophilia in chronic bronchitis during exacerbations. Am J Respir Crit Care Med 1994; 150:1646–1652.

18. Grashoff WFH, Sont JK, Sterk PJ, Hiemstra PS, deBoer WI, Stolk J, Han J, van Krieken JM. Chronic obstructive pulmonary disease: Role of bronchiolar mast cells and macrophages. Am J Pathol 1997; 151:1785–1790.

19. Taube C, Holz O, Mucke M, Jerres RA, Magnussen H. Airway response to inhaled hypertonic saline in patients with moderate to severe chronic obstructive pulmonary disease. Am J Respir Crit Care Med 2001; 164:1810–1815.

20. Rutgers SR, Timens W, Kauffman HF, Postma DS. Markers of active airway inflammation and remodelling in chronic obstructive pulmonary disease. Clin Exp Allergy 2001; 31:193–205.

21. Chanez P, Vignola AM, O'Shaugnessy T, Enander I, Li D, Jeffery PK, et al. Corticosteroid reversibility in COPD is related to features of asthma. Am J Respir Crit Care Med 1997; 155:1529–1534.

22. Pizzichini E, Pizzichini MMM, Gibson P, Parameswaran K, Gleich GJ, Berman L, Dolovich J, Hargreave FE. Sputum eosinophilia predicts benefit from prednisone in smokers with chronic obstructive bronchitis. Am J Respir Crit Care Med 1998; 158:1511–1517.

23. Fujimoto K, Kibo K, Yamamoto H, Yamaguchi S, Matsuzawa Y. Eosinophilic inflammation in the airway is related to glucocorticoid reversibility in patients with pulmonary emphysema. Chest 1999; 115:679–702.

24. Callahan CM, Dittus RS, Katz BP. Oral corticosteroid therapy for patients with stable chronic obstructive pulmonary disease. A meta-analysis. Ann Int Med 1991; 114:216–223.

25. Burge PS, Calverley PMA, Jones PW, Spencer S, Anderson JA. Prednisolone response in patients with chronic obstructive pulmonary disease: results from the ISOLDE study. Thorax 2003; 58:654–658.

26. Senderovitz T, Vestbo J, Fradsen J, Maltbaek N, Norgaard M, Nielsen C, Kampmann JP. Steroid reversibility test followed by inhaled budesonide or

placebo in outpatients with stable chronic obstructive pulmonary disease. The Danish Society of Respiratory Medicine. Respir Med 1999; 93:715–718.

27. Davies L, Nisar M, Pearson MG, Costello RW, Earis JE, Calverly Pm. Oral corticosteroid trials in the management of stable chronic obstructive pulmonary disease. QJM 1999; 92:395–400.

28. Postma DS, Peters I, Steenhuis IJ, Sluiter HJ. Moderately severe chronic airflow obstruction. Can corticosteroids slow down Progression? Eur Respir J 1988; 1:22–26.

29. Postma DS, Steenhuis EJ, Van der Weele LT, Sluiter HJ. Severe chronic airflow obstruction: can corticosteroids slow down progression? Eur J Respir Dis 1985; 67:56–64.

30. Decramer M, Lacquet LM, Fagard R, Rogiers P. Corticosteroids contribute to muscle weakness in chronic airflow obstruction. Am J Respir Crit Care Med 1994; 150:11–16.

31. Decramer M, Stas KJ. Corticosteroid-induced myopathy involving respiratory muscles in patients with chronic obstructive pulmonary disease or asthma. Am Rev Respir Dis 1992; 146:800–802.

32. Gosselink R, Troosters T, Decramer M. Peripheral muscle weakness contributes to exercise limitation in COPD. Am J Respir Crit Care Med 1996; 153:976–980.

33. Decramer M, de Bock V, Dom R. Functional and histologic picture of steroid-induced myopathy in chronic obstructive pulmonary disease. Am J Respir Crit Care Med 1996; 153:1958–1964.

34. Strom K. Oral corticosteroid treatment during long-term oxygen therapy in chronic obstructive pulmonary disease: a risk factor for hospitalization and mortality in women. Respir Med 1998; 92:50–56.

35. Thompson WH, Nielson CP, Carvalho P, Charan NB, Crowley JJ. Controlled trial of oral prednisone in outpatients with acute COPD exacerbation. Am J Respir Crit Care Med 1996; 154:407–412.

36. Niewoehner DE, Erbland ML, Deupree RH, Collins D, Gross NJ, Light RW, Anderson P, Morgan NA and for the Department of Veteran Affairs Cooperative Study Group. Effect of systemic glucocorticoids on exacerbations of chronic obstructive pulmonary disease. N Engl J Med 1999; 340:1941–1947.

37. Davies L, Angus RM, Calverley RM. Oral corticosteroids in patients admitted to hospital with exacerbations of chronic obstructive pulmonary disease: a prospective randomized controlled trial. Lancet 1999; 354:456–460.

38. Aaron SD, Vandemheen KL, Hebert P, Dales R, Stiell IG, Ahuja J, Dickinson G, Brison R, Rowe BH, Dreyer J, Yetisir E, Cass D, Wells G. Outpatient oral prednisone after emergency treatment of chronic obstructive pulmonary disease. N Engl J Med 2003; 348:2618–2625.

39. Weir DC, Burge PS. Effects of high dose inhaled beclomethasone dipropionate, 750 micrograms and 1500 micrograms twice daily, and 40 mg per day oral prednisolone on lung function, symptoms, and bronchial hyperresponsiveness

in patients with non-asthmatic chronic airflow obstruction. Thorax 1993; 48:309–316.

40. Auffarth B, Postma DS, De Monchy JG, van der Mark TW, Boorsma M, Koeter GH. Effects of inhaled budesonide on spirometric values, reversibility, airway responsiveness, and cough threshold in smokers with chronic obstructive lung disease. Thorax 1991; 46:372–377.

41. Wilcke JTR, Dirksen A. The effect of inhaled glucocorticosteroids in emphysema due to alpha(1)-antitrypsin deficiency. Respir Med 1997; 91:275–279.

42. Bourbeau J, Rouleau MY, Boucher S. Randomised controlled trial of inhaled corticosteroids in patients with chronic obstructive pulmonary disease. Thorax 1998; 53:477–482.

43. Weiner P, Zamir D, Beckerman M. [Inhaled budesonide for chronic obstructive pulmonary disease]. Harefuah 1997; 132:756–759,823.

44. Paggiaro PL, Dahle R, Bakran I, Frith L, Hollingworth K, Efthimiou J. Multicentre randomized placebo-controlled trial of inhaled fluticasone propionate in patients with chronic obstructive pulmonary disease. Lancet 1998; 351:773–780.

45. Szafranski W, Cukier A, Ramirez A, Menga G, Sansores R, Nahabedian S, Peterson S, Olsson H. Efficacy and safety of budesonide/formoterol in the management of chronic obstructive pulmonary disease. Eur Respir J 2003; 21:74–81.

46. Calverley P, Pauwels R, Vestbo J, Jones P, Pride N, Gulsvik A, Anderson J, Maden C. Combined salmeterol and fluticasone in the treatment of chronic obstructive pulmonary disease: a randomised controlled trial. Lancet 2003; 361:449–456.

47. Pauwels RA, Lofdahl CG, Laitinen LA, Schouten JP, Postma DS, Pride NB, Ohlsson SV. Long-term treatment with inhaled budesonide in persons with mild chronic obstructive pulmonary disease who continue smoking. European Respiratory Society Study on Chronic Obstructive Pulmonary Disease. N Engl J Med 1999; 340:1948–1953.

48. Dompeling E, van Schayck CP, van Grunsven PM, van Herwaarden CL, Akkermans R, Molema J, Folgering H, van Weel C. Slowing the deterioration of asthma and chronic obstructive pulmonary disease observed during bronchodilator therapy by adding inhaled corticosteroids. A 4-year prospective study. Ann Intern Med 1993; 118:770–778.

49. Dompeling E, van Schayck CP, Molema J, Folgering H, van Grunsven PM, van Weel C. Inhaled beclomethasone improves the course of asthma and COPD. Eur Respir J 1992; 5:945–952.

50. Renkema TEJ, Schouten JP, Koeter GH, Postma DS. Effects of long-term treatment with corticosteroids in COPD. Chest 1996; 109:1156–1162.

51. vanGrunsven PM, vanSchayck CP, Derenne JP, Kerstjens HAM, Renkema TEJ, Postma DS, Similowski T, Akkermans RP, PaskerdeJong PCM, Dekhuijzen PNR, vanHerwaarden CLA, van Weel C. Long term effects of inhaled corticosteroids in chronic obstructive pulmonary disease: a meta-analysis. Thorax 1999; 54:7–14.

52. Vestbo J, Sorensen T, Lange P, Brix A, Torre P, Viskum K. Long-term effect of inhaled budesonide in mild and moderate chronic obstructive pulmonary disease: a randomised controlled trial. Lancet 1999; 353:1819–1823.
53. Johnell O, Pauwels R, Lofdahl CG, Laitinen LA, Postma DS, Pride NB, Ohlsson SV. Bone mineral density in patients with chronic obstructive pulmonary disease treated with budesonide Turbuhaler. Eur Respir J 2002; 19:1058–1063.
54. Altose MD, Redline S, Deitz CD, Quinlan KJ, Eichenhorn MS, Conway WA, Lung Health Study Research Group. Effect of inhaled triamcinolone on the decline in pulmonary function in chronic obstructive pulmonary disease. N Engl J Med 2000; 343:1902–1909.
55. Pauwels RA, Buist AS, Calverley PM, Jenkins CR, Hurd SS. Global strategy for the diagnosis, management, and prevention of chronic obstructive pulmonary disease. NHLBI/WHO Global Initiative for Chronic Obstructive Lung Disease (GOLD) Workshop summary. Am J Respir Crit Care Med 2001; 163:1256–76.
56. Sin DD, Tu JV. Inhaled corticosteroids and the risk of mortality and readmission in elderly patients with chronic obstructive pulmonary disease. Am J Respir Crit Care Med 2001; 164:580–584.

18

Antibiotics in COPD

NIKOLAOS SIAFAKAS, ELENI TZORTZAKI, and M. TSOUMAKIDOU

University Hospital of Heraklion Crete
Department of Thoracic Medicine
Heraklion, Crete, Greece

I. Introduction

Antibiotics are today an accepted mode of therapy in the management of chronic obstructive pulmonary disease (COPD) (1–6). Since the beginning of this century, scientists have postulated that exacerbations of chronic bronchitis were caused by infectious microorganisms (7). In the 1950s it was reported that there was an association between exacerbation of chronic bronchitis and the recovery of *Haemophilus influenzae* and *Streptococcus pneumoniae* from the sputum (8).

The introduction of antibiotics in the early 1950s revolutionized the therapy of chronic bronchitis with positive initial reports. Almost all classes of antibiotics have been studied for the treatment of COPD.

However, despite the long clinical experience and the great number of clinical trials, the role of antibiotics in COPD remains controversial. Some of the methodological problems involved changes in the definition of COPD (inclusion/exclusion of asthma) as well as the lack of precise definition of an acute exacerbation of COPD. In addition, lack of microbiological data and subjective interpretation of improvement as "symptom-driven" or patient "self-reports" or "investigator's clinical impression" mean that most clinical studies lack evidence-based standards (7). Thus, there are still unanswered questions, such as which is the best antibiotic agent, what is the optimal duration, is microbiological confirmation necessary before starting treatment, is it appropriate to instruct the patient to self-administer antibiotics, etc.

In this chapter we will review clinical trials investigating the efficacy of antibiotic therapy in COPD with emphasis on the methodological and interpretive difficulties and on the consensus guidelines for the management of the disease. We will review the "prophylactic" use of antibiotics in stable COPD and the use of antibiotics in acute exacerbations of the disease.

II. General Approach

A. Common Pathogens in COPD Exacerbations

A purulent sputum is not *associated* with bacterial infection *only*, since other conditions, such as allergic inflammation, could have the same appearance. Sputum Gram's stain showing neutrophils and not eosinophils suggests bacterial infection, but it is rarely performed in clinical practice. Furthermore, sputum cultures are contaminated from the upper respiratory tract flora and frequently are not in agreement with those taken by protected methodologies (9). Since sputum culture has many limitations, empirical therapy with antibiotics is recommended by all recent guidelines (1–6). However, in difficult cases attempts to obtain uncontaminated samples from the respiratory tract may be justified. This could be done by stopping antimicrobial treatment for 48–72 hours before performing a bronchoscopy with protected bronchoalveolar lavage or protected brush to avoid oropharyngeal contamination (10).

Potential bacterial pathogens are cultured from respiratory secretions in approximately two thirds of all acute exacerbations of COPD (AECOPD) (11). The three most common bacterial pathogens isolated during acute AECOPD are *Haemophilus influenzae, Streptococcus pneumoniae*, and *Moraxella catarrhalis* (12–17). In 1959 it was found that these three bacteria are present in sputum cultures, singly or jointly, in 75% of COPD patients. *H. influenzae* was isolated most commonly, being found in 54% of patients who had bacterial presence compared with pneumococci in 32% and mixed cultures of these two pathogens in 11% (16). In a recent study, intracellular *H influenzae* was found in 13 of 15 acutely ill chronic bronchitis patients (18).

Recently, *M. catarrhalis* has been recognized as a frequent pathogen (19,20). Airway inflammation has been associated with isolation of *H. influenzae* and *M. catarrhalis*, supporting an etiological role of these pathogens in acute exacerbations of chronic bronchitis (21). However, *H. influenzae* is the pathogen most widely studied (22–26). It has been shown that the ability of a COPD patient to react against *H. influenzae* infection depends partly on the ability of his or her T cells to recognize P6 (an outer membrane lipoprotein highly conserved among strains of *H. influenzae*) (27).

It has been found experimentally that *H. influenzae* produces an IgA protease enzyme that inactivates secretory IgA in bronchi, permeating in this manner the pathogen to adhere to epithelium (23–25). Also, the major outer membrane proteins of *H. influenzae* change over time, making the antibodies from previous infection inactive and permitting the development of new infection. However, the reports on this issue are conflicting (28,29), probably reflecting differences in disease severity and methodology. In addition to sputum cultures, more invasive techniques, including transtracheal lung aspiration and protected specimen brush technique, have been employed in an attempt to minimise upper airway contamination.

It is remarkable that the same common pathogens (*H. influenzae*, *S. pneumoniae*, and *M. catarrhalis*) have been isolated over the last 40 years in mild nonhospitalized COPD patients during exacerbations. The only significant change observed during these years is the increase in resistant strains. In a recent study it has been found that β-lactamase activity is often detected in sputum specimens from patients with acute exacerbation of chronic bronchitis (30). Thus, knowledge of local resistance patterns is very useful in directing empirical antibiotic therapy. In addition, recent studies reported that *Chlamydia pneumoniae* might be the cause of at least 4% of AECOPD (31,32). Also, in a serologically based study, atypical bacteria, such as *Legionella* spp. *Mycoplasma pneumoniae*, and *Coxiella burnetti*, were identified more often than classic bacteria (33).

Other gram-negative bacteria, e.g., *Pseudomonas aeruginosa*, are isolated from patients with more severe COPD (34). Patients with the greatest degree of functional impairment during an exacerbation, as measured by FEV_1, present a higher probability of having an isolation of *P. aeruginosa* of *H. influenzae* in significant concentrations in sputum (35). Fagon et al. (36) studied 54 patients with severe AECOPD needing mechanical ventilation. In half of them, bacterial infection was found on bronchoscopic protected specimen. This important study supports the opinion that not all AECOPD are of bacterial origin and that antibiotics should be prescribed only in severe exacerbations. The most common isolates were *H. parainfluenzae* (25%), *S. pneumoniae* (16%), and

H. influenzae (14%). Other isolates included *M. catarrhalis, P. aeruginosa, Proteus mirabilis,* and *Staphylococcus aureus.* Thus, gram-bacteria could be the cause of a severe exacerbation in patients with frequent hospital admissions, particularly in those treated in the ICU with low FEV_1 (34–37).

B. Bacterial Colonization in Stable COPD

A number of COPD patients are permanently colonized by bacteria between exacerbations (38) and the bacterial burden increases during exacerbation (39,40). In one study it was found using bronchoscopic protected brush specimen that 10 of 40 COPD patients were colonized by bacteria when in stable condition. During an exacerbation the percentage of infected samples, mostly by the three most common bacteria, reached 50% (41). Bacterial colonization of distal airways in stable COPD patients has been related to the degree of airflow obstruction and cigarette smoking (42,43).

Bronchial infections usually remains localized in the mucosa, and many resolve spontaneously without antibiotic treatment (44). Persistence of bacterial infection reflects the severity of impairment of respiratory defenses rather than the virulence of the microorganism, It is believed that the damage produced by the host inflammatory response to chronic bacterial infection may be more important than the damage by the bacteria (44,45). The role of infection in COPD had been reviewed by Wilson (46).

III. Antibiotics in Stable COPD

The prophylactic use of antibiotics in COPD was tested in large-scale controlled studies in the 1950s and 1960s (47–50). In one classic study contracted by the Medical Research Council (49), patients with "early" chronic bronchitis were treated in a double-blind, placebo-controlled fashion with oxytetracycline (2 g/day per os) and placebo for prophylaxis in a 5-year period. Patients who had "mild disability," were defined clinically (no more than two chest infections in the preceding 3 years) and spirometrically (FEV_1 exceeding 1.4 L). It was found that treated patients had no benefit from antibiotic prophylaxis and no difference in the number of exacerbations and FEV_1 decline over 5 years. Another study by Johnston et al. examined the efficacy of winter prophylaxis over a maximum period of 5 years (51). They used four regimens: placebo, tetracycline 500 mg bid for 2 winters and then placebo for 3 winters, placebo for 2 winters and then tetracycline for 3 winters, or tetracycline for 5 winters. They also concluded that there was no significant benefit for prophylactic use of antibiotics in COPD. Few studies in the 1970s or 1980s were performed on prophylaxis in COPD (52–55). The clinical trials of antibiotic prophylaxis in stable COPD are summarized in Table 1. Based on the above evidence, none of the recent guidelines for COPD is in favor of prophylactic use of antibiotics in stable COPD (1–6).

Table 1 Placebo-Controlled Studies on Antibiotic Prophylaxis in COPD

No. of patients	Antibiotic and dose	Results	Ref.
226	Tetracycline 250 mg PO b.i.d. vs. placebo	Frequency of acute exacerbations comparable in all groups: number of days lost from work decreased for antibiotic group	46
519	Four Regimens: A. Placebo maintenance, penicillin for exacerbations (312 mg PO b.i.d.) B. Tetracycline maintenance (250 mg b.i.d.) placebo for exacerbations C. Maintenance penicillin, placebo for exacerbations D. Maintenance placebo, tetracycline for exacerbations	Frequency of exacerbations decreased somewhat for regimens B, C, D: no differ-ence between intermittent and continuous tetracycline (B and D are the same)	47
373	Oxytetracycline (500 mg q.d. to 1 g b.i.d.) during winter months over 5 y vs. placebo	Frequency of exacerbations not improved with antibiotics	48
79	Four regimens: A. Placebo for 5 winters B. Tetracycline (500 mg b.i.d.) × 2 winters, then placebo × 3 winters C. Placebo × 2 winters, then tetracycline × 3 winters D. Tetracycline × 5 winter	Frequency of exacerbations comparable for all groups: possible benefit reported for antibiotic in high-risk patient, ignored in original study design	50
24	Trimethoprim (300 mg PO q.d.) vs. placebo	No benefit with antibiotic prophylaxis	54

Source: Modified from Ref. 7.

IV.   Antibiotics in Acute Exacerbation of COPD

A.   Introduction

The use of antibiotics in the treatment of AECOPD is universally accepted (1–6,56). However, significant methodological clinical issues make studies with antibiotics in AECOPD difficult to interpret. There is not a commonly accepted definition of an AECOPD. Furthermore, it is well known that more than 50% of AECOPD may be caused by factors other than bacterial infection (25). A significant confounding factor is viral infection with a prevalence rating from 4.4 to 63%, which may mimick bacterial infection (57). In addition, the lack of radiographic signs cannot exclude bacterial infection of the lower airways (tracheobronchitis). A computerized research of the literature showed a large number of hits for "COPD" and "antibiotics." However, only 46 comply with "placebo," of which only 18 were relevant (7 are reviews, one is a meta-analysis, 6 investigate one drug versus placebo, and 4 investigated combinations).

A meta-analysis of randomized trials on the effectiveness of antibiotics in treating exacerbations of COPD included nine studies and showed that the overall summary effect size was 0.22, indicating a small benefit in the antibiotic group (58). In addition, the overall change in peak expiratory flow rate was 0.19 (summary effect size) in favor of antibiotics (Fig. 1). The authors concluded that there is a small but significant improvement from antibiotic therapy in patients with exacerbations of COPD and that this improvement may be clinically significant, especially in patients with low

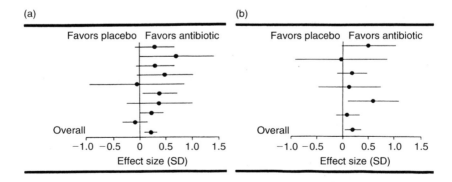

Figure 1   Results of meta-analysis of the effects of antibiotics on AECOPD. (a) A mean outcome in the antibiotic and placebo groups and overall estimate in favor of antibiotics. (b) Peak expiratory flow rate effects, and overall estimate that favors antibiotics (Modified from Ref. 58.).

baseline flow rates. One recent study comparing ofloxacin to placebo in severe exacerbation of COPD showed the effectiveness of the antibiotic (59). Besides patients with severe functional impairment, those with a high number of exacerbations per year gain the greatest benefit from antibiotic treatment (60). Additionally, it has been found that patients with AECOPD treated with antibiotics have significantly lower relapse rates than those who did not receive antibiotics (61).

B. Penicillin

The majority of clinical trials of antibiotics on COPD were performed using a penicillin class agent. More than 250 studies have been reported with ampicillin (219 studies) and amoxicillin (112 studies) the antibiotics most commonly tested. In addition, other agents of penicillin origin were studied for COPD, such as methicillin (14 studies), oxacillin (7 studies), piperacillin (6 studies), tricarcillin, and dicloxacillin. Of the 250 studies, very few had a placebo arm and were randomized. These few studies were performed using ampicillin, amoxicillin, or amoxicillin/clavulanate as the prime antibiotics. Only three of these reports were included in the recent meta-analysis by Saint et al. (58). These were the study of Elmes et al. in 1965 using ampicillin in 56 inpatients with COPD (62), the study of Anthonisen et al. in 310 outpatients using amoxicillin in combination with sulfamethoxazole/trimethoprim (63), and the study of Jorgensen et al. with amoxicillin in 262 outpatients with COPD (64). Two of the above studies showed an effect size favoring the antibiotic, but the study of Jorgensen et al. favors placebo (58). Thus, ampicillin, amoxicillin, or amoxicillin/clavulanate are effective on the most common pathogens causing acute exacerbation of COPD, and these agents are considered today as first-line antibiotics for AECOPD.

C. Chloramphenicol

Forty-one studies used chloramphenicol as the prime antibiotic to treat AECOPD. From these studies, only one had a placebo arm and was included in the meta-analysis of Saint et al. (58). This study of Petersen et al. was performed in 19 patients admitted into the hospital and showed a small overall effect in favor of placebo versus the active drug (65). Thus, chloramphenicol is no longer considered as a first-line antibiotic in COPD.

D. Trimethoprim-Sulfamethoxazole

The computerized research of the literature showed 83 hits on the above antibiotic in COPD. From those, only 3 used a placebo arm and only one, the study of Anthonisen et al. (63), was randomized, and this was included in the meta-analysis. In this study the combination of trimethoprim/ sulfamethoxazole plus amoxicillin or doxycycline was studied versus placebo. The study was performed in 310 outpatients with AECOPD. This study showed positive results in favor of the active drugs versus placebo. In addition, Anthonisen et al.'s study showed the greater effect of antibiotics on the peak expiratory flow rates (PEFR) in relation to the other studies included in the meta-analysis (58) (Fig. 1).

E. Tetracyclines

There are many studies using agents of this class of antibiotics to treat AECOPD (133 studies). Six of these studies had a placebo arm and were randomized and included in the meta-analysis (58). These early studies were performed in outpatients using oxytetracycline (66–68). The total number of subjects was 265, and all three studies came up with results in favor of oxytetracycline. Two more studies investigated tetracycline in hospitalized patients with acute AECOPD (69,70). The total number of patients was 189, and both studies showed results favoring the use of tetracycline versus placebo in inpatients with COPD. In addition, the Anthonisen et al. study used doxycycline as an alternative to amoxicillin and showed an equivalent efficacy when those antibiotics were added to trimethoprim (63). Therefore, tetracyclines are considered as first-line antibiotics for AECOPD.

F. Macrolides

A number of studies (98 studies) investigated macrolides in COPD patients. All major macrolides, such as erythromycin (77 studies), clarithromycin ($n = 26$), azithromycin ($n = 16$), and dirithromycin ($n = 12$), were studied in AECOPD. However, only four of the above studies were randomized (69–72), and none was placebo controlled. The majority of the studies, especially those testing the newer macrolides, are comparable to those using other antibiotics. The common message of those studies is that newer macrolides are as effective as erythromycin or amoxicillin in the treatment of AECOPD.

G. Aminoglycosides

Twenty-nine studies included aminoglycosides in the treatment of COPD. Only one had a placebo arm and showed efficacy of this class of antibiotics in severe hospitalized patients (75).

H. Cephalosporins

One hundred and seventy studies investigated the effect of cephalosporins on COPD patients. Most of these studies compared cephalosporins with common antibiotics, such as amoxicillin, tetracycline, or macrolides. Very few used a placebo arm (59), and four were randomized (76–79). All generations of cephalosporins were studied, and the general conclusion is that cephalosporins are as effective as the first-line antibiotics.

I. Quinolones

Sixteen studies were found to investigate quinolones in COPD with positive results. Most were comparative studies between quinolones and other commonly used antibiotics (80). However, quinolones should be used as second-line agents when the simple ones fail to treat AECOPD (63).

J. Imipenem

Three are 11 studies using imipenem in COPD. Only one was randomized (81). Those studies showed that imipenem is effective in COPD but should be used only in severe hospitalized patients (81).

K. Recent Comparative Studies

Since a recent meta-analysis of the use of antibiotics in AECOPD (58), there are few randomized studies investigating antibiotics in acute exacerbations of COPD. Most compare the effect of two agents and lack a placebo arm. The majority of these studies compare "classical" antibiotics such as amoxicillin + clavulanic acid or macrolides with newer cephalosporines or quinolones (71–74, 81–106). The common finding of all these studies was that newer antibiotics are as effective as the first-line inexpensive ones.

V. Cost-Effectiveness

There are very few studies on the cost-effectiveness of antibiotics in AECOPD. In 1997, a pharmacoeconomic analysis by Quenzer et al. showed significant differences among various antibiotics in AECOPD, e.g., $307 for clarithromycin in $612 for cefaclor (107). Grossman et al. investigated the cost-effectiveness of ciprofloxacin versus usual antibiotics and concluded that ony in severe cases with at least four acute exacerbations within the previous year did ciprofloxacin offer economic benefits (89). However, de Klerk et al. compared ceftriaxone with usual therapy and showed a lower cost with ceftriaxone (108). Finally, Destache et al. in 1999 studied the clinical and economic considerations in the treatment of AECOPD and found that the cost was lower with first-line agents, but that newer more expensive drugs reduced the failure rates (109). It is obvious that more studies investigating the cost-effectiveness are needed to validate the proper use of antibiotics in AECOPD from an economic point of view (110,112).

VI. Clinical Recommendations

A. Antibiotic Selection

Recently Schentag and Tillotson proposed seven parameters to be taken into account when selecting an antibiotic in AECOPD (113): 1) local common pathogens and local susceptibility, 2) spectrum of the antibiotic and mode of action, 3) tissue penetration, 4) drug tolerability, 5) frequency and route of administration, 6) drug metabolism and excretion, and 7) cost-effective treatment. Although all of the above factors have excellent theoretical value, only the first two could have a significant effect on the outcomes.

B. Classification of Infectious Exacerbations in COPD

An important issue to be taken into account before choosing an antibiotic is the severity of the exacerbation. Anthonisen et al. used basic symptoms such as cough and sputum, sputum purulence, and dyspnea to categorize patient with AECOPD (63). They concluded that if the patient had all three symptoms, he or she was more likely to benefit from antibiotic therapy (63). More recently, Wilson et al. proposed a four-category classification scheme (46). They included in the first category previously healthy patients with postviral tracheobronchitis without underlying structural disease. The second category included patients with mild bronchial obstruction and bronchial infection by one of the three most common bacteria in almost half of the cases. In this category, amoxicillin, doxycyline or TMP-SMX is usually sufficient. In the third category, COPD patients with bronchial infection have a significant degree of bronchial obstruction, comorbid conditions, and usually ≥4 exacerbations per year. The bacterial pathogens are the same but resistance to β-lactam is common. Therefore, it is preferable to prescribe a β-lactam with a β-lactamase inhibitor or a newer macrolide as the first-line antibiotic. In the fourth category, patients have severe bronchial obstruction, chronic bronchial suppuration (bronchiectasis), usually infected, despite the above common pathogens, with gram-negative bacteria *Enterobacter* spp., *Pseudomonas aeruginosa*, etc.). They have comorbidity and are on oral steroids for long periods (46).

Since infectious exacerbations in COPD are difficult to distinguish from noninfectious ones, recent guidelines for the management of COPD adopt a more simplistic approach to categorize the severity of an exacerbation. Two major categories have been proposed (1–6): mild exacerbations that can be treated at home, and severe exacerbations that require hospital admission. The assessment of severity of an acute episode is based on 1) the condition of the patient before the exacerbation, 2) symptoms and physical examination (signs), and 3) laboratory measurements (2,56).

C. International Guidelines for the Management of AECOPD

When to Use Antibiotics During an AECOPD

All recent guidelines for the management of COPD recommend the use of antibiotics in the management of AECOPD. However, when to use them is not clear. The European guidelines as well as the recent GOLD guidelines (6) recommend antibiotics when there are clinical signs of an exacerbation and purulent sputum (2), while American guidelines specify a change in sputum color and/or consistency for the outpatients and in all cases of hospitalized patients (1). Canadian guidelines suggest antibiotics when two or more symptoms of increased cough/sputum, sputum purulence, and dyspnea are present (4). The recent British guidelines recommend antibiotics when two or more symptoms of increased breathlessness, increased sputum volume, and development of purulent sputum coexist (3).

Sputum Analysis

Initial sputum analysis is not recommended by most guidelines. Only the Canadian ones suggest an initial sputum culture when FEV_1 is < 30% of predicted, age is <65 years, or there are more than four exacerbations per year (4). All guidelines recommend a sputum analysis when the response to initial (empiric) therapy is poor or there is deterioration (1–6). ATS guidelines recommend sputum culture in patients living in nursing homes (1).

First-Line Antibiotics

The ERS guidelines indicate amoxicillin, tetracycline derivatives, and amoxicillin/clavulanic acid as antibiotics for initial empirical therapy (2). ATS guidelines recommend tetracycline, doxycycline, amoxicillin, erythromycin, trimethoprim-sulfamethoxazole, cefaclor (1), and the Canadian ones aminopenicillin, tetracycline, or trimethoprim-sulfamethoxazole (4). The GOLD guidelines recommend that the choice of agents should reflect local patters of antibiotic sensitivity among *S. pneumoniae, H. influenzae,* and *M. catarrhalis* (6).

Second-Line Antibiotics

If first-line drugs fail or in cases of severe hospitalized patients, a second-line antibiotic should be used. In these include the newer cephalosporines, macrolides, and quinolones (2), in the United States broad-spectrum penicillins and cephalosporines (1), and in Canada the cephalosporines (second/third-generation) amoxicillin/clavulanic acid, newer macrolides, and quinolones (4).

Route of Administration

The British guidelines comment that oral rather than IV routes should be used (3). Other guidelines state that intravenous routes should be used in severe hospitalized cases (1,2). Finally, the efficacy of aerosolized antibiotics in AECOPD is not known, and this route is not recommended (2).

Duration of Treatment

There is not universal agreement on the duration of antibiotic treatment for an AECOPD. ERS guidelines recommended 7–14 days (2), the British Thoracic Society states that 7 days treatment is sufficient (3), but the more recent Finnish guidelines recommend a course of 10–20 days (5).

The above differences and similarities in international guidelines have been reviewed by Ball and Make (114). The value of antibiotics and outcomes of therapy in exacerbations of COPD have been recently reviewed (115,116).

VII. Conclusions

1. The prophylactic use of antibiotics in stable COPD is not recommended.
2. Knowledge of local microbiological data and resistance rates is useful in choosing empirical antibiotic therapy in AECOPD.
3. The most common bacteria responsible for AECOPD are *Streptococcus pneumoniae, Haemophilus influenzae*, and *Moraxella catarrhalis*. However, *Chlamydia* species in mild cases or gram-bacteria in hospitalized patients may be causative agents of an AECOPD.
4. Sputum culture is usually not required before starting antibiotic therapy in mild cases. It may be of importance in hospitalized severe patients, those with frequent exacerbations, or nursing home residents.

5. Begin antibiotic therapy when cough/sputum and dyspnea increase and sputum becomes purulent.
6. In most areas of the world, inexpensive antibiotics (amoxycillin, tetracycline, amoxycillin/calvulanic acid, erythromycin, trimethoprim/sulfamethoxazole) are effective and considered as first-line agents in AECOPD.
7. Newer antibiotics (cephalosporines, macrolides, quinolones, imipenem) should be used in severe cases or in case of treatment failure.
8. The duration of treatment should be 7–14 days.
9. More cost-effective studies are needed to validate the use of antibiotics in AECOPD.

References

1. ATS Statement. Standards for the diagnosis and care of patients with chronic obstructive pulmonary disease. Am J Respir Crit Care Med 1955; 152:S77–S120.
2. Saifakas NM, Vermeire P, Pride NB, Paoletti P, Gibson J, Howard P, Yernault JC, Decramer M, Higenbottam T, Postma DS, et al. ERS Consensus Statement. Optimal assessment and management of chronic obstructive pulmonary disease (COPD). Eur Respir J 1995; 8:1398–1420.
3. The COPD Guidelines Group of the Standards of Care Committee of the BTS. BTS Guidelines for the Management of Chronic Obstructive Pulmonary Disease. Thorax 1997; 52:S1–S28.
4. Balter MS, Ryland RH, Low DE, et al. Recommendations on the management of chronic bronchitis: a practical guide for Canadian physicians. Can Med Assoc J 1994; 151(10 suppl):8–23.
5. Laitinen LA, Koskela K, and the Expert Advisory Group Listed in the foreword. Chronic bronchitis and chronic obstructive pulmonary disease: Finnish National Guidelines for prevention and treatment 1998–2007. Respir Med 1999; 93:297–332.
6. Pauwels RA, Buist AS, Ma P, Jenkins CR, Hurd SS. Global strategy for the diagnosis, management, and prevention of chronic obstructive pulmonary disease: National Heart, Lung, and Blood Institute and World Health Organization Global Initiative for Chronic Obstructive Lung Disease (GOLD): executive summary. Respir Care 2001; 46(8):798–825.
7. Isada CM, Stoller JK. Chronic bronchitis: role of antibiotics. In: Nederman MS, Sarosi GA, Glassroth J, eds. Respiratory Infections. A Scientific Basis for Management. Philadelphia: W. B. Saunders, 1994:621–633.
8. May JR. The bacteriology of chronic bronchitis. Lancet 1953; 2:534–537.
9. Niederman MS. Respiratory infections: an opportunity for integrated disease management (ed). Chest 1996; 109:1133–1134.

10. Hosker H, Cooke NJ, Hawkey P. Antibiotics in chronic obstructive pulmonary disease. Br Med J 1994; 308:871–872.

11. Connors AF Jr, Dawson NV, Thomas C, Harrell FE Jr, Desbiens N, Fulkerson WJ, Kussin P, Bellamy P, Goldman L, Knaus WA. Outcomes following acute exacerbations of severe chronic obstructive lung disease. Am J Respir Crit Care Med 1996; 154:959–967.

12. Chodosh S. Acute bacterial exacerbations in bronchitis and asthma. Am J Med 1987; 82(suppl 4A):154–163.

13. Ball P, Tillotson G, Wilson R. Chemotherapy for chronic bronchitis controversies. Presse Med 1995; 24:184–194.

14. MacFarlane JT, Colville A, Guion A, Macfarlane RM, Rose DH. Prospective study of aetiology and outcome of adult lower respiratory tract infections in the community. Lancet 1993; 341:511–514.

15. Sportel JH, Koeter GH, van Altena R, Lowenberg A, Boersma WG. Relation between b-lactamase producing bacteria and patient characteristics in chronic obstructive pulmonary disease (COPD). Thorax 1995; 50:249–253.

16. Lees AW, McNaught W. Bacteriology of lower respiratory tract secretions, sputum and upper respiratory tract secretions in normals and chronic bronchitics. Lancet 1959; 2:1112–1115.

17. Sethi S, Murphy TF. Bacterial infection in chronic obstructive pulmonary disease in 2000: a state-of-the-art review. Clin Microbiol Rev 2001; 14(2):336–363.

18. Bandi V, Apicella MA, Mason E, Murphy TF, Siddiqi A, Atmar RL, Greenberg SB. Nontypeable *Haemophilus influenzae* in the lower respiratory tract of patients with chronic bronchitis. Am J Respir Crit Care Med 2001; 164(11):2114–2119.

19. McLeod DT, Ahmad F, Power JT, Calder MA, Seaton A. Bronchopulmonary infection due to *Branhamella catarrhalis*. Br Med J 1983; 287:1446–1447.

20. Slevin NJ, Airken J, Thornley PE. Clinical and microbiological features of *Branhamella catarrhalis* bronchopulmonary infections. Lancet 1984; 1:782–783.

21. Sethi S, Muscarella K, Evans N, Klingman KL, Grant BJ, Murphy TF. Airway inflammation and etiology of acute exacerbations of chronic bronchitis. Chest 2000; 118(6):1557–1565.

22. Murphy TF, Apicella MA. Nontypable *Haemophilus influenzae*: a review of clinical aspects, surface antigens, and the human response to infection. Rev Infect Dis 1987; 9:1–15.

23. Groeneveld K, van Alphen L, Eijk PP, Jansen HM, Zanen HC. Change in outer membrane proteins of nontypable *Haemophilus influenzae* in patients with COPD. J Infect Dis 1988; 158:360–365.

24. Turk DC. The pathogenicity of *Haemophilus influenzae*. J Med Microbiol 1984; 18:1–16.

25. Loeb MR, Smith DH. Outer membrane protein composition in disease isolates of *Haemophilus influenzae*: pathogenic and epidemiological implications. Infect Immun 1980; 30:709–717.

26. Clancy R, Cripps A, Murree-Allen K, Yeung S, Engel M. Oral immunization with killed *Haemophilus influenzae* for protection against acute bronchitis in chronic obstructive lung disease. Lancet 1985; 2:1395–1397.

27. Abe Y, Murphy TF, Sethi S, Faden HS, Dmochowski J, Harabuchi Y, Thanavala YM. Lymphocyte proliferative response to P6 of *Haemophilus influenzae* is associated with relative protection from exacerbations of chronic obstructive pulmonary disease. Am J Respir Crit Care Med 2002; 165(7):967–971.

28. Tager I, Speizer FE. Role of infection in chronic bronchitis. N Engl J Med 1975; 292:563–571.

29. Irwin RS, Corrao WM, Erickson AD, et al. Characterization by transtracheal aspiration of the tracheobronchial microflora during acute exacerbations of chronic obstructive bronchitis (abstr). Am Rev Respir Dis 1980; 121:150–151.

30. Brook I, Frazier EH. Bacteriology and beta-lactamase activity in acute exacerbation of chronic bronchitis. Int J Infect Dis 2001; 5(2):74–77.

31. Blasi F, Legnani D, Lombardo VM, Negretto GG, Magliano E, Pozzoli R, Chiodo F, Fasoli A, Allegra L. *Chlamydia pneumoniae* infection in acute exacerbations of COPD. Eur Respir J 1993; 6:19–22.

32. Mogulkoc N, Karakurt S, Isalska B, Bayindir U, Celikel T, Korten V, Colpan N. Acute purulent exacerbation of chronic obstructive pulmonary disease and *Chlamydia pneumoniae* infection. Am J Respir Crit Care Med 1999; 160:349–353.

33. Lieberman D, Lieberman D, Ben-Yaakov M, Lazarovich Z, Hoffman S, Ohana B, Friedman MG, Dvoskin B, Leinonen M, Boldur I. Infectious etiologies in acute exacerbation of COPD. Diagn Microbiol Infect Dis 2001; 40(3):95–102.

34. Eller J, Ede A, Schaberg T, Niederman MS, Mauch H, Lode H. Infective exacerbations of chronic bronchitis: relation between bacteriologic etiology and lung function. Chest 1998; 113(6):1542–1548.

35. Miravitlles M, Espinosa C, Fernandez-Laso E, Martos JA, Maldonado JA, Gallego M. Relationship between bacterial flora in sputum and functional impairment in patients with acute exacerbations of COPD. Study Group of Bacterial Infection in COPD. Chest 1999; 116(1):40–46.

36. Fagon JY, Chastre J, Trouillet JL, et al. Characterization of distal bronchial microflora during acute exacerbation of chronic bronchitis: use of the protected specimen brush technique in 54 mechanically ventilated patients. Am Rev Respir Dis 1990; 142:1004–1008.

37. Miravitlles M, Espinosa C, Fernandez-Laso E, Martos JA, Maldonado JA, Gallego M. Relationship between flora in sputum and functional impairment in patients with acute exacerbations of COPD. Study Group of Bacterial Infection in COPD. Chest 1999; 116:40–46.

38. Groeneveld K, van Alphen L, Eijk PP, Visschers G, Jansen HM, Zanen HC. Endogenous and exogenous reinfections by *Haemophilus influenzae* in patients with chronic obstructive pulmonary disease: the effect of antibiotic treatment on persistence. J Infect Dis 1990; 161:512–517.

39. Fisher M, Akhtar AJ, Calder MA, Moffat MA, Stewart SM, Zealley H, Crofton JW. Pilot study of factors associated with exacerbations in chronic bronchitis. Br Med J 1969; 4:197–199.
40. Bandi V, Apicella MA, Mason E, Murphy TF, Siddiqi A, Atmar RL, Greenberg SB. Nontypeable *Haemophilus influenzae* in the lower respiratory tract of patients with chronic bronchitis. Am J Respir Crit Care Med 2001; 164(11):2114–2119.
41. Monso E, Ruiz J, Rosell A, Manterola J, Fiz J, Morera J, Ausina V. Bacterial infection in chronic obstructive airways disease: a study of stable and exacerbated outpatients using the protected specimen brush. Am J Respir Crit Care Med 1995; 152:1316–1320.
42. Monso E, Rosell A, Bonet G, Manterola J, Cardona PJ, Ruiz J, Morera J. Risk factors for lower airway bacterial colonization in chronic bronchitis. Eur Respir J 1999; 13(2):338–342.
43. Zalacain R, Sobradillo V, Amilibia J, Barron J, Achotegui V, Pijoan JI, Llorente JL. Predisposing factors to bacterial colonization in chronic obstructive pulmonary disease. Eur Respir J 1999; 13(2):343–843.
44. Murphy TF, Sethi S. Bacterial infection in chronic obstructive pulmonary disease. Am Rev Respir Dis 1992; 46:1067–1083.
45. Wilson R, Dowling RB, Jackson AD. The biology of bacterial colonization and invasion of the respiratory mucosa. Eur Respir J 1996; 9:1523–1530.
46. Wilson R. The role of infection in COPD. Chest 1998; 113:242S–248S.
47. Francis RS, Spicer CC. Chemotherapy in chronic bronchitis: influence of daily penicillin and tetracycline on exacerbations and their cost. A report to the research committee of the British Tuberculosis Association by their chronic bronchitis subcommittee. Br Med J 1960; 1:297–303.
48. Francis RS, May JR, Spicer CC. Chemotherapy of bronchitis: influence of penicillin and tetracycline administered daily, or intermittently, for exacerbations. Br Med J 1961; 2:979–985.
49. Fletcher CM, Ball JD, Carstairs LW, et al. Value of chemoprophylaxis and chemotherapy in early chronic bronchitis: A report to the Medical Research Council by their Working Party on Trials of Chemotherapy in early chronic bronchitis. Br Med J 1996; 1:1317–1322.
50. Murdoch JM, Leckie WJH, Doenie J. An evaluation of continuous antibiotic therapy in chronic bronchitis. Br Med J 1959; 2:1277–1285.
51. Johnston RN, McNeill RS, Smith DH, et al. Five-year winter chemoprophylaxis for chronic bronchitis. Br Med J 1969; 265–269.
52. Pines A. Cephalexin in the prevention of purulent exacerbations of chronic bronchitis. Br J Clin Pract 1972; 26:209–210.
53. Pines A. Trimethoprim-sulfamethoxazol in the treatment and prevention of purulent exacerbations of chronic bronchitis. J Infect Dis 1973; 128(suppl): S706–S709.
54. Cooper J, Inman JS, Currie WJC. Prophylactic treatment of chronic bronchitis comparing co-trimoxazole and amoxicilline. Br J Clin Pract 1975; 29:307–310.

55. Liipo K, Pelliniemi TT, Letho H. Trimethroprim prophylaxis in acute exacerbations of COPD. Acta Med Scand 1987; 221:455–459.

56. Siafakas NM, Bouros D. Management of acute exacerbation of chronic obstructive pulmonary disease. In: Postma DS, Siafakas NM, eds. Management of Chronic Obstructive Pulmonary Disease. Vol. 7. Eur Respir Monograph, UK, Sheffield, 1998:264–277.

57. Sachs FL. Chronic bronchitis. In: Pennington JE (ed). Respiratory Infections: Diagnosis and Management. New York: Raven Press, 1989; 142–158.

58. Saint S, Bent S, Vittinghoff E, Grady D. Antibiotics in chronic obstructive pulmonary disease exacerbations. A meta-analysis. JAMA 1995; 273(12):957–960.

59. Nouira S, Marghli S, Belghith M, Besbes L, Elatrous S, Abroug F. Once daily oral ofloxacin in chronic obstructive pulmonary disease exacerbation requiring mechanical ventilation: a randomised placebo-controlled trial. Lancet 2001; 358(9298):2020–2025.

60. Allegra L, Blasi F, de Bernardi B, Cosentini R, Tarsia P. Antibiotic treatment and baseline severity of disease in acute exacerbations of chronic bronchitis: a re-evaluation of previously published data of a placebo-controlled randomized study. Pulm Pharmacol Ther 2001; 14(2):149–155.

61. Adams SG, Melo J, Luther M, Anzueto A. Antibiotics are associated with lower relapse rates in outpatients with acute exacerbations of COPD. Chest 2000; 117(5):1345–1352.

62. Elmes PC, King TK, Langlands JH, Mackay JA, Wallace WF, Wade OL, Wilson TS. Value of ampicillin in the hospital treatment of exacerbations of chronic bronchitis. Br Med J 1965; 2:904–908.

63. Anthonisen NR, Harding GKM, Nelson NA. Antibiotic therapy in exacerbations of chronic obstructive pulmonary disease. Ann Intern Med 1987; 106:196–204.

64. Jorgensen AF, Coolidge J, Pedersen PA, Petersen KP, Waldorff S, Widding E. Amoxicillin in treatment of acute uncomplicated exacerbations of chronic bronchitis. Scand J Prim Heath Care 1992; 10:7–11.

65. Petersen ES, Esmann V, Honcke P, Munkner C. A controlled study of the effect of treatment on chronic bronchitis: an evaluation using pulmonary function tests. Acta Med Scand 1967; 182:293–305.

66. Elmes PC, Fletcher CM, Dutton AAC. Prophylactic use of oxytetracycline for exacerbations of chronic bronchitis. Br Med J 1957; 2:1272–1275.

67. Berry DG, Fry J, Hindley CP, Hodson JM, Horder EJ, Horder JP, Marien EA, Rea JN, Ryle A, Curwen MP, Tomlinson AJ. Exacerbations of chronic bronchitis treatment with oxytetracycline. Lancet 1960; 1:137–139.

68. Fear EC, Edwards G. Antibiotic regimes in chronic bronchitis. Br J Dis Chest 1962; 56:153–162.

69. Pines A, Raafat H, Greenfield JSB, Linsell WD, Solari ME. Antibiotic regimens in moderately ill patients with purulent exacerbations of chronic bronchitis. Br J Dis Chest 1972; 66:107–115.

70. Nicotra MB, Rivera M, Awe RJ. Antibiotic therapy of acute exacerbations of chronic bronchitis. Ann Intern Ned 1982; 97:18–21.
71. Martinot JB, Carr WD, Cullen S, Heredia Budo JL, Bauer K, MacLeod C, Sanguinetti CM, van Veldhuizen WC. A comparative study of clarithromycin modified release and amoxicillin/clavulanic acid in the treatment of acute exacerbation of chronic bronchitis. Adv Ther 2001; 18(1):1–11.
72. Adler JL, Jannetti W, Schneider D, Zhang J, Palmer R, Notario G. Phase III, randomized, double-blind study of clarithromycin extended-release and immediate-release formulations in the treatment of patients with acute exacerbation of chronic bronchitis. Clin Ther 2000; 22(12):1410–1420.
73. McCarty JM, Pierce PF. Five days of cefprozil versus 10 days of clarithromycin in the treatment of an acute exacerbation of chronic bronchitis. Ann Allergy Asthma Immunol 2001; 87(4):327–334.
74. Martinot JB, Carr WD, Cullen S, Heredia Budo JL, Bauer K, MacLeod C, Sanguinetti CM, van Veldhuizen WC. A comparative study of clarithromycin modified release and amoxicillin/clavulanic acid in the treatment of acute exacerbation of chronic bronchitis. Adv Ther 2001; 18(1):1–11.
75. Pines A, Raafat H, Plucinski K, Greenfield JSB, Solari M. Antibiotic regimens in severe and acute purulent exacerbations of chronic bronchitis. Br Med J 1968; 2:735–738.
76. Periti P, Novelli A, Schildwachter G, Schmidt-Gayk H, Ryo Y, Zuck P. Efficacy and tolerance of cefpodoxime proxetil compared with co-amoxiclav in the treatment of exacerbations of chronic bronchitis. J Antimicrob Chemother 1990; 26(suppl E):63–69.
77. Behler PG, et al. Amoxicillin/clavulanic acid vs cefetamet pivoxil in the treatment of acute exacerbation of chronic bronchitis (AECB) in adults. J Chemother 1995; 7:16–20.
78. Bint AJ, Cefai C, McGhie D, Perera BS. A randomised, prospective, single-blind comparison of cefadroxil and amoxycillin in the treatment of acute exacerbations of chronic bronchitis. Br J Clin Pract 1989; 43:19–23.
79. McCarty JM, Pierce PF. Five days of cefprozil versus 10 days of clarithromycin in the treatment of an acute exacerbation of chronic bronchitis. Ann Allergy Asthma Immunol 2001; 87(4):327–334.
80. Grossman RF. The role of fluoroquinolones in respiratory tract infections. J Antimicrob Chemother 1997; 40(suppl A):59–62.
81. Harmacher J, et al. Treatment of acute bacterial exacerbations of chronic obstructive pulmonary disease in hospitalised patients a comparison of meropenem and imipenem/cialtatin. COPD Study Group. J Antimicrob Chemother 1995; 36(suppl A):121–133.
82. Cazzola M, Vinciguerra A, Beghi GF, Paizis G, Giura R, Madonini V, Fiorentini F, Consigli GF, Tonna M, Casalini A, et al. Comparative evaluation of the clinical and microbiological efficacy of co-amoxislav vs cefixime or ciprofloxacine in bacterial exacerbation of chronic bronchitis. J Chemother 1995; 7(5):432–441.

83. Allegra L, Konietzko N, Leophonte P, Hosie J, Pawels R, Guyen JN, Petitpertz P. Comparative safety and efficacy of sparfloxacin in the treatment of acute exacerbations of chronic obstructive pulmonary disease: a double blind, randomised, parallel, mulitcenter study. J Antimicrob Chemother 1996; 37(suppl A):93–104.

84. Anzueto A, Niederman MS, Haverstock DC, Tillotson GS. Efficacy of ciprofloxacin and clarithromycin in acute bacterial exacerbations of complicated chronic bronchitis: interim analysis. Bronchitis Study Group. Clin Ther 1997; 19(5):989–1001.

85. Langan CE, Cranfield R, Breisch S, Pettit R. Randomized, double blind study of grepafloxacin versus amoxycillin in patients with acute bacterial exacerbations of chronic bronchitis. J Antimicrob Chemother 1997; 40(suppl A):63–72.

86. Hoepelman IM, Mollers MJ, van Schie MH, Greefhorst AP, Schlosser NJ, Sinninghe Damste EJ, van de Moosdijk CN, Dalinghaus WH, Eland ME, Mol SJ, Rozenberg-Arska M. A short (3-day) course of azithromycin tablets versus a ten day course of amoxycilline-calvulanic acid (co-amoxiclav) in the treatment of adults with lower respiratory tract infections and effects on long-term outcome. Int J Antimicrob Agents 1997; 9(3):141–146.

87. Mc Adoo Ma, Rice K, Gordon GR, Sahn SA. Comparison of ceftibuten once daily and amoxicillin-clavulanate three times daily in the treatment of acute exacerbations of chronic bronchitis. Clin Ther 1998; 20(1):88–100.

88. Ziering W, McElvaine P. Randomized comparison of once-daily ceftibuten and twice-daily clarithromycin in the treatment of acute exacerbation of chronic bronchitis. Infection 1998; 26(1):68–75.

89. Grossman R, Mukherjee J, Vaughan D, Eastwood C, Cook R, LaForge J, Lampron N. A 1-year community-based health economic study of ciprofloxacin vs usual antibiotic treatment in acute exacerbations in chronic bronchitis. Chest 1998; 113(1):131–140.

90. DeAbate CA, Henry D, Bensch G, Jubran A, Chodosh S, Harper L, Tipping D, Talbot GH. Sparfloxacin vs ofloxacin in the treatment of acute bacterial exacerbations of chronic bronchitis: a multicentre, double-blind, randomized, comparative study. Sparfloxacin multicentre ABECB study group. Chest 1998; 114(1):120–130.

91. Langan C, Clecner B, Cazzola CM, Brambilla C, Holmes CY, Staley H. Short-course cefuroxime axetil therapy in the treatment of acute exacerbations of chronic bronchitis. Int J Clin Pract 1998; 52(5):289–297.

92. O'Doherty B, Daniel R. Treatment of acute exacerbations of chronic bronchitis: comparison of trovafloxacin and amoxicillin in a multicentre, double-blind, double-dummy study. Trovlafloxacin bronchitis study group. Eur J Clin Microbiol Infect Dis 1998; 17(6):441–446.

93. Chodosh S, McCarty J, Farkas S, Drehoble M, Tosiello R, Shan M, Aneiro L, Kowalski S. Randomized, double-blind study of ciprofloxacin and cefuroxime axetil for treatment of acute bacterial exacerbations of chronic bronchitis. The Bronchitis Study Group. Clin Infect Dis 1998; 27(4):772–729.

94. Chodosh S, Schreurs A, Siami G, Barkman HW, Anzueto A, Shan M, Moesker H, Stack T, Kowalski S. Efficacy of oral ciprofloxacin vs. clarithromycin for treatment of acute bacterial exacerbations of chronic bronchitis. The Bronchitis Study Group. Clin Infect Dis 1998; 27(4):730–738.

95. DeAbate CA, Bettis R, Munk ZM, Fleming H, Munn NJ, Riffer E, Bagby B, Giguere G, Collins JJ. Effectiveness of short-course therapy (5 days) with grepafloxacin in the treatment of acute bacterial exacerbations of chronic bronchitis. Clin Ther 1999; 21(1):172–188.

96. Ball P, Wilson R, Mandell L, Brown J, Henkel T. Efficacy of gemifloxacin in acute exacerbations of chronic bronchitis: a randomised, double-blind comparison with trovafloxacin. J Chemother 2001; 13(3):288–298.

97. Martinot JB, Carr WD, Cullen S, Heredia Budo JL, Bauer K, MacLeod C, Sanguinetti CM, van Veldhuizen WC. A comparative study of clarithromycin modified release and amoxicillin/calvulanic acid in the treatment of acute exacerbation of chronic bronchitis. Adv Ther 2001; 18(1):1–11.

98. Gotfried MH, DeAbate CA, Fogarty C, Mathew CP, Sokol WN. Comparison of 5-day, short-course gatifloxacin therapy with 7-day gatifloxacin therapy and 10-day clarithromycin therapy for acute exacerbation of chronic bronchitis. Clin Ther 2001; 23(1):97–107.

99. Paste RZ, McAdoo MA, Keyserling CH, Nemeth MA, Tack KJ, Griffin TJ. A comparison of a five-day regimen of cefdinir with a seven-day regimen of loracarbef for the treatment of acute exacerbations of chronic bronchitis. Int J Clin Pract 2000; 54(5):293–299.

100. Fogarty CM, Bettis RB, Griffin TJ, Keyserling CH, Nemeth MA, Tack KJ. Comparison of 5 day regimen of cefdinir with a 10 day regimen of cefprozil for treatment of acute exacerbations of chronic bronchitis. J Antimicrob Chemother 2000; 45(6):851–858.

101. Anzueto A, Fisher CL Jr, Busman T, Olson CA. Comparison of the efficacy of extended-release clarithromycin tablets and amoxicillin/clavulanate tablets in the treatment of acute exacerbation of chronic bronchitis. Clin Ther 2001; 23(1):72–86.

102. Masterton RG, Burley CJ. Randomized, double-blind study comparing 5- and 7-day regimens of oral levofloxacin in patients with acute exacerbation of chronic bronchitis. Int J Antimicrob Agents 2001; 18(6):503–512.

103. Lipsky BA, Unowsky J, Zhang H, Townsend L, Talbot GH. Treating acute bacterial exacerbations of chronic bronchitis in patients unresponsive to previous therapy: sparfloxacin versus clarithromycin. Clin Ther 1999; 21(6):954–965.

104. Haczynski J, Chyczewska E, Grzelewska-Rzymowska I, Malolepszy J, Marcinkowska-Suchowierska E, Milanowski J, Oklek K, Plusa T, Slominski J, Szmygin K, Rek M. Comparative study of cefaclor AF vs. cefuroxime axetil in acute exacerbations of chronic bronchitis. Med Sci Monit 2002; 8(1):PI1–7.

105. Shah PM, Maesen FP, Dolmann A, Vetter N, Fiss E, Wesch R. Levofloxacin versus cefuroxime axetil in the treatment of acute exacerbation of chronic

bronchitis: results of a randomized, double-blind study. J Antimicrob Chemother 1999; 43(4):529–539.

106. Umut S, Tutluoglu B, Aydin Tosun G, Musellim B, Erk M, Yildirim N, Vahapoglu H, Yilmaz N, Arseven O, Turker H, Erelel M, Ilvan A, Goylusun V, Yilmaz Kuyucu T, Kosar F, Soysal F, Gur A, Unutmaz S, Ozturk S, Akman M. Determination of the etiological organism during acute exacerbations of COPD and efficacy of azithromycin ampicillin-sulbactam, ciprofloxacin and cefaclor. Turkish Thoracic Society COPD Working Group. J Chemother 1999; 11(3):211–214.

107. Quenzer RW, Pettit KG, Arnold RJ, Kaniecki DJ. Pharmacoeconomic analysis of selected antibiotics in lower respiratory tract infection. Am J Manag Care 1997; 3(7):1027–1036.

108. de Klerk GJ, van Steijn JH, Lobatto S, Jaspers CA, van Veldhuizen WC, Hensing CA, Bunnik MC, Geraedts WH, Dofferhof AS, Van Den Berg J, Melis JH, Hoepelman AI. A randomised, multicentre study of ceftriaxone versus standard therapy in the treatment of lower respiratory tract infections. Int J Antimicrob Agents 1999; 12(2):121–127.

109. Destache CJ, Dewan N, O'Donodhue WJ, Campbell JC, Angelillo VA. Clinical and economic considerations in the treatment of acute exacerbations of chronic bronchitis. J Antimicrob Chemother 1999; 43(suppl A):107–113.

110. Grossman R. How do we achieve cost-effective options in lower respiratory tract infection therapy? Chest 1998; 113:205S–210S.

111. Grossman RF. Cost-effective therapy for acute exacerbations of chronic bronchitis. Semin Respir Infect 2000; 15(1):71–81.

112. Pechere JC, Lacey L. Optimizing economic antibiotic therapy of patients with acute bacterial exacerbations of chronic bronchitis. J Antimicrob Chemother 2000; 45:19–24.

113. Schentag JJ, Tillotson GS. Antibiotic selection and dosing for the treatment of acute exacerbations of COPD. Chest 1997; 112:314S–319S.

114. Ball P, Make B. Acute exacerbations of chronic bronchitis. An international comparison. Chest 1998; 113(3):199S–204S.

115. Reynolds HY. Antibiotic treatment of bronchitis and chronic lung disease. In: Cherniack NS, ed. Chronic Obstructive Pulmonary Disease. Philadelphia: W. B. Saunders, 1991; 456–461.

116. Grossman R. The value of antibiotics and the outcomes of antibiotic therapy in exacerbations of COPD. Chest 1998; 113:249S–255S.

19

Long-Term Intervention Studies: α_1-Antitrypsin Substitution

ROBERT A. STOCKLEY

University of Birmingham NHS Trust
Queen Elizabeth Hospital
Edgbaston, Birmingham, England

I. Introduction

α_1-Antitrypsin deficiency is one of the most common inherited genetic defects of Caucasians. It is associated with an increased incidence of lung disease, neonatal liver disease and cirrhosis, the vasculitides, and rarer conditions such as necrotizing panniculitis. α_1-Antitrypsin is a 52 kDa glycoprotein of 394 residues with three asparagine-linked carbohydrate side chains. The gene is located at q32.1 on chromosome 14, and both alleles are usually expressed. The protein is polymorphic with many nucleotide substitutions, most of which are consistent with the protein functioning entirely normally. The polymorphisms can be identified by isoelectric focusing, and over 80 phenotypes have been identified. In the majority the function of the α_1-antitrypsin is retained, but some lead to a reduction in the antiproteinase inhibitory capacity of the plasma and hence the lung (see below).

Defective antiproteinase activity is associated with dysfunctional protein such as in the F phenotype, reductions in concentration due to increased catabolism as in the S phenotype, and markedly decreased

α_1-antitrypsin levels as in the Z phenotype. Finally, the protein may be absent altogether, as in the null phenotypes where transcription of the gene is defective (1).

II. α_1-Antitrypsin Deficiency

α_1-Antitrypsin deficiency was first described in 1963, and of the five patients identified, three were found to have severe emphysema at an early age (2). Subsequent studies confirmed that the deficiency was inherited, and in most of the early studies emphysema and chronic bronchitis were common features (3). The deficiency was shown to be associated with a marked reduction in the ability of the plasma to inhibit the serine proteinase trypsin, and later studies showed that this also reflected an inability of the serum to inhibit the enzyme neutrophil elastase.

Human neutrophil elastase was shown to produce both emphysema and chronic bronchial disease in animal models (4). This led to the concept that patients with severe α_1-antitrypsin deficiency had a reduced capacity to control this enzyme once it was released in the lung. The resultant effect was destruction of the lung by the enzyme leading to features of chronic bronchitis and emphysema. This concept was supported by clinical studies, which demonstrated that α_1-antitrypsin was the main inhibitor of neutrophil elastase in the lower airways and subjects with α_1-antitrypsin deficiency had low concentrations of the protein in this region of the lung (5). Furthermore, this deficiency was associated with an almost complete absence of elastase inhibitory capacity in the secretions lining the peripheral airways and alveoli. These experiments and observations led to the establishment of the proteinase/antiproteinase theory of the development of emphysema. In patients with α_1-antitrypsin deficiency, it is thought that the low concentration in the lung is insufficient to control neutrophil elastase released by migrating neutrophils. The enzyme is then able to digest lung elastin, leading to the development of pathological disease.

The concentration of α_1-antitrypsin in the lungs of deficient patients is low predominantly because the majority of α_1-antitrypsin is derived from the plasma by simple protein transudation. Although alveolar macrophages have been shown to produce α_1-antitrypsin, it is likely that this represents a small proportion of the total lung α_1-antitrypsin and may only play a role in the immediate vicinity of the lung macrophage. In normal subjects, therefore, virtually all of the lung α_1-antitrypsin has been derived from serum, and during episodes of acute lung inflammation the concentrations rise due to increased protein leakage as well as the increased acute phase response (6). These simple processes determine the concentrations of

α_1-antitrypsin both within the interstitium of the lung (where elastin degradation takes place) and in the secretions lining the airways.

In normal subjects the average serum concentration of α_1-antitrypsin is approximately 30 µmol and the concentration in epithelial lining fluid has been shown to be 2–5 µmol (7), representing a significant concentration gradient. In patients with α_1-antitrypsin deficiency, the serum level is markedly reduced to approximately 5 µmol, and a similar reduction is found in the epithelial lining fluid with an average concentration of approximately 0.5 µmol.

III. Replacement Strategies

With the observations outlined above and the belief that a local reduction in α_1-antitrypsin concentration was the key to the development of emphysema, it seemed logical to develop strategies to increase the serum α_1-antitrypsin leading to an appropriate increase in α_1-antitrypsin in the lung interstitium and epithelial lining fluid (8).

A. Acute Phase Response

α_1-Antitrypsin is an acute phase protein that is known to increase its serum concentrations during pregnancy and periods of systemic inflammation between two- and fourfold. Because anabolic steroids were known to increase the concentration of another serum proteinase inhibitor, C1 esterase inhibitor, early studies were conducted to determine whether pharmacological intervention could lead to an increase in α_1-antitrypsin release from the liver. Studies showed that danazol (9) and tamoxifen (10) were able to increase serum α_1-antitrypsin levels, although the response was small and nonuniform.

However, in these early studies the mechanism that led to α_1-antitrypsin deficiency in patients with the PIZ phenotype was unknown. Subsequent studies indicated that a single base change in the codon for glutamic acid at position 348 resulted in the production of a protein with lysine at this site. This leads to increased mobility of the active site loop and an opening of the A sheets facilitating polymerization of the protein causing accumulation of the protein in the endoplasmic reticulum of the hepatocyte inhibiting protein secretion (11). Thus, even stimulation of the acute phase response resulting in more protein production would, most likely, result in an increase in protein retention, restricting the serum acute phase response. Indeed, studies of deficient patients with acute exacerbations due to infection where a natural acute phase response should occur (Fig. 1) results in a minimal change in α_1-antitrypsin concentration (12). Thus, in retrospect

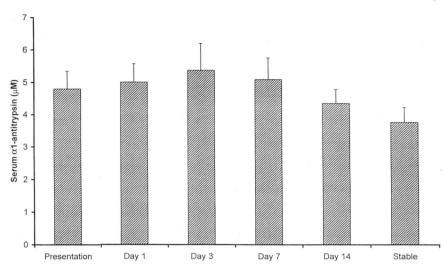

Figure 1   Acute phase response during exacerbations in α_1-antitrypsin deficiency. The vertical axis is the concentration of α_1-antitrypsin, and the histograms are mean with standard error. Data are shown for a group of patients at presentation with an acute bronchial exacerbation of their disease, for the 14 days following antibiotic therapy, and finally in a stable clinical state 2 weeks after the episode had resolved.

the failure of danazol or tamoxifen therapy to significantly increase the α_1-antitrypsin levels was predictable, and long-term therapy was more likely to produce side effects than any potential beneficial effect.

Studies have shown that it is possible to prevent the polymerization of the Z variant of α_1-antitrypsin (13), which should facilitate its secretion. At present these strategies would also lead to impairment of α_1-antitrypsin function, thereby abrogating any potential benefit to the lung.

B.   Replacement Therapy

The most logical way of treating α_1-antitrypsin deficiency seemed to be to adopt the strategy used in immunoglobulin deficiency, namely replacement therapy. The concentration of α_1-antitrypsin in normal plasma is high enough to facilitate a reasonable yield by protein purification. Early studies showed that it was possible to infuse the α_1-antitrypsin into the plasma of deficient subjects and that this would result in an increase in the concentration of α_1-antitrypsin in the lung lining fluid, indicating that diffusion from plasma had taken place (8). This led to the development of a variety of strategies to increase circulating α_1-antitrypsin. Epidemiological studies had indicated that subjects who were heterozygous for α_1-antitrypsin deficiency appeared to be at no greater risk of developing lung disease than subjects who had normal α_1-antitrypsin (14). In addition, subjects with the SZ phenotype where the plasma concentration was typically 11–14 µmol also appeared to be at little or no extra risk for developing lung disease (15). On the basis of these studies, it was felt that a serum α_1-antitrypsin concentration of 11 µmol or more was likely to be protective, thereby preventing neutrophil elastase–mediated lung destruction. On this basis it was argued that infusion of α_1-antitrypsin should lead to a significant increase in the plasma concentration of deficient subjects and that repeated infusions should be administered just prior to the plasma concentration falling below this putative protective threshold.

Initial studies (Fig. 2) showed that weekly infusions of 60 mg/kg of α_1-antitrypsin achieved these goals (16). Because of the inconvenience of weekly infusions, some patients have been treated on a biweekly basis (17), and finally studies showed that large infusions on a monthly basis could also be protective for most of the interval between treatments (18). On the basis

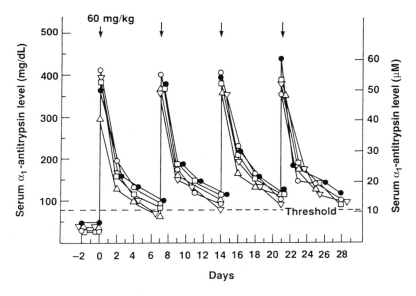

Figure 2 Serum concentration of α_1-antitrypsin following replacement therapy 60 mg/kg on a weekly basis. The results show that after the first infusion the patient's serum α_1-antitrypsin is maintained above the "protective threshold" for the 7 days preceding the next infusion. (From Ref. 16.) The individual symbols represent results from a single patient.

of these studies, FDA approved α_1-antitrypsin therapy on a weekly basis for patients with genetic deficiency associated with the PIZ or PI null phenotypes. Nevertheless, the National Heart, Lung and Blood registry indicated that a variety of regimens were in current use (19), and to date no clinical studies have been carried out to determine which is the most appropriate. Replacement therapy by this mechanism, however, has been shown to be acceptable to patients and apparently safe.

C. Inhaled Therapy

Because of the general shortage and expense of α_1-antitrypsin replacement therapy, strategies involving the inhaled route have been considered. Inhalation of either native or genetically engineered α_1-antitrypsin has been shown to increase its concentration in epithelial lining fluid (20). Twice-daily inhalation of 100 µg of protein leads to an increase in epithelial lining fluid concentration (on average) to just above the "normal" concentration. Such a strategy is clearly more acceptable to patients, more sparing of the product, and is currently under intense consideration as an alternative strategy.

IV. Mechanisms of Tissue Destruction in α_1-Antitrypsin Deficiency

Development of intervention strategies have to date been largely conceptual and hampered by a lack of understanding of the exact mechanisms involved in the development of emphysema in deficient subjects. It is thought that the process central to the development of emphysema is degradation of lung elastin within the interstitium. Because α_1-antitrypsin in the most effective naturally occurring inhibitor of neutrophil elastase and is normally present in high concentrations, it is believed that neutrophil elastase is the key to tissue destruction in patients with α_1-antitrypsin deficiency. The major source of human neutrophil elastase is the neutrophil, and the enzyme is made during cell differentiation and packaged into the azurophil granules. As the cells become activated, these granules are exocytosed, releasing the enzyme into the surrounding environment. This is thought to be an important physiological process, which allows the neutrophil to digest connective tissue as part of the process of migration from the vascular space into the airways. The neutrophil facilitates its passage through the compact connective tissue matrix by effectively generating its own "hole." Studies have shown that this process is largely elastase dependent and once the neutrophil is activated and adherent to a connective tissue substrate, the process of tissue degradation cannot be prevented by specific inhibitors, although it can be significantly limited (21).

Studies in patients with α_1-antitrypsin deficiency have shown that the number of neutrophils in the airways is markedly increased even in subjects with normal lung function (22). The major reason for this was an increase in the concentration of leukotriene B_4 (LTB4) within the airways (see later). The resultant migration of this large number of neutrophils is thought to be central to the development of connective tissue damage leading to the development of emphysema. As indicated above, studies have shown that α_1-antitrypsin can only partially prevent connective tissue degradation by activated neutrophils, and initially it was felt that this was predominantly because of exclusion of the protein from the microenvironment between the cell membrane and the connective tissue (23). More recently, however, studies have described the process of quantum proteolysis that demonstrates both theoretically (24) and practically (25) the reason for connective tissue degradation in the presence of elastase inhibitors.

The average concentration of elastase within the azurophil granule is approximately 5 mmol, and therefore its concentration close to the azurophil granule greatly exceeds that of normal α_1-antitrypsin. As the azurophil granule is released from the cell, elastase diffuses away and its concentration decreases until it equals that of the inhibitors when it becomes inactive as an enzyme. This process has been modeled mathematically, indicating the expected concentration of elastase at various distances from the source, i.e. the azurophil granule. The model predicts the radius of tissue destruction that would occur depending on the concentration of the surrounding inhibitor. The theory suggests that the concentration of the inhibitor would be critical and that at concentrations above 10 µmol a degree of degradation would always occur, but that within the normal physiological range for α_1-antitrypsin deficiency even wide variations in concentration would make little difference. For a concentration below 10 µmol, it is predicted that the area of continued enzyme activity would increase exponentially.

The theory was shown to be correct by studies using varying concentrations of a variety of natural and synthetic inhibitors of neutrophil elastase (25). More recently this has been extended to show that serum from subjects who are heterozygous for α_1-antitrypsin deficiency (i.e., the SZ and MZ phenotypes) as well as normal phenotypes are virtually identical in their ability to control the area of connective tissue destruction produced by an activated neutrophil. However, when serum from α_1-antitrypsin–deficient subjects is used, there is a 10-fold increase in the area of connective tissue damage (26). These studies have confirmed that the concentration of α_1-antitrypsin surrounding migrating neutrophils is directly responsible for

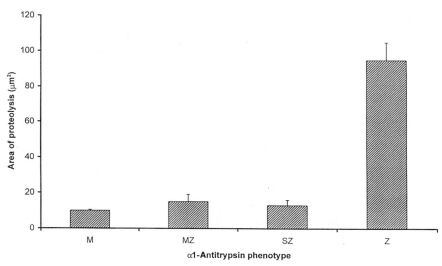

Figure 3 The area of proteolytic degradation of connective tissue is shown on the vertical axis. The results are mean plus standard deviation for neutrophils in the presence of serum obtained from patients with different α_1-antitrypsin phenotypes as indicated on the horizontal axis. The results indicate a significant increase in the area of damage produced by neutrophils in the presence of serum from patients with a PiZ phenotype. Note, serum from SZ patients has very little effect on the area of damage and may therefore explain the relatively low risk for this phenotype. (From Ref. 26.)

the degree of connective tissue destruction that would occur (Fig. 3). With this as a background, it is possible to review the potential replacement strategies to determine whether such approaches could be expected to lead to a significant reduction in connective tissue damage and hence progression of emphysema.

A. Intravenous Route

As indicated previously, there is a concentration gradient from the plasma into the airways. Studies have shown that most of the restriction of protein movement into the airways resides at the epithelial surface (27) and the concentration of albumin within the interstitium is approximately 80% of that in plasma. Since α_1-antitrypsin is essentially the same size as serum albumin, it would be expected to move through the endothelium and epithelial layers in the same manner. Thus, in a normal

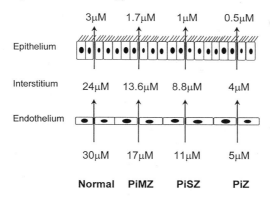

Figure 4 Projected concentrations of α₁-antitrypsin in the interstitium of the lung in subjects with different phenotypes. Concentrations in the epithelial lining fluid are taken from clinical studies for the PiM and PiZ phenotypes, whereas those for MZ and SZ phenotypes are predicted using the same concentration gradients. (Results derived from Ref. 27.)

subject with a serum concentration of 30 µmol it would be expected that the interstitial concentration should be approximately 24 µmol (Fig. 4). Thereafter there is a further 5- to 10-fold reduction in concentration, resulting in an epithelial lining fluid concentration of between 2 and 5 µmol. In α₁-antitrypsin deficiency the plasma concentration is 5 µmol but would follow the same pattern of concentration changes as normal subjects. The interstitial concentration would therefore be expected to be approximately 4 µmol, with a further 10-fold reduction leading to an epithelial lining fluid concentration of 0.5 µmol, consistent with clinical studies (20).

The same calculations can be applied to the PISZ and PIMZ phenotypes, where the plasma (and hence interstitial and airway) concentration is thought to be protective. It would be noted from this concept that if interstitial concentration of α₁-antitrypsin is 8.5 µmol or above, it is likely to be protective, which is consistent with the theory and practical demonstrations of Liou and colleagues exploring the theory of quantum proteolysis (24,25).

Thus, if replacement therapy is to be effective in protecting connective tissue in the interstitial space, maintenance of a plasma concentration above 11 µmol would be expected to provide concentrations in the interstitium similar to that found in the SZ phenotype (predicted to be 8.5 µmol or above), and these concentrations are able to control most tissue degradation by the activated neutrophil (27).

Unfortunately, to date no clinical trial has been carried out to demonstrate that management based on theory is effective. This is largely because the major outcome measure that has been considered to monitor progress in α_1-antitrypsin deficiency is the decline in FEV_1. Power calculations have shown that a large number of patients would need to be studied over several years to demonstrate a clear effect on FEV_1 decline, and the cost would make this prohibitive.

There have been attempts to generate information that at least superficially supports the role of intravenous replacement therapy. Some studies are based on historical data demonstrating that the decline in lung function in patients receiving intravenous therapy was less than the decline observed prior to the availability of replacement therapy (28). Clearly such historical data cannot be flawless, but do provide some circumstantial evidence of efficacy.

In the United States the NHLBI has maintained a registry of α_1-antitrypsin–deficient subjects for many years. A proportion of these patients has received IV therapy, albeit for varying periods of time and using different regimens. Comparison of survival and lung function decline has shown that subjects who have occasionally, intermittently, or always received IV therapy on a weekly, twice-weekly, or monthly basis have better survival and possibly less FEV_1 decline than subjects who never received therapy (19). However, as emphasized by the authors, this was not a controlled clinical trial and subjects who had never received therapy would have been exposed to fewer health care resources and represented a different socioeconomic group. These two factors could be of major importance in determining progression of lung disease and survival, so once again although the data is tantalizing it remains far from convincing.

Finally, recent data from a small controlled trial conducted in Denmark and Holland (29) have shown that although conventional lung function testing is not influenced by replacement therapy, progression of emphysema visualized by CT scanning was reduced by replacement therapy, although this failed to reach conventional statistical significance ($p = 0.07$). This study was not intended to monitor this outcome, but CT scanning is becoming recognized as a tool for the accurate identification and quantitation of emphysema in life (30). It could be predicted that the pathological changes would be detected by sensitive techniques long before measurable changes in variable lung function, such as effort-dependent FEV_1. Further development and assessment of high-resolution CT scan is more likely to lead to the realistic development of financially viable and academically sound controlled clinical trials to confirm the efficacy of replacement therapy.

B. Inhaled Therapy

The concept of α_1-antitrypsin replacement is based upon raising the concentration in the epithelial lining fluid to normal. Whereas initially this was believed to be important in protecting the lung, it became clear that passage of α_1-antitrypsin into the interstitium was critical in the prevention of emphysema. Circumstantial evidence that this occurred following α_1-antitrypsin inhalation was provided by studying patients with the PI null phenotype and demonstrated that inhaled α_1-antitrypsin was detectable in the serum (20). By implication it was suggested that this indicated that concentrations were increased in the interstitium reaching the serum via the lymph. Studies with sheep demonstrated that α_1-antitrypsin did indeed pass from the epithelial surface into the lymphatic system, supporting this concept (31). However, the studies indicated that the concentration in the lymph fluid itself was several orders of magnitude below that on the epithelium. This would clearly be consistent with the concept that the epithelium restricts protein movements to a major degree (27). In addition, the volume of distribution in the interstitium is large, and it could be predicted that a large quantity of α_1-antitrypsin would have to be delivered to the epithelial surface at high concentrations in order to have a significant effect on the concentrations in the interstitium (Fig. 5).

In addition to this problem, many patients with α_1-antitrypsin deficiency have abnormal lungs and ventilation is patchy, as demonstrated by inhalation studies (32). The results indicated that it is difficult to target

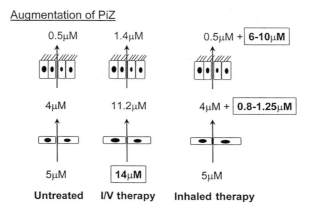

Figure 5 The predicted effect of augmentation therapy on α_1-antitrypsin levels in the interstitium and airway. Results are given from lowest average concentrations in the serum just prior weekly infusions of α_1-antitrypsin (IV therapy). Predicted results are also given from inhalation studies using values obtained as described in Ref. 20.

abnormal regions of the lung by inhalation therapy to have a protective effect. This does not, however, negate the possibility that a protective effect could be achieved in relatively normal areas of the lung, thereby preserving their function. Nevertheless, as indicated above, even good distribution in subjects with relatively normal lungs is unlikely to provide high enough concentrations to protect the interstitium.

It may not be necessary to provide direct protection at this site. As indicated previously, the numbers of neutrophils are increased in the airways of patients with α_1-antitrypsin deficiency, and the migration of these cells is likely to be central to the interstitial tissue damage leading to emphysema. The high concentration of LTB4 found in the epithelial lining fluid is thought to be the main factor causing neutrophil migration (22). The authors argued that the source of the LTB4 was airway macrophages and demonstrated that neutrophil elastase could stimulate these cells to release LTB4. The authors suggested that the low concentrations of α_1-antitrypsin in the epithelial lining fluid failed to inhibit the elastase released by neutrophils in the airway, and this elastase in turn stimulated the macrophages to release LTB4, thereby recruiting more neutrophils and amplifying interstitial damage (Fig. 6). On the basis of this concept, the blockage of elastase by inhaled α_1-antitrypsin would remove the effect of this enzyme on macrophages and thereby reduce the LTB4 released by the cells. This in turn would result in a reduction of neutrophil migration in response to the LTB4, and the reduction in migration of neutrophils through the interstitium would decrease the interstitial damage. Thus, inhalation of α_1-antitrypsin is more likely to have an indirect effect in protecting the interstitium, rather than a direct effect by penetrating the interstitial space. Nevertheless, if this strategy is to be effective, then clearly α_1-antitrypsin has to be distributed throughout the airways, particularly to the more peripheral airways and alveoli, which are the sites of tissue damage in emphysema. Clearly further studies are necessary, including careful monitoring to determine that a reduction in airways inflammation does not lead to continued unchecked progression of the emphysematous change in the lung periphery and interstitium.

V. Airways Disease

Approximately 30% of all patients with lung disease related to α_1-antitrypsin deficiency have a clear history of chronic bronchitis (33). Studies have shown that bronchial disease has a major effect on lung defenses and the presence of bronchial disease is associated with a more rapid progression of airflow obstruction in patients with COPD not due to α_1-antitrypsin

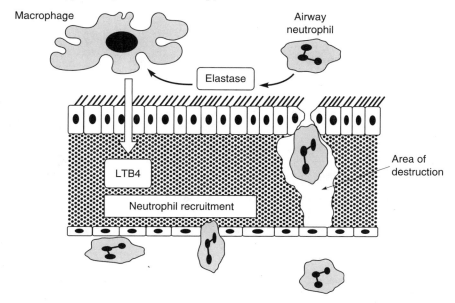

Figure 6 Diagrammatic representation of amplification of tissue damage occurring in α_1-antitrypsin deficiency. Neutrophils recruited to the airways release elastase and in doing so produce an area of connective tissue destruction. Because of α_1-antitrypsin deficiency, the elastase is also inadequately inhibited in the airway, and this stimulates alveolar macrophages to release LTB4, which results in further neutrophil recruitment, thereby amplifying the effect. (From Ref. 22.)

deficiency (34). Furthermore, neutrophil elastase has been shown to generate all the features of airways disease, suggesting that antielastases in the airways are also important in disease progression. The concentration of active elastase in the airways of α_1-antitrypsin–deficient subjects is increased compared to age- and lung function–matched COPD patients with no deficiency (Fig. 7). In addition, the amount of elastase activity is increased by the presence and size of the colonizing bacterial load within the airways (35), which is more likely where the airways and host defenses are damaged. Finally, the inflammation and amount of elastase released in the airways is increased during acute bacterial exacerbations, and this is also amplified (Fig. 7) by the increase in neutrophil recruitment and the failure of the α_1-antitrypsin acute phase response in patients with α_1-antitrypsin deficiency (12).

Increased concentrations of α_1-antitrypsin can be achieved by either the intravenous route or the inhaled route. In patients with bronchial disease

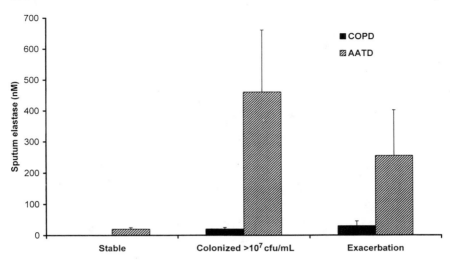

Figure 7 Concentration of sputum, neutrophil elastase is shown for COPD patients and α_1-antitrypsin–deficient patients with a similar degree of airflow obstruction. The histograms are mean plus standard error, and data are shown for both groups of patients in a stable clinical state. Neutrophil elastase activity is rarely found in ordinary COPD patients in this state in the absence of bacterial colonization. Data are also shown for patients in a stable state, but where the airways are colonized by greater than 10^7 CFU/mL of a putative pathogen. Finally, data are also shown for acute infective exacerbations in both groups of patients.

this would be expected to decrease the active elastase concentration in the airway. This, theoretically, should have a beneficial effect by reducing the LTB4 released by airway macrophages (as suggested above), and this, in turn, would downregulate inflammation, leading to less neutrophil recruitment. The net result would be indirect protection of the interstitium and direct protection of the airways by α_1-antitrypsin therapy. Clearly further studies are indicated to determine 1) whether this occurs and 2) whether such changes have an influence on the morbidity and mortality associated with α_1-antitrypsin deficiency.

In theory, α_1-antitrypsin deficiency is a direct cause of accelerated lung damage due to the release of neutrophil elastase in several compartments of the lung. Studies have shown that replacement therapy can return the α_1-antitrypsin levels to "normal," although at present there are no studies demonstrating clearly that such a strategy works. Undoubtedly α_1-antitrypsin replacement therapy does have some beneficial effects on patients with panniculitis, showing a clear and obvious superficial clinical response (36). As the pathogenic processes leading to lung damage become clarified, it is hoped that appropriate studies with α_1-antitrypsin replacement will demonstrate not only a normalization of lung α_1-antitrypsin, but also beneficial effects on lung inflammation and tissue damage. Further studies are indicated and should lead to more logical and feasible approaches to demonstrate both short- and long-term clinical benefit.

VI. Future Therapies

The concepts underlying α_1-antitrypsin replacement therapy can similarly be applied to therapies with other inhibitors. Recombinant secretory leukoproteinase inhibitor has been given to patients by inhalation. This inhibitor is better than α_1-antitrypsin at protecting connective tissue from degradation by neutrophils, perhaps because of its ability to bind ionically to the substrate (21). The role of chemical inhibitors remains unknown, although the small molecular size of these agents suggests that penetration into the interstitium may be greater than for the native proteins, and again strategies for parenteral, oral, or inhaled therapy need to be explored. The role of other anti-inflammatory therapies remains even more contentious, although in COPD in general, corticosteroids have been shown to have beneficial effect on lung inflammation in the stable state (37) and on recovery from exacerbations (38). Finally, gene therapy has remained an important concept in increasing lung α_1-antitrypsin. Studies have shown that it is possible to transfect airway cells with the α_1-antitrypsin gene leading to production of α_1-antitrypsin. In particular, studies have also shown vectoral secretion of the α_1-antitrypsin (39), suggesting that this is a potential strategy for targeting the protein to the interstitium. However, at present gene transfection remains an unproven and potentially harmful procedure using the currently available vectors, and transfectional efficiency remains low. Liver transplantation corrects the defect in the plasma entirely, although clearly such an approach is only appropriate for patients with end-stage liver disease. Clinical studies have suggested that patients with liver disease only rarely have lung disease and vice versa (40), thus it would be even more difficult to determine whether liver transplantation influences the progression of lung disease. Nevertheless, this would remove any need for replacement therapy.

Much has been learned about the function of α_1-antitrypsin and its deficiency. Increasing the effective amount of elastase inhibitors in the lung interstitium remains a therapeutic target. Better ways of monitoring disease progression makes it likely that clinical trials will be undertaken to translate theory into proven fact.

References

1. Stockley RA. α1-Antitrypsin deficiency. In: Molecular Biology of the Lung. Vol. 1. Emphysema and Infection. Stockley RA, ed. Basel: Birkhauser Verlag. 1999:37–53.

2. Laurell C, Eriksson S. The electophoretic a1-globulin pattern of serum in a1-antitrypsin deficiency. Scand J Clin Lab Invest 1963; 15:132–140.

3. Eriksson S. Studies in a-1 antitrypsin deficiency. Act Med Scand 1965; 177(suppl 432):1–85.

4. Snider GL, Stone PJ, Lucey EC, Breuer R, Colore JD, Seshadri T, Cantonase A, Maschler R, Schnebli HP, Eglin C. A polypeptide derived from the medicinal leech prevents human neutrophil elastase induced emphysema and bronchial secretory cell metaplasia. Am Rev Respir Dis 1985; 132:1155–1161.

5. Gadek JE, Fells GA, Zimmerman RL, Rennard SI, Crystal RG. Anti-elasatases of human alveolar structures. Implications for the protease-antiprotease theory of emphysema. J Clin Invest 1981; 68:889–898.

6. Stockley RA. Measurement of soluble proteins in lung secretions. Thorax 1984; 39:241–247.

7. Hubbard RC, Brantly ML, Sellars SC, Mitchell ME, Crystal RG. Anti-neutrophil elastase defences of the lower respiratory tract in α1-antitrypsin deficiency, direct augmentation with aerosol α1-antitrypsin. Ann Intern Med 1989; 111:206–212.

8. Gadek JE, Klein HG, Holland PV, Crystal RG. Replacement therapy of alpha-1-antitrypsin deficiency reversal of protease–anti-protease balance within alveolar structures of PiZ subjects. J Clin Invest 1981; 68:1158–1165.

9. Gadek JE, Fulmer JD, Gelfand JA, Frank MM, Petty TL, Crystal RG. Danazol induced augmentation of serum α1 antitrypsin levels in individuals with marked deficiency of this anti-protease. J Clin Invest 1980; 66:82–87.

10. Wewers MD, Brantley ML, Casolaro MA, Crystal RG. Evaluation of tamoxifen as a therapy to augment alpha-1-antitrypsin concentrations in Z homozygous alpha-1-antitrypsin deficient subjects. Am Rev Respir Dis 1987; 135:401–402.

11. Lomas DA, Evans DL, Finch JT, Carrell RW. The mechanism of Z α1-antitrypsin accumulation in the liver. Nature 1992; 357:605–607.

12. Hill AT, Campbell EJ, Bayler DL, Hill SL, Stockley RA. Evidence for excessive bronchial inflammation during acute exacerbation of COPD in patients with alpha-1-antitrypsin deficiency (PiZ). Am J Respir Crit Care Med 1999; 160: 1968–1975.

13. Lomas DA, Evans DL, Stone SR, Chang W-SW, Carol RW. The effect of the Z mutation on the physical and inhibitory properties of α1 antitrypsin. Biochemistry 1993; 32:500–508.

14. Bruce RM, Cohen BH, Diamond EL, Fallat RJ, Knudson RJ, Lebowitz MD, Mittman C, Patterson CD, Tochman MS. Collaborative study to assess risk of lung disease in PiMZ phenotype subjects. Am Rev Respir Dis 1984; 130:386–390.

15. Turino GM, Barker AF, Brantly ML, Cowan AB, Connelly RP, Crystal RG, Eden E, Schluchter MD, Stoller JK. Clinical features of individual PiSZ phenotype of alpha1-antitrypsin deficiency. Alpha-1-antitrypsin deficiency registry study group. Am J Respir Crit Care Med 1996; 154:1718–1725.

16. Wewers MD, Casolaro MA, Sellers S, Swayze SC, McPhaul KM, Wittes JT, Crystal RG. Replacement therapy for alpha-1-antitrypsin deficiency associated with emphysema. N Engl J Med 1987; 316:1055–1062.

17. McElvaney NG, Crystal RG. Therapy of a1 AT deficiency. In: Crystal R, ed. Alpha 1-Antitrypsin Deficiency. New York: Marcel Dekker, 1995:319–331.

18. Hubbard RC, Sellars S, Czerski D, Stephens L, Crystal RG. Biochemical efficacy and safety of monthly augmentation therapy for α1-antitrypsin deficiency. JAMA 1988; 260:1259–1264.

19. The Alpha-1-Antitrypsin Deficiency Registry Study Group. Survival and decline in individuals with severe deficiency of α1-antitrypsin. Am J Respir Crit Care Med 1988; 49–59.

20. Hubbard RC, Crystal RG. Strategies for aerosol therapy α1-antitrypsin deficiency via the aerosol route. Lung 1990; 168(suppl) 565–578.

21. Llewellyn-Jones CG, Lomas DA, Stockley RA. Potential role of recombinant secretory leukoprotease inhibitor in the prevention of neutrophil mediated matrix degradation. Thorax 1994; 49:567–572.

22. Hubbard RC, Fells G, Gadek J, Pacholok S, Humes J, Crystal RG. Neutrophil accumulation in the lung in alpha-1-antitrypsin deficiency: spontaneous release of leukotrine B4 from alveolar macrophages. J Clin Invest 1991; 88:891–897.

23. Campbell EJ, Senior RM, McDonald JA, Cox DW. Proteolysis by neutrophils. Relative importance of cell-substrate contact and oxidative inactivation of protease inhibitors in-vitro. J Clin Invest 1982; 70:745–752.

24. Liou TG, Campbell EJ. Non-isotropic enzyme–inhibitor interactions: a novel non-oxidative mechanism for quantum proteolosis by human neutrophils. Biochemistry 1995; 34:16171–16177.

25. Liou TG, Campbell EJ. Quantum proteolysis resulting from release of single granules by human neutrophils. J Immunol 1996; 157:2624–2631.

26. Campbell EJ, Campbell MA, Boukedes SS, Owen CA. Quantum proteolosis by neutrophils; implications for pulmonary emphysema and alpha-1-antitrypsin deficiency. J Clin Invest 1999; 104:337–344.

27. Gorin AB, Stuart PA. Differential Permeability of endothelial and epithelial barriers to albumin flux. J Appl Physiol 1979; 47:1315–1324.

28. Wencker M, Banik N, Buhl R, Seidel R, Konietzko N. Long-term treatment of α1-antitrypsin deficiency–related pulmonary emphysema with human α1-antitrypsin. Eur Respir J 1998; 11:428–433.

29. Dirksen A, Dijkman JA, Flemming M, Stoel B, Hutchinson DCS, Ulrik CS, Skongaard LT, Kok-Jensen A, Rudolphus A, Seersholm N, Vrooman HA,

Keiber JHC, Honsen NC, Heckscher T, Viskumk, Stalk J. A randomised placebo-control trial of alpha-1-antitrypsin augmentation therapy in patients with severe alpha-1-antitrypsin deficiency and emphysema. Am J Respir Crit Care Med 1999; 160:1468–1472.

30. Muller NL, Staples CA, Miller RR, Abboud RT. "Density mask." An objective method to quantitate emphysema using computed tomography. Chest 1988; 94:782–787.

31. Smith M, Traber LD, Traber DL, Spragg RG. Pulmonary deposition and clearance of aerosolised alpha-1-protease inhibitor administered to dogs and to sheep. J Clin Invest 1989; 84:1145–1154.

32. Stolk J, Camps J, Fetsma HIJ, Hermans J, Dijkman JH, Pauwels EKJ. Pulmonary deposition and disappearance of aerosolised secretory leukocyte protease inhibitor. Thorax 1995; 50:645–650.

33. Brantley ML, Paul LD, Miller BH, Falk RT, Wu M, Crystal RG. Clinical features and history of the destructive lung disease associated with α1-antitrypsin deficiency of adults with pulmonary symptoms. An Rev Respir Dis 1988; 138:327–366.

34. Vestbo J, Prescott E, Lange P. Association of chronic mucus hypersecretion with FEV_1 decline and chronic obstructive pulmonary disease morbidity. Am J Respir Crit Care Med 1996; 153:1530–1535.

35. Hill A, Campbell EJ, Hill SL, Bayley DL, Stockley RA. Association between airway bacterial load and markers of airway inflammation in patients with stable chronic bronchitis. Am J Med 2000; 109:288–295.

36. Pittelkow MR, Smith KC, Su WPD. Alpha-1-antitrypsin deficiency and panniculitis. Perspectives on disease relationship in replacement therapy. Am J Med 1988; 84(suppl 6a):80–86.

37. Vogelmeier C, Buhl, R, Hoyt RF, Wilson E, Fells GA, Hubbard RC, Schnebli HP, Thompson RC, Crystal RG. Aerosolisation of recombinant SLPI to augment anti-neutrophil elastase protection of pulmonary epithelium. J Appl Physiol 1990; 69:1843–1848.

38. Wiggins J, Elliot JA, Stevenson RD, Stockley RA. The effects of corticosteroids on sputum sol phase protease inhibitors in chronic obstructive pulmonary disease. Thorax 1982; 37:652–656.

39. Thompson WH, Neilson CP, Carvalho P, Charan NB, Crowley JJ. Control trial of oral prednisolone in outpatients with acute COPD exacerbation. Am J Respir Crit Care Med 1996; 154:407–412.

40. Dhami R, Zay K, Gilkes B, Porter S, Wright JL, Churg A. Pulmonary epithelial expression of human alpha 1 antitrypsin in transgenic mice results in delivery of α1 antitrypsin protein to the interstitium. J Mol Med 1999; 77:377–385.

41. Crystal RG. α1 antitrypsin deficiency, emphysema, and liver disease: genetic basis and strategies for therapy. J Clin Invest 1990; 85:1343–1352.

20

Surgery and Transplantation for COPD

JOHN R. PEPPER

National Heart and Lung Institute
Imperial College
and Royal Brompton Hospital
London, England

I. Introduction

In the early days of thoracic surgery a variety of procedures were attempted to help patients with emphysema. These included tracheostomy, pneumoperitoneum, autonomic denervation, costochondrectomy, and bullectomy. Only bullectomy has survived as an effective operation for a small minority of patients with large emphysematous bullae. In 1950, Brantigan (1) introduced lung volume reduction, referred to as pneumoplasty, for patients with end-stage, generalized emphysema. He reported encouraging preliminary results, but the early mortality of 27% was high and the procedure was not adopted. It remained forgotten until the reintroduction of single lung transplantation in the 1980s. In a few instances where the hyperinflated, unoperated lung was found to be compressing the transplanted lung in the early postoperative stage, nonanatomical resection of a portion of the native lung proved life-saving (2). In 1991 Wakabayashi et al. (3) reported encouraging results following unilateral laser pneumoplasty via an endoscopic approach in 500 procedures performed on 443 patients. Unfortunately the study was flawed due to inadequate documentation of objective measures of lung function and quality of life. In 1995 Cooper et al. (4) reported on bilateral lung volume reduction surgery (LVRS) in 20 patients in whom 20–30% of the volume of each lung had been removed through a midline sternotomy. The mean FEV_1 improved by 20%, and total lung capacity (TLC), residual volume (RV), and trapped gas were significantly reduced.

By this time single lung transplantation had become the most common form of lung transplant performed worldwide, and emphysema the most common indication. The goals of lung transplantation for emphysema are to restore normal lung function, prolong life, and limit morbidity from both the procedure and immunosuppression. In contrast, LVRS aims to relieve symptoms and improve exercise capacity. Because of the scarcity of donor organs, lung transplantation is performed for survival and not for quality of life alone. This is an issue in emphysema patients because statistically, patients with relatively severe disease can survive for several years. Therefore, transplantation should be reserved for patients with FEV_1 of less than 20% of their predicted value. LVRS is not a true alternative to transplantation, but it does not preclude subsequent lung transplant (5).

II. Rationale for Lung Volume Reduction

LVRS is an operation designed to improve the mechanics of lung function, but it is unlikely to improve alveolar gas exchange and particularly arterial oxygen tension. A smaller thoracic volume returns the chest wall to a more favorable position on its pressure-volume curve. Reduction in positive alveolar pressure will reduce the inspiratory loading of the respiratory muscles. The diaphragm is returned to a more normal position with improved length-tension relationships and a reduced radius of curvature. Overall elastic recoil may be improved with subsequent improvement in maximal expiratory flow. This should improve dyspnea beyond the improvement achieved by reducing thoracic volume alone. It is conceivable that the removal of an "overwhelming volume" of emphysematous lung might affect alveolar gas exchange depending upon the prior distribution of perfusion to the area removed. Alveolar gas exchange could be expected to become more efficient with a reduction in alveolar dead space and venous admixture. Improvement in lung elastic recoil pressure could also affect pulmonary blood flow, either regionally or globally. The resultant capillary recruitment and tethering in areas of reexpanded lung could improve blood flow and overall ventilation-perfusion ratios of the lung, leading to improved alveolar gas exchange. Homan and colleagues (6) measured lung function tests in 36 consecutive patients undergoing LVRS in the same laboratory. They analyzed ventilated lung alveolar volume (VA) from the gas transfer measurements used as a proxy for effective lung volume. The mean VA increased by 0.674 L from 4.04 to 4.72 ($p < 0.0001$; $n = 34$). The change in FEV_1 correlated well with the change in VA ($R = 0.63$), and in those patients whose VAs did not increase ($n = 7$), there was no significant change in FEV_1. They concluded that the increase in VA reflected an increase in ventilating lung volume, and it was associated with an improvement in spirometry.

Furthermore, pulmonary vascular resistance could decrease leading to a fall in right ventricular afterload. Restored negative intrathoracic pressure could augment right ventricular preload and improve right ventricular function. Mineo et al. (7) used fast-thermistor thermodilution measurement of cardiac output at rest and during submaximal upright exercise in 12 patients before and 6 months after bilateral LVRS. Preoperatively, all patients had severe airflow obstruction, with a mean FEV_1 of 0.69 L and an RV : TLC ratio of 0.67. Six months after LVRS, significant improvements occurred in respiratory function (+0.39 L in FEV_1, $p < 0.002$; ±0.15 in RV/TLC ratio, $p < 0.002$). Significant changes also occurred in right ventricular function measured at rest (+0.21 L in cardiac index, $p < 0.01$; +3.0 mL in stroke volume index, $p < 0.01$) and on exercise [+0.9 L in cardiac index, $p < 0.002$; +10.0 mL in stroke volume index, $p < 0.002$; +20% in RV ejection fraction (RVEF), $p < 0.002$]. A significant correlation was found between perioperative changes in RVEF response to exercise and changes in the RV/TLC ratio ($R = -0.68$; $p = 0.01$). So it seems that a significant improvement in right ventricular performance, particularly during exercise, can occur 6 months after bilateral LVRS.

III. Patient Selection for LVRS

In the majority of case series reported, about 25% of patients with severe emphysema are judged to be candidates for LVRS after preoperative evaluation. In the NETT study (8) only 32% of those who began to undergo screening were ultimately determined to be eligible. In general lung function testing should show evidence of severe nonreversible airflow obstruction with an FEV_1 in the range of 15–35% of predicted, and evidence of hyperinflation and air trapping should also be present as shown by TLC greater than 100% of predicted and RV greater than 150% of predicted. The chest radiograph and high-resolution computed tomography (CT) should show parenchymal emphysematous changes and hyperinflation.

Exclusion criteria include age over 75, smoking within 6 months of preoperative evaluation, hypercapnia ($PaC_{O_2} > 55$ mmHg) and moderate to severe pulmonary hypertension (mean PA systolic pressure >50 mmHg), and other significant comorbidity, such as heart valve disease or impaired renal function. Patients who are obese ($BMI > 32$ kg/m^2) and who are ventilator dependant are usually excluded, but there are exceptions (9).

The experience of Cooper and colleagues (10) from their first consecutive series of 84 patients undergoing LVRS revealed that advanced age and hypercapnia were associated with increased operative mortality. Keenan et al. (11) studied 57 patients who had lung resected via thoracoscopy with a stapler. Analysis showed that elevated pCO_2 and decreased lung-diffusing capacity for carbon monoxide (DLCO) were each significantly associated with prolonged hospital stay and higher early mortality. Conversely, O'Brien and coworkers have shown that patients with moderate to severe hypercapnia show a significant improvement in spirometry, gas exchange, and quality of life after bilateral LVRS (12). Although hypercapnic patients had lower preoperative FEV_1, diffusion capacity of carbon monoxide, ratio of arterial oxygen pressure (Pa_{O2}) to fraction of inspired oxygen (Fi_{O_2}), and 6MWT distance were comparable to normocapnic patients; the percentage improvements in FVC, FEV_1, TLC, RV, and RV/TLC were comparable to normocapnic patients.

McKenna et al. (13) studied 166 patients who underwent thoracoscopic unilateral or bilateral surgery and demonstrated that the initial elevated RV correlated with improved outcome in terms of lung function at 6 months after operation. The weight of tissue resected was correlated with improvement in FEV_1 ($R = 0.55$; $p < 0.0001$). No other authors have confirmed these findings, and how much lung tissue should be removed has been very difficult to establish. The amount of lung removed is difficult to measure in a meaningful way. If too much lung is removed, troublesome bronchopleural fistulae causing prolonged air leak may result. Alternatively, removal of too small an amount of tissue will compromise the result. At the moment this aspect of the procedure relies heavily on surgical judgment. In a study of 29 patients from Boston (14), only preoperative lung resistance during inspiration predicted changes in expiratory flow rates after surgery. Inspiratiory lung resistance correlated significantly and inversely with improvement in postoperative FEV_1 ($R = -0.63$; $p < 0.001$).

In general, imaging studies have so far proved more useful than lung function tests in identifying those patients who will obtain the greatest benefit from LVRS. Gierada and colleagues (15) carried out a retrospective analysis of 50 patients after LVRS. On the basis of inspiratory and expiratory CT scans, they concluded that upper lobe predominance of emphysematous disease, a greater degree of parenchymal compression, a higher amount of regional heterogeneity, and a larger percentage of normal or mildly emphysematous lung best predicted improvement after operation. Fischer et al. (16) correlated preoperative perfusion lung scans, including quantitative measures of perfusion distribution, with postoperative functional studies. Significantly greater improvement in outcome was found with heterogeneity, a larger percentage of maximally perfused lung, upper lobe predominance of decreased perfusion, and a higher degree of matched ventilation and perfusion.

IV. Surgical Techniques in Lung Volume Reduction Surgery

The operative technique has been controversial, but there has been clarification of some issues. The goal of LVRS is targeted resection of 30–40% of the severely emphysematous lung as identified on the preoperative CT scan, quantitative ventilation/perfusion scan, and intraoperative findings. Favorable results have been obtained by both VATS (17) or median sternotomy approaches (10). McKenna and colleagues (18) compared the efficacy of neodymium:yttrium-aluminium-garnet (Nd:YAG) laser surgery with stapled resection in 72 patients who underwent unilateral LVRS. There was no difference in postoperative morbidity and mortality between the two groups. But patients who underwent stapled lung resection had a significantly greater improvement in lung function compared with the laser ablation group ($FEV_1 = 33\%$ vs. 13%, $p < 0.01$).

Bilateral LVRS is preferred over unilateral LVRS because of a greater improvement in postoperative lung function with similar preoperative mortality (19). Furthermore, bilateral LVRS via VATS has better 2-year survival rates than unilateral LVRS. In a study of 260 patients (20) who underwent LVRS via VATS (bilateral VATS = 159, unilateral = 110), the overall survival rate at 2 years was 86.4% after bilateral LVRS compared with 72.6% after unilateral LVRS ($p = 0.001$). But a further study involving 673 patients who underwent LVRS showed no survival advantage for patients who underwent bilateral LVRS compared with the unilateral approach (21). In general, bilateral LVRS is the preferred approach because the function outcome is better. A targeted approach to the individual patient is probably the ideal. A recent report of 65 patients examined the medium-term results of unilateral versus bilateral LVRS at 2-year follow-up (22). They found no benefit from bilateral simultaneous LVRS and preferred unilateral LVRS because of the lower morbidity, resulting in earlier discharge and slower decline in physiological benefit.

The morbidity of the surgical approach remains significant (23). A recent preliminary report (24) of an endoscopic approach to achieve volume reduction using valve implants at the segmental or subsegmental level is encouraging.

V. Results of Lung Reduction

Criner and colleagues (25) reported a randomized trial of 37 of 200 patients with nonbullous emphysema. Of the 18 patients enrolled in the medical arm, 15 completed 3 additional months of pulmonary rehabilitation. Thirty-two patients underwent bilateral LVRS via sternotomy. In 28 patients who underwent LVRS, FEV_1 increased significantly (0.69 ± 0.2 L to 0.90 ± 0.3 L; $p < 0.001$), and there was a significant decrease in TLC (6.3 ± 1.2 L vs. 7.2 ± 1.7 L; $p < 0.001$). There was also a significant increase in 6-minute walking distance (6-MWD) (337 ± 99 m vs. 282 ± 100 m; $p < 0.001$) and maximum oxygen consumption (13.8 ± 4 mL/Kg/min vs. 12.0 ± 3 mL/Kg/min; $p < 0.01$).

Geddes et al. (26) reported a randomized controlled trial of LVRS versus medical treatment in 48 of 178 patients who were screened as potential candidates. Of the 48 patients, 24 were randomized to the medical arm and 24 to the LVRS arm. For patients who underwent bilateral LVRS, the mean FEV_1 increased by 70 mL at 6 months, whereas patients who were randomized to the medical arm had an 80 mL decrease in mean FEV_1 over the same period. Similarly the 6MWD increased by 50 m in the surgical group, whereas the medical group had a 20 m decline at 6 months follow-up. Quality of life, as measured by SF-36, significantly improved 6 months after surgery. There were 4 early deaths (17%) in the surgical group due to postoperative respiratory failure, and 3 patients (12%) in the medical group died. Five of the first 15 patients died during the early part of the trial, which prompted the investigators to modify the study entry criteria to exclude patients with a diffusion capacity of less than 30% of predicted and shuttle walk distance of less than 150 m. The mortality rate after the modified entry criteria were used was 6%.

More recently results from the much-heralded National Emphysema Treatment Trial (NETT) were reported (8). After exclusion of 140 patients with a high risk of death from surgery according to an interim analysis (27), the 538 patients who were randomly assigned to surgery were more likely than the 540 assigned to medical treatment to have improvements in exercise capacity and quality of life, but there was no reduction in mortality during an average of 29 months of follow-up. Secondary analyses showed that the effects of surgery on mortality varied markedly among subgroups defined according to the presence or absence of predominantly upper lobe emphysema and whether the patient had high or low exercise capacity at baseline. Among patients with predominantly upper lobe emphysema and low exercise capacity, the risk ratio for death in the surgery group as compared with the medical group was 0.47 ($p = 0.005$), indicating a significant benefit of surgery. Among patients with predominantly upper lobe emphysema and high exercise capacity, the risk ratio was 0.98 ($p = 0.70$), and among those with non–upper lobe emphysema and low exercise capacity, the risk ratio was 0.81 ($p = 0.49$). Finally, among patients with non–upper lobe emphysema and high exercise capacity, the risk ratio was 2.06 ($p = 0.02$). These results suggest that surgery may reduce the risk of death among patients with upper lobe emphysema and low exercise capacity, increase the risk among patients with non–upper lobe emphysema and high exercise capacity, and have little effect on the risk of death in the other two groups. This is explored further in an excellent review by Ware (28).

A nonrandomized but prospective comparison of LVRS and medical treatment was reported by Wilkens et al. (29). The patients were divided into two groups according to their own decision. There were no significant differences in lung function between the two groups at baseline, but a tendency toward better functional status in the medical group. Model-based comparisons were used to estimate the differences between the two groups over 18 months. Significant improvements were seen in the LVRS group compared to the medical group. The estimated difference in FEV_1 was 33% (95% CI 13–58%; $p > 0.0001$), in TLC 12.9% (95% CI 7.9–18.8%; $p < 0.0001$), in RV 60.9% (95% CI 32.6–89.2%; $p < 0.0001$), in 6-minute walking distance 230 m (95% CI 138–322 m; $p < 0.01$) and in Modified Medical Research Council (MMRC) dyspnea score 1.17 (95% CI 0.79–1.55; $p < 0.0001$). They concluded that LVRS was more effective than conservative treatment for the improvement of dyspnea, lung function, and exercise capacity in selected patients with severe emphysema.

Reports of long-term studies are beginning to appear in the literature. Yusen and coworkers (30) used a prospective cohort study design to assess the first 200 patients undergoing bilateral LVRS from 1993 to 1998 with a median follow-up of 4 years. The 90-day postoperative mortality was 4.5%. Annual Kaplan-Meier survival through the 5 years after surgery was 93, 88, 83, 74, and 63%, respectively. During follow-up, 15 patients underwent subsequent lung transplantation. The FEV_1 was improved in 92% (6 months), 72% (3 years), and 58% (5 years) of patients. They concluded that the duration of improvement was at least 5 years in the majority of survivors.

Fujimoto and colleagues (31) reported on a case series of 88 patients who underwent LVRS between 1994 and 1998. The overall survival rate at 5 years was 71% with a mean length of follow-up of 54.2 months. The survival difference was statistically significant between patients with a preoperative FEV_1 of $\geq 28.5\%$ and those with FEV_1 of 28.5% ($p = 0.0152$).

Bloch et al. (32) followed 115 patients with a median FEV_1 27% of predicted value who underwent LVRS. The follow-up extended over a median of 37 months. They examined the functional effect of the operation on different patterns of emphysema. FEV_1 improvement peaked within 6 months postoperatively. The subsequent decline was most rapid in the first year and slowed down in succeeding years according to an exponential decay and was similar for all morphological patterns of disease.

VI. Transplantation for Emphysema

Lung transplantation is an accepted treatment for end-stage emphysema. In fact, emphysema remains the leading indication for lung transplantation. Single lung transplant is an attractive option for several reasons. Most patients do not have adhesions, so that extraction of the lung is straightforward. The large pleural space provides excellent exposure for implantation. The 1-year survival rate of 85% (33) for this procedure exceeds that for other etiologies and for other forms of lung transplantation. A major cause of postoperative morbidity is the unpredictable occurrence of ischemia-reperfusion injury, which manifests as a radiographically confirmed infiltrate on the side of the allograft usually in the first 48 hours after transplantation. The cause of this injury is unclear because the incidence of ischemia-reperfusion injury does not correlate well with ischemic time of the donor organ, method of organ preservation, or other donor-related factors (33). Nevertheless, patients with emphysema tend to have the least complicated postoperative course compared to other groups undergoing single lung transplantation. The time spent on a ventilator, days in the ICU, the intensity of ventilator support, use of inotropic drugs, and the days required on supplemental oxygen are the least of all patient groups. Early gas exchange and hemodynamics are significantly better. Why is this so? Blood flow is distributed more evenly, with an average of two thirds of the cardiac output perfusing the transplanted lung. In conjunction with lower pulmonary pressures, the amount of edema in the transplanted lung is lower in this patient group.

The postoperative FEV_1 is generally $>50\%$ of predicted but not as high as that achieved with bilateral lung transplant, although no difference in exercise tolerance following bilateral transplantation has been reported.

The 5-year survival is slightly better in bilateral recipients than in their single lung counterparts (33). This may be because there is a greater reserve of lung parenchyma to preserve function against the development of obliterative bronchiolitis. Most transplant centers now apply single lung transplant to emphysema patients without bullous disease who are of smaller stature or older age who might be less tolerant of the bilateral procedure.

Hosenpud et al. analyzed the survival benefit of lung transplantation for different etiologies (34). While the clearest survival benefit occurred in the cystic fibrosis group, no survival benefit was apparent in the emphysema group. Data was analyzed for all patients listed for transplantation in the United States for emphysema, cystic fibrosis, or pulmonary fibrosis in the years 1992–1994. In the emphysema group the risks of transplantation relative to remaining on the waiting list were 2.76, 1.12, and 1.10 at 1 month, 6 months, and 1 year, respectively, and the relative risk did not decrease to below 1.0 during 2 years of follow-up. The authors concluded that lung transplantation for patients with emphysema is difficult to justify on the grounds of survival benefit alone. The impact of LVRS is difficult to assess at present, but if patients on the transplant list are treated by LVRS, the transplant waiting list mortality will increase, as the early mortality rate for patients such as these undergoing LVRS is around 10%.

VII. Bridge to Transplantation

LVRS may be used as a "bridge" to lung transplantation for patients who have rapidly deteriorating lung function. Until recently it was unclear which group of COPD patients awaiting lung transplantation would benefit from LVRS and which group would do badly after LVRS and therefore be better served by lung transplantation as a first option. In a study from the University of Pittsburgh involving 95 patients with end-stage emphysema assessed for lung transplantation, 45 (47%) met the criteria for both lung transplantation and LVRS (35). Fifteen patients who underwent sequential LVRS (including 11 unilateral, 4 bilateral LVRS) and lung transplantation (ipsilateral in 7 and contralateral in 8) on average 28 months *apart* (median 27.4 months, range 3.7–61.7 months) without significantly increasing posttransplant morbidity or mortality. They also found that bilateral LVRS bridged the time to transplantation to a greater extent than unilateral LVRS (34.9 ± 29.8 months vs. 25.4 ± 16.3; $p = 0.2$.). Myers et al. (36) retrospectively studied 99 of 200 patients following bilateral LVRS who were eligible for lung transplantation. The age at transplantation was 58 ± 5 years, with transplantation occurring 3.8 ± 1.1 years after LVRS. There were 4 operative deaths and 17 late deaths. Two- and 5-year survival after evaluation for LVRS was 92 and 75%, respectively. They concluded that the preliminary use of LVRS did not appear to jeopardize the chances for subsequent successful transplantation.

Thus, LVRS is a viable alternative to lung transplantation in selected patients with end-stage emphysema. Patients with α_1-antitrypsin deficiency and hypercapnia should undergo lung transplantation rather than LVRS.

VIII. Outcome After Transplantation

The causes of mortality after lung transplantation are common to the different types of transplant. Transplant-specific problems occur occasionally, such as severe hyperinflation of the unoperated lung in single lung transplantation for COPD. Infection remains the major cause of early mortality, especially cytomegalovirus infection, and accounts for 35% of early deaths. Primary graft failure, cardiac dysfunction, anastomotic breakdown, and hemorrhage less commonly prove fatal. Primary graft failure is usually a consequence of graft ischemia-reperfusion injury. Other causes of early graft dysfunction are severe volume overload, occlusion of the pulmonary venous anastomosis, and aspiration. Treatment is supportive, relying mainly on mechanical ventilation. Independent lung ventilation, inhaled nitric oxide, and extracorporeal membrane oxygenation have been used as extra measures (37,38). Multiorgan failure typically occurs in the setting of sepsis and primary graft dysfunction. Acute rejection is an uncommon cause of early death, accounting for 5% of early deaths.

Chronic rejection, in the form of obliterative bronchiolitis (BOS) is responsible for approximately 30% of late deaths (39). BOS has an incidence of up to 40% at 2 years posttransplant and is responsible for mortality in 50% of affected patients. Sepsis accounts for 30% of late deaths but often occurs in the presence of BOS. Malignancy accounts for 6% of late deaths.

IX. Quality-of-Life Studies

Several prospective studies have described the quality of life (QOL) of lung transplant candidates and recipients, but none have studied emphysema patients in isolation. Squier et al. (40) examined the predictive value of a baseline measure of health-related QOL (HRQOL) on the survival of patients in the San Diego lung transplant program. They found that HRQOL varied according to the indications for transplant with COPD patients during assessment for transplant, scoring, on average, worse than cystic fibrosis (CF) patients. The situation was different after transplant, patients with COPD tended to enjoy better survival than CF patients. Within each transplant category, those with higher baseline HRQOL had a better chance of survival. Such indicators may, in the future, help to refine the candidate selection process in the setting of donor organ scarcity. A report by Gross et al. (41) showed a positive impact of lung transplantation on the dimensions of physical function, health perception, social function, and role function using a medical outcomes study health survey, the MOS-20 Health Profile. The benefits were maintained for 5 years unless obliterative bronchiolitis supervened.

A report on 39 consecutive patients who underwent LVRS for diffuse emphysema and were followed up for 2 years concluded that the operation had positive effects on HRQOL (42). A recent study from Canada (43) followed in a prospective manner patients less than 75 years of age with severe COPD randomized to surgical or control groups. They all received pulmonary rehabilitation and were monitored at 3-month intervals for 12 months with no crossover between groups. LVRS resulted in important benefits in disease-specific quality of life compared with medical treatment, which were sustained at 12 months after treatment. A major cost-effectiveness study was carried out as part of the NETT trial and reported separately (44). Long-term studies are ideal for this type of analysis, but the follow-up period for this study was 3 years, and the authors used mathematical modeling to extrapolate the data and arrive at 10-year estimates. Over the observation period the cost-effectiveness ratio for surgery as compared with medical treatment was unfavorable because of the costs of the operation, the number of adverse outcomes, and very long stays in both hospitals and nursing homes during the first few months after surgery. They concluded that LVRS may be cost-effective if benefits can be maintained over time.

X. Conclusion

The most appropriate surgical treatment of patients with severe emphysema is controversial. Patients with diffuse disease, low FEV_1, hypercapnia, and associated pulmonary hypertension are considered for transplantation.

Although the results of single lung transplant for emphysema, in terms of early survival, are better than for any other form of lung transplant, it has been difficult to demonstrate a survival benefit for emphysema as against other forms of parenchymal disease. It may be that for subsets of emphysema such as α_1-antitrypsin deficiency, transplantation does show benefit, but this information is not available. In the context of declining donor lung availability, to achieve an equitable distribution of organs is difficult.

It has been clear for some time from case series that some patients derive considerable benefit from lung volume reduction, but to identify these patients, who represent only 20–25% of the entire emphysema population, can be very difficult. Patients with favorable features for LVRS show hyperinflation, heterogeneous distribution of disease, $FEV_1 > 20\%$ of predicted, and normal PC_{O_2}. The recent publication of the NETT trial is helpful but also raises many questions. Two factors were identified as having an important role in predicting benefit from LVRS. Those factors are the anatomical distribution of the emphysema and the capacity of the patient to perform physical work. Long-term follow-up is required particularly to understand the cost-effectiveness of this procedure. Meanwhile, new less invasive endoscopic procedures are being developed and will need to be carefully scrutinized before they are widely applied.

References

1. Brantigan O, Mueller E. Surgical treatment of pulmonary emphysema. Ann Surg 1957; 23:789–804.
2. Khaghani A, Al-Khattan KM, Tadjkarimi S, Banner N, Yacoub M. Early experience with single lung transplantation and volume reduction. Eur J Cardiothorac Surg 1997; 11:604–608.
3. Wakabayashi A, Brenner M, Kayaleh R. Thoracoscopic carbon dioxide laser treatment of bullous emphysema. Lancet 1991; 337:881–883.
4. Cooper J, Trulock E, Triantafillou A, Patterson GA, Pohl MS, Deloney PA, Sundaresan RS, Roper CL. Bilateral pneumectomy (volume reduction) for chronic obstructive pulmonary disease. J Thorac Cardiovasc Surg 1995; 109:106–119.
5. Zenati M, Keenan RJ, Landreneau RJ, Lung reduction as a bridge to lung transplantation in pulmonary emphysema. Ann Thorac Surg 1995; 59:1581–1583.
6. Homan S, Porter S, Peacock M, Saccoia N, Southcott AM, Ruffin R. Increased effective lung volume following lung volume reduction surgery in emphysema. Chest 2001; 120:1157–1162.
7. Mineo TC, Pompeo E, Rogliani P, Dauri M, Turani F, Bollero P, Magliocchetti N. Effect of lung volume reduction surgery for severe emphysema on right ventricular function. Am J Respir Crit Care Med 2002; 165:489–494.
8. National Emphysema Treatment Trial Group. A randomized trial comparing lung-volume-reduction surgery with medical therapy for severe emphysema. N Engl J Med 2003; 348:2059–2073.
9. Murtuza B, Keogh B, Simonds AK, Pepper JR. Lung volume reduction surgery in a ventilated patient with severe pulmonary emphysema. Ann Thorac Surg 2001; 71:1037–1038.

10. Yusen R, Trulock E, Phol M, Biggar DG. Results of lung volume reduction surgery in patients with emphysema. Semin Thorac Cardiovasc Surg 1996; 8:99–109.
11. Keenan R, Landreneau R, Sciurba F. Unilateral thoracoscopic surgical approach for diffuse emphysema. J Thorac Cardiovasc Surg 1996; 110:308–316.
12. O'Brien G, Furukawa S, Kuzma AM. Improvements in lung function, exercise, and quality of life in hypercapnic COPD patients after lung volume reduction surgery. Chest 1999; 115:75–84.
13. McKenna R, Brenner M, Fischel R. Should lung volume reduction surgery for emphysema be unilateral or bilateral? J Thorac Cardiovasc Surg 1996; 112:1331–1339.
14. Ingenito EP, Evans RB, Loring SH, Kaczka DW, Rodenhouse JD, Body SC, Sugarbaker DJ, Mentzer SJ, DeCamp MM, Reilly JJ. Relation between preoperative inspiratory lung resistance and the outcome of lung volume-reduction surgery for emphysema. N Engl J Med 1998; 338:1181–1185.
15. Gierada D, Slone RM, Bae KT, Yusen RD, Lefrak SS, Cooper JD. Pulmonary emphysema: comparison of preoperative quantitative CT and physiologic index values with clinical outcome following lung volume reduction surgery. Radiology 1997; 205:235–242.
16. Fischer K, Slone R, Gierada D, Yusen RD, Cooper JD. Scintigraphic markers of outcome after lung volume reduction surgery as assessed with preoperative lung scans. Am J Roent 1996; 166(suppl.):74–82.
17. Stammberger U, Thurnheer R, Bloch KE, Zollinger A, Schmid RA, Russi EW, Weder W. Thoracoscopic bilateral lung volume reduction for diffuse pulmonary emphysema. Eur J Cardiothorac Surg. 1997; 11:1005–1010.
18. McKenna R, Brenner M, Gelb A, Fischel R. A randomized prospective trial of stapled lung reduction versus laser bullectomy for diffuse emphysema. J Thorac Cardiovasc Surg 1996; 111:317–322.
19. Klepetko W. Surgical aspects and techniques of lung volume reduction for severe emphysema. Eur Respir J 1999; 13:919–925.
20. Serna DL, Brenner M, Osann KE. Survival after unilateral versus bilateral lung volume reduction surgery for emphysema. J Thorac Cardiovasc Surg 1999; 118:1101–1109.
21. Naunheim KS, Kaiser LR, Bavaria JE. Long-term survival after thorascopic lung volume reduction: a multi-institutional review. Ann Thorac Surg 1999; 68:2026–2032.
22. Oey IF, Waller DA, Bal S, Singh SJ, Spyt TJ, Morgan MDL. Lung volume reduction surgery—a comparison of the long term outcome of unilateral vs. bilateral approaches. Eur J Cardiothorac Surg 2002; 22:610–614.
23. Toma TP, Goldstraw P, Geddes DM. Lung volume reduction surgery. Thorax 2002; 57:5.
24. Toma TP, Hopkinson NS, Hillier J, Hansell DM, Morgan C, Goldstraw P, Polkey MI, Geddes DM. Bronchoscopic volume reduction with valve implants in patients with severe emphysema. Lancet 2003; 361:931–933.

25. Criner GJ, Cordova FC, Furukawa S. Prospective randomized trial comparing bilateral lung volume reduction surgery to pulmonary rehabilitation in severe chronic obstructive pulmonary disease. Am J Respir Crit Care Med 1999; 160:2018–2027.

26. Geddes D, Davies M, Koyama H, Hansell D, Pastorino U, Pepper J, Agent P, Cullinan P, MacNeill SJ, Goldstraw P. Effect of lung-volume-reduction surgery in patients with severe emphysema. N Engl J Med 2000; 343:239–245.

27. National Emphysema Treatment Trial Research Group. Patients at high risk of death after lung-volume-reduction surgery. N Engl J Med 2001; 345:1075–1083.

28. Ware JH. The National Emphysema Treatment Trial — how strong is the evidence? N Engl J Med 2003; 348:2055–2056.

29. Wilkens H, Demertzis S, Konig J, Leitnaker CK, Schafers HJ, Sybrecht GW. Lung volume reduction surgery versus conservative treatment in severe emphysema. Eur Respir J 2000; 16:1043–1049.

30. Yusen RD, Lefrak SS, Gierada DS, Davis GE, Meyers BF, Patterson GA, Cooper JD. A prospective evaluation of lung volume reduction surgery in 200 consecutive patients. Chest 2003; 123:1026–1037.

31. Fujimoto T, Teschler H, Hillejan L, Zaboura G, Stamatis G. Long-term results of lung volume reduction surgery. Eur J Cardiothorac Surg 2002; 21:483–488.

32. Bloch KE, Georgescu CL, Russi EW, Weder W. Gain and subsequent loss of lung function after lung volume reduction surgery in cases of severe emphysema with different morphologic patterns. J Thorac Cardiovasc Surg 2002; 123:845–854.

33. Hertz MI, Taylor DO, Trulock EP, Boucek MM, Mohacsi PJ, Edwards LB, Keck BM. The registry of the international society for heart and lung transplantation: nineteenth official report—2002. J Heart Lung Transplant 2002; 21:950–970.

34. Hosenpud JD, Bennett LE, Keck BM, Edwards EB, Novick RJ. Effect of diagnosis on survival benefit of lung transplantation for end-stage lung disease. Lancet 1998; 351:24–27.

35. Burns KE, Keenan RJ, Grgurich WF, Manzetti JD, Zenati MA. Outcomes of lung volume reduction surgery followed by lung transplantation: a matched cohort study. Ann Thorac Surg 2002; 73:1587–1593.

36. Meyers BF, Yusen RD, Guthrie TJ, Davis G, Pohl MS, Lefrak SS, Patterson GA, Cooper JD. Outcome of bilateral lung volume reduction in patients with emphysema potentially eligible for lung transplantation. J Thorac Cardiovasc Surg 2001; 122:10–17.

37. Christie JD, Bavaria JE, Palevsky HI. Primary graft failure after lung transplantation. Chest 1998; 114:51–60.

38. Glassman IR, Keenan RJ, Fabrizio MC. Extracorporeal membrane oxygenation as adjunct treatment for primary graft failure in adult lung transplant recipients. J Thorac Cardiovasc Surg 1995; 110:723–727.

39. Cooper JD, Billingham M, Egan T. A working formulation for the standardization of nomenclature and for clinical staging of chronic dysfunction in lung allografts. J Heart Lung Transplant 1993; 12:713–716.

40. Squier HC, Ries AL, Kaplan RM. Quality of well-being predicts survival in lung transplantation candidates. Am J Respir Crit Care Med 1995; 152:2032–2039.

41. Gross CR, Savil K, Bolman RM, Hertz MI. Long-term health status and quality of life outcomes of lung transplant recipients. Chest 1995; 108:1587–1593.

42. Hamacher J, Buchi S, Georgescu CL, Stammberger U, Thurnheer I, Bloch KE, Weder W, Russi EW. Improved quality of life after lung volume reduction surgery. Eur Respir J 2002; 19:54–60.

43. Goldstein RS, Todd TR, Guyatt G, Keshavjee S, Dolmage TE, VanRooy S, Frip B, Maltais F, LeBlanc P, Pakhale S, Waddell TK. Influence of lung volume reduction surgery (LVRS) on health related quality of life in patients with chronic obstructive pulmonary disease. Thorax 2003; 58:405–410.

44. National Emphysema Treatment Trial Research Group. Cost-effectiveness of lung-volume-reduction surgery for patients with severe emphysema. N Engl J Med 2003; 348:2092–2102.

21

New Therapies for COPD

PETER J. BARNES

National Heart and Lung Institute
Imperial College
London, England

I. Introduction

There is a pressing need to develop new treatments for chronic obstructive pulmonary disease (COPD), as no currently available drug has been shown to reduce the relentless progression of the disease. There is a particular need to develop drugs that suppress the underlying inflammatory and destructive processes that underlie this disease. These drugs are important for long-term intervention in COPD. Yet there have been disappointingly few therapeutic advances in the drug therapy of COPD, in contrast to the enormous advances made in asthma management that reflect a much better understanding of the underlying disease (1–3). Although COPD is commonly treated with drugs developed for asthma, this is often inappropriate as the inflammatory process in COPD differs markedly from that in asthma (4,5). Recognition of the global importance and rising prevalence of COPD and the absence of effective therapies has led to a concerted effort to develop new drugs for this disease (6,7).

Rational therapy depends on understanding the underlying disease process, and there have been recent advances in understanding the cellular and molecular mechanisms that may be involved. COPD involves a chronic inflammation in small airways and lung parenchyma, with the involvement of neutrophils, macrophages, and T lymphocytes, with a predominance of cytotoxic T cells (CD8+) (8,9). This inflammation is associated with fibrosis and narrowing of small airways (chronic obstructive bronchiolitis) and with lung parenchymal destruction due to the action of various proteases, such as neutrophil elastase and matrix metalloproteinases (emphysema). This inflammation is quite different from that seen in asthma, indicating that different treatments are likely to be needed (4).

There are several reasons why drug development in COPD has proved difficult. Only recently has there been any research interest in the molecular and cell biology of COPD in order to identify new therapeutic targets (10). Animal models of COPD for early drug testing are not satisfactory (11,12). There are uncertainties about how to test drugs for COPD, which may require long-term studies (>3 years) in relatively large numbers of patients. Many patients with COPD may have comorbidities, such as ischemic heart disease and diabetes, which may exclude them from clinical trials of new therapies. There is little information about surrogate markers, e.g., biomarkers in blood, sputum, or breath, to monitor the short-term efficacy and predict the long-term potential of new treatments. However, progress is underway, and several classes of drug are now in preclinical and clinical development (7,13).

II. Smoking Cessation

Cigarette smoking is the major cause of COPD worldwide, and smoking cessation is the only therapeutic intervention so far shown to reduce disease progression. Nicotine addiction is the major problem, and treatment should be directed at dealing with this addictive state. The major approaches have involved behavioral and nicotine replacement therapy, but the overall rates of quitting are small (5–15%) (14). An important advances has been the discovery that the antidepressant bupropion, given as a short course (6–9 weeks), is an effective treatment, with sustained quit rates of 18% at 12 months, compared with 9% for nicotine skin patches and 6% for placebo (15). Results in patients with COPD are similar (16). This does not appear to be a general effect of antidepressants, although nortriptyline has some effect (17). Bupropion is well tolerated apart from sleeplessness, but epileptic fits occur in approximately 0.1% patients, predominantly those with previous epilepsy (18). In the future, more effective drugs may arise from a greater understanding of the neural mechanisms involved in nicotine addiction, such as dopaminergic pathways in the nucleus accumbens (19).

III. New Bronchodilators

Since bronchodilators are the mainstay of current management, a logical approach is to improve existing bronchodilators. Several once-daily inhaled β_2-agonists are now in clinical development, but the once-daily inhaled anticholinergic tiotropium has recently become available in several countries.

A. Long-Acting Anticholinergics

Tiotropium bromide is a long-acting anticholinergic drug that has a unique kinetic selectivity, with very slow dissociation from M_1 and M_3 muscarinic receptors (20,21). Clinical studies in COPD indicate that inhaled tiotropium once daily is an effective bronchodilator in patients with COPD and more effective than conventional ipratropium bromide four times a day (22,23). Long-term studies with tiotropium bromide have demonstrated significant improvement in symptoms and improvement in quality of life, as well as an unexpected reduction in exacerbations (24,25). Tiotropium is likely to become the bronchodilator of first choice in COPD and may have additive effects with long-acting β_2-agonists. However, it is unlikely that tiotropium will change the course of the disease, as it does not deal with the underlying inflammatory process.

Several other long-acting anticholinergics are now in clinical development, including LAS 34273 (26).

B. Long-Acting β_2-Agonists

The long-acting β_2-agonists salmeterol and formoterol have proved to be very useful bronchodilators in COPD, and it is likely that they will now be combined with long-acting anticholinergic drugs in fixed-combination inhalers (27). Inhaled β_2-agonists with longer duration that are suitable for once-daily dosing are now in clinical development, so it is likely that these will be combined with tiotropium and other long-acting anticholinergics as the bronchodilator treatment of choice in COPD.

IV. Mediator Antagonists

Several inflammatory mediators are likely to be involved in COPD, as many inflammatory cells and structural cells are activated and there is an ongoing inflammatory process, even in patients who have given up smoking (28).

Table 1   Mediator Antagonists for COPD

LTB$_4$ antagonists (LY 29311, SC-53228, CP-105,696, SB 201146, BIIL284)
5'-Lipoxygenase inhibitors (zileuton, Bay x1005)
Chemokine inhibitors
    Interleukin-8 antagonists (CXCR2 antagonists, e.g., SB 225002)
    MCP antagonists (CCR2 antagonists)
    CXCR3 receptor antagonists
TNF inhibitors (monoclonal antibodies, soluble receptors, TNF-α converting
    enzyme inhibitors)
TGF-β inhibitors (TGF-β receptor kinase inhibitors)
EGF receptor kinase inhibitors (e.g., geftinib)
Antioxidants (e.g., stable glutathione analogues)
iNOS inhibitors (e.g., L-NIL)

LTB$_4$, leukotriene B$_4$; MCP, monocyte chemotactic protein; TNF, tumor necrosis factor; TGF, transforming growth factor; EGF, epithelium-derived growth factor; COX, cyclooxygenase; iNOS, inducible nitric oxide synthase; L-NIL, L-N^6-(1-iminoethyl)-lysine-HCl.

The profile of mediators in COPD differs from that in asthma, so that different mediator antagonists are likely to be effective. Since COPD is characterized by a neutrophilic inflammation, attention has largely focused on mediators involved in recruitment and activation of neutrophils or on reactive oxygen species in view of the increased oxidative stress in COPD (Table 1). Many chemokines and cytokines have now been implicated in COPD, several of which are targets for the development of new therapies (29).

A.   Leukotriene B$_4$ Inhibitors

Leukotriene B$_4$ (LTB$_4$) is a potent chemoattractant of neutrophils and is increased in the sputum and exhaled breath of patients with COPD (30,31). It is probably derived from alveolar macrophages as well as neutrophils and may be synergistic with IL-8. Two subtypes of receptor for LTB$_4$ have been described; BLT$_1$ receptors are mainly expressed on granulocytes and monocytes, whereas BLT$_2$ receptors are expressed on T lymphocytes (32). BLT$_1$ antagonists, such as LY29311, have now been developed for the treatment of neutrophilic inflammation (33). LY293111 and another antagonist, SB225002, inhibit the neutrophil chemotactic activity of sputum from COPD patients, indicating the potential clinical value of such drugs (34,35). Several selective BLT$_1$ antagonists are now in development. LTB$_4$ is synthesized by 5'-lipoxygenase (5-LO), of which there are several inhibitors, although there have been problems in the clinical development of drugs in this class because of side effects. A recent pilot study in COPD patients with a $5'$-lipoxygenase inhibitor BAYx1005 showed only a modest reduction in sputum LTB_4 concentrations but no effect on neutrophil activation markers (36).

B. Chemokine Inhibitors

Several chemokines are involved in neutrophil chemotaxis and belong mainly to the CXC family, of which the most prominent member is interleukin (IL)-8. IL-8 levels are markedly elevated in the sputum of patients with COPD and are correlated with disease severity (37). Blocking antibodies to IL-8 and related chemokines inhibit certain types of neutrophilic inflammation in experimental animals and reduce the chemotactic response of neutrophils to sputum from COPD patients (30,35). A human monoclonal antibody to IL-8 blocks the chemotactic response of neutrophils to IL-8 and is effective in animal models of neutrophilic inflammation (38). This antibody is now in clinical trials for COPD, but it may be less effective than drugs that block the common receptor for other members of the CXC chemokine family. IL-8 activates neutrophils via a specific low-affinity G-protein–coupled receptor (CXCR1) coupled to activation and degranulation and high-affinity receptor (CXCR2), shared with other members of the CXC family, which is important in chemotaxis (39). Other CXC chemokines, such as growth-related oncoprotein-α (GRO-α), are also elevated in COPD (40), and therefore a CXCR2 antagonist is likely to be more useful than a CXCR1 antagonist, particularly as CXCR2 are also expressed on monocytes. Indeed, inhibition of monocyte chemotaxis may prevent the marked increase in macrophages found in the lungs of patients with COPD that may drive the inflammatory process. Small molecule inhibitors of CXCR2, such as SB225002, have now been developed and are entering clinical trials (41,42).

CC-chemokines are also involved in COPD. There is increased expression of monocyte chemotactic protein-1 (MCP-1) and its receptor CCR2 in macrophages and epithelial cells from COPD patients, and this may play a role in recruitment of blood monocytes to the lungs of COPD patients (43). This suggests that CCR2 antagonists may be of use, and small molecule inhibitors are in clinical development.

Chemokine receptors are also important for the recruitment of CD82+ T cells, which predominate in COPD airways and lungs and might contribute to disease pathophysiology. CD8+ cells show increased expression of CXCR3, and there is upregulation of CXCR3 ligands, such as CXCL10, in peripheral airways of COPD patients (44). This suggests that CXCR3 antagonists might be useful.

C. TNF-α Inhibitors

Tumor necrosis factor (TNF)-α levels are raised in the sputum of COPD patients (37). TNF-α induces IL-8 and other chemokines in airway cells via activation of the transcription factor nuclear factor-κB (NF-κB). The severe wasting in some patients with advanced COPD might be due to skeletal muscle apoptosis, resulting from increased circulating TNF-α. COPD patients with cachexia have increased release of TNF-α from circulating leukocytes (45). Humanized monoclonal TNF antibody (such as infliximab) and soluble TNF receptors (etanercept) that are effective in other chronic inflammatory diseases, such as rheumatoid arthritis and inflammatory bowel disease, should also be effective in COPD, particularly in patients who have systemic symptoms (46,47). Trials of anti-TNF therapies in COPD are currently underway. There may be problems with long-term administration of proteins because of the development of blocking antibodies and repeated injections are inconvenient. TNF-α converting enzyme (TACE), which is required for the release of soluble TNF-α, may be a more attractive target, as it is possible to discover small molecule TACE inhibitors, some of which are also matrix metalloproteinase inhibitors (48,49). General anti-inflammatory drugs such as phosphodiesterase inhibitors and p38 MAP kinase inhibitors also potently inhibit TNF-α expression.

D. TGF-β Inhibitors

Transforming growth factor-β1 (TGF-β1) is highly expressed in airway epithelium and macrophages of small airways in patients with COPD (50,51). It is a potent inducer of fibrosis, partly via the release of the potent fibrogenic mediator connective tissue growth factor, and may be important in inducing the fibrosis and narrowing of peripheral airways in COPD. TGF-β1 also activates MMP-9, whereas MMP-9 activates TGF-β, thus providing a link between small airway fibrosis and emphysema in COPD (9). TGF-β also downregulates β2-adrenoceptors and thus may impair responses to β2-agonists in peripheral airways (52). Inhibition of TGF-β signaling may therefore be a useful therapeutic strategy in COPD. Small molecule antagonists that inhibit TGF-β1 receptor kinase are now in development (53), although the long-term safety of such drugs might be a problem, particularly as TGF-β affects tissue repair and is a potent anti-inflammatory mediator.

E. Antioxidants

Oxidative stress is increased in patients with COPD (54,55), particularly during exacerbations, and reactive oxygen species contribute to its pathophysiology (56). This suggests that antioxidants may be of use in the therapy of COPD. *N*-Acetyl cysteine (NAC) provides cysteine for enhanced production of the antioxidant glutathione (GSH) and has antioxidant effects in vitro and in vivo. Recent systematic reviews of studies with oral NAC in COPD suggest a small but significant reduction in exacerbations (57,58). More effective antioxidants, including stable glutathione compounds, analogues of superoxide dismutase, and selenium-based drugs, are now in development for clinical use (56,59).

F. iNOS Inhibitors

Oxidative stress and increased nitric oxide release from expression of inducible nitric oxide synthase (iNOS) may result in the formation of peroxynitrite, which is a potent radical and may nitrate proteins, resulting in altered function. 3-Nitrotyrosine may indicate peroxynitrite formation and is markedly increased in sputum macrophages of patients with COPD (60). Selective inhibitors of iNOS are now in development (61), and one of these—L-N^6-(1-iminoethyl)lysine (L-NIL)—gives a profound and long-lasting reduction in the concentrations of nitric oxide in exhaled breath (62).

V. New Anti-Inflammatory Treatments

COPD is characterized by chronic inflammation of the respiratory tract, even in ex-smokers, with increased numbers of macrophages, neutrophils, and cytotoxic (CD8+) T lymphocytes in airways and lung parenchyma (1,5). This suggests that anti-inflammatory treatments may be of value, and there are several possible approaches (Fig. 1).

A. Resistance to Corticosteroids

Because there is chronic inflammation in COPD airways, it was argued that inhaled corticosteroids might prevent the progression of the disease. However, four large controlled trials of 3 years duration of inhaled corticosteroids have demonstrated no reduction in disease progression (63–66). This might be predicted by the demonstration that neither inhaled nor oral corticosteroids have any significant effect on neutrophil counts, granule proteins, inflammatory mediators or proteases in induced sputum (67–69). Inhaled corticosteroids do not inhibit neutrophilic inflammation induced by ozone in humans (70), and this may reflect that corticosteroids

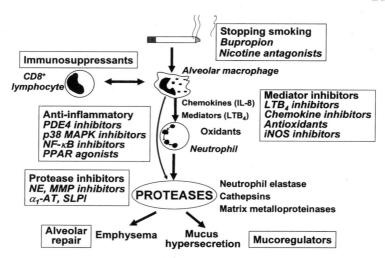

Figure 1 Targets for COPD therapy based on current understanding of the inflammatory mechanisms. Cigarette smoke and other irritants activate macrophages in the respiratory tract that release neutorphil chemotactic factors, including interleukin-8 (IL-8) and leukotriene B₄ (LTB₄). These cells then release proteases that break down connective tissue in the lung parenchyma, resulting in emphysema, and also stimulate mucus hypersecretion. These enzymes are normally counteracted by protease inhibitors, including α_1-antitrypsin, secretory leukoprotease inhibitor (SLPI), and tissue inhibitor of matrix metalloproteinases (TIMP). Cytotoxic T cells (CD8+) may also be involved in the inflammatory cascade.

prolong neutrophil survival (71). There may also be an active resistance to corticosteroids due to an inhibitory effect of cigarette smoke on histone deacetylation, which is required for corticosteroids to switch off inflammatory genes (72). The disappointing action of corticosteroids in COPD suggests that novel types of nonsteroidal anti-inflammatory treatment may be needed. Alternatively, therapeutic strategies that unlock the molecular mechanism of resistance might be possible. For example, drugs that increase histone deacetylase activity may resensitize cells to the effects of corticosteroids. For example, theophylline in low concentrations increases the activation of HDACs and increases the responsiveness to corticosteroids (73). This effect is mediated via a molecular mechanism distinct from those causing side effects, raising the possibility that novel theophylline-like drugs with a greater safety profile might be developed in the future (74). There are several other new approaches to anti-inflammatory treatment in COPD (Table 2).

Table 2 New Anti-inflammatory Drugs for COPD

Phosphodiesterse-4 inhibitors (SB 207499, CP 80633, CDP-840)
NF-κB inhibitors (proteasome inhibitors, IKK-2 inhibitors, IκB-α gene transfer)
Adhesion molecule inhibitors (anti CD11/CD18, anti-ICAM-1, E-selectin inhibitors)
Interleukin-10 and analogs
p38 MAP kinase inhibitors (SB203580, SB 220025, RWJ 67657)
PI3 kinase-γ inhibitors
PPAR activators
Resveratrol

NF-κB, nuclear factor-κB; IκB, inhibitor of NF-κB; IKK, IκB kinase; MAP, mitogen-activated protein; PI, phosphoinositide; PPAR, peroxisome proliferation activated receptor.

B. PDE4 Inhibitors

Phosphodiesterase (PDE)-4 is the predominant PDE expressed in neutrophils, CD8+, cells and macrophages (75), suggesting that PDE4 inhibitors would be effective in controlling inflammation in COPD. Selective PDE4 inhibitors, such as cilomilast and roflumilast, are active in animal models of neutrophil inflammation (76,77). Cilomilast has some beneficial clinical effect in COPD patients (78), and larger studies are currently underway. Roflumilast appears to be well tolerated at doses that significantly inhibit TNF-α release from peripheral blood monocytes (79). PDE4 inhibitors have been limited by side effects, particularly nausea and other gastrointestinal effects, but it might be possible to develop isoenzyme subtype selective inhibitors in the future which are less likely to be dose-limited by adverse effects.

Several steps may be possible to overcome the limitation of side effects. It now seems likely that vomiting is due to inhibition of a particular subtype of PDE4. At least four human PDE4 genes have been identified, and each has several splice variants (80). This raises the possibility that subtype-selective inhibitors may be developed that may preserve the anti-inflammatory effect, while having less propensity to side effects. PDE4D appears to be of particular importance in nausea and vomiting and is expressed in the chemosensitive trigger zone in the brain stem (81), and in mice deletion of the gene for PDE4D prevents a behavioral equivalent of emesis (82). This isoenzyme appears to be less important in anti-inflammatory effects and gene knockout studies in mice indicate that PDE4B is more important than PDE4D in inflammatory cells (83). PDE4B-selective inhibitors may therefore have a greater therapeutic margin and theoretically might be effective anti-inflammatory drugs. Cilomilast is the PDE4 inhibitor that has been most fully tested in clinical studies, particularly in COPD, but this drug is selective for PDE4D and therefore has a propensity to cause emesis. Roflumilast, which is nonselective for PDE4 isoenzymes, looks more promising, as it has a more favorable therapeutic ratio (84). Several PDE4 inhibitors with an improved therapeutic ratio are now in clinical development for COPD.

C. NF-κB Inhibitors

NF-κB regulates the expression of IL-8 and other chemokines, TNF-α and other inflammatory cytokines, and some matrix metalloproteinases. NF-κB is activated in macrophages and epithelial cells of COPD patients, particularly during exacerbations (85,86). There are several possible approaches to inhibition of NF-κB, including gene transfer of the inhibitor of NF-κB (IκB), a search for inhibitors of IκB kinase (IKK), NF-κB–inducing kinase (NIK), and IκB ubiquitin ligase, which regulate the activity of NF-κB, and the development of drugs that inhibit the degradation of IκB (87). The most promising approach may be the inhibition of IKK-2 by small molecule inhibitors which are now in development (88). A small molecule IKK-2 inhibitor suppresses the release of inflammatory cytokines and chemokines from alveolar macrophages (89) and might be effective in COPD when alveolar macrophages appear to be resistant to the anti-inflammatory actions of corticosteroids (90). One concern about long-term inhibition of NF-κB is that effective inhibitors may result in immune suppression and impair host defenses, since mice that lack NF-κB genes succumb to septicemia. However, there are alternative pathways of NF-κB activation that might be more important in inflammatory disease (91).

D. Adhesion Molecule Blockers

Recruitment of neutrophils, monocytes, and cytotoxic T cells into the lungs and respiratory tract is dependent on adhesion molecules expressed by these cells and on endothelial cells in the pulmonary and bronchial circulations. Several adhesion molecules can now be inhibited pharmacologically. For example, E-selectin on endothelial cells interacts with sialyl-Lewis[x] on neutrophils. A mimic of sialyl-Lewis[x], TBC1269, blocks selectins and inhibits granulocyte adhesion, with preferential effects on neutrophils (92). However, there are concerns about this therapeutic approach for a chronic disease, as an impaired neutrophilic response may increase the susceptibility to infection. The expression of Mac-1 (CD11b/CD18) is increased on neutrophils of patients with COPD, suggesting that targeting this adhesion molecule, which is also expressed on monocytes and macrophages, might be beneficial (93).

E. Interleukin-10

IL-10 is a cytokine with a wide spectrum of anti-inflammatory actions. It inhibits the secretion of TNF-α and IL-8 from macrophages, but tips the balance in favor of antiproteases, by decreasing the expression of matrix metalloproteinases, while increasing the expression of endogenous tissue inhibitors of matrix metalloproteinases (TIMP). IL-10 concentrations are reduced in induced sputum from patients with COPD, so that this may be a mechanism of amplifying lung inflammation (94). IL-10 is currently in clinical trials for other chronic inflammatory diseases (inflammatory bowel disease, rheumatoid arthritis, and psoriasis), including patients with steroid resistance, but IL-10 may cause hematological side effects (95). Treatment with daily injections of IL-10 over several weeks has been well tolerated. IL-10 may have therapeutic potential in COPD, especially if a selective activator of IL-10 receptors or unique signal transduction pathways can be developed in the future.

F. p38 MAP Kinase Inhibitors

Mitogen-activated protein (MAP) kinases play a key role in chronic inflammation, and several complex enzyme cascades have now been defined (96). One of these, the p38 MAP kinase pathway, is involved in expression of inflammatory cytokines, including IL-8, TNF-α, and MMPs (97). Non-peptide inhibitors of p38 MAP kinase, such as SB 203580, SB 239063, and RWJ 67657, have now been developed, and these drugs have a broad range of anti-inflammatory effects (98). SB 239063 reduces neutrophil infiltration after inhaled endotoxin and the concentrations of IL-6 and MMP-9 in bronchoalveolar lavage fluid of rats, indicating its potential as an anti-inflammatory agent in COPD (99). It is likely that such a broad-spectrum anti-inflammatory drug will have some toxicity, but inhalation may be a feasible therapeutic approach.

G. Phosphoinositide 3-Kinase Inhibitors

PI-3Ks are a family of enzymes that lead to the generation of lipid second messengers that regulate a number of cellular events. A particular isoform, PI-3Kγ, is involved in neutrophil recruitment and activation. Knock-out of the PI-3Kγ gene results in inhibition of neutrophil migration and activation, as well as impaired T-lymphocyte and macrophage function (100). This suggests that selective PI-3Kγ inhibitors may have relevant anti-inflammatory activity in COPD, and small molecule inhibitors of PI-3Kγ and PI-3Kδ are now in development (101).

H. PPAR Activators

Peroxisome prliferator–activated receptors (PPARs) are a family of ligand-activated nuclear hormone receptors belonging to the steroid receptor superfamily, and the three recognized subtypes—PPAR-α, -γ and -δ—are widely expressed. There is evidence that activation of PPAR-α and PPAR-δ may have anti-inflammatory and immunomodulatory effects. For example, PPARγ agonists, such as troglitazone, inhibit the release of inflammatory cytokines from monocytes and induce apoptosis of T lymphocytes (102,103), suggesting that they may have anti-inflammatory effects in COPD.

I. Resveratrol

Resveratrol is a phenolic component of red wine that has anti-inflammatory and antioxidant properties. It has a marked inhibitory effect on cytokine release from alveolar macrophages from COPD patients that show little or no response to corticosteroids (104). The molecular mechanism for this action is currently unknown, but identification of the cellular target for resveratrol may lead to the development of a novel class of anti-inflammatory compounds. Resveratrol itself has a very low oral bioavailability, so related drugs will need to be developed.

VI. Protease Inhibitors

There is compelling evidence for an imbalance between proteases that digest elastin (and other structural proteins) and antiproteases the protect against this. This suggests that either inhibiting these proteolytic enzymes or increasing endogenous antiproteases may be beneficial and theoretically should prevent the progression of airflow obstruction in COPD (Fig. 1). Considerable progress has been made in identifying the enzymes involved in elastolytic activity in emphysema and in characterizing the endogenous antiproteases that counteract this activity (105,106).

A. Endogenous Antiproteases

One approach is to give endogenous antiproteases (α_1-antitrypsin, secretory leukoprotease inhibitor, elafin, tissue inhibitors of MMP), either in recombinant form or by viral vector gene delivery. These approaches are unlikely to be cost-effective, as large amounts of protein have to be delivered and gene therapy is unlikely to provide sufficient protein.

B. Protease Inhibitors

A more promising approach is to develop small molecule inhibitors of proteinases, particularly those that have elastolytic activity. Small molecule inhibitors, such as ONO-5046 and FR901277, have been developed which have high potency (107,108). These drugs inhibit neutrophil elastase–induced lung injury in experimental animals, whether given by inhalation or systematically, and also inhibit the other serine proteases released from neutrophils cathepsin G and proteinase-3. Small molecule inhibitors of neutrophil elastase are now entering clinical trials, but there is concern that neutrophil elastase may not play a critical role in emphysema and that other proteases are more important in elastolysis. Inhibitors of elastolytic cysteine proteases, such as cathepsins K, S, and L, that are released from macrophages (109) are also in development (110). Matrix metalloproteinases with elastolytic activity (such as MMP-9) may also be targets for drug development (Fig. 1), although nonselective MMP inhibitors, such as marimastat, appear to have considerable side effects. It is possible that side effects could be reduced by increasing selectivity for specific MMPs or by targeting delivery to the lung parenchyma. MMP-9 is markedly over-expressed by alveolar macrophages from patients with COPD and is the major elastolytic enzyme released by these cells (111), so a selective inhibitor might be useful in the treatment of emphysema.

VII. Remodeling Agents

Since a major mechanism of airway obstruction in COPD is loss of elastic recoil due to proteolytic destruction of lung parenchyma, it seems unlikely that this could be reversible by drug therapy, although it might be possible to reduce the rate of progression by preventing the inflammatory and enzymatic disease process.

A. Retinoic Acid

Retinoic acid increases the number of alveoli in developing rats and, remarkably, reverses the histological and physiological changes induced by elastase treatment of adult rats (112,113). However, this is not observed in other species (114). Retinoic acid activates retinoic acid receptors, which act as transcription factors to regulate the expression of many genes involved in growth and differentiation. The molecular mechanisms involved and whether this can be extrapolated to humans is not yet known. Several retinoic acid receptor subtype agonists have now been developed that may have a greater selectivity for this effect and therefore a lower risk of side effects. The receptor mediating the effect on alveoli appears to be the RAR-γ receptor. A short-term trial of all-*trans*-retinoic acid in patients with emphysema did not show may improvement in clinical parameters (115), but a longer study is currently underway. This approach is unlikely to be successful as adult human lung, unlike rat lung, has no potential for repair.

B. Stem Cells

Another approach to repairing damaged lung in emphysema is the use of stem cells to seed the lung (116). Type 2 pneumocytes and Clara cells might be suitable for alveolar repair, and that is currently an active area of research.

VIII. Mucoregulators

Mucus hypersecretion is commonly seen in cigarette smokers and is not necessarily associated with airflow obstruction (chronic bronchitis). It may accelerate the decline in lung function in patients with COPD, however, by increasing the frequency of exacerbations. This suggests that reducing mucus hypersecretion may have therapeutic benefit, although suppression of the normal airway mucus secretion may be detrimental. Several approaches to inhibiting mucus hypersecretion are currently being explored (3). Mucus hypersecretion appears to be driven in COPD by the neutrophil inflammatory response, so that effective anti-inflammatory treatments would be expected to reduce mucus secretions. Of particular interest are two novel approaches.

A. EGF Receptor Inhibitors

Epidermal growth factor (EGF) plays a critical role in airway mucus secretion from goblet cells and submucosal glands and appears to mediate the mucus secretory response to several secretagogues, including oxidative stress, cigarette smoke, and inflammatory cytokines (117). Small molecule inhibitors of EGF receptor kinase, such as gefitinib, have now been developed for clinical use. There has been some concern about interstitial lung disease in some patients with small-cell lung cancer treated with gefitinib, but it is not yet certain if this is related to EGF inhibition (118).

B. Chloride Channel Activators

Another novel approach involves inhibition of calcium-activated chloride channels (CACC), which are important in mucus secretion from goblet cells. Activation of human hCLCA1 induces mucus secretion and mucus gene expression and may therefore be a target for inhibition. Small molecule inhibitors of CACC, such as niflumic acid and MSI 1956, have been developed (119).

IX. Drug Delivery

Bronchodilators are currently given as metered dose inhalers or dry powder inhalers that have been optimized to deliver drugs to the respiratory tract in asthma. But in emphysema the inflammatory and destructive process is localized to the lung parenchyma, and in chronic obstructive bronchitis the predominant irreversible changes are in the small airways. This implies that if a drug is to be delivered by inhalation, it should have a lower mass median diameter so that there is preferential deposition in the lung periphery. It may be more appropriate to give therapy parenterally as it will reach the lung parenchyma and terminal airways via the pulmonary circulations, but parenteral administration may increase the risk of systemic side effects. Targeted delivery of drugs to particular cell types is another approach to limit toxicity. For example, alveolar macrophages may be targeted by molecules that are packaged to be phagocytosed by these cells. Another important concept is the idea of disease activation of drugs; for example, in COPD, active drugs that are released from inactive prodrugs by elastases might be considered. This would concentrate the active drug at the site of disease activity and reduce systematic exposure.

X. Future Directions

New drugs for the treatment of COPD are greatly needed. While preventing and quitting smoking is the obvious preferred approach, this has proved to be very difficult in the majority of patients, and even with bupropion only ~15% of patients are sustained quitters. In addition, it is likely that the inflammatory process initiated by cigarette smoking may continue even when smoking has ceased (28). Furthermore, COPD may be due to other environmental factors (cooking fumes, pollutants, passive smoking, other inhaled toxins) or developmental changes in the lungs (120).

A. Identification of Novel Therapeutic Targets

It is important to identify the genetic factors that determine why only 10–20% of smokers develop COPD (121,122). Identification of genes that predispose to the development of COPD in smokers may identify novel therapeutic targets. Powerful techniques, including high-density DNA arrays (gene chips), are able to identify multiple polymorphisms. Differential display may identify the expression of novel genes, whereas proteomics identifies expression of novel proteins.

B. Surrogate Markers

It will be difficult to demonstrate the efficacy of novel treatments as determination of the effect of any drug on the rate of decline in lung function will require large studies over at least 2 and preferably 3 years. There is a need to develop surrogate markers, such as analysis of sputum parameters (cells, mediators, enzymes) or exhaled condensates (lipid mediators, reactive oxygen species, cytokines) (123), that may predict the clinical usefulness of such drugs. More research on the basic cellular and molecular mechanisms of COPD is urgently needed to aid the logical development of new therapies for this common and important disease for which no effective preventative treatments currently exist. It may also be important to more accurately define the presence of emphysema versus small airway obstruction using improved imaging techniques, as some drugs may be more useful for preventing emphysema, whereas others may be more effective against the small airway inflammatory-fibrosis process.

References

1. Barnes PJ. Chronic obstructive pulmonary disease. N Engl J Med 2000; 343:269–280.
2. Hogg JC. Chronic obstructive pulmonary disease: an overview of pathology and pathogenesis. Novartis Found Symp 2001; 234:4–19.
3. Barnes PJ. Current and future therapies for airway mucus hypersecretion. Novartis Found Symp 2002; 248:237–249.
4. Barnes PJ. Mechanisms in COPD: differences from asthma. Chest 2000; 117:10S–14S.
5. Saetta M, Turato G, Maestrelli P, Mapp CE, Fabrri LM. Cellular and structural bases of chronic obstructive pulmonary disease. Am J Respir Crit Care Med 2001; 163:1304–1309.
6. Barnes PJ. New treatments for chronic obstructive pulmonary disease. Curr Opin Pharmacol 2001; 1:217–222.
7. Barnes PJ. New treatments for COPD. Nature Rev Drug Disc 2002; 1:437–445.
8. Barnes PJ. New concepts in COPD. Ann Rev Med 2003; 54:113–129.
9. Barnes PJ. Shapiro SD, Pauwels RA. COPD: molecular and cellular mechanisms. Eur Respir J 2003; 2:672–688.
10. Barnes PJ. Novel approaches and targets for treatment of chronic obstructive pulmonary disease. Am J Respir Crit Care Med 1999; 160:S72–S79.
11. Shapiro SD. Animal models for COPD. Chest 2000; 117:223S–227S.

12. Dawkins PA, Stockley RA. Animal models of chronic obstructive pulmonary disease. Thorax 2001; 56:972–977.
13. Barnes PJ. New treatments for COPD. Thorax 2003; 58:803–880.
14. Lancaster T, Stead L, Silagy C, Sowden A. Effectiveness of interventions to help people stop smoking: findings from the Cochrane Library. Br Med J 2000; 321:355–358.
15. Jorenby DE, Leischow SJ, Nides MA, Rennard SI, Johnston JA, Hughes AR, et al. A controlled trial of sustained-release bupropion, a nicotine patch, or both for smoking cessation. N Engl J Med 1999; 340:685–691.
16. Tashkin DP, Kanner R, Bailey W, Buist S, Anderson P, Nides MA, et al. Smoking cessation in patients with chronic obstructive pulmonary disease: a double-blind, placebo controlled, randomised trial. Lancet 2001; 357:1571–1575.
17. Hughes JR, Stead LF, Lancaster T. Antidepressants for smoking cessation (Cochrane Review). Cochrane Database Syst Rev 2000; 4:CD000031.
18. Holm KJ, Spencer CM. Bupropion: a review of its use in the management of smoking cessation. Drugs 2000; 59:1007–1024.
19. Dani JA. Roles of dopamine signaling in nicotine addiction. *Mol Psychiatry* 2003; 8:255–256.
20. Disse B, Speck GA, Rominger KL, Witek TJ, Hammer R. Tiotropium (Spiriva): mechanistical considerations and clinical profile in obstructive lung disease. Life Sci 1999; 64:457–464.
21. Barnes PJ. The pharmacological properties of tiotropium. Chest 2000; 117:63S–66S.
22. Littner MR, Ilowite JS, Tashkin DP, Friedman M, Serby CW, Menjoge SS, et al. Long-acting bronchodilation with once-daily dosing of tiotropium (Spiriva) in stable chronic obstructive pulmonary disease. Am J Respir Crit Care Med 2000; 161:1136–1142.
23. Hansel TT, Barnes PJ. Tiotropium bromide: a novel once-daily anticholinergic bronchodilator for the treatment of COPD. Drugs Today 2002; 38:585–600.
24. Casaburi R, Mahler DA, Jones PW, Wanner A, San PG, Zu Wallack RL, et al. A long-team evaluation of once-daily inhaled tiotropium in chronic obstructive pulmonary disease. Eur Respir J 2002; 19:217–224.
25. Vincken W, van Noord JA, Greefhorst AP, Bantje TA, Kesten S, Korducki L, et al. Improved health outcomes in patients with COPD during 1 yr's treatment with tiotropium. Eur Respir J 2002; 19:209–216.
26. Schelfhout VJ, Joos GF, Ferrer P, Luria X, Pauwels RA. Activity of LAS 34273, a new long-acting anticholinergic antagonist. Am Resp Crit Care Med 2003; 167:A93.
27. Tennant RC, Erin EM, Barnes PJ, Hansel TT. Long-acting β$_2$-adrenoceptor agonists or tiotropium bromide for patients with COPD: is combination therapy justified? Curr Opin Pharamcol 2003; 3:270–276.
28. Rutgers SR, Postma DS, ten Hacken NH, Kauffman HF, Van der Mark TW, Koeter GH, et al. Ongoing airway inflammation in patients with COPD who do not currently smoke. Thorax 2000; 55:12–18.

29. Barnes PJ. Cytokine modulators as novel therapies for airway disease. Eur Respir J Suppl 2001; 34:67s–77s.

30. Hill AT, Bayley D, Stockley RA. The interrelationship of sputum inflammatory markers in patients with chronic bronchitis. Am J Respir Crit Care Med 1999; 160:893–898.

31. Montuschi P, Kharitonov SA, Ciabattoni G, Barnes PJ. Exhaled leukotrienes and prostaglandins in COPD. Thorax 2003; 58:585–588.

32. Yokomizo T, Kato K, Terawaki K, Izumi T, Shimizu T. A second leukotriene B_4 receptor BLT2. A new therapeutic target in inflammation and immunological disorders. J Exp Med 2000; 192:421–432.

33. Silbaugh SA, Stengel PW, Cockerham SL, Froelich LL, Bendele AM, Spaethe SM, et al. Pharmacologic actions of the second generation leukotriene B_4 receptor antagonist LY29311: in vivo pulmonary studies. Nnaunyn Schmied Arch Pharamacol 2000; 361:397–404.

34. Crooks SW, Bayley DL, Hill SL, Stockley RA. Bronchial inflammation in acute bacterial exacerbations of chronic bronchitis: the role of leukotriene B_4. Eur Respir J 2000; 15:274–280.

35. Beeh KM, Kornmann O, Buhl R, Culpitt SV, Giembyez MA, Barnes PJ. Neutrophil chemotactic activity of sputum from patients with COPD: role of interleukin 8 and leukotriene B_4. Chest 2003; 123:1240–1247.

36. Gompertz S, Stockley RA. A randomized, placebo-controlled trial of a leukotriene synthesis inhibitor in patients with COPD. Chest 2002; 122:289–294.

37. Keatings VM, Collins PD, Scott DM, Barnes PJ. Differences in interleukin-8 and tumor necrosis factor-α in induced sputum from patients with chronic obstructive pulmonary disease or asthma. Am J Respir Crit Care Med 1996; 153:530–534.

38. Yang XD, Corvalan JR, Wang P, Roy CM, Davis CG. Fully human anti-interleukin-8 monoclonal antibodies: potential therapeutics for the treatment of inflammatory disease states. J Leukoc Biol 1999; 66:401–410.

39. Rossi D, Zlotnik A. The biology of chemokines and their receptors. Annu Rev Immunol 2000; 18:217–242.

40. Traves SL, Culpitt S, Russell REK, Barnes PJ, Donnelly LE. Elevated levels of the chemokines GRO-α and MCP-1 in sputum samples from COPD patients. Thorax 2002; 57:590–595.

41. White JR, Lee JM, Young PR, Hertzberg RP, Jurewicz AJ, Chaikin MA, et al. Identification of a potent, selective non-peptide CXCR2 antagonist that inhibits interleukin-8-induced neutrophil migration. J Biol Chem 1998; 273:10095–10098.

42. Hay DWP, Sarau HM. Interleukin-8-receptor antagonists in pulmonary diseases. Curr Opin Pharmacol 2001; 1:242–247.

43. de Boer WI, Sont JK, van Schadewijk A, Stolk J, van Krieken JH, Hiemstra PS. Monocyte chemoattractant protein 1, interleukin 8, and chronic airways inflammation in COPD. J Pathol 2000; 190:619–626.

44. Saetta M, Mariani M, Panina-Bordignon P, Turato G, Buonsanti C, Baraldo S, et al. Increased expression of the chemokine receptor CXCR3 and its ligand

CXCL10 in peripheral airways of smokers with chronic obstructive pulmonary disease. Am J Respir Crit Care Med 2002; 165:1404–1409.

45. de Godoy I, Donahoe M, Calhoun WJ, Mancino J, Rogers RM. Elevated TNF-alpha production by peripheral blood monocytes of weight-losing COPD patients. Am J Respir Crit Care Med 1996; 153:633–637.

46. Markham A, Lamb HM. Infliximab: a review of its use in the management of rheumatoid arthritis. Drugs 2000; 59:1341–1359.

47. Jarvis B, Faulds D. Etanercept: a review of its use in rheumatoid arthritis. *Drugs* 1999; 57:945–966.

48. Barlaam B, Bird TG, Lambert-Van DB, Campbell D, Foster SJ, Maciewicz R. New alpha-substituted succinate-based hydroxamic acids as TNFα convertase inhibitors. J Med Chem 1999; 42:4890–4908.

49. Rabinowitz MH, Andrews RC, Becherer JD, Bickett DM, Bubacz DG, Conway JG, et al. Design of selective and soluble inhibitors of tumor necrosis factor-α converting enzyme (TACE). J Med Chem 2001; 44:4252–4267.

50. de Boer WI, van Schadewijk A, Sont JK, Sharma HS, Stolk J, Hiemstra PS, et al. Transforming growth factor beta and recruitment of macrophages and mast cells in airways in chronic obstructive pulmonary disease. Am J Respir Crit Care Med 1998; 158:1951–1957.

51. Takizawa H, Tanaka M, Takami K, Ohtoshi T, Ito K, Satoh M, et al. Increased expression of transforming growth factor-beta1 in small airway epithelium from tobacco smokers and patients with chronic obstructive pulmonary disease (COPD). Am J Respir Crit Care Med 2001; 163:1476–1483.

52. Mak JC, Rousell J, Haddad EB, Barnes PJ. Transforming growth factor-β1 inhibits β_2-adrenoceptor gene transcription. Naunyn Schemied Arch Pharmacol 2000; 362:520–525.

53. Yakymovych I, Engstrom U, Grimsby S, Heldin CH, Souchelnytskyi S. Inhibition of transforming growth factor-β signaling by low molecular weight compounds interfering with ATP- or substrate-binding sites of the TGFβ type I receptor kinase. Biochemistry 2002; 41:11000–11007.

54. Montuschi P, Collins JV, Ciabattoni G, Lazzeri N, Corradi M, Kharitonov SA, et al. Exhaled 8-isoprostane as an *in vivo* biomarker of lung oxidative stress in patients with COPD and healthy smokers. Am J Respir Crit Care Med 2000; 162:1175–1177.

55. Paredi P, Kharitonov SA, Leak D, Ward S, Cramer D, Barnes PJ. Exhaled ethane, a marker of lipid peroxidation, is elevated in chronic obstructive pulmonary disease. Am J Respir Crit Care Med 2000; 162:369–373.

56. Macnee W. Oxidants/Antioxidants and COPD. Chest 2000; 117:303S–317S.

57. Grandjean EM, Berthet P, Ruffmann R, Leuenberger P. Efficacy of oral long-term N-acetylcysteine in chronic bronchopulmonary disease: a meta-analysis of published double-blind, placebo-controlled clinical trials. Clin Ther 2000; 22:209–221.

58. Poole PJ, Black PN. Oral mucolytic drugs for exacerbations of chronic obstructive pulmonary disease: systematic review. Br Med J 2001; 322:1271–1274.

59. Cuzzocrea S, Riley DP, Caputi AP, Salvemini D. Antioxidant therapy: a new pharmacological approach in shock, inflammation, and ischemia/reperfusion injury. Pharmacol Rev 2001; 53:135–159.

60. Ichinose M, Sugiura H, Yamagata S, Koarai A, Shirato K. Increase in reactive nitrogen species production in chronic obstructive pulmonary disease airways. Am J Respir Crit Care Med 2000; 160:701–706.

61. Hobbs AJ, Higgs A, Moncada S. Inhibition of nitric oxide synthase as a potential therapeutic target. Annu Rev Pharmacol Toxicol 1999; 39:191–220.

62. Hansel TT, Kharitonov SA, Donnelly LE, Erin EM, Currie MG, Moore WM, et al. A selective inhibitor of inducible nitric oxide synthase inhibits exhaled breath nitric oxide in healthy volunteers and asthmatics. FASEB J 2003; 17:1298–1300.

63. Vestbo J, Sorensen T, Lange P, Brix A, Torre P, Viskum K. Long-term effect of inhaled budesonide in mild and moderate chronic obstructive pulmonary disease: a randomised controlled trial. Lancet 1999; 353:1819–1823.

64. Pauwels RA, Lofdahl CG, Laitinen LA, Schouten JP, Postma DS, Pride NB, et al. Long-term treatment with inhaled budesonide in persons with mild chronic obstructive pulmonary disease who continue smoking. N Engl J Med 1999; 340:1948–1953.

65. Burge PS, Calverley PMA, Jones PW, Spencer S, Anderson JA, Maslen T. Randomised, double-blind, placebo-controlled study of fluticasone propionate in patients with moderate to severe chronic obstructive pulmonary disease; the ISOLDE trial. Br Med J 2000; 320:1297–1303.

66. Lung Health Study Research Group. Effect of inhaled triamcinolone on the decline in pulmonary function in chronic obstructive pulmonary disease. New Engl J Med 2000; 343:1902–1909.

67. Barnes PJ. Inhaled corticosteroids are not helpful in chronic obstructive pulmonary disease. Am J Respir Crit Care Med 2000; 161:342–344.

68. Keatings VM, Jatakanon A, Worsdell YM, Barnes PJ. Effects of inhaled and oral glucocorticoids on inflammatory indices in asthma and COPD. Am J Respir Crit Care Med 1997; 155:542–548.

69. Culpitt SV, Nightingale JA, Barnes PJ. Effect of high dose inhaled steroid on cells, cytokines and proteases in induced sputum in chronic obstructive pulmonary disease. Am J Respir Crit Care Med 1999; 160:1635–1639.

70. Nightingale JA, Rogers DF, Chung KF, Barnes PJ. No effect of inhaled budesonide on the response to inhaled ozone in normal subjects. Am J Respir Crit Care Med 2000; 161:479–486.

71. Meagher LC, Cousin JM, Seckl JR, Haslett C. Opposing effects of glucocorticoids on the rate of apoptosis in neutrophilic and eosinophilic granulocytes. J Immunol 1996; 156:4422–4428.

72. Ito K, Lim S. Caramori G, Chung KF, Barnes PJ, Adcock IM. Cigarette smoking reduces histone deacetylase 2 expression, enhances cytokine expression and inhibits glucocorticoid actions in alveolar macrophages. FASEB J 2001; 15:1100–1102.

73. Ito K, Lim S, Caramori G, Cosio B, Chung KF, Adcodk IM, et al. A molecular mechanism of action of theophylline: Induction of histone deacetylase activity to decrease inflammatory gene expression. Proc Natl Acad Sci USA 2002; 99:8921–8926.

74. Barnes PJ. Theophylline: new perspectives on an old drug. Am J Respir Crit Care Med 2003; 167:813–818.

75. Souness JE, Aldous D, Sargent C. Immunosuppressive and anti-inflammatory effects of cyclic AMP phosphodiesterase (PDE) type 4 inhibitors. Immunopharmacology 2000; 47:127–162.

76. Spond J, Chapman R, Fine J, Jones H, Kreutner W, Kung TT, et al. Comparison of PDE 4 inhibitors, rolipram and SB 207499 (ariflo), in a rat model of pulmonary neutrophilia. Pulm. Pharmacol Ther 2001; 14:157–164.

77. Bundschuh DS, Eltze M, Barsing J, Wollin L, Hatzelmann A, Beume R. In vivo efficacy in airway disease models of roflumilast, a novel orally active PDE4 inhibitor. J Pharmacol Exp Ther 2001; 297:280–290.

78. Compton CH, Gubb J, Nieman R, Edelson J, Amit O, Bakst A, et al. Cilomilast, a selective phosphodiesterase-4 inhibitor for treatment of patients with chronic obstructive pulmonary disease: a randomised, dose-ranging study. Lancet 2001; 358:265–270.

79. Timmer W, Leclerc V, Birraux G, Neuhauser M, Hatzelmann A, Bethke T, et al. The new phosphodiesterase 4 inhibitor roflumilast is efficacious in exercise-induced asthma and leads to suppression of LPS-stimulated TNF-alpha ex vivo. J Clin Pharmacol 2002; 42:297–303.

80. Muller T, Engels P, Fozard J. Subtypes of the type 4 cAMP phosphodiesterase: structure, regulation and selective inhibition. Trends Pharmacol Sci 1996; 17:294–298.

81. Lamontagne S, Medows E, Luk P, Normandin D, Muise E, Boulet L, et al. Localization of phosphodiesterase-4 isoforms in the medulla and nodose ganglion of the squirrel monkey. Brain Res 2001; 920:84–96.

82. Robichaud A, Stamatiou PB, Jin SL, Lachance N, MacDonald D, Laliberte F, et al. Deletion of phosphodiesterase 4D in mice shortens alpha(2)-adrenoceptor-mediated anesthesia, a behavioral correlate of emesis. J Clin Invest 2002; 110: 1045–1052.

83. Jin SL, Conti M. Induction of the cyclic nucleotide phosphodiesterase PDE4B is essential for LPS-activated TNF-alpha responses. Proc Natl Acad Sci USA 2002; 99:7628–7633.

84. Reid P. Roflumilast. Curr Opin Invest Drugs 2002; 3:1165–1170.

85. Di Stefano A, Caramori G, Capelli A, Lusuardi M, Gnemmi I, Ioli F, et al. Increased expression of NF-κB in bronchial bioipsies from smokers and patients with COPD. Eur Respir J 2002; 20:556–563.

86. Caramori G, Romagnoli M, Casolari P, Bellettato C, Casoni G, Boschetto P, et al. Nuclear localisation of p65 in sputum macrophages but not in sputum neutrophils during COPD exacerbations. Thorax 2003; 58:348–351.

87. Delhase M, Li N, Karin M. Kinase regulation in inflammatory response. Nature 2000; 406:367–368.

88. Kishore N, Sommers C, Mathialagan S, Guzova J, Yao M, Hauser S, et al. A selective IKK-2 inhibitor blocks NF-κB-dependent gene expression in IL-1β stimulated synovial fibroblasts. J Biol Chem 2003; 277:13840–13847.

89. Jazrawi E, Cosio BG, Barnes PJ, Adcock IM. Inhibition of IKK2 and JNK differentially regulates GM-CSF and IL-8 release in epithelial cells and alveolar macrophages. Am J Resp Crit Care Med 2003; 167:A798.

90. Culpitt SV, Rogers DF, Shah P, de Matos C, Russell RE, Donnelly LE, et al. Impaired inhibition by dexamethasone of cytokine release by alveolar macrophages from patients with chronic obstructive pulmonary disease. Am J Respir Crit Care Med 2003; 167:24–31.

91. Nasuhara Y, Adcock IM, Catley M, Barnes PJ, Newton R. Differential IKK activation and IκBα degradation by interleukin-1β and tumor necrosis factor-α in human U937 monocytic cells: evidence for additional regulatory steps in κB-dependent transcription. J Biol Chem 1999; 274:19965–19972.

92. Davenpeck KL, Berens KL, Dixon RA, Dupre B, Bochner BS. Inhibition of adhesion of human neutrophils and eosinophils to P-selectin by the sialyl Lewis antagonist TBC1269: preferential activity against neutrophil adhesion in vitro. J Allergy Clin Immunol 2000; 105:769–775.

93. Noguera A, Batle S, Miralles C, Iglesias J, Busquets X, Macnee W, et al. Enhanced neutrophil response in chronic obstructive pulmonary disease. Thorax 2001; 56:432–437.

94. Takanashi S, Hasegawa Y, Kanehira Y, Yamamoto K, Fujimoto K, Satoh K, et al. Interleukin-10 level in sputum is reduced in bronchial asthma, COPD and in smokers. Eur Respir J 1999; 14:309–314.

95. Fedorak RN, Gangl A, Elson CO, Rutgeerts P, Schreiber S, Wild G, et al. Recombinant human interleukin 10 in the treatment of patients with mild to moderately active Crohn's disease. Gastroenterology 2000; 119:1473–1482.

96. Johnson GL, Lapadat R. Mitogen-activated protein kinase pathways mediated by ERK, JNK, and p38 protein kinases. Science 2002; 298:1911–1912.

97. Meja KK, Seldon PM, Nasuhara Y, Ito K, Barnes PJ, Lindsay MA, et al. p38 MAP kinase and MKK-1 co-operate in the generation of GM-CSF from LPS-stimulated human monocytes by an NF-κB-independent mechanism. Br J Pharmacol 2000; 131:1143–1153.

98. Lee JC, Kumar S, Griswold DE, Underwood DC, Votta BJ, Adams JL. Inhibition of p38 MAP kinase as a therapeutic strategy. Immunopharmacology 2000; 47:185–201.

99. Underwood DC, Osborn RR, Bochnowicz S, Webb EF, Rieman DJ, Lee JC, et al. SB 239063, a p38 MAPK inhibitor, reduces neutrophilia, inflammatory cytokines, MMP-9, and fibrosis in lung. Am J Physiol Lung Cell Mol Physiol 2000; 279:L895–L902.

100. Sasaki T, Irie-Sasaki J, Jones RG, Oliveria dSA, Stanford WL, Bolon B, et al. Function of PI3Kgamma in thymocyte development, T cell activation, and neutrophil migration. Science 2000; 287:1040–1046.

101. Ward S, Sotsios Y, Dowden J, Bruce I, Finan P. Therapeutic potential of phosphoinositide 3-kinase inhibitors. Chem Biol 2003; 10:207–213.

102. Jiang C, Ting AT, Seed B. PPAR-γ agonists inhibit production of monocyte inflammatory cytokines. Nature 1998; 391:82–86.

103. Harris SG, Phipps RP. Induction of apoptosis in mouse T cells upon peroxisome proliferator-activated receptor gamma (PPAR-γ) binding. Adv Exp Med Biol 2002; 507:421–425.

104. Culpitt SV, Rogers DF, Barnes PJ, Donnelly LE. Resveratrol has a greater inhibitory effect than corticosteroids in inhibiting alveolar macrophages from COPD patients. Am J Resp Crit Care Med 2003: 167:A91.

105. Stockley RA. Neutrophils and protease/antiprotease imbalance. Am J Respir Crit Care Med 1999; 160:S49–S52.

106. Shapiro SD, Senior RM. Matrix metalloproteinases. Matrix degradation and more. Am J Respir Cell Mol Biol 1999; 20:1100–1102.

107. Kawabata K, Suzuki M, Sugitani M, Imaki K, Toda M, Miyamoto T. ONO-5046, a novel inhibitor of human neutrophil elastase. Biochem Biophys Res Commun 1991; 1717:814–820.

108. Fujie K, Shinguh Y, Yamazaki A, Hatanaka H, Okamoto M, Okuhara M. Inhibition of elastase-induced acute inflammation and pulmonary emphysema in hamsters by a novel neutrophil elastase inhibitor FR901277. Inflamm Res 1999; 48:160–167.

109. Punturieri A, Filippov S, Allen E, Caras I, Murray R, Reddy V, et al. Regulation of elastinolytic cysteine proteinase activity in normal and cathepsin K-deficient macrophages. J Exp Med 2000; 192:789–800.

110. Leung-Toung R, Li W, Tam TF, Karimian K. Thiol-dependent enzymes and their inhibitors: a review. Curr Med Chem 2002; 9:979–1002.

111. Russell RE, Culpitt SV, DeMatos C, Donnelly L, Smith M, Wiggins J, et al. Release and activity of matrix metalloproteinase-9 and tissue inhibitor of metalloproteinase-1 by alveolar macrophages from patients with chronic obstructive pulmonary disease. Am J Respir Cell Mol Biol 2002; 26:602–609.

112. Massaro G, Massaro D. Retinoic acid treatment abrogates elastase-induced pulmonary emphysema in rats. Nat Med 1997; 3:675–677.

113. Belloni PN, Garvin L, Mao CP, Bailey-Healy I, Leaffer D. Effects of all-trans-retinoic acid in promoting alveolar repair. Chest 2000; 117:235S–241S.

114. Lucey EC, Goldstein RH, Breuer R, Rexer BN, Ong DE, Snider GL. Retinoic acid does not affect alveolar septation in adult FVB mice with elastase-induced emphysema. Respiration 2003; 70:200–205.

115. Mao JT, Goldin JG, Dermand J, Ibrahim G, Brown MS, Emerick A, et al. A pilot study of all trans-retinoic acid for the treatment of human emphysema. Am J Respir Crit Care Med 2002; 165:718–723.

116. Otto WR. Lung epithelial stem cells. J Pathol 2002; 197:527–535.

117. Nadel JA, Burgel PR. The role of epidermal growth factor in mucus production. Curr Opin Pharmacol 2001; 1:254–258.

118. Inoue A, Saijo Y, Maemondo M, Gomi K, Tokue Y, Kimura Y, et al. Severe acute interstitial pneumonia and gefitinib. Lancet 2003; 361:137–139.

119. Zhou Y, Shapiro M, Dong Q, Louahed J, Weiss C, Wan S, et al. A calcium-activated chloride channel blocker inhibits goblet cell metaplasia and mucus overproduction. Novartis Found Symp 2002; 248:150–165.
120. Smith KR. Inaugural article: national burden of disease in India from indoor air pollution. Proc Natl Acad Sci USA 2000; 97:13286–13293.
121. Barnes PJ. Molecular genetics of chronic obstructive pulmonary disease. Thorax 1999; 54:245–252.
122. Limas DA, Silverman EK. The genetics of chronic obstructive pulmonary disease. Respir Res 2001; 2:20–26.
123. Kharitonov SA, Barnes PJ. Exhaled markers of pulmonary disease. Am J Respir Crit Care Med 2001; 163:1693–1772.

INDEX